2019

PREP® Self-Assessment

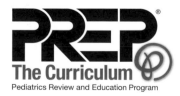

PREP®
The Curriculum
Pediatrics Review and Education Program

2019 PREP Self-Assessment Editorial Board

The AAP gratefully acknowledges the contributions of the
PREP Self-Assessment Editorial Board.

2019 PREP Self-Assessment Editorial Board (continued)

Principal Staff – PREP® Self-Assessment

Hilary M. Haftel, MD, MHPE, FAAP
Sr. Vice President, Department of Education

Susan Piscoran
Managing Editor
Pediatrics Review and Education Program Publications
E-Learning

Carolyn Mahler
Copy Editor
Pediatrics Review and Education Program Publications
E-Learning

Acknowledgments

The American Academy of Pediatrics (AAP) gratefully acknowledges the contributions of the PREP Self-Assessment Editorial Board.

PREP® The Curriculum Objectives

The AAP Pediatrics Review and Education Program (PREP) The Curriculum is a coordinated continuing medical education program and includes the PREP Self-Assessment and the journal *Pediatrics in Review*. Designed to provide continuous professional development, the program objectives of PREP The Curriculum are to assist pediatricians and other healthcare practitioners:

- acquire the knowledge and skills needed to provide health supervision and manage acute and chronic illnesses in infants, children, adolescents, and young adults
- identify and address gaps in their knowledge and clinical practice
- assess their knowledge and identify their own continuing education needs using evidence-based information

PREP The Curriculum is based on the Content Specifications, or knowledge statements important to the practice of pediatric medicine, provided to the AAP by the American Board of Pediatrics (ABP). Most Content Specifications will be addressed in the PREP Self-Assessment within a 4-year period, providing pediatricians with an educational program that is ideal for lifelong learning, as well as for preparing for the ABP Maintenance of Certification™ Assessment for Pediatrics (MOCA-Peds examination).

How to Use PREP Self-Assessment – Requirements for Claiming CME and MOC Credits

Subscribers may review the PREP Self-Assessment using the print or online versions via computer, tablet, or mobile device. Physicians should review the front matter that includes the program objectives and disclosure grid, read all questions and critiques either online in learning mode or in print, achieve all completion requirements (below), and claim CME and MOC credit. All others who successfully complete the program may request a certificate of completion.

The 2019 edition, available January 1, 2019, offers 291 multiple-choice questions. The critiques describe the rationale behind each preferred answer and reasons that the other 3 answers are not the best choices. Answers in the online versions are retained so that the PREP Self-Assessment can be completed at the user's convenience; an estimated 40 hours is required to complete.

How to access your PREP Self-Assessment Online

Follow these steps to access PREP Self-Assessment:
- Go to http://www.PediaLink.org
- In the upper-right corner, enter your AAP login and password. Click the Submit Button.
- Quick launch the 2019 PREP Self-Assessment by clicking the "LAUNCH" button

Recommended Browsers:

It is recommended that learners use one of the latest two versions of Internet Explorer, Mozilla Firefox, or Google Chrome for Windows-based PCs, and Safari on OS X based computers.

PREP Self-Assessment Print

Questions start at page Q-1: Critiques start at page C-1. Learners who prefer to study the print edition may record answers on the answer sheet provided at the end of the book. Transfer all responses online in the Answer Sheet link located in the 2019 PREP-Self-Assessment menu. It is not necessary to click through every question and critique to record these responses. Paper answer sheets are not accepted.

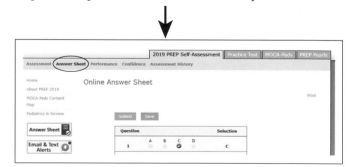

Completion requirements: To successfully complete the 2019 PREP Self-Assessment for *AMA PRA Category 1 Credit*™ or MOC part II points, learners must achieve the following 3 steps:

1. *Minimum performance level* — demonstrate a minimum performance level of 70% or higher on this assessment, which measures achievement of the educational purpose and objectives of this activity; if you score less than 70%, you will be redirected to incorrectly answered questions that can be reset and answered until a passing score is achieved.
2. *Learning mode (default mode)* — answer all the questions and record all answers using the online program in Pedia-Link. Answers recorded in the Practice Test are not eligible for credit claiming.
3. *Complete course* — confirm that every question has been answered and click the "Complete Assessment" button to mark your assessment as completed.

After meeting these requirements, both *AMA PRA Category 1 Credit*™ and/or MOC part II points can be claimed by clicking the claim credit link (left navigation column) from within the Self-Assessment program online in Pedia-Link. **The date recorded is when you first attempt to claim credit. MOC and CME credit can be claimed at different times within the 3-year lifespan of this activity and according to a learner's specific needs; however, dates cannot be changed once credit claiming has been initiated.**

Transmitting completion to the ABP:

Real-time transmission of completion data occurs after clicking the claim ABP MOC Credit "Submit" button. The transmission is stamped with the time and date when you initiate the transmission.

In order to confirm that MOC completion data has been successfully transmitted to the ABP, learners should check their portfolio by logging into their account at www.abp.org. If transmission to the ABP fails, you may reinitiate notice of completion to the ABP by accessing "CME Transcript" at http://transcript.aap.org. If you encounter issues claiming your CME or MOC credit using the transcript tool, you may contact the AAP's Transcript department by filling out the discrepancy form for additional assistance.

Optimize Your Use of PREP with Features to Enhance Your Learning

- **NEW - MOCA-Peds** content mapping identifies PREP questions and *Pediatrics in Review* articles tied to the 2019 ABP learning objectives. Online learners will be able to easily access bonus 2019 learning objective questions from previous editions of PREP.
- **NEW - Practice Test** allows learners to simulate timed examinations based on user selected content areas (ie, by MOCA-Peds learning objectives or subspecialty category). A dashboard will display historical progress on the practice tests. *(Note, neither CME nor MOC credit can be claimed if only the practice test is completed.)*
- **PREP Alerts** (accessed by clicking on the "PREP alerts" link on the left navigation) deliver questions via SMS (text-message) or email notification. Choose when you wish to receive questions from several options and keep PREP as close as your mobile device.
- **Peer-performance results** are presented as unique data sets for practitioner and nonpractitioner learners. Results can be seen within each critique (right side at the top of the critique box; the blue "View Peer Results" displays a histogram of all peer answer responses) or by specialty category from the "Performance" tab. Each learner's first attempt (baseline score) and current score is recorded to illustrate learning progress. Review performance by topic and identify areas for further study.
- **Confidence ratings** help learners hone their test taking skills. Instead of clicking on "submit" after answering each question, learners can select 100%, 50%, or 0% options based on their confidence in answering each question. (100% = I know I'm right; 50% = I think I'm right; 0% = I'm guessing.) Updated confidence rating reports allow learners to create reports by Confidence Category or by one of the major Specialty Categories. Content with the highest confidence rating and the lowest score represents the greatest knowledge gaps.
- **PREP Pearls** at the end of each critique summarize key practice points. All PREP Pearls are aggregated by specialty category and can be viewed from the "PREP Pearls" tab, providing a useful review tool prior to examinations.
- **Suggested reading** lists provide opportunities for further study and learning. The online version links directly to the most salient related content including relevant review articles in *Pediatrics in Review* for PREP the Curriculum subscribers.

About the Questions and Critiques

Each question represents an incomplete statement that requires the selection of the SINGLE BEST ANSWER. The Critique is the educational component of the PREP Self-Assessment. Learners can reset and retake the self-assessment as often as desired and compare their most recent performance to their baseline initial score.

No product-specific advertising of any type, or links to product web sites, appear in this educational activity.

Learning or Practice Mode:

The learning mode is the default mode. CME and MOC credit may only be claimed after all the questions have been answered and a score of 70% or greater has been achieved in the learning mode.

The practice test allows learners to create a timed examination in the content area of their choice and assess their knowledge before studying for high-stakes testing. Learners should complete their timed practice test in one online session. The 2017 and 2018 online MOCA-Peds bonus questions are accessible in the practice test and by clicking on the MOCA-Peds tab at the top of the screen.

Note the exam mode is no longer offered in the 2019 PREP Self-Assessment.

Information About CME Credit for the 2019 PREP Self-Assessment:

The American Academy of Pediatrics (AAP) is accredited by the Accreditation Council for Continuing Medical Education (ACCME) to provide continuing medical education for physicians.

The AAP designates this enduring material for a maximum of 40.00 AMA PRA Category 1 Credits™. Physicians should claim only the credit commensurate with the extent of their participation in the activity.

This activity is acceptable for a maximum of 40.00 AAP credits. These credits can be applied toward the AAP CME/CPD* Award available to Fellows and Candidate Members of the AAP.

The American Academy of Physician Assistants (AAPA) accepts certificates of participation for educational activities certified for AMA PRA Category 1 Credit™ from organizations accredited by ACCME. Physician assistants may receive a maximum of 40.00 hours of Category 1 credit for completing this program.

This program is accredited for 40.00 NAPNAP CE contact hours of which 6.5 contain pharmacology (Rx) content, (0.00 related to psychopharmacology) (0.00 related to controlled substances), per the National Association of Pediatric Nurse Practitioners Continuing Education Guidelines.

National AAP Members and PediaLink subscribers can record their AMA PRA Category 1 Credits™ directly in their AAP transcript files at www.pedialink.org. Nonmembers may choose to access their transcripts for a fee.

The 2019 PREP Self-Assessment is approved for 40 Points by the ABP through the AAP MOC Portfolio Program for MOC Part 2: Lifelong Learning and Self-Assessment. All approved activities must be completed by the MOC credit approval end date. All deadlines and MOC point values should be confirmed on the ABP's web site and within each physician's ABP portfolio.

For Learners in Canada:

"This activity is an Accredited Self-Assessment Program (Section 3) as defined by the Maintenance of Certification Program of The Royal College of Physicians & Surgeons of Canada, and approved by the Canadian Paediatric Society. You may claim a maximum of 40 hours (credits are automatically calculated)."

2019 Transcript Deadline: December 31, 2019

For AAP members and PediaLink subscribers to have credit summarized on the 2019 CME transcript, the CME credit claiming deadline is 11:59 pm EST on December 31, 2019. CME credit claiming requests submitted after December 31, 2019 will be reflected on the following year's transcript.

Expiration of Credit: December 31, 2021

Credit for the 2019 PREP Self-Assessment expires on December 31, 2021 at 11:59 pm EST. Subscribers can only request credit using the online format. Print users can record their responses on the online answer form and "sign" the attestation that the program was completed as intended. Duplicate claims will not be accepted.

Customer Service

If you have a question, suggestion, or comment about the PREP Self-Assessment or an address change, please contact the AAP Customer Service Center at: csc@aap.org.

*Continuing Professional Development

ACGME Core Competency Icons

The Accreditation Council for Graduate Medical Education (ACGME) and the 24 American Board of Medical Specialties (ABMS) certifying Boards have identified 6 core competencies that they consider to be the foundation of high-quality medical care.

To assist PREP Self-Assessment users in identifying when ACGME core competencies and the Institute of Medicine's physician attributes are addressed in a question/critique, icons have been added as noted below. Since medical knowledge and patient care are routinely addressed in PREP Self-Assessment questions/critiques, these competencies are not referenced with an icon.

 Interpersonal and Communication Skills result in effective information exchange and teaming with patients, families, and other health professionals

 Professionalism manifested through a commitment to professional responsibilities, adherence to ethical principles, and sensitivity to a diverse patient population

 Practice-Based Learning and Improvement involves investigation and evaluation of one's own patient care, appraisal, and assimilation of scientific evidence, and improvements of patient care

 Systems-Based Practice demonstrates an awareness of and responsiveness to the larger context and system of health care and effectively calls on system resources to provide care that is of optimal value

 Safety

 Interdisciplinary Teams

Privacy and Confidentiality Statement

At the AAP, we take the issue of privacy very seriously. We do not sell, distribute, barter, or transfer personally identifiable information obtained from a user to a third party without your consent. Any information collected on the web site is only used for the purpose stated.

The AAP list is only for important AAP communications, and your e-mail address will not be sold or provided to third parties. You will not receive advertising or promotional material on this list.

The AAP may use "cookie" technology to obtain non-personal information from its online visitors. We do not extract personal information in this process nor do we provide this information to third parties. We also do not contact you based on the information in your cookie file.

The AAP has taken steps to make all information received from our online visitors as secure as possible against unauthorized access and use. All information is protected by our security measures, which are periodically reviewed.

AAP PREP Editorial Board and Staff

Disclosure of Financial Relationships and Resolution of Conflicts of Interest for AAP CME Activities Grid

No commercial support is associated with this CME activity.

The AAP CME/CPD program develops, maintains, and improves the competence, skills, and professional performance of pediatricians and pediatric healthcare professionals by providing quality, relevant, accessible, and effective educational experiences that address gaps in professional practice. The AAP CME/CPD program strives to meet the educational needs of pediatricians and pediatric healthcare professionals and support their lifelong learning with a goal of improving care for children and families. *(AAP CME/ CPD Program Mission Statement, May 2015)*

The AAP recognizes that there are a variety of financial relationships between individuals and commercial interests that require review to identify possible conflicts of interest in a CME activity. The "AAP Policy on Disclosure of Financial Relationships and Resolution of Conflicts of Interest for AAP CME Activities" is designed to ensure quality, objective, balanced, and scientifically rigorous AAP CME activities by identifying and resolving all potential conflicts of interest prior to the confirmation of service of those in a position to influence and/or control CME content. The AAP has taken steps to resolve any potential conflicts of interest.

All AAP CME activities will strictly adhere to the *Accreditation Council for Continuing Medical Education (ACCME) Standards for Commercial Support: Standards to Ensure the Independence of CME Activities*. In accordance with these Standards, the following decisions will be made free of the control of a commercial interest: identification of CME needs, determination of educational objectives, selection and presentation of content, selection of all persons and organizations that will be in a position to control the content, selection of educational methods, and evaluation of the CME activity.

The purpose of this policy is to ensure all potential conflicts of interest are identified and mechanisms to resolve them prior to the CME activity are implemented in ways that are consistent with the public good. The AAP is committed to providing learners with commercially unbiased CME activities.

Activity Title: 2019 PREP Self-Assessment
Activity Dates: January 1, 2019 through December 31, 2021

Disclosure of Financial Relationships

All individuals in a position to influence and/or control the content of AAP CME activities are required to disclose to the AAP and subsequently to learners that the individual either has no relevant financial relationships or any financial relationships with the manufacturer(s) of any commercial product(s) and/or provider(s) of commercial services discussed in CME activities. Listed below are the disclosures provided by individuals in a position to influence and/or control CME activity content.

* A commercial interest is defined as any entity producing, marketing, re-selling, or distributing health care goods or services consumed by, or used on, patients.

No commercial support is associated with this CME activity.

Name	Role	Relevant Financial Relationship (Please indicate Yes, or No)	Name of Commercial Interest(s)* (Please list name(s) of entity) AND Nature of Relevant Financial Relationship(s) (Please list: Research Grant, Speaker's Bureau, Stock/Bonds excluding mutual funds, Consultant, Other - identify)	Disclosure of Off-Label (Unapproved)/ Investigational Uses of Products AAP CME faculty are required to disclose to the AAP and to learners when they plan to discuss or demonstrate pharmaceuticals and/or medical devices that are not approved by the FDA and/or medical or surgical procedures that involve an unapproved or "off-label" use of an approved device or pharmaceutical. (Do intend to discuss or Do not intend to discuss)
Berkow, Roger L.	Editor	No	None	I do not intend to discuss an unapproved/investigative use of a commercial product/device
Carl, Rebecca	Author	No	None	I do not intend to discuss an unapproved/investigative use of a commercial product/device
Duryea, Teresa K.	Author	Yes	Wolters Kluwer Health, Inc. (Royalties)	I do not intend to discuss an unapproved/investigative use of a commercial product/device
Fish, Jonathan D.	Author	Yes	AstraZeneca (Data Safety Monitoring Board) Daiichi Sankyo (Paid consultant – Data Safety Monitoring Board)	I do not intend to discuss an unapproved/investigative use of a commercial product/device
Frale, Kathleen	Staff	No	None	I do not intend to discuss an unapproved/investigative use of a commercial product/device
Guill, Margaret F.	Author	No	None	I do intend to discuss an unapproved/investigative use of a commercial product/device
Guralnick, Susan	Editor	No	None	I do intend to discuss an unapproved/investigative use of a commercial product/device
Jaffe, David	Staff/ Disclosure Reviewer & Resolver	No	None	I do not intend to discuss an unapproved/investigative use of a commercial product/device
Kapur, Gaurav	Author	Yes	Alexion (Research Grant)	I do not intend to discuss an unapproved/investigative use of a commercial product/device
King, Joanna	Staff	No	None	I do not intend to discuss an unapproved/investigative use of a commercial product/device
Krowchuk, Daniel P.	Author	No	None	I do not intend to discuss an unapproved/investigative use of a commercial product/device and will disclose such references to learners
Larson, Ilse	Author	No	None	I do not intend to discuss an unapproved/investigative use of a commercial product/device
LaTuga, Mariam Susan	Author	No	None	I do not intend to discuss an unapproved/investigative use of a commercial product/device
Liu, Yi Hui	Author	No	None	I do intend to discuss an unapproved/investigative use of a commercial product/device
Louden, Kathleen	Copy editor	No	None	I do not intend to discuss an unapproved/investigative use of a commercial product/device
Mahler, Carolyn	Copy editor	No	None	I do not intend to discuss an unapproved/investigative use of a commercial product/device
Marquez, Lucila	Author	Yes	Cempra, Inc (Research Grant)	I do intend to discuss an unapproved/investigative use of a commercial product/device
Maxwell, Lisbeth	Copy editor	No	None	I do not intend to discuss an unapproved/investigative use of a commercial product/device
McBride, Mary Eileen	Author	No	None	I do not intend to discuss an unapproved/investigative use of a commercial product/device
Montez, Kimberly	Author	Yes	Boston Scientific (Stocks and Bonds); Valeant Pharmaceuticals (Stocks and Bonds); Alexion Pharmaceuticals (Stocks and Bonds); Regeneron Pharmaceuticals (Stocks and Bonds); Novo Nordisk (Stocks and Bonds)	I do not intend to discuss an unapproved/investigative use of a commercial product/device

Name	Role	Relevant Financial Relationship (Please indicate Yes or No)	Name of Commercial Interest(s)* (Please list name(s) of entity) AND Nature of Relevant Financial Relationship(s) (Please list: Research Grant, Speaker's Bureau, Stock/Bonds excluding mutual funds, Consultant, Other - identify)	Disclosure of Off-Label (Unapproved)/ Investigational Uses of Products AAP CME faculty are required to disclose to the AAP and to learners when they plan to discuss or demonstrate pharmaceuticals and/or medical devices that are not approved by the FDA and/or medical or surgical procedures that involve an unapproved or "off-label" use of an approved device or pharmaceutical. (Do intend to discuss or Do not intend to discuss)
Morita, Denise	Author	Yes	Taylor and Francis Group (Royalties)	I do intend to discuss an unapproved/investigative use of a commercial product/device and will disclose such references to learners
Needham, Heather	Author	No	None	I do not intend to discuss an unapproved/investigative use of a commercial product/device and will disclose such references to learners
Parsley, L. Kristin	Author	No	None	I do not intend to discuss an unapproved/investigative use of a commercial product/device
Piscoran, Susan	Staff/Disclosure Reviewer & Resolver	No	None	I do not intend to discuss an unapproved/investigative use of a commercial product/device
Rao, Beena	Copy Editor	No	None	I do not intend to discuss an unapproved/investigative use of a commercial product/device
Rose, Jerri A.	Author	No	None	I do not intend to discuss an unapproved/investigative use of a commercial product/device
Sarnaik, Ajit	Author	No	None	I do not intend to discuss an unapproved/investigative use of a commercial product/device
Shetty, Avinash K.	Author	No	None	I do not intend to discuss an unapproved/investigative use of a commercial product/device
Sullivan, Jillian	Author	Yes	Cystic Fibrosis Foundation (Research Grant)	I do not intend to discuss an unapproved/investigative use of a commercial product/device
Van Cleave, Jeanne Marie	Author	No	None	I do not intend to discuss an unapproved/investigative use of a commercial product/device
Vogt, Karen S.	Author	No	None	I do not intend to discuss an unapproved/investigative use of a commercial product/device

Editors and Authors = Planners

2019

PREP® Self-Assessment
Questions and Images

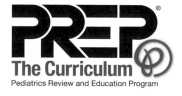

Item 1

A 14-year-old boy is being evaluated for back pain. He describes bilateral low back pain that began 9 months ago. The pain is intermittent, and is worse after physical activity or prolonged sitting. He does not recall a preceding acute injury or incident. He denies radiation of pain, fever, rash, joint swelling, weakness, and bowel or bladder changes. The boy was evaluated for the pain at an urgent care facility 3 months ago. Radiographs obtained at that visit were reportedly normal. On physical examination, the boy has pain with lumbar flexion and bilateral rotation. He is tender to palpation along the lumbar paraspinal muscles and has tightness of his hamstring and calf muscles. Full neurologic examination findings are normal.

Of the following, the MOST appropriate next step in this boy's evaluation and management is

A. bone scintigraphy with single-photon emission computed tomography

B. magnetic resonance imaging of the lumbar spine

C. physical therapy for core stabilization

D. rest from sports and physical education class

Item 2

A mother brings her 5-year-old son to the clinic for evaluation of a harsh cough. The child has a 2-day history of clear rhinorrhea and cough, without fever or respiratory distress. The mother is demanding a prescription for an albuterol inhaler because she is concerned her child's condition will worsen over the next few days. She also requests a doctor's note to excuse the child from school for the entire upcoming week. The resident seeing the patient believes that the boy has a mild viral upper respiratory illness and he does not feel that the mother's requests are medically indicated.

The boy's vital signs are normal. His physical examination findings are unremarkable other than mild clear rhinorrhea. In particular, the lung examination finds no wheezing or focal findings.

The child's medical history helps with understanding the mother's concerns. The boy was born late preterm and stayed in the hospital for 2 weeks for observation and phototherapy. At 11 months of age, he required hospitalization for 3 days for bronchiolitis. He has been seen often for mild viral illnesses, but has no documented history of wheezing. However, the mother admits that she sometimes gives the patient his brother's albuterol when he is coughing a lot. The boy has been diagnosed and treated for otitis media twice, but has no history of pneumonia. He has received all his routine health maintenance care, including immunizations. He has normal growth and development, but has some behavioral problems at school.

Of the following, the MOST appropriate next step in management is to

A. discuss with the mother her parental perception of vulnerability to illness

B. perform laboratory tests to evaluate the boy for an underlying immunodeficiency

C. reassure the mother and provide the requested doctor's note for school

D. refer the boy to a pulmonary specialist for pulmonary function testing

Item 3

A 1-year-old boy with fever and cough has a history of multiple bacterial infections, including pneumonia, otitis media, and a skin abscess. His parents describe multiple malodorous stools daily and a chronic diaper rash. He has a temperature of 38.5°C, heart rate of 140 beat/min, respiratory rate of 20 breaths/min, blood pressure of 90/60 mm Hg, weight of 7.5 kg (< third percentile for age), and length of 71 cm (third percentile for age). His weight-for-length percentile is 3%. He is fatigued and thin. His lung examination reveals left-sided crackles. His abdomen is distended but soft and nontender. He has an erythematous and ulcerated perianal rash.

Laboratory data are shown:

Laboratory Test	Result
White blood cell count	5,000/µL (5.0 × 10^9/L)
Absolute neutrophil count	700/µL (0.7 × 10^9/L)
Hemoglobin	8.8 g/dL (88 g/L)
Hematocrit	27.3%
Platelet count	112 × 10^3/µL (112 × 10^9/L)
Pancreatic elastase	< 50 µg/g stool
Fecal fat (spot)	42%

Ultrasonography of the abdomen demonstrates fatty replacement of the pancreas.

Of the following, the MOST likely diagnosis is

A. chronic pancreatitis

B. cystic fibrosis

C. Fanconi anemia

D. Shwachman-Diamond syndrome

Item 4

A 4-year-old boy has behavioral problems. His foster mother states that when he is upset, he will have a tantrum, throw toys, and hit anyone near him. He was dismissed from preschool because of concerns for the safety of his classmates. The boy was recently placed in the care of his foster mother who does not know the circumstances leading to his removal from his biological family. She asks about possible contributors to his aggressive behaviors.

Of the following, the MOST accurate response is that these behaviors have been associated with

A. an authoritative parenting style
B. decreased dopamine and serotonin levels
C. a lower number of siblings
D. prenatal exposure to cocaine

Item 5

A 12-year-old girl is brought to the emergency department for new-onset clumsiness. Her parents report that over the past week she has been tripping over small things, like steps into their house or curbs. The girl says it is especially hard to walk up stairs. Her lower back aches all over, but there is no shooting pain into her legs or pain in her calves or feet. Her feet feel a little numb and tingly, but her hands and arms feel normal. She denies urinary or stool incontinence. She had a fever and cough 2 weeks ago, and missed several days of school, but otherwise has been well. The girl's vital signs are normal. Her neurologic examination shows normal eye movements, and she can puff out her cheeks and purse her lips normally. She has full strength in both upper extremities. She is able to rise from a chair quickly without using her hands, but has difficulty standing on her tiptoes and on her heels. She can feel light touch on her face, arms, and legs, and all over her back. No reflexes are elicited from her arms or legs. When walking, she lifts her thighs up high; her little brother says she looks like a pony when she walks. The remainder of her physical examination findings are unremarkable. A negative inspiratory force measurement is obtained, and it is normal.

Of the following, the next BEST management step for this girl is to

A. obtain a creatine kinase level
B. perform a lumbar puncture
C. provide reassurance
D. start intravenous methylprednisolone

Item 6

A 3-year-old boy has an intensely itchy rash of 7 weeks' duration. The lesions come and go but do not last for more than 24 hours before new lesions develop. During this time, he has also experienced a few episodes of sudden lip swelling that took 48 hours to subside. The family is unaware of any triggering factors. No other family members have a similar rash, and there is no family history of atopy. He has been otherwise healthy without fever and is not taking any medications. The rash consists of circumscribed, raised, blanching erythematous papules, some of which have central pallor, located on the trunk and extremities. The face (Item Q6) and scalp are involved, but the mucous membranes and the palms and soles are spared. The remainder of the examination findings are normal.

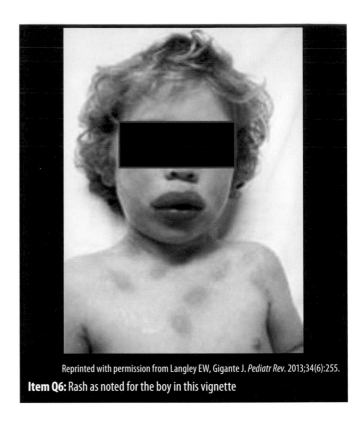

Reprinted with permission from Langley EW, Gigante J. *Pediatr Rev.* 2013;34(6):255.

Item Q6: Rash as noted for the boy in this vignette

Of the following, the laboratory value MOST likely to be abnormal in this child is

A. antinuclear antibodies
B. rheumatoid factor
C. thyroid-stimulating hormone
D. tissue transglutaminase antibodies

Item 7

A 2-year-old African American boy is brought to the emergency department by his parents because of excessive fatigue and "funny breathing." He had been well until 2 days ago when he was seen by his pediatrician for cellulitis on his thumb, for which he was prescribed trimethoprim-sulfamethoxazole. He received the first dose just over 24 hours ago. He has not been taking any other medications, vitamins, or supplements, and he has had normal growth and development.

He is at the 55th percentile for height and the 60th percentile for weight. He has a heart rate of 122 beats/min, blood pressure of 100/75 mm Hg, temperature of 37°C, respiratory rate of 30 breaths/min, and oxygen saturation of 99% on room air. He appears pale and fatigued, but his examination findings are otherwise unremarkable.

Laboratory data are shown:

Laboratory Test	Result
White blood cell count	6,700 /μL (6.7 × 10⁹/L)
Hemoglobin	5.1 g/dL (51 g/L)
Platelet count	640 × 10³ /μL (640 × 10⁹/L)
Reticulocytes	37%

A peripheral blood smear is remarkable for the presence of "blister" cells and polychromatic macrocytes.

Of the following, this child's disease is MOST likely caused by an

A. acquired antibody-mediated hemolytic anemia

B. autosomal dominant red cell membranopathy

C. autosomal recessive hemoglobinopathy

D. X-linked red cell enzymopathy

Item 8

A local Emergency Medicine Services (EMS) agency calls to request medical direction for a 2-year-old girl they are preparing to transport to the emergency department. Fifteen minutes ago, the girl was injured when her teenage brother, while giving her a "piggyback ride" down the front steps, lost his balance and fell, pinning the girl's left leg underneath his body. Her aunt witnessed the event and immediately called 911, because the girl's left leg appeared deformed and she was screaming in pain.

The girl is alert and interactive, but has been crying incessantly. Her left femur is significantly deformed and bruised, and she refuses to move her left leg. Her neurologic status appears to be intact. The EMS team has made 4 attempts to place an intravenous line without success. They are requesting your guidance on the most appropriate pain control regimen for this girl, who is being transported an approximately 30-minute drive from her home. You advise the EMS team to immobilize the girl's left lower extremity.

Of the following, the BEST next step in this girl's management is to provide

A. intranasal fentanyl

B. oral ibuprofen

C. oral 25% sucrose solution

D. distraction techniques during transport

Item 9

A previously healthy 7-year-old boy is brought to the emergency department (ED) for evaluation. He has had diarrhea for the last 8 days and bloody diarrhea for 2 days. He has become increasingly listless over the past several hours. He has no known previous medical problems. There is no history of similar illness in other family members. A week ago the boy visited an apple orchard on a school trip. His family does not know if any other children on the trip had similar symptoms. Physical examination reveals an ill-appearing child, with marked pallor and periorbital edema. His temperature is 38.4°C, heart rate is 120 beats/min, respiratory rate is 28 breaths /min, and blood pressure is 90/50 mm Hg. He has normal growth parameters.

Of the following, the test MOST likely to confirm the boy's diagnosis is

A. complete blood cell count with smear

B. serum electrolyte panel

C. stool culture

D. urinalysis

Item 10

An 8-year-old boy who is a new patient is brought for a health supervision visit. He and his mother have no concerns. His vital signs are unremarkable except for a blood pressure in the right arm of 160/80 mm Hg. His physical examination findings are remarkable for a delayed right femoral pulse relative to the right brachial pulse. He is referred to a pediatric cardiologist.

Of the following, the BEST next step in management for this child's hypertension is

A. adoption of healthy diet and exercise

B. initiation of amlodipine

C. initiation of enalapril

D. surgical or transcatheter repair

Item 11

A 17-year-old adolescent boy is seen for a health supervision visit. He has a history of attention-deficit/hyperactivity disorder and type 1 diabetes mellitus. He is not always compliant with taking his methylphenidate. His parents are very involved in his medical care. He is in 11th grade and is discussing the universities he and his parents plan to tour during spring break. All of the schools are out of state.

Of the following, the BEST next step in preparation for more independent care is to

A. discuss his medications with his mother

B. discuss readiness to establish care with an adult provider

C. inquire about medication adverse effects

D. update his immunizations

Item 12

A 6-year-old girl is being evaluated 5 days after she suffered a severe traumatic brain injury. She underwent decompressive craniectomy and placement of an external ventricular drain, and has been receiving mechanical ventilation. Elevated intracranial pressures have been treated with sedation, mannitol, maintenance of normocarbia, and cerebrospinal fluid drainage. She has been tolerating nasogastric tube feeds of a standard pediatric formula at 50 mL/hour. Her weight is 20 kg. On physical examination, the girl is intubated and sedated. She does not open her eyes spontaneously and withdraws all extremities equally upon pain stimuli. Pupils are 4 mm, equal, and sluggishly reactive. Her mucous membranes are moist, and she has periorbital and soft tissue edema. Urine output over the past 24 hours was 240 mL.

Urine studies show the following:

Laboratory Test	Result
Specific gravity	1.015
Sodium	50 mEq/L (50 mmol/L)
Potassium	20 mEq/L (20 mmol/L)
Creatinine	4.0 mg/dL (353.6 μmol/L)
Urine urea nitrogen	6 mg/dL (2.1 mmol/L)

Of the following, the girl's MOST likely serum electrolyte disturbance is

A. hyperchloremia
B. hyperkalemia
C. hypocalcemia
D. hyponatremia

Item 13

A 3-year-old boy is being evaluated for fever and rash. He has had daily fevers for the past 15 days; fevers occur in the late afternoon or early evening and his temperatures are routinely between 39°C and 40°C. During the day, the boy has had slightly decreased energy and has occasionally reported fatigue, but he has been well enough to attend daycare. He has an evanescent rash on his trunk that is most notable when he is febrile. On physical examination a rash is noted (Item Q13) as well as small effusions of his right knee and left elbow. His liver edge is palpable 3 cm below the right costal margin.

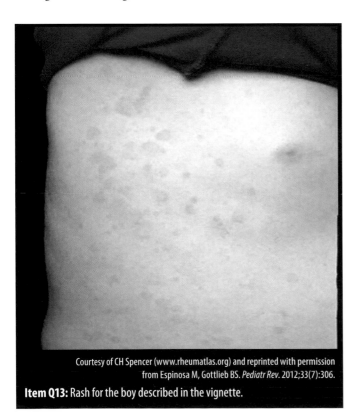

Courtesy of CH Spencer (www.rheumatlas.org) and reprinted with permission from Espinosa M, Gottlieb BS. *Pediatr Rev.* 2012;33(7):306.
Item Q13: Rash for the boy described in the vignette.

Of the following, the laboratory abnormality MOST likely to be associated with the suspected diagnosis is

A. elevated antinuclear antibody titer
B. elevated erythrocyte sedimentation rate
C. leukopenia
D. positive rheumatoid factor

Item 14

A 20-month-old, previously healthy girl is preparing to go on a 5-week trip to Lagos, Nigeria, as part of an organized church group trip. Her mother is concerned about their risk of acquiring poliomyelitis in Nigeria. The child was born in the United States and received inactivated polio vaccination at 2, 4, and 15 months of age. Her mother was also born in the United States and received her complete polio vaccination series as a child. The girl's physical examination findings are normal.

Of the following, the MOST appropriate management to minimize the risk of infection of both the child and mother is to administer inactivated polio vaccine in

A. 1 dose to the child and none to the mother
B. 1 dose to the mother and none to the child
C. 1 dose to both the mother and child
D. 2 doses to both the mother and child (4 weeks apart)

Item 15

A neonate with petechiae is being evaluated 15 hours after birth. She was born vaginally, at term, 20 hours after rupture of membranes, to a 26-year-old gravida 2, para 0 woman whose noninvasive prenatal screening was positive for trisomy 21. She had declined confirmatory testing. Group B *Streptococcus* screening was negative. On physical examination, the neonate has facial features consistent with trisomy 21, normal respiratory effort, mild generalized hypotonia, and 10 petechiae scattered over the abdomen. No murmur is heard. A complete blood cell count from a central sample shows a white blood cell count of 16,000/μL (16 × 10⁹/L), hemoglobin of 23 g/dL (230 g/L), hematocrit of 69%, and platelet count of 125 × 10³/μL (125 × 10⁹/L). She has breastfed 3 times and taken 15 mL of formula. Her mother reports 1 stool and 1 wet diaper.

Of the following, the BEST next management step for this neonate is to

A. infuse 10 mL/kg of normal saline
B. infuse 10 mL/kg of platelets
C. observe closely
D. perform partial exchange transfusion

Item 16

A 10-year-old boy has a chronic cough. His mother notes that he coughs at night several times each week, enough to wake her but it does not seem to bother him. He has trouble keeping up with peers in sports activities and gym class; he says he runs out of breath easily and has to stop and rest. There is a family history of asthma in a paternal uncle, cystic fibrosis in a maternal cousin, and seasonal allergies in both parents. Physical examination findings are normal, including growth parameters and vital signs.

Of the following, the BEST next step in his evaluation is to perform

A. chest radiography
B. methacholine inhalation
C. spirometry
D. sweat chloride testing

Item 17

A 16-year-old adolescent boy is being evaluated for a lesion on his back. He reports that the lesion appeared 5 or 6 weeks ago as a "small red bump" and has grown since then. He has no history of trauma and no associated symptoms. The physical examination findings are unremarkable with the exception of a lesion on the upper right side of the back (Item Q17).

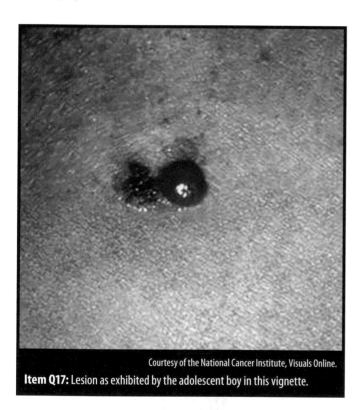

Courtesy of the National Cancer Institute, Visuals Online.

Item Q17: Lesion as exhibited by the adolescent boy in this vignette.

Of the following, the MOST appropriate next step is to

A. advise the patient that the lesion will resolve without intervention
B. apply mupirocin and reevaluate in 4 weeks
C. cauterize the lesion with silver nitrate
D. refer the patient to a dermatologist for excision of the lesion

Item 18

A 14-year-old adolescent girl is admitted to the pediatric intensive care unit for diabetic ketoacidosis. She was diagnosed with type 1 diabetes at 8 years of age. This admission is her third in the past year for diabetic ketoacidosis. Her diabetes is managed with 22 units of insulin glargine subcutaneously at bedtime and bolus doses of rapid-acting insulin. During the 12 hours prior to admission, she had diffuse abdominal pain and vomiting without fever. She weighs 45 kg.

Laboratory data at the time of admission are shown:

Laboratory Test	Result
Glucose	486 mg/dL (27 mmol/L)
Serum bicarbonate	8 mEq/L (8 mmol/L)
Venous pH	7.15
White blood cell count	17,000/μL (17.0 × 10⁹/L)

Of the following, the MOST likely precipitating factor of her diabetic ketoacidosis is

A. excessive carbohydrate intake
B. gastroenteritis
C. inadequate basal insulin dose
D. insulin omission

Item 19

A neonate with multiple anomalies is being evaluated in the newborn nursery. Her physical examination findings are remarkable for bilateral iris colobomas, bilateral choanal atresia, and unilateral facial palsy, as well as facial dysmorphology, which includes a square/flat midface, broad, prominent forehead, and broad nasal bridge. The ears are low set and asymmetric with a prominent antihelix and clipped-off helix. On auscultation, a cardiac murmur is detected. Echocardiography reveals an atrioventricular canal defect. In addition, the neonate failed her hearing screen bilaterally.

Of the following, the neonate's MOST likely diagnosis is

A. 22q11.2 deletion
B. branchio-oto-renal syndrome
C. CHARGE syndrome
D. Treacher Collins syndrome

Item 20

A 5-year-old girl is seen for a health supervision visit. The child and her siblings have had multiple missed appointments and a history of elevated social needs. The mother states that the girl is being seen today for "shots and a school note."

The girl was last seen at 3.9 years of age, at which time food insecurity, poor weight gain, and early caries were documented, and age-appropriate nutrition recommendations were reviewed. Referrals were made to the federal supplemental nutrition program and a dental clinic. However, the girl's medical record documents multiple attempts by the care coordinator and the dental clinic staff to contact the mother with no response. A 2-month follow-up visit was scheduled but not kept.

Today, the mother reports that she never received those calls, although she verified that her phone number is correct. She states that she does not want to apply for food stamps and that her daughter has not been to the dentist because of "stuff going on." She requests a letter excusing 30 days of missed school for illnesses this year. The girl's weight has fallen from the 15th percentile to the 1st percentile. She has brown spots on multiple teeth, suggesting worsening tooth decay.

Of the following, the MOST appropriate response to this mother's behavior pattern is to

A. arrange for the care coordinator to meet with the mother in person after your visit

B. provide the school excuse on the condition that she attends a dental visit within 3 weeks

C. report her to the state child welfare agency for suspected neglect

D. threaten to report her to the state child welfare agency if she does not attend a dental visit within 3 weeks

Item 21

A 2-year-old boy with no significant medical history is brought to the emergency department with a limp. The limp began 2 days ago and has been associated with fever. His parents are unable to localize the pain. One week prior to this illness, he had nasal congestion and rhinorrhea and fell, resulting in abrasions to his knee and elbow. He has a temperature of 39.1°C, heart rate of 162 beats/min, respiratory rate of 30 breaths/min, and blood pressure of 106/51 mm Hg. He appears ill and grimaces with movement of the right hip.

Laboratory data are shown:

Laboratory Test	Result
White blood cell count	16,600/μL (16.6 × 10⁹/L)
Neutrophils	51%
Bands	20%
Lymphocytes	19%
Monocytes	10%
Hemoglobin	11.8 g/dL (118 g/L)
Platelet count	237 × 10³/μL (237 × 10⁹/L)
C-reactive protein	6.9 mg/dL (657 nmol/L)
Erythrocyte Sedimentation rate	29 mm/h

Radiographs of the hip are concerning for a right-sided effusion.

Of the following, the clinical findings BEST support a diagnosis of

A. juvenile idiopathic arthritis

B. pyogenic arthritis

C. transient synovitis

D. traumatic effusion

Item 22

A 16-year-old boy presents for a sports preparticipation physical examination before his junior year in high school. He would like to join his school's wrestling and baseball teams this year. The boy wears glasses and contact lenses for myopia. His corrected vision is 20/20 on the left and 20/70 on the right.

Of the following, the MOST appropriate recommendation for this boy is that he may participate in

A. baseball with appropriate sports goggles, but not wrestling

B. baseball with appropriate sports goggles, and wrestling without special requirement

C. neither baseball nor wrestling

D. wrestling, but not baseball

Item 23

A parent needs to administer 125 mg of oral amoxicillin liquid (250 mg/5 mL) to their young child.

Of the following, the method MOST likely to reduce the likelihood of a dosing error is to administer the medication using a

A. medication cup labeled in 2.5-mL increments

B. medication cup labeled in ½-teaspoon increments

C. medication cup labeled in ½-teaspoon and 2.5-mL increments

D. syringe labeled in 0.5-mL increments

Item 24

A 15-year-old Native American adolescent girl has concerns of bloating, flatulence, and diarrhea. These symptoms began 12 to 18 months ago and are not improving. She reports that certain foods, specifically ice cream and pizza, make her symptoms worse. Her diarrhea is nonbloody and can occur up to 3 to 5 times per day. Other adults in her family have similar symptoms. She appears well nourished and is in no acute distress. She has a weight of 52 kg (50th percentile), height of 163 cm (50th percentile), and body mass index of 19.3 kg/m² (45th percentile). Her abdomen is distended but soft and nontender. The remainder of the physical examination findings are normal.

Of the following, the MOST likely diagnosis is

A. galactosemia
B. hereditary fructose intolerance
C. primary lactase deficiency
D. sucrase-isomaltase deficiency

Item 25

A 10-year-old boy is seen for behavioral concerns. His parents are concerned about his high energy and impulsivity. They describe him as periodically irritable. He can become quite angry, aggressive, and out of control. Sometimes, he is in a great mood and his hyperactivity seems more pronounced. For the past week, he has been up most of the night building models of aircraft. Despite sleeping only a few hours, he is not tired during the day. When you speak with the boy, he is talkative and excited to tell you how he is designing the fastest plane in the world and will be earning millions when he sells his design. The boy's parents are worried that he will become like his aunt who has had difficulty keeping steady employment because of frequent disappearances to go on shopping sprees.

Of the following, the MOST likely diagnosis is

A. attention-deficit/hyperactivity disorder
B. bipolar disorder
C. disruptive mood dysregulation disorder
D. oppositional defiant disorder

Item 26

A 16-year-old boy is brought to the emergency department (ED) for altered consciousness. He had been at a party at a friend's house where no adults were present. His friends found him unconscious in an empty room and immediately drove him to the ED. In the ED, he seems sleepy and confused, but his symptoms improve during his stay. He remembers being at the party and then feeling "weird," so he went into the room to be alone. He does not remember anything after that. He denies taking any medications or drugs. He has never had an episode like this before. His vital signs and general physical examination findings are normal. There are no signs of injury. His neurologic examination shows improving mental status over the course of the ED visit, and symmetrically brisk deep tendon reflexes. Electrolyte levels, renal and liver function tests, complete blood cell count with differential, and toxicology screening results are all normal. Results of electrocardiography and computed tomography of the head are also normal.

Of the following, the test MOST likely to reveal the boy's underlying diagnosis is

A. electroencephalography
B. lumbar puncture
C. magnetic resonance imaging of the brain
D. serum ammonia level

Item 27

A 4-day-old term neonate born via spontaneous vaginal delivery is readmitted to the hospital with symptoms of vomiting, lethargy, poor feeding, and decreased urine output. He has been exclusively breastfed and was feeding normally the first 2 days after birth. Since discharge at 48 hours after birth, he has had vomiting and lethargy that has progressively gotten worse. His weight today is 2.7 kg, and his birthweight was 3.0 kg. He has a temperature of 38.4°C, heart rate of 165 beats/min, and respiratory rate of 55 breaths/min. He has jaundice in the lower extremities, a bulging anterior fontanelle, abdominal distention, a liver edge palpable 3 cm below the right costal margin, and hypotonia.

Laboratory data are shown.

Laboratory Test	Result
White blood cell count	26,000/μL (26 × 10⁹/L)
Neutrophils	55%
Band neutrophils	20%
Lymphocytes	15%
Monocytes	10%
Hemoglobin	10.2 g/dL (102 g/L)
Platelet count	90 × 10³/μL (90 × 10⁹/L)
Total bilirubin	18.2 mg/dL (311.3 μmol/L)
Direct bilirubin	2.8 mg/dL (47.9 μmol/L)
Alanine aminotransferase	355 U/L
Aspartate aminotransferase	460 U/L
Urine culture	> 100,000 colony-forming units of *Escherichia coli*
Urine reducing substances	Positive

Of the following, the MOST common ophthalmologic finding associated with this neonate's condition is

A. aniridia
B. cataract
C. coloboma
D. glaucoma

Item 28

A previously healthy 10-year-old boy is brought to the emergency department with a 2-week history of worsening exercise intolerance, orthopnea requiring 2 pillows to sleep at night, and a 2-day history of facial swelling. He is thin and in mild respiratory distress with suprasternal retractions. His face is slightly swollen with a subtle red coloration. He has a temperature of 38.8°C, heart rate of

110 beats/min, blood pressure of 104/76 mm Hg, respiratory rate of 28 breaths/min, and oxygen saturation of 97% on room air. A chest radiograph is obtained (Item Q28).

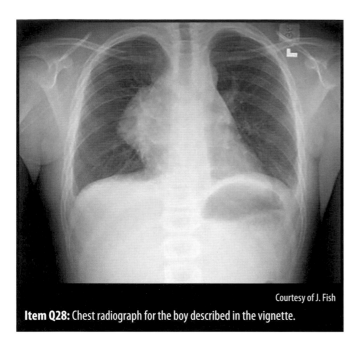

Courtesy of J. Fish

Item Q28: Chest radiograph for the boy described in the vignette.

Of the following, the MOST appropriate next step in managing this patient is to

A. consult a surgeon for an emergency biopsy

B. obtain urgent chest computed tomography with the patient lying supine

C. secure the airway via elective intubation

D. support the airway via noninvasive positive pressure

Item 29

A 4-year-old boy is brought to the emergency department (ED) because of fever and trouble breathing that developed over the past 3 to 4 hours. He initially complained of a sore throat about 12 hours ago, and did not want to eat breakfast this morning. He has not had any cough or nasal congestion. His mother denies any history of choking episodes and notes he seemed unusually restless today. The boy was born full-term at home. He has had no hospitalizations, and takes no medications. He has no allergies, and has never received any immunizations.

On arrival to the ED, the boy's temperature is 39.8°C, heart rate is 150 beats/min, respiratory rate is 40 breaths/min, and pulse oximetry measurement is 95% on room air. He is sitting upright on the bed with his torso leaning forward and neck hyperextended. He is drooling, toxic-appearing, and seems anxious. While his lungs are clear bilaterally with good aeration, he is tachypneic, has suprasternal retractions, and there is intermittent inspiratory stridor. There is marked tenderness to palpation over his anterior neck. You note no other abnormal findings on physical examination. A portable radiograph of the boy's neck is obtained (Item Q29).

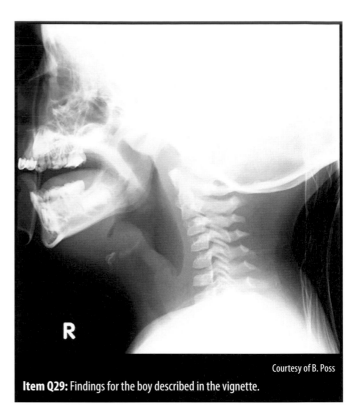

Courtesy of B. Poss

Item Q29: Findings for the boy described in the vignette.

Of the following, the BEST next step in this boy's management is to administer

A. albuterol by nebulizer

B. ceftriaxone and vancomycin, intravenously

C. dexamethasone, intramuscularly

D. 100% humidified oxygen

Item 30

A 7-year-old boy is undergoing a health supervision visit. His urinalysis 1 year ago, performed during a routine health supervision visit, had shown microscopic hematuria (>100 red blood cells per high-power field [hpf]) with no other abnormalities. Because of transient insurance issues, the family did not follow up as scheduled. Today, the boy's temperature is 37.7°C, heart rate is 76 beats/min, respiratory rate is 20 breaths/min, and blood pressure is 110/70 mm Hg. His physical examination findings are normal. His urinalysis demonstrates light amber urine with a specific gravity of 1.025, pH of 6.0, 3+ blood, 3+ protein, with no leukocyte esterase or nitrites. On urine microscopy, there are more than 100 red blood cells/hpf, and no white blood cells, crystals, or bacteria. The boy denies dysuria, frequency, urgency, flank pain, or trauma. Blood tests show normal serum creatinine, electrolyte, and complement levels. Family history includes a maternal uncle with deafness and renal failure and a paternal grandmother with kidney problems.

Of the following, the boy's MOST likely diagnosis is

A. Alport syndrome

B. immunoglobulin A nephritis

C. lupus nephritis

D. myoglobinuria

Item 31

A 1-day-old full-term neonate born by spontaneous vaginal delivery has been doing well by nursing and parent reports. The maternal history is unremarkable, and the mother is expected to be discharged this afternoon. The neonate appears to be latching well. The neonate has age-appropriate vital signs and completely benign physical examination findings. Per newborn nursery protocol, the neonate undergoes critical congenital heart disease (CCHD) screening, which reads 88% with good waveform on the right hand and 99% also with good waveform on the right foot. The test has been repeated 3 times with similar results.

Of the following, the cardiac defect MOST likely to be present in this neonate is

A. Ebstein anomaly

B. hypoplastic left heart syndrome

C. pulmonary atresia

D. transposition of the great arteries

Item 32

A 16-year-old adolescent girl with morbid obesity is seen for a health supervision visit. Her mother is concerned that she is failing 3 classes. During a HEADSS (home and environment; education, employment, and eating; activities; drugs; sexuality; suicide, depression, and safety) assessment, with her mother out of the room, the patient discloses that she is teased at school about her weight and that she feels alone because she does not have many friends. She reports that she has no suicidal thoughts. She has acanthosis nigricans on her neck and both axillae and several superficial well-healed scars on her left wrist.

Of the following, the BEST next step in this patient's evaluation and management would be to

A. order hemoglobin A1C and fasting plasma glucose tests

B. provide information on adolescent weight loss programs

C. refer her to a dietitian for nutrition counseling

D. refer her to a psychologist for counseling

Item 33

A 6-month-old previously healthy boy was brought to the emergency department (ED) by his parents because of altered mental status and blue discoloration around the lips. He and his mother were sleeping in the same bed. When she awoke, she noted that he was breathing irregularly and was difficult to awaken. Upon arrival at the ED, the boy's vital signs are as follows: temperature, 37°C; heart rate, 95 beats/min; blood pressure, 105/60 mm Hg; and respiratory rate, 18 breaths/min. On pulse oximetry, his oxygen saturation is 85% on room air, and improves to 100% on a nonrebreather face mask with 15 L/min oxygen flow. On physical examination, the boy is obtunded. Upon pain stimulus, he withdraws without posturing, does not open his eyes, and moans. His pupils are 4 mm and sluggishly reactive. He exhibits gurgling and a weak cough and gag. He is breathing slowly, deeply, and with occasional pauses that last about 5 seconds. His

lungs are clear to auscultation. He is warm and well-perfused with strong pulses, and his heart sounds are regular, with no murmurs, rubs, or gallops. His abdomen is soft, nontender, and nondistended. There are no external signs of trauma. Point-of-care capillary blood gas analysis shows a pH of 7.15, partial pressure of carbon dioxide of 50 mm Hg, bicarbonate of 18 mEq/L (18 mmol/L), and blood glucose level of 80 mg/dL (4.4 mmol/L).

Of the following, the BEST next management step for this boy is

A. hypertonic saline

B. positive pressure ventilation

C. sodium bicarbonate

D. therapeutic hypothermia

Item 34

A 6-month-old female infant is seen for a health supervision visit. Her parents are concerned that her right eye occasionally turns inward when she is playing with toys. She is developing normally; she sits with assistance, babbles, transfers toys from hand to hand, and appears to enjoy watching older children at her daycare. Her growth parameters are normal and she appears well. Her pupils are equal, round, and reactive to light bilaterally, and her eye shape is normal. Her red reflexes are present and symmetrical. A thorough cover-uncover test (also known as an alternating cover test) cannot be performed because she is fussy during this portion of the examination.

Of the following, the MOST appropriate next step in management is

A. reassurance that this is a normal finding at this age

B. referral to an ophthalmologist for further evaluation and management

C. referral to an ophthalmologist only if there is a family history of childhood visual impairment

D. repeat ocular examination at the next health supervision visit

Item 35

A neonate who has developed conjunctivitis is being evaluated in the neonatal intensive care unit (NICU). During the past 2 weeks, 3 premature infants in the NICU were diagnosed with conjunctivitis after a routine evaluation by the ophthalmologic consultant team for retinopathy of prematurity. One week later, 2 of the nursing staff and a pediatric resident caring for some of the NICU infants developed red eyes with watery discharge, photophobia, and a gritty sensation in their eyes. Infection control was consulted and identified an additional 8 infants in the NICU with conjunctivitis.

Of the following, the MOST likely pathogen causing this outbreak is

A. adenovirus

B. *Chlamydia trachomatis*

C. herpes simplex virus

D. respiratory syncytial virus

Item 36

A 34-week-gestation neonate is admitted to the neonatal intensive care unit. Maternal history is significant for a urinary tract infection and premature prolonged rupture of membranes at 18 weeks. He was delivered via cesarean section because of maternal preeclampsia. The neonate required intubation in the delivery room for respiratory failure. Physical examination findings include compressed facies (Item Q36A), large auricles, and reducible left ankle held in dorsiflexed position (Item Q36B).

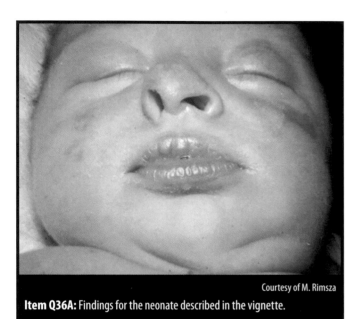

Courtesy of M. Rimsza

Item Q36A: Findings for the neonate described in the vignette.

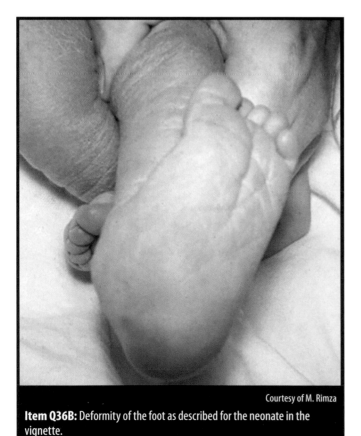

Courtesy of M. Rimsza

Item Q36B: Deformity of the foot as described for the neonate in the vignette.

Of the following, the MOST likely explanation for this neonate's physical examination findings is

A. amniotic band sequence

B. maternal urinary tract infection

C. oligohydramnios sequence

D. prematurity

Item 37

A 15-year-old adolescent girl is playing soccer for the first time on her high school team. She has been physically active in the past, but not at the level required for competitive soccer. She is concerned that she gets short of breath more quickly than her peers when running. She has to stop and rest after a very short period of intense exercise but can walk for long distances and run at a slow jogging pace for more than 30 minutes without respiratory compromise. She reports tightness in her upper chest and difficulty taking in a good breath. She makes what she describes as a wheezing noise when she is having difficulty breathing.

She does not have problems with cough or shortness of breath under any other circumstances. There is no history of asthma or allergies, and no family history of respiratory problems.

She has a history of menorrhagia, for which she takes birth control pills.

She is comfortable at rest with normal vital signs and growth parameters. Pulse oximetry is 99% on room air at rest. There is no increased work of breathing. Breath sounds are clear, with good air entry and no adventitious sounds. The remainder of her examination findings are normal. An exercise provocation test shows an oxygen saturation of 99% on room air throughout the study and postexercise monitoring. Pre-exercise spirometry is normal, and the maximum decrease in forced expiratory volume in 1 second is 5% at 10 minutes after completion of exercise. Her symptom of shortness of breath was reproduced in the study and was the limiting factor in her running.

The flow volume loop at the completion of the 6-minute exercise period is shown (Item Q37):

Item Q37. Spirometry results for the adolescent described in the vignette.

Result	Predicted	Best	% Predicted
FVC (L)	3.72	3.79	102%
FEV1 (L)	3.30	3.33	101%
FEV1/FVC	0.89	0.88	99%
FEF25-75% (L/s)	3.86	4.08	105%
PEFR (L/s)	---	5.89	---

FVC, Forced Vital Capacity (liters); FEV 1, Forced Expiratory Volume in 1 second (liters); FEF 25/75, Forced Expiratory Flow between 25% and 75% of FVC (liters/sec); PEFR, Peak Expiratory Flow Rate (liters/second); % pred, actual value as a percent of the predicted value for age and height

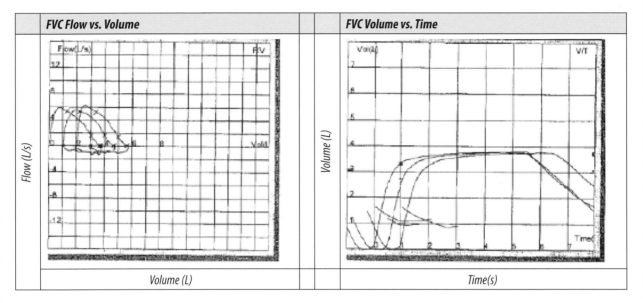

FVC Flow vs. Volume	FVC Volume vs. Time
Volume (L)	Time(s)

Courtesy of M. Guill

Of the following, the MOST likely explanation for her exercise intolerance is

A. anemia

B. cardiomyopathy

C. exercise-induced asthma

D. vocal cord dysfunction

Item 38

During a health supervision visit for a 3-year-old boy, a "bump" on his lateral forehead that has been present since birth is evaluated (Item Q38). The lesion has grown slightly over time and there are no associated symptoms. On palpation, the lesion is firm and mobile; it is not tender and is not compressible.

Of the following, the MOST likely diagnosis is

A. dermoid cyst

B. epidermal cyst

C. infantile hemangioma

D. juvenile xanthogranuloma

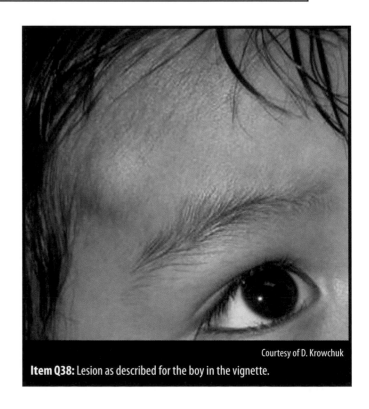

Courtesy of D. Krowchuk

Item Q38: Lesion as described for the boy in the vignette.

Item 39

A 14-year-old previously healthy adolescent girl is brought for follow-up after sustaining a head injury the day prior. She was evaluated in the emergency department after a fall during cheerleading practice that was associated with a brief loss of consciousness. Computed tomography of the head showed no intracranial abnormality, but it did show a nodule in her right thyroid lobe measuring 1.5 cm in greatest diameter. There is no family history of thyroid disease. Physical examination of her thyroid is normal, and the nodule is not palpable. There is no cervical lymphadenopathy. The remainder of her physical examination findings are unremarkable. The results of thyroid function tests are normal. Thyroid ultrasonography confirms a hypoechoic 1.5-cm nodule in the right lobe.

Of the following, the BEST next step in evaluating this patient's incidental finding is to

A. obtain nuclear thyroid scintigraphy

B. reassure her that no additional testing is indicated

C. refer her for a fine needle aspiration biopsy

D. repeat thyroid ultrasonography in 6 months

Item 40

An 8-year-old boy with a known history of myopia was recently diagnosed with upward dislocation of the lens. He has a tall stature, long arms, pectus excavatum, arachnodactyly, flat feet, and reduced elbow extension. His face is long and narrow with deep-set eyes and a receding chin (Item Q40). His mother has a similar appearance and body habitus, as well as a history of mitral valve prolapse and myopia. The maternal grandfather died in his 50s of a sudden cardiac death.

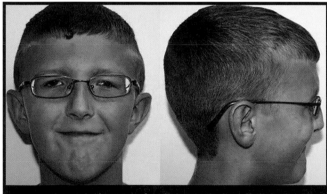

Reprinted with permission from the American Academy of Pediatrics Committee on Genetics. Specific genetic conditions. In: Saul RA, ed. *Medical Genetics in Pediatric Practice*. Elk Grove Village, IL: American Academy of Pediatrics; 2013:204-205.

Item Q40: Boy described in the vignette.

Of the following, the boy's MOST likely diagnosis is

A. Ehlers Danlos syndrome

B. Loeys Dietz syndrome

C. Marfan syndrome

D. Sotos syndrome

Item 41

A 4-year-old boy is seen for a health supervision visit. He was diagnosed with autism spectrum disorder at the age of 2 years. He is receiving applied behavioral analysis therapy and is in a special education preschool program through his local school district. His mother states that his behavior is an occasional problem, with some behavioral outbursts and aggression toward her. She also reports that he sleeps poorly. The boy often does not fall asleep until 10 or 11 PM. His bedtime routine consists of teeth brushing, watching a video, and having his mother lie in bed with him coaxing him to sleep. He naps inconsistently, between 2 and 5 times per week for 20 minutes to 3 hours at a time. His mother reports that he does not snore or cough during sleep. He takes polyethylene glycol for constipation and a daily multivitamin with iron. He has one soft bowel movement per day.

Of the following, the MOST effective next step to assist this family with their child's problems is to

A. initiate a sleep education program

B. obtain a serum ferritin level

C. obtain a sleep study

D. prescribe melatonin

Item 42

An 11-year-old girl with no significant medical history is seen for a health supervision visit. Two months ago, she was evaluated in an urgent care clinic for chronic cough and tested positive for pertussis by polymerase chain reaction. The case was reported to the local health department, and all household members received azithromycin. The girl has a temperature of 37.1°C, heart rate of 82 beats/min, respiratory rate of 16 breaths/min, and blood pressure of 105/62 mm Hg. She is well nourished and in no distress. Lung examination reveals good air entry and no adventitious sounds. Age-appropriate immunizations, including MenACWY and HPV, are given.

Of the following, the additional vaccine that is MOST appropriate at this time is

A. DT

B. DTaP

C. Td

D. Tdap

Item 43

A 12-year-old girl is being followed up 2 days after a fall onto the front of her left knee during a soccer game. She initially had pain over the anterior aspect of the knee, which has resolved. She was seen at an urgent care facility shortly after her injury. The family scheduled a follow-up appointment, because the urgent care physician noted an "abnormality" on the radiographs obtained there. On physical examination, the girl has full range of motion of the knee and hip, and very mild tenderness over the patella. The remainder of her examination findings are normal. The radiographs of the girl's knee are available for review (Item Q43).

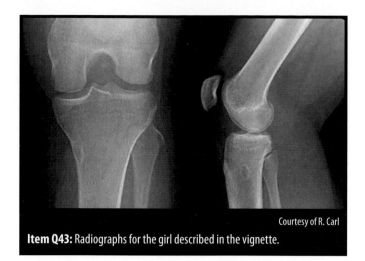

Item Q43: Radiographs for the girl described in the vignette.

Courtesy of R. Carl

Of the following, the MOST appropriate next management step for this girl is

A. monitoring of the lesion with radiography every 6 months

B. reassurance that no treatment is needed for this benign lesion

C. referral to oncology for evaluation

D. referral to orthopaedic surgery for curettage and bone grafting

Item 44

A group of prospective foster parents wish to learn about the epidemiology of sexual abuse. They are seeking information about the psychosocial and environmental factors that place children and adolescents at greater risk for becoming victims. The participants feel that this information may increase their awareness and help them to be better parents to survivors of child sexual abuse.

Of the following, the factor MOST correlated with a victim's risk is

A. ethnicity

B. family structure

C. number of strangers encountered

D. socioeconomic status

Item 45

A 16-year-old adolescent boy has diarrhea that began 5 days ago; his stools float in the toilet and are described as foul-smelling and watery. Bowel movements occur 4 to 5 times daily and are associated with significant abdominal cramping. There is no blood in the stool. His friends who recently accompanied him on a camping trip have had similar symptoms. He appears fatigued. Vital signs are normal for age. His abdomen is soft but distended. There are no palpable masses. Digital rectal examination findings are normal, and the hemoccult test result is negative.

Of the following, the stool study that is MOST likely to establish his diagnosis is a(n)

A. *Clostridium difficile* toxin

B. ova and parasite examination

C. pancreatic elastase

D. stool culture or polymerase chain reaction for bacterial pathogens

Item 46

A 6-year-old girl is seen for evaluation of behavioral concerns. Her parents were contacted by her teacher regarding poor concentration and an apparent lack of motivation. Her parents report that their daughter has lost interest in play-dates and family activities. She became quite tearful and complained about stomach aches when her parents brought her to a friend's backyard barbecue party. She is jumpy whenever she hears an unexpected noise. She has been having difficulty falling asleep and has been having frequent nightmares. She is unable to tell her parents what the nightmares are about. She has been struggling since the family was evacuated from their home in the middle of the night 2 months ago because of wildfires. She witnessed several houses burn down.

Of the following, the MOST appropriate initial intervention to recommend is

A. an α-adrenergic agonist

B. parent-child interaction therapy

C. a selective serotonin reuptake inhibitor

D. trauma-focused cognitive behavioral therapy

Item 47

A clinic has received feedback that patients are frustrated because providers are "always running late" for their appointments. Clinicians are working with the outpatient clinic manager to identify ways to improve the clinic workflow, so that patients can see their providers more quickly. Based on the Langley Model for Improvement, the following aim, measurement, and possible changes are defined:

Aim	• Decrease average time from check-in to ready-to-be-seen from 15 minutes to 10 minutes over the next 6 months
Measurement	• Time from patient check-in at the front desk to the time the medical assistant enters their vital signs (which is when the patient is ready to be seen) as recorded in the electronic medical record
Changes that may lead to an improvement	• Patients will verify their demographics and insurance online before the appointment • Medical assistants will obtain vital signs in the clinic room instead of at the medical assistant's station, where there is space for only 1 patient at a time • The number of medical assistants will be increased

Before permanently implementing any of the changes for the whole clinic, a pilot test will be run on a smaller scale. The clinic uses the Plan-Do-Study-Act model, and arranges for a few of the medical assistants to obtain vital signs in the clinic rooms for the next 2 weeks. At the end of the 2-week period, the clinician and the office manager review the time data collected, which demonstrates that the average time from check-in to entry of vital signs has increased from 15 to 17 minutes. The office manager notes that it is the beginning of winter, and many patients are now wearing coats and boots. More time is required for them to take the extra clothes off.

Of the following, the MOST accurate statement regarding this project is that

A. implementation on a large scale would have been more effective in creating change leading to improvement

B. obtaining vital signs in the clinic room was an ineffective method of creating change leading to improvement

C. the best next step is to change the Aim statement

D. the best next step is to do another Plan-Do-Study-Act cycle

Item 48

A 17-year-old adolescent boy is a new patient who did not bring any records from prior health care facilities. He reports a history of severe obesity for which he underwent bariatric surgery 2 years ago. He does not remember the details of his surgery and was lost to follow-up after multiple moves. He takes no medications and has no allergies. He reports that he has lost 75 lbs since his surgery and maintains an active and healthy lifestyle. Today his main concerns are hair thinning on the scalp, eyebrows, and eyelashes; areas of dry, red, and scaling skin; sores on the side of his mouth; and changes in his ability to taste.

Of the following, the mineral MOST likely to be deficient in this patient is

A. chromium

B. copper

C. magnesium

D. zinc

Item 49

A radiograph (Item Q49) is obtained of a congenital anomaly in a 6-hour-old neonate.

Of the following, the management of this neonate will MOST likely include

A. extracorporeal membrane oxygenation

B. packed red blood cell transfusions

C. platelet transfusions

D. renal dialysis

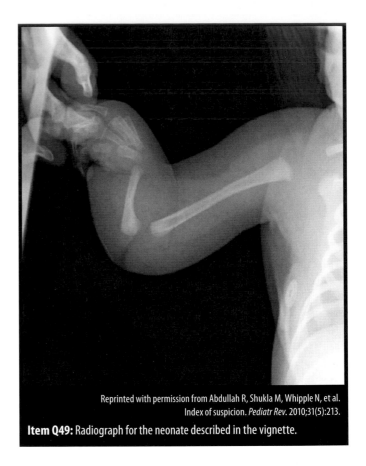

Item Q49: Radiograph for the neonate described in the vignette.

Item 50

A 3-year-old girl is being seen at a new patient visit. One week ago, she was removed from her mother's custody and placed into the custody of her aunt (who brought her to the pediatrician to establish a new medical home). The patient's mother, who has a history of substance abuse, has been charged with child neglect and endangerment.

The girl was born full-term. She has a history of failure to thrive, an elevated blood lead level, and speech delay. She was hospitalized 6 months ago after ingesting a household substance that resulted in extensive esophageal burns. She has had 2 subsequent hospital stays for management of esophageal strictures that developed as a complication of this injury.

Of the following, the household substance the girl MOST likely ingested is

A. drain cleaner

B. household bleach

C. insecticide

D. lamp oil

Item 51

A 15-year-old girl presents to the emergency department with sudden-onset excruciating right flank pain radiating to the groin, that has persisted for the last 6 hours. The girl also complains of nausea that began 1 hour ago. She reports difficulty with urination and red urine that morning. On physical examination she is clearly uncomfortable. Her temperature is 38.0°C, heart rate is 100 beats/min, respiratory rate is 28 breaths/min, and blood pressure is 140/90 mm Hg. There is evidence of mild dehydration. She refuses to allow her abdomen to be examined. Urinalysis demonstrates a specific gravity of 1.030, a pH of 6.0, 1+ protein, 3+ blood, and no leukocyte esterase or nitrites. Urine microscopy shows more than 100 red blood cells per high-power field (hpf), less than 5 white blood cells/hpf, and no crystals or bacteria.

Of the following, the metabolic abnormality MOST commonly associated with this girl's suspected diagnosis is

A. hypercalciuria

B. hypercitraturia

C. hyperoxaluria

D. hyperuricosuria

Item 52

A 7-year-old boy is seen for a health supervision visit as a new patient. He and his mother have no concerns. He is growing well, developing appropriately, and doing well in school. His physical examination findings are unremarkable. His mother recently learned that she has high cholesterol (total cholesterol, 300 mg/dL [7.77 mmol/L]). In adherence to the most recent guidelines, a fasting lipid profile panel is ordered; it reveals an elevated triglyceride level.

Of the following, the BEST next step in management of this boy is to

A. counsel on diet and exercise

B. initiate therapy with atorvastatin

C. initiate therapy with clofibrate

D. repeat fasting lipid profile

Item 53

A 16-year-old adolescent girl has recently become sexually active. Her mother would like to discuss contraceptive options. The patient reports that she does not want to become pregnant, but does not want to start a birth control method because her friends have experienced adverse effects. She and her boyfriend have been using the withdrawal method, and she has not become pregnant.

Of the following, the BEST next step in management is to

A. discuss all forms of birth control and their side effects

B. provide her with condoms

C. schedule a follow-up visit in 3 months to reassess her thoughts about birth control

D. test for gonorrhea, chlamydia, HIV, and syphilis

Item 54

A 10-year-old girl with cardiogenic shock is being treated in the pediatric intensive care unit. She is sedated and receiving mechanical ventilation. She is receiving diuretics, continuous inotropic medications, and afterload reducing agents. Because of concerns about her cardiac output, she was given a bolus of 5% albumin solution. The effect of this therapy on her cardiac output is being monitored with blood oxygen saturation measurements.

Of the following, this information would BEST be obtained with blood samples from a(n)

A. antecubital venous catheter

B. capillary fingerstick

C. internal jugular venous catheter

D. radial artery catheter

Item 55

A 15-month-old girl with a history of epilepsy treated with phenobarbital is being evaluated for a rash. For the past several days she has had a low-grade fever, decreased energy and appetite, and an increase in her baseline seizure frequency. Her eyes have been slightly red and itchy, and she developed several small sores inside her mouth the day before the visit. This morning, she awoke with a widespread, red rash. She is fussy and refusing to eat or drink. She had 1 wet diaper overnight, but has not voided yet today. She appears ill. She has a temperature of 38.4°C, heart rate of 185 beats/min, and respiratory rate of 16 breaths/min. She has bilateral nonpurulent conjunctival injection, cracking of her lips, multiple shallow ulcerations on her buccal and gingival mucosa, and a diffuse rash (Item Q55).

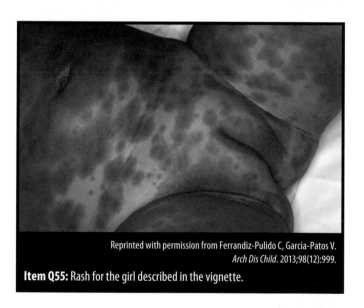

Reprinted with permission from Ferrandiz-Pulido C, Garcia-Patos V. *Arch Dis Child*. 2013;98(12):999.

Item Q55: Rash for the girl described in the vignette.

Of the following, the intervention MOST highly associated with an improved clinical outcome for this patient is prompt

A. administration of broad-spectrum antibiotics

B. administration of high-dose corticosteroids

C. administration of intravenous immunoglobulin

D. discontinuation of phenobarbital

Item 56

A 5-year-old boy presents with a 1-day history of vomiting and watery diarrhea without blood or mucus. Several of his school friends have become ill with diarrhea. He and his friends had recently visited a large city park with a wading pool. Further inquiry reveals that the health department is currently investigating a community outbreak of watery diarrhea among individuals who had visited that pool. The boy's temperature is 37°C, and his vital signs are normal. His physical examination is notable only for evidence of mild dehydration. Laboratory investigation reveals the presence of fecal leukocytes, but heme-negative stools.

Of the following, the MOST likely cause of this boy's diarrheal illness is

A. *Bacillus cereus*

B. *Campylobacter jejuni*

C. enterotoxigenic *Escherichia coli*

D. *Shigella sonnei*

Item 57

A 10-year-old girl with a genetic mutation leading to spasticity, poor trunk control, seizures, and cognitive disability is seen for a routine health supervision visit. Over the last 2 to 3 years she has developed worsening scoliosis (Item Q57). She has had 3 episodes of pneumonia in the last year and prolonged time for recovery from viral upper respiratory

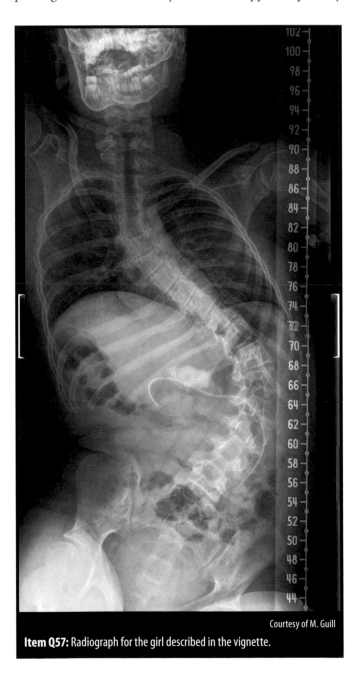

Item Q57: Radiograph for the girl described in the vignette.

Courtesy of M. Guill

infections. She requires the use of a wheelchair. She smiles in response to her mother's voice but has little other meaningful interaction. She has rotoscoliosis and difficulty with trunk control. Breath sounds are distant and diminished on the right; cardiac sounds are displaced to the left. There are no rales or wheezes.

Of the following, the MOST likely mechanism for her recurrent respiratory infections is

A. airway hyperreactivity

B. bronchiectasis

C. hypogammaglobulinemia

D. ineffective cough

Item 58

A 9-year-old girl is evaluated for concerns about her lack of growth. The girl has not been outgrowing her clothes, and her sister, who is 2 years younger, is catching up to her in height. She has no significant medical history and takes no medication. A review of systems reveals worsening vision over the past month. She has also been having intermittent headaches at school that her mother attributes to her vision problems. Her adjusted midparental height is at the 60th percentile. Her mother had menarche at 12 years of age, and her father had delayed puberty. She has a temperature of 37°C, blood pressure of 100/65 mm Hg, and heart rate of 72 beats/min. Her visual acuity is 20/100 bilaterally. Her growth curve is shown (Item Q58). The remainder of the physical examination findings are unremarkable.

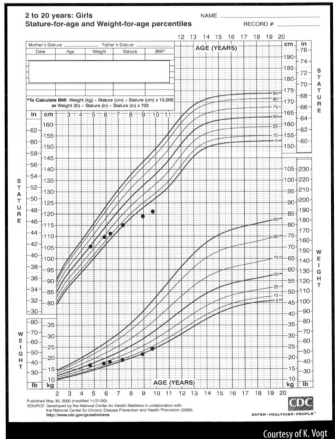

Item Q58: Growth chart for the girl described in the vignette.

Courtesy of K. Vogt

Of the following, the test MOST likely to reveal the diagnosis is

A. bone age radiography
B. brain magnetic resonance imaging
C. a karyotype
D. a thyroid-stimulating hormone level

Item 59

The mother of a 5-year old girl, adopted 2 years ago from Eastern Europe, is concerned that the girl is small for her age and continues to have significant global delays despite appropriate therapy. She has behavioral problems including hyperactivity, decreased attention, and poor memory. Distinctive physical features include microcephaly, smooth philtrum, short palpebral fissures, low nasal bridge, thin upper lip, and fifth finger clinodactyly. Pregnancy and family histories are unknown.

Of the following, the girl's findings are MOST consistent with

A. Angelman fragile X syndrome
B. fetal alcohol syndrome
C. Noonan syndrome
D. Rett syndrome

Item 60

The parents of a 16-hour-old term neonate have noticed a small "divot" in front of his left ear, and their internet searching suggests it is a preauricular pit. The pregnancy and delivery were uncomplicated, and the neonate is feeding well and acting normally. He passed the newborn hearing screen. There is no family history of ear anomalies, deafness, or renal malformations. Prior to their son being examined, the parents ask if renal ultrasonography is needed.

Of the following, the MOST appropriate response to the parents' question is that renal ultrasonography is

A. always recommended for neonates with the finding noted by the parents in this vignette
B. not recommended for neonates with the finding noted by the parents in this vignette
C. recommended if there are any other congenital anomalies found on examination
D. recommended only if other urogenital anomalies (eg, hypospadias) are found on examination

Item 61

A 7-year-old boy is brought to the emergency department for evaluation of fever and malaise. He has been ill for 3 days and has had associated headache and neck pain. Ten days ago he traveled to North Carolina where he played in fields and hiked in wooded areas. Vital signs show a temperature of 39.3°C, heart rate of 110 beats/min, respiratory rate of 44 breaths/min, and blood pressure of 97/58 mm Hg. He has pain on neck flexion and a generalized exanthem involving the palms (Item Q61).

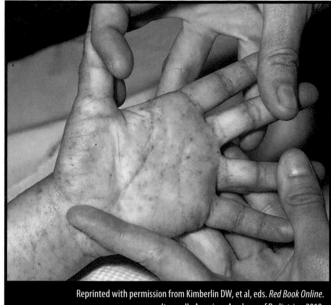

Reprinted with permission from Kimberlin DW, et al, eds. *Red Book Online*. Itasca, IL: American Academy of Pediatrics; 2018.

Item Q61: Rash for the boy described in the vignette.

Laboratory data are shown:

Laboratory Test	Result
White blood cell count	5,900/µL (5.9 × 10^9/L)
Neutrophils	72%
Lymphocytes	25%
Monocytes	3%
Hemoglobin	11.3 g/dL (113 g/L)
Platelet count	103 × 10^3/µL (103 × 10^9/L)
Aspartate aminotransferase	218 U/L
Alanine aminotransferase	204 U/L

Of the following, the antimicrobial that will BEST treat this patient's illness is

A. ampicillin
B. azithromycin
C. ceftriaxone
D. doxycycline

Item 62

A 2-week-old male infant is at a health supervision visit. He was delivered at term by vaginal delivery and was discharged from the hospital after 2 days. His mother reports that prenatal testing was normal. On physical examination in the newborn nursery, it was noted that his left foot was turned inward. The remainder of his examination findings were normal. The boy is otherwise healthy. Physical examination reveals a left foot deformity (Item Q62). The foot can be passively stretched almost to the midline, but it is not possible to dorsiflex the ankle to a neutral position.

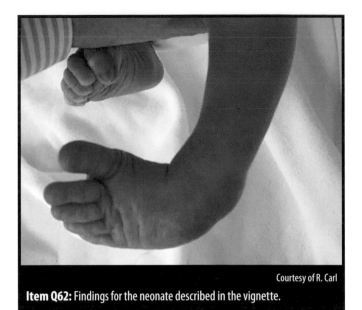

Courtesy of R. Carl

Item Q62: Findings for the neonate described in the vignette.

Of the following, the BEST next management step for this neonate is

A. bracing with reverse last shoes

B. home stretching exercises with reevaluation at age 6 months

C. immediate referral to orthopaedic surgery for casting

D. referral to orthopaedic surgery for surgical reconstruction at age 6 months

Item 63

A 5-week-old male infant is being evaluated for vomiting. He was born via spontaneous vaginal delivery at 39 weeks' gestation. There were no perinatal complications. His birthweight was 3.4 kg. At his 2-week routine health maintenance visit, he weighed 3.6 kg. At that time, his mother reported that he was breastfeeding well, with some mild regurgitation after feedings. Today she reports that although he continues to breastfeed well, he has been vomiting large amounts immediately after every feeding for the past 2 days. She has noted fewer wet diapers today so she is concerned that he may be dehydrated. The vomiting is reported as nonbilious and nonbloody. The infant has no history of fever or diarrhea. His newborn screening results are normal. His weight is 4 kg, temperature is 37°C, and heart rate is 150 beats/min. His length and frontal-occipital head circumference measurements are at the 50th percentile. On physical examination, the boy is alert and actively sucking on his pacifier. He appears thin, but in no acute distress. His abdomen is soft and nontender. You suspect a diagnosis of hypertrophic pyloric stenosis, which is confirmed on abdominal ultrasonography. A chemistry panel is obtained.

Of the following, the MOST likely blood chemistry findings in this case are

A. hyperchloremic hyperkalemic metabolic alkalosis

B. hyperchloremic hypernatremic metabolic acidosis

C. hypochloremic hypokalemic metabolic alkalosis

D. hypochloremic hyponatremic metabolic acidosis

Item 64

A 7-year-old boy has recurrent bright red blood per rectum. His mother reports intermittently seeing blood in the toilet for the last year. She states that she has occasionally seen a mass coming from his rectum that looks like a raspberry. He has daily, soft stools, without straining. He reports no abdominal pain, pallor, fatigue, or weight loss. There is no family history of early colon cancer. He has a weight of 25.4 kg (60th percentile), height of 122 cm (35th percentile), and body mass index of 17 kg/m² (75th percentile). He appears healthy and in no acute distress. He has no rash or mucocutaneous hyperpigmentation. His abdomen is soft, nontender, and nondistended. On digital rectal examination, a 1- to 2-cm nontender mass is palpated.

He is referred to a pediatric gastroenterologist. A colonoscopy is performed, and 8 polyps are removed. Item Q64 shows a representative lesion.

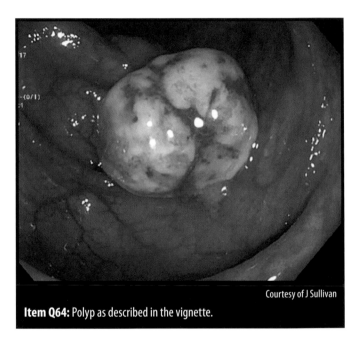

Courtesy of J Sullivan

Item Q64: Polyp as described in the vignette.

Histopathologic examination of the polyps reveals that they are juvenile polyps.

Of the following, the BEST next step in management is

A. referral for genetic testing

B. referral to a colorectal surgeon for colectomy

C. repeat colonoscopy only if rectal bleeding recurs

D. thyroid ultrasonography

Item 65

A 12-year-old boy presents with back pain of 6 months' duration. The pain is in a specific spot in his middle back, just to the right of midline. At onset the pain was intermittent, but now is constant. He reports that over the past week, his right leg has started to buckle; he has to move carefully now so that he does not fall. He cannot run normally because of back pain and the fear of falling because his "legs might give out." He denies incontinence, but complains that he feels like he has to urinate all the time but cannot completely empty his bladder. He has been purposefully drinking less fluids to avoid any accidents. The boy's vital signs and general physical examination results are normal. A neurologic examination shows normal cranial nerve function, upper extremity strength and reflexes, and response to light touch on his arms and legs. There is an oval area of numbness, just to the right of midline, in the location of his midback pain. His right hip flexion is slightly weak, but otherwise he has normal strength in his lower extremities. Reflexes are 2/4 in his biceps and 3/4 in his patellae; on plantar stroking, his right toe extends and his left toe flexes. When standing with his eyes closed, he breaks stance and falls to the side.

Of the following, the BEST next diagnostic step for this boy is

A. electromyography/nerve conduction study

B. magnetic resonance imaging of the brain, with and without contrast

C. magnetic resonance imaging of the spine, with and without contrast

D. urodynamic studies

Item 66

An 18-month-old child is seen for a health supervision visit. The fingerstick hemoglobin measurement is 11.8 g/dL (118 g/L), and the lead concentration is 6 µg/dL (0.3 µmol/L).

Of the following, the next BEST step for this patient is to

A. follow-up at the next health supervision visit

B. obtain a venous lead level

C. recheck a fingerstick lead level in 3 months

D. start ferrous sulfate therapy

Item 67

A 20-hour-old male neonate is examined because his nurses report that he looks pale. He was born at an estimated 39 weeks' gestation to a 19-year-old woman who did not receive prenatal care. This was her first live birth, although she reported having had a pregnancy loss in the third trimester 2 years ago.

The neonate's Apgar scores were 9 at 1 minute and 9 at 10 minutes. He is vigorously crying and appears jaundiced. His heart rate is 182 beats/min. His heart, lung, and abdominal examination findings are normal, and his umbilical stump appears normal. An initial set of laboratory data is shown:

Laboratory Test	Result
Hemoglobin	7.2 g/dL (72 g/L)
Reticulocytes	23%
Total bilirubin	14.3 mg/dL (244.6 µmol/L)
Direct bilirubin	0.3 mg/dL (5.1 µmol/L)

Of the following, the set of laboratory values MOST consistent with this presentation is

	Maternal Blood Type	Newborn Blood Type	Neonatal Direct Antibody Test
A.	A+	A–	Negative
B.	AB–	A+	Positive
C.	A+	O–	Positive
D.	AB–	B+	Negative

Item 68

A 3-year-old previously healthy girl presents to your office for evaluation of bleeding from her right naris. Her nose has been bleeding frequently from the right naris over the past 2 weeks. The mother reports that there is thick yellow discharge mixed with the blood at times. The girl has had no history of bruising, rashes, or bleeding from sites other than her nose. She has had no cough and no history of vomiting. Her vital signs are normal for age. On physical examination, she is well appearing and in no respiratory distress. Dried blood is visible below her right naris but she has no active bleeding. Her breath is foul-smelling.

Of the following, the MOST likely explanation for this girl's epistaxis is

A. juvenile angiofibroma

B. nasal foreign body

C. rhinitis sicca

D. von Willebrand disease

Item 69

A 15-year-old girl presents with a 1-week history of pain and swelling in her fingers and wrists. She also complains of generalized fatigue and a rash for the last 3 weeks. Her rash seems to be exacerbated by sun exposure. Her medical history is not significant otherwise. Her family history is significant for an aunt with rheumatoid arthritis and a grandmother with thyroid disease. On physical examination, the girl's temperature is 38°C, heart rate is 66 beats/min, respiratory rate is 16 breaths/min, and blood pressure is 112/60 mm Hg. She is alert and cooperative. She has an erythematous maculopapular rash over the bridge of her nose, erythema of the hard palate, and a few shallow gingival ulcers. There is mild swelling, tenderness to palpation, and pain with range of motion in the proximal interphalangeal joints of several of her fingers and both wrists. The remainder of her physical examination findings are normal. Urinalysis demonstrates a specific gravity of 1.035, pH of 6.0, 3+ blood, 4+ protein, 2+ leukocyte esterase, no glucose, and no nitrites. Urine microscopy shows more than 100 red blood cells/high-power field (hpf), 10 to 20 white blood cells/hpf, no crystals, and no bacteria.

Of the following, the MOST likely diagnosis for the girl in the vignette is

A. antineutrophil cytoplasmic antibody vasculitis

B. juvenile idiopathic arthritis

C. systemic lupus erythematosus

D. Sjögren syndrome

Item 70

A 9-year-old girl with a history of dilated cardiomyopathy is seen for a health supervision visit. She is followed closely by the heart failure service at the local pediatric hospital. Her growth has started to plateau, and she is less active than she had been. Her mother reports that her cardiologist is concerned that they may have to consider heart transplantation. The girl is often thirsty. The mother asks for suggestions to help with her thirst, which is known to be associated with heart failure.

Of the following, the beverage that would be MOST likely to help her fluid intake is

A. juice

B. nutritional protein supplement

C. sports drink with sodium replacement

D. water

Item 71

A 15-year-old adolescent girl is seen for evaluation of nausea and headache after being sent home from school. She has had intermittent headaches over the past month that resolve with rest. She has not had any associated vomiting, fever, or visual changes. Her mother is concerned because her daughter recently quit the cheerleading team, she is failing 2 classes, and she has been spending a lot of time alone in her room. Her mother discloses that she is getting a divorce.

Of the following, the BEST next step in management is to

A. order a complete blood cell count and comprehensive metabolic panel

B. order magnetic resonance imaging of the brain

C. prescribe a trial of a nonsteroidal anti-inflammatory drug

D. screen for nonsuicidal self-injury

Item 72

A 2-year-old boy developed respiratory failure after he drank the oil from a plug-in air freshener. In the emergency department, he was hemodynamically stable, awake, and alert, but anxious. He became progressively more tachypneic and hypoxic. He underwent intubation, was started on mechanical ventilation, and was transferred to the intensive care unit. He is currently sedated and not breathing above the mechanical ventilator rate. On physical examination, his lungs have scattered rales bilaterally, and breath sounds are diminished in dependent regions and at the bases. He is receiving pressure-controlled, synchronized intermittent mandatory ventilation, at a rate of 24 breaths/min, inflation pressure of 30 cm H_2O, positive end-expiratory pressure of 5 cm H_2O, mean airway pressure 12 cm H_2O, and fraction of inspired oxygen 90%. Exhaled tidal volumes are 6 mL/kg of body weight. An arterial blood gas shows a pH of 7.40, partial pressure of carbon dioxide of 40 mm Hg, partial pressure of oxygen of 50 mm Hg, and 85% oxygen saturation. His chest radiograph is shown in Item Q72.

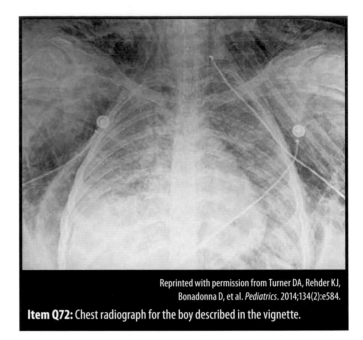

Reprinted with permission from Turner DA, Rehder KJ, Bonadonna D, et al. *Pediatrics.* 2014;134(2):e584.

Item Q72: Chest radiograph for the boy described in the vignette.

Of the following, the BEST next step in management is to

A. increase peak inflation pressure

B. increase positive end-expiratory pressure

C. refer for extracorporeal membrane oxygenation

D. start helium-oxygen mixture

Item 73

A 6-month-old female infant is being evaluated at a health supervision visit. She has been exclusively breastfed and her parents have questions about the introduction of complementary foods. Both parents eat a strict vegetarian diet and plan to raise their daughter with the same dietary restrictions.

Of the following, the vitamin MOST likely to be deficient in this infant's diet is

A. cobalamin

B. niacin

C. riboflavin

D. thiamine

Item 74

A previously healthy 6-year-old boy with a 4-day history of varicella presents to the emergency department with fever and severe pain with rapidly progressive swelling over his left upper arm. There are no sick contacts, no pets at home, and no recent travel. He is home-schooled and has not received many of his routine childhood vaccinations due to parental concerns about vaccine-related adverse effects. On arrival, the boy is ill-appearing with a temperature of 39.2°C, heart rate of 150 beats/min, respiratory rate of 46 breaths/min, and blood pressure of 73/32 mm Hg. His physical examination findings are remarkable for diffuse swelling and erythema of the left upper extremity. The overlying skin has a mottled appearance with several small bullous lesions. Laboratory data are notable for a white blood cell count of 26,000/μL

([26×10⁹/L], 95% neutrophils), a hemoglobin of 11.1 g/dL (111 g/L), and a platelet count of 80×10³/μL (80×10⁹/L). After surgical consultation, he underwent emergency surgical debridement.

Of the following, the MOST likely organism isolated from surgical tissue specimens is

A. *Clostridium perfringens*

B. *Clostridium septicum*

C. group A *Streptococcus*

D. methicillin-resistant *Staphylococcus aureus*

Item 75

A 1-month-old infant born at term presents for a health supervision visit. She was delivered via emergency cesarean section because of placental abruption. Delivery room resuscitation included intubation, chest compressions, and fluid resuscitation. Apgar scores were 0, 4, 5, and 7 at 1, 5, 10, and 15 minutes, respectively. The parents ask about the predictive value of this infant's Apgar scores.

Of the following, these scores correlate MOST closely with

A. neurodevelopmental scores

B. physiologic state at birth

C. probability of cerebral palsy

D. risk of mortality at 1 year

Item 76

A 5-year-old boy is brought to the emergency department for wheezing with a viral respiratory infection that has been present for the last 4 days. This is his third visit this year to emergency or urgent care services for the same symptoms. He uses an albuterol inhaler without a holding chamber when he has audible wheezing, but his mother says it never completely stops his symptoms. He has had 3 courses of oral prednisolone in the last year. He wheezes only with viral illnesses, but does cough at night several times weekly. His teacher has said that he frequently seems short of breath when playing at recess or in gym class.

He has a temperature of 37.2°C, heart rate of 135 beats/min, respiratory rate of 30 breaths/min, and oxygen saturation of 94% on room air. He looks uncomfortable and has intercostal and suprasternal retractions. Breath sounds are generally diminished, and there is a faint end-expiratory wheeze heard throughout his chest. Cardiovascular examination findings are normal, and his skin is warm and well perfused. There is concern that the boy has previously unrecognized persistent asthma triggered by viral respiratory infections.

His acute symptoms are managed with bronchodilators and systemic steroids.

Of the following, the BEST long-term approach to his care would be to begin an

A. inhaled anticholinergic agent

B. inhaled corticosteroid

C. oral antihistamine

D. oral leukotriene receptor antagonist

Item 77

A 6-year-old girl is being evaluated for a 4-month history of a perineal rash accompanied by intermittent pruritus and discomfort, painful urination and defecation, and constipation. She is well in other respects. She has an unremarkable medical history and normal growth at the 25th percentile for height and weight. Physical examination findings are normal except for the perineum (Item Q77).

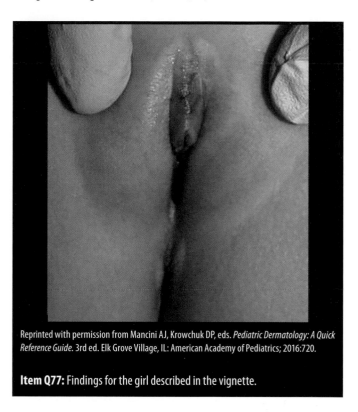

Reprinted with permission from Mancini AJ, Krowchuk DP, eds. *Pediatric Dermatology: A Quick Reference Guide*. 3rd ed. Elk Grove Village, IL: American Academy of Pediatrics; 2016:720.

Item Q77: Findings for the girl described in the vignette.

Of the following, the MOST likely diagnosis is

A. irritant contact dermatitis

B. lichen sclerosus et atrophicus

C. sexual abuse

D. vulvovaginitis

Item 78

An 8-year-old girl is seen for a health supervision visit. Her mother is concerned about her small size. She was born at term with a birth weight of 2.3 kg. She has been healthy except for recurrent episodes of acute otitis media for which she underwent tympanostomy tube placement at the age of 2 years. She takes no medication. She is in the second grade and requires extra help in math. Her adjusted mid-parental height is at the 50th percentile. Her mother had menarche at 11 years of age, and her father had average timing of puberty. Her growth curve is shown (Item Q78). Physical examination findings are significant for bilateral epicanthal folds, a high-arched palate, and multiple benign-appearing nevi.

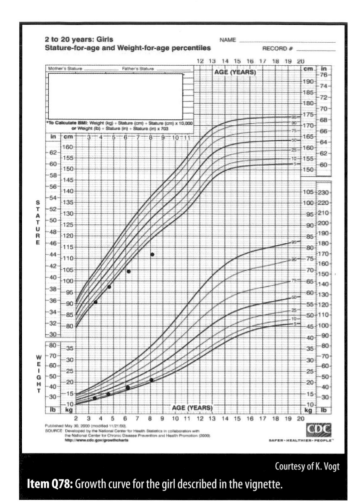

Item Q78: Growth curve for the girl described in the vignette.

Courtesy of K. Vogt

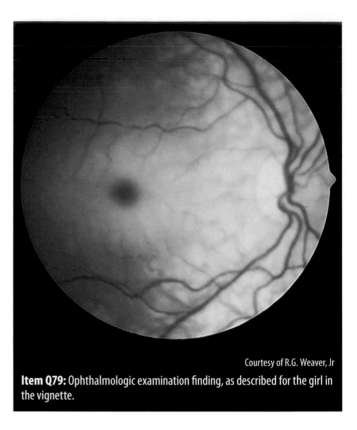

Item Q79: Ophthalmologic examination finding, as described for the girl in the vignette.

Courtesy of R.G. Weaver, Jr

Of the following, the test MOST likely to reveal the diagnosis is

A. brain magnetic resonance imaging

B. an insulin-like growth factor-1 level

C. a karyotype

D. a thyroid-stimulating hormone level

Item 79

A 9-month-old girl presents to the emergency department (ED) with seizures. Her history is significant for developmental regression. Her mother states that the girl was completely normal at birth. Between 3 and 6 months of age, she developed decreased visual attentiveness, an exaggerated startle response, progressive motor weakness, and myoclonic jerks. The girl's pediatrician had referred her for an ophthalmology assessment that revealed an unusual finding (Item Q79). Physical examination in the ED reveals mild macrocephaly, a normal-sized liver and spleen, generalized muscular hypotonia, and hyperreflexia. Complete metabolic panel, urine organic acids, serum amino acids, copper, ceruloplasmin, and complete blood cell count are within normal limits. Leukocyte enzyme testing reveals the etiology of her signs and symptoms.

Of the following, based on her history, physical examination, and laboratory findings, the girl's MOST likely diagnosis is

A. Gaucher disease

B. mucopolysaccharidosis type I

C. Tay-Sachs disease

D. Wolman disease

Item 80

The "practice champion" for a countywide effort to improve developmental screening in all pediatric primary care practices is speaking at the monthly provider meeting to discuss implementing workflow changes to enable screening all children for developmental problems with formal tools at 9, 18, and 24 or 30 months, and specifically for autism at 18 and 24 months. Examples of screening tools used by neighboring practices are distributed. One of the providers expresses reservations about participating in this effort, stating that the tools seem "hokey" and he feels that after 3 decades in practice, he can "spot a developmentally delayed child a mile away."

Of the following, the MOST accurate statement regarding this initiative is that

A. the assessment tools can be completed by caregivers in 2 minutes or less in most cases

B. few Medicaid programs reimburse primary care practices for using developmental assessment tools

C. scoring the tools can be complicated; thus, this task can be delegated to nursing staff but not medical assistants

D. surveillance by experienced pediatricians has equivalent specificity but lower sensitivity compared to validated developmental assessment tools

Item 81

A 6-week-old male infant born at 32 weeks' gestation has been hospitalized in the neonatal intensive care unit since birth. The hospital course has been complicated by necrotizing enterocolitis managed conservatively and an episode of *Escherichia coli* bacteremia. Two days ago, he developed respiratory distress and underwent an evaluation for an invasive infection. A chest radiograph revealed new bilateral airspace opacities. He currently has a temperature of 38°C, heart rate of 170 beats/min, respiratory rate of 46 breaths/min, and blood pressure of 80/45 mm Hg. Coarse breath sounds are auscultated bilaterally. His abdomen is distended but nontender.

Laboratory data are shown:

Laboratory Test	Result
White blood cell count	24,000/µL (24.0 × 10⁹/L)
Neutrophils	16%
Band neutrophils	44%
Lymphocytes	33%
Monocytes	7%
Hemoglobin	10.5 g/dL (105 g/L)
Platelet count	75 × 10³/µL (75 × 10⁹/L)
Aspartate aminotransferase	200 U/L
Alanine aminotransferase	206 U/L
Blood culture	Negative
Urine culture	Negative
Cerebrospinal fluid culture	Negative
Cytomegalovirus quantitative polymerase chain reaction (urine)	2,600,000 IU/mL

Of the following, the BEST isolation precaution to use when caring for this patient is

A. airborne

B. contact

C. droplet

D. universal

Item 82

A 4-year-old girl is being evaluated at a health supervision visit. Her medical history is remarkable for frequent episodes of otitis media and torticollis, for which she received physical therapy. On physical examination, the girl has a short neck with decreased cervical motion, and her head is tilted slightly laterally to the left. Cervical spine radiographs show vertebral fusions at C1/C2 and C3/C4.

Of the following, the MOST appropriate next studies to order would be

A. echocardiography and magnetic resonance imaging (MRI) of the cervical spine

B. thoracolumbar spine radiography and MRI of the entire spine

C. thoracolumbar spine radiography and renal ultrasonography

D. vertebral artery ultrasonography and echocardiography

Item 83

A full-term large-for-gestational age neonate who is 4 hours of age is being evaluated in the normal newborn nursery. The infant was born via spontaneous vaginal delivery, vertex presentation, to a primigravida mother after 28 hours of labor. The neonate's vital signs are normal and his physical examination findings are remarkable only for a soft mass that covers the crown of the head with overlying ecchymoses.

Of the following, this condition is MOST likely associated with

A. cranial molding

B. falling hematocrit

C. linear skull fracture

D. low platelet count

Item 84

An 11-month-old male infant is brought for follow-up after an emergency department visit for diarrhea and vomiting. The diarrhea began acutely 3 days ago and is described as 6 to 8 watery and nonbloody bowel movements per day. For the first 24 hours, the child had frequent nonbilious nonbloody emesis and was seen in the emergency department for dehydration. Intravenous fluid was administered, and stool testing was performed. Over the last 48 hours, his vomiting has resolved, and he has tolerated liquids. His diarrhea has continued, although the stool frequency has decreased. He has no other significant medical history, and has not recently received antibiotics. He attends day care, and several children are ill with similar symptoms. He is alert and has normal vital signs. His abdomen is soft, nontender, and nondistended.

Stool reverse-transcriptase polymerase chain reaction for norovirus and polymerase chain reaction for *Clostridium difficile* from his emergency department visit have positive results.

Of the following, the BEST next step in management is

A. loperamide

B. metronidazole

C. supportive care

D. vancomycin

Item 85

A 17-year-old adolescent boy is seen for a health supervision visit. In response to a question about substance use, he admits to drinking alcohol at parties and alone. He sometimes rides in a car driven by friends after they have been drinking. He has forgotten things when drinking and has found that he needs to drink more to relax. His grades have worsened. His girlfriend has suggested that he drink less, but he has had difficulty doing so. He reports that he does not use any other substances.

Of the following, the sign or symptom that would be MOST consistent with withdrawal from the substance of concern is

A. dizziness

B. increased heart rate

C. loss of balance

D. lower body temperature

Item 86

A 5-year-old boy with myclomeningocele has a ventriculo peritoneal shunt that was last revised when he was 1 year old. He has epilepsy that is well-controlled with levetiracetam. He ambulates with forearm crutches. Over the past 2 months, the boy has been complaining that his legs and back hurt, and he refuses to walk longer distances. On physical examination, he has weak and atrophic lower extremities with diminished reflexes, and bilateral pes cavus. The remainder of his examination findings are normal. Computed tomography of the head without contrast shows his shunt tubing in appropriate position and ventricles unchanged in size from the previous imaging 18 months ago.

Of the following, the MOST likely cause of his new symptoms is

A. chronic urinary tract infection

B. expected progression of myelomeningocele

C. shunt failure

D. tethered cord

Item 87

A 9-year-old girl has a 2-month history of foul-smelling right ear discharge and difficulty hearing. She has a history of recurrent suppurative otitis media infections that were treated with oral antibiotics, the last course of which was 1 month ago. She reports no fever, rhinorrhea, ear pain, or cough. An otoscopic image of her right ear is shown in Item Q87.

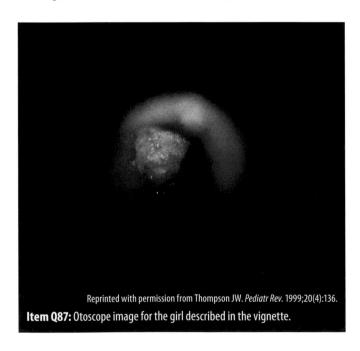

Reprinted with permission from Thompson JW. *Pediatr Rev.* 1999;20(4):136.

Item Q87: Otoscope image for the girl described in the vignette.

Of the following, the treatment MOST likely to resolve this patient's underlying condition is

A. ear lavage

B. oral antibiotics

C. surgery

D. topical antibiotic ear drops

Item 88

A 17-year-old adolescent girl is brought to the emergency department for increasing fatigue and pallor. For the last year she has had increasingly heavy menstrual cycles. Her latest cycle has been ongoing for the last 8 days. She has not had any obvious clots, but has had to use double pads throughout the day. She reports that she has never been sexually active. Her medical history is otherwise unremarkable with no other bleeding symptoms. Her physical examination findings are normal.

The patient's mother reports having a similar history of heavy menstrual bleeding. She also needed a packed red blood cell transfusion following the birth of her daughter.

A laboratory evaluation reveals:

Laboratory Test	Result
Hemoglobin	6.9 g/dL (69 g/L)
Mean corpuscular volume	68 fL
Platelet count	$290 \times 10^3/\mu L$ (290×10^9/L)
Prothrombin time	13 s (reference range, 11-13.5 s)
Partial thromboplastin time	34 s (reference range, 25-35 s)
Blood type	A-Positive
Urine β-human chorionic gonadotropin	Negative
Von Willebrand factor antigen	34% (reference range, 50%-200%)
Von Willebrand factor activity	36% (reference range, 50%-200%)

Of the following, the MOST likely cause of the patient's heavy menstrual bleeding is a deficiency of a

A. factor in the common coagulation pathway

B. factor in the extrinsic coagulation pathway

C. factor in the intrinsic coagulation pathway

D. protein involved in platelet adhesion to collagen

Item 89

A 6-year-old boy presents an hour after he lost control of his scooter and fell onto his outstretched arm. His physical examination findings are significant for mild swelling and tenderness over the middle portion of his forearm. A radiograph of his forearm is shown (Item Q89).

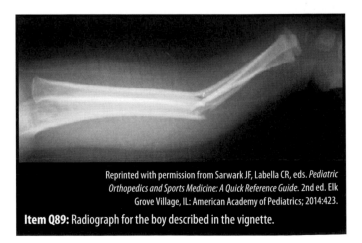

Reprinted with permission from Sarwark JF, Labella CR, eds. *Pediatric Orthopedics and Sports Medicine: A Quick Reference Guide.* 2nd ed. Elk Grove Village, IL: American Academy of Pediatrics; 2014:423.

Item Q89: Radiograph for the boy described in the vignette.

Of the following, the boy's injury is BEST described as a

A. greenstick fracture

B. metaphyseal corner fracture

C. Salter Harris type 1 fracture

D. Salter Harris type 4 fracture

Item 90

A 14-year-old boy presents for a health supervision visit. The patient has been healthy, with normal growth parameters and development. He has no significant medical or surgical history. His physical examination findings and vital signs are unremarkable. His parents are concerned because their son was noted to have protein in his urine 6 months ago when he had presented to an urgent care center with high fever. A urinalysis in the office reveals a specific gravity of 1.020, a pH of 6.0, 2+ protein, and no blood, leukocyte esterase, or nitrites.

Of the following, the best next step in management for this boy is

A. evaluation by a pediatric nephrologist

B. urinalysis on a first-morning sample

C. 24-hour quantitative urine protein measurement

D. renal ultrasonography

Item 91

An 8-year-old boy is seen for follow-up after a visit to a local urgent care center last week for upper respiratory infection symptoms. At the urgent care center, he was noted to be hypertensive with a documented blood pressure of 130/80 mm Hg. There is concern that improper technique may have been used in obtaining the blood pressure. A medical student on rotation asks how to properly measure blood pressure.

Of the following, the MOST correct response is

A. the cuff bladder width should be 40% of the arm circumference

B. the cuff should be deflated faster than 1 mm Hg per second

C. the cuff should be inflated 60 mm Hg above the point where the radial pulse disappears

D. the cuff should cover 50% of the length of the upper arm

Item 92

A 16-year-old adolescent boy has lost weight after previously being overweight. He has been eating healthier and limits his intake to 1,200 cal/day. He has exercised 5 days per week for the past 3 months. He is bradycardic (heart rate of 45 beats/min), has orthostatic changes with standing, and has lost 20% of his total body weight since his last visit 4 months ago. His pediatrician suspects an eating disorder and recommends an evaluation in the emergency department. The patient's mother speaks only Spanish, but the patient speaks both Spanish and English. The patient translates the concerns about an eating disorder. His mother becomes upset and replies that he just needs to eat more of the meals she prepares at home.

Of the following, the BEST next step in management is to

A. order a comprehensive metabolic panel, erythrocyte sedimentation rate, and thyroid-stimulating hormone level

B. refer him to a psychiatrist to evaluate for an eating disorder

C. review supplement options to increase his daily caloric intake

D. use an interpreter to discuss the medical complications of an eating disorder

Item 93

A previously healthy 2-month-old boy was brought to the emergency department by his mother. Approximately 15 minutes after a feeding, he had an episode in which he suddenly started choking, gagging, and arching his back. His skin color turned red, then dusky. He then appeared to stop breathing for approximately 10 seconds, after which he was briefly gasping then resumed his normal breathing pattern. After about 1 more minute, his color returned to normal and he was appropriately responsive. The boy has no history of similar episodes. He was born at 35 weeks of gestation to a gravida 1, para 0 mother. There were no illnesses or infections during the pregnancy, and no concerns in the perinatal period. The boy has not had any recent illnesses, fever, or difficulty breathing. He does not breathe noisily or snore. He has been gaining weight appropriately, and takes 4 ounces of formula every 3 hours, requiring about 5 minutes to finish a feeding. When he is burped after every feed, a small amount of formula dribbles out of his mouth. The boy's vital signs are as follows: temperature, 37°C; blood pressure (right arm), 80/45 mm Hg; blood pressure (left leg), 75/40 mm Hg; respiratory rate, 25 breaths/min; and heart rate, 130 beats/min. Physical examination reveals a well-nourished infant with no external signs of trauma. While sleeping, the boy has occasional periods of apnea lasting about 6 seconds, which are followed by a few second-long periods of rapid, shallow breathing. He then resumes a normal breathing pattern. He arouses appropriately with examination. His lungs are clear, pulses are equal and strong, and his heart has a normal S1 and S2 which is variably split with breathing, with no rubs, gallops, or murmurs. His abdomen is soft, nontender, and nondistended, with no masses or organomegaly.

Of the following, the MOST likely explanation for this event is

A. anomalous left coronary artery

B. brief resolved unexplained event (BRUE)

C. periodic breathing

D. seizure

Item 94

A 4-year-old boy is being evaluated for eye pain. He was playing at the park when another child threw a handful of sand toward his face. The boy cried immediately and has been reporting eye pain and refusing to open his right eye since then. He is visibly uncomfortable. His right eye is tearing excessively and there is diffuse erythema of the bulbar conjunctiva. Upon eversion of his eyelid no foreign body is visible. After application of fluorescein, examination with a Wood lamp confirms a 2-mm linear area of enhancement in the corneal region (Item Q94).

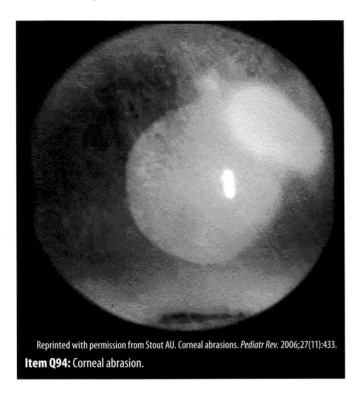

Reprinted with permission from Stout AU. Corneal abrasions. *Pediatr Rev.* 2006;27(11):433.

Item Q94: Corneal abrasion.

Of the following, the MOST appropriate treatment for his condition is

A. anesthetic ophthalmic drops

B. antibiotic ophthalmic drops

C. corticosteroid ophthalmic drops

D. patching of the right eye

Item 95

A 17-year-old college student presents with a 1-day history of right testicular pain and swelling. He was well until 5 days ago when he developed low-grade fever, malaise, sore throat, and bilateral submaxillary swelling. He has 1 female sexual partner and reports consistent condom use. Two of his college roommates recently developed a similar illness, 1 of whom also developed meningitis. On physical examination, the boy is alert and appropriately interactive. He is febrile (38.4°C) with normal vital signs. His left testicle is swollen, warm, erythematous, and exquisitely tender to palpation.

Of the following, the MOST likely cause of this boy's illness is

A. *Chlamydia trachomatis*

B. *Haemophilus influenzae* type b

C. mumps

D. *Neisseria gonorrhoeae*

Item 96

A 30-week-gestation male neonate dies of hyperkalemia in your neonatal intensive care unit. Analysis of the total parenteral nutrition (TPN) being administered at the time of death reveals a potassium dose 10 times higher than the dose ordered by the medical team. The medical error is disclosed to the family by the supervising physician.

Of the following, the BEST next step for the medical team is

A. changing the TPN ordering guidelines

B. disciplinary action

C. supportive counseling

D. education on TPN components

Item 97

A 6-month-old white infant is seen in the emergency department for concerns of turning blue. His mother reports intermittent blueness on the backs of his hands and his cheeks. It may be worse when he is cold, but she is unsure if there are other triggers. She has not noticed blue lips or earlobes, but she has noticed that his nail beds are sometimes bluish. The infant appears well and has normal growth parameters, heart rate, and respiratory rate. Peripheral oxygen saturation obtained by pulse oximetry is 98%. His oral mucosa and tongue are pink. The cardiorespiratory examination findings are normal. There is no hepatosplenomegaly and no digital clubbing. His extremities are cool and his nail beds are dusky.

Of the following, the MOST appropriate next step in the care of this infant is to

A. admit to the hospital for telemetric monitoring of cardiovascular status and pulse oximetry

B. consult with child protective services regarding suspected child abuse

C. counsel the mother regarding causes of peripheral cyanosis in infants and young children

D. obtain an electrocardiogram and chest radiograph

Item 98

A 15-year-old adolescent boy is being evaluated for light spots on his face, which appeared several weeks ago. The areas are itchy at times and flaky. He also reports flaking of his scalp. The patient is well in other respects and has an unremarkable medical history. The physical examination findings are normal except for the alar creases, which reveal mild erythema, hypopigmentation, and scaling (Item Q98).

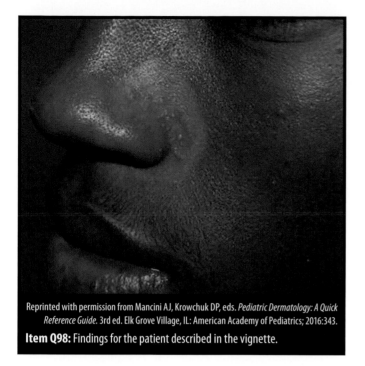

Reprinted with permission from Mancini AJ, Krowchuk DP, eds. *Pediatric Dermatology: A Quick Reference Guide*. 3rd ed. Elk Grove Village, IL: American Academy of Pediatrics; 2016:343.

Item Q98: Findings for the patient described in the vignette.

Of the following, the MOST likely diagnosis is

A. atopic dermatitis
B. periorificial dermatitis
C. seborrheic dermatitis
D. tinea corporis

Item 99

An 8-year-old boy with trisomy 21 is seen for a health supervision visit. His mother has no concerns. He has a history of an atrioventricular septal defect that was repaired in infancy. His only medication is a daily multivitamin. He is doing well in the second grade with an Individualized Education Program. A review of systems is unremarkable. He has a temperature of 37°C, heart rate of 62 beats/min, and blood pressure of 102/64 mm Hg. His weight and height are at the 50th percentile on syndrome-specific growth curves. His thyroid appears enlarged. There is no cervical lymphadenopathy. The remainder of his physical examination findings are unremarkable.

Of the following, the MOST likely cause of his examination findings is

A. Graves disease
B. Hashimoto thyroiditis
C. multinodular goiter
D. simple colloid goiter

Item 100

A 5-day-old breastfed nondysmorphic neonate presents with poor feeding, vomiting, failure to thrive, hypoglycemia, jaundice, hepatomegaly, elevated liver function tests, and a bleeding diathesis. A workup for infection reveals *Escherichia coli* sepsis, for which antibiotics are initiated. The newborn screening results are abnormal, confirming that this neonate has an inborn error of metabolism. A change is immediately implemented in the neonate's diet.

Of the following, the diet required to ABATE this neonate's symptoms is

A. gluten-free
B. lactose-restricted
C. phenylalanine-free
D. protein-restricted

Item 101

A 12-month-old girl is seen for a health supervision visit. There were no concerns identified at her previous visit 3 months ago. When asked about her development, her father replies that she is cruising along furniture, crawling up stairs, and walking when supported, but she is not yet taking independent steps. She is stringing consonant sounds together (eg, "dadadada") but it is not clear whether she is directing the sounds toward her father. She plays peek-a-boo and is wary with strangers, but she does not point to things she wants and does not point to get others' attention. She is banging 2 objects together and is using a pincer grasp but does not yet hold a crayon to scribble. She is starting to drink from a sippy cup but is not yet using a spoon.

Of the following, the aspect of her history that is MOST concerning for a developmental delay is that

A. she does not yet hold a crayon to scribble
B. she does not yet point to things she wants or to get others' attention
C. she is not yet taking steps independently
D. she is not yet using a spoon

Item 102

A 3-year-old Chinese girl is brought to an international adoption clinic for evaluation. She has been in the custody of her adoptive family for 2 weeks and has been in good health during that time. Her medical history is limited, but it is known that her mother had chronic hepatitis B infection and that the girl did not receive hepatitis B virus immunization at birth. She has a temperature of 37.2°C, heart rate of 110 beats/min, respiratory rate of 22 breaths/min, and blood pressure of 98/51 mm Hg. She is in no distress. Her abdomen is mildly distended but there is no tenderness or hepatomegaly.

Laboratory data are shown:

Laboratory Test	Result
Hepatitis B surface antigen	Positive
Hepatitis B core antibody	Positive
Hepatitis B e antigen	Positive
Hepatitis B e antibody	Negative
Hepatitis B quantitative DNA	25,000 IU/mL

Of the following, this patient is MOST at risk for

A. biliary carcinoma
B. hepatic sarcoma
C. hepatoblastoma
D. hepatocellular carcinoma

Item 103

An 18-month-old girl is undergoing a health supervision visit. Her parents are concerned about their daughter's intoed gait. They report that she intoes mainly on the left and that she trips frequently. Physical examination reveals that when the girl stands with the patellae in a neutral position, the left foot points inward. Hip rotation is symmetric, with internal rotation of 55 degrees and external rotation of 45 degrees bilaterally. Observation of her gait reveals intoeing on the left.

Of the following, the BEST next management step for this girl is

A. day and night bracing with reverse last shoes
B. nighttime bracing with shoes connected by a bar
C. physical therapy
D. reassurance

Item 104

A 9-year-old boy with autism is being evaluated for abdominal pain. He has a history of chronic constipation that is managed with diet and occasional laxative use. The boy's appetite and stool frequency have decreased in the past 2 weeks. He has had no fever, vomiting, or diarrhea, but today he is more irritable and refusing to eat. His last stool, 2 days ago, was hard, small, and nonbloody. He is not able to communicate about his pain. Physical examination is difficult to perform because of poor cooperation, but a general fullness and mild tenderness to palpation without rebound is noted in the right lower quadrant. Plain radiographs of the abdomen are shown (Item Q104).

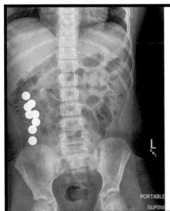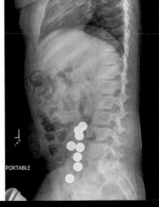

Reprinted with permission from Green SS. Ingested and aspirated foreign bodies. *Pediatr Rev.* 2015;(10):430-437.

Item Q104: Radiographs for the boy described in the vignette.

After viewing the radiographs, the mother is asked if she recalls whether the boy may have ingested magnets. She remembers that he was found playing with a desktop magnet toy intended for adults a few weeks ago.

Of the following, the MOST appropriate next step in management for this boy is

A. hospital admission for serial abdominal radiography
B. performance of a mineral oil enema in the office
C. prescription of a laxative and close observation of stools at home
D. referral for an urgent surgical consult

Item 105

An 8-hour-old male neonate in the newborn nursery has had multiple episodes of nonbloody, yellowish-green emesis. He was born at 39 weeks' gestation via spontaneous vaginal delivery. The pregnancy was remarkable for polyhydramnios. He has breastfed since delivery, and he passed meconium at 6 hours after birth. He has a temperature of 37.5°C and heart rate of 160 beats/min. He has upslanting palpebral fissures and a flat nasal bridge. His abdomen is scaphoid, and epigastric fullness is present. Bowel sounds are hypoactive. Rectal examination reveals a normally appearing anus. Extremities are warm and well perfused. There is a sandal gap between his first and second toes.

An abdominal radiograph (Item Q105) is shown.

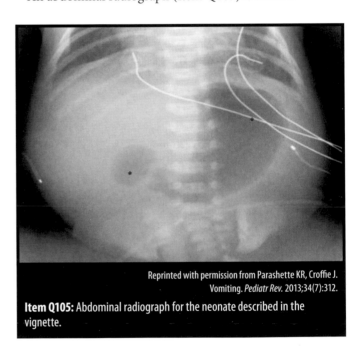

Reprinted with permission from Parashette KR, Croffie J. Vomiting. *Pediatr Rev.* 2013;34(7):312.

Item Q105: Abdominal radiograph for the neonate described in the vignette.

Of the following, the MOST likely diagnosis is

A. cow milk protein allergy
B. duodenal atresia
C. gastroesophageal reflux disease
D. Hirschsprung disease

Item 106

A 9-year-old girl is seen for problems at school. Her parents report that she has had no academic struggles before starting fourth grade this year. She has variable performance in each of her class subjects. She tells you that she does her homework but sometimes cannot find it when it is time to turn it in. The girl's softball coach has moved her from the outfield because she sometimes does not notice when the ball has been pitched. She has lost several notebooks. Results of standardized rating scales from both parents and teacher confirm the suspected diagnosis. Behavior management strategies and classroom accommodations are implemented. After treatment with a long-acting methylphenidate is initiated, the parents are pleased with the degree of improvement in symptoms but are concerned that their daughter seems emotional in the late afternoon. They would like to continue with the same medication if possible, but are willing to switch if necessary.

Of the following, the MOST appropriate next step is to

A. add an afternoon dose of short-acting methylphenidate

B. change to a morning dose of short-acting methylphenidate

C. replace the medication with an α-adrenergic agonist

D. switch to a mixed salts of amphetamine preparation

Item 107

At a routine health supervision visit, a 10-year-old girl reports frequent nosebleeds, but she is otherwise healthy. She is a good student and plays on a local soccer team. The girl's mother has migraines. Her father had a stroke due to a hemorrhage from an arteriovenous malformation. Her paternal grandmother died of a brain abscess caused by a pulmonary arteriovenous malformation. The girl's physical examination findings are normal.

Of the following, the BEST next step in this girl's evaluation is to

A. perform pulmonary function tests

B. perform transthoracic echocardiography

C. refer her for dermatology evaluation

D. refer her for genetics evaluation

Item 108

A 16-year-old adolescent boy noticed a lump in his left scrotum 1 week ago. He reports a feeling of heaviness in his left scrotum, and his left lower abdomen feels achy. He reports no fever, dysuria, or urethral discharge. He is sexually active with 1 female partner and does not use condoms. His medical history is significant for left cryptorchidism corrected by orchiopexy at age 2 years. His sexual maturity rating is stage 5. A nontender, firm mass that is not reducible is palpated in his left scrotum.

Of the following, the MOST helpful next diagnostic step is

A. α-fetoprotein level

B. scrotal ultrasonography

C. testosterone level

D. urine gonorrhea/chlamydia test

Item 109

A 16-year-old adolescent girl is seen for evaluation of a lump in her neck. She had been well with normal growth and development until approximately 2 weeks ago when she noticed a lump just below the angle of her right mandible.

It has not changed since she first noticed it. She has not had fevers, weight loss, or night sweats.

She is at the 45th percentile for height and the 65th percentile for weight. She has a temperature of 37°C, heart rate of 72 beats/min, and blood pressure of 114/82 mm Hg. She is in no distress. There is a 1.5-cm ovoid, firm but freely movable nodule on her neck just inferior to the mandibular angle on the right. There is no overlying erythema on the nodule. It is mildly tender to palpation. The remainder of her physical examination findings are unremarkable other than facial acne vulgaris, with a conspicuous, inflamed pimple lateral to the right nares.

Of the following, this patient's presentation is MOST consistent with

A. infectious lymphadenitis caused by Epstein-Barr virus

B. infectious lymphadenitis caused by *Staphylococcus aureus*

C. malignant lymphadenopathy caused by Hodgkin lymphoma

D. reactive lymphadenopathy caused by *Staphylococcus aureus*

Item 110

A 17-year-old previously healthy boy is being evaluated for a painful lesion on his left ankle. Last evening he and a friend went camping, using a tent that had been stored in the family garage. This morning he complained of pain in his left ankle, and his parents noticed the lesion. He does not recall any trauma, and he has had no recent fevers. He has no history of allergies, and his immunizations are up to date. The boy's father found a dead spider in the tent this morning (Item Q110).

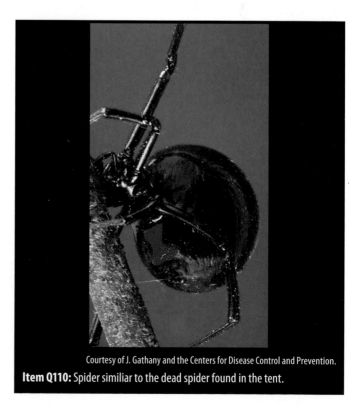

Courtesy of J. Gathany and the Centers for Disease Control and Prevention.

Item Q110: Spider similiar to the dead spider found in the tent.

On physical examination, the boy's vital signs are normal for his age. He is well-appearing. There is a 1-cm blanched circular patch, with surrounding erythema and central punctum on his left ankle. The ankle is slightly tender at the site of the lesion, but he has no tenderness proximally. He is able to ambulate without difficulty. The rest of the boy's physical examination findings, including a complete neurologic assessment, are unremarkable. He washed the lesion with soap and water before coming for his evaluation.

Of the following, the BEST next step in the boy's management is

A. prescription of an oral analgesic and antibiotic therapy

B. prescription of an oral analgesic and corticosteroid therapy

C. prescription of an oral analgesic only

D. referral to the emergency department for *Latrodectus* antivenin therapy

Item 111

A male neonate with severe respiratory distress is being evaluated in the newborn nursery. The 2.0-kg neonate was delivered vaginally by a 34-year-old gravida 2, para 1 woman. Physical examination findings are significant for pseudoepicanthus, flattened ears, and bilateral club feet (Item Q111). His vital signs include a temperature of 37°C, heart rate of 160 beats/min, respiratory rate of 60 breaths/min, and oxygen saturation of 92% by pulse oximetry on 4L oxygen by nasal cannula. Abdominal ultrasonography reveals bilaterally enlarged echogenic kidneys with poor corticomedullary differentiation; there are no cysts or hydronephrosis. The liver, spleen, pancreas, and gallbladder are reported to be normal. After reviewing the findings, further inquiry reveals no family history of renal failure.

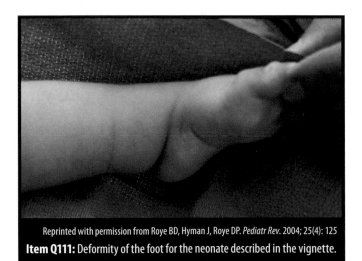

Reprinted with permission from Roye BD, Hyman J, Roye DP. *Pediatr Rev.* 2004; 25(4): 125

Item Q111: Deformity of the foot for the neonate described in the vignette.

Of the following, the MOST likely cause of this neonate's symptoms is

A. chromosomal abnormality

B. maternal hypertension

C. maternal substance abuse

D. oligohydramnios

Item 112

An 8-year-old boy is seen for a health supervision visit as a new patient. He feels well and is doing well in school. His parents have no concerns. His father had a myocardial infarction at the age of 45 years. The family shares that they are meticulous in maintaining a heart healthy diet and that they engage in physical activity as a family. All of the boy's growth parameters are at the 45th percentile, and the remainder of his physical examination findings are unremarkable.

In addition to continuing the heart healthy diet and exercise, the BEST next step in management is to perform a comprehensive assessment of serum lipid and lipoprotein levels

A. now

B. at age 18 years

C. at age 25 years

D. at age 40 years

Item 113

A 15-year-old adolescent girl with a history of migraine headaches (with aura) is seen for a health supervision visit. For the past 6 months, she has been missing 1 to 2 days of school per month because of severe menstrual cramps. She also experiences bloating, diarrhea, and lower back pain during her cycle. She had menarche at age 13 years, and her periods have been regular and last 5 days. She takes 600 mg of ibuprofen 3 times a day during the first 2 days of her period, which provides minimal relief of her symptoms. Her migraine headaches are well controlled with propranolol. She is not sexually active.

Of the following, the BEST next treatment in the management of this patient would be a trial of

A. combined oral contraceptive pills

B. a contraceptive patch

C. prescription-dose naproxen

D. progestin-only contraceptive pills

Item 114

A 5-month-old infant born at 26 weeks' gestation was admitted to the intensive care unit and underwent intubation for respiratory failure. His 4-month-long neonatal intensive care course was complicated by intubation and mechanical ventilation for a period of 3 months, grade III intraventricular hemorrhage requiring a ventriculoperitoneal shunt, and necrotizing enterocolitis requiring resection of approximately 30 cm of small intestine. The boy underwent extubation at 3 months of age, but required reintubation within several hours. He underwent successful extubation and was placed on oxygen by nasal noninvasive continuous positive airway pressure 1 week after the first attempt. He was gradually weaned to oxygen by nasal cannula, and discharged from the hospital on 0.5 L/min of oxygen. His home medications include chlorothiazide, furosemide, and multivitamins.

The boy had been doing well at home for 2 weeks, when he developed progressive difficulty breathing over the course of 1 week. There were no intercurrent illnesses. He was brought to the emergency department, where a physical examination revealed a respiratory rate of 30 breaths/min, with severe respiratory distress marked by deep retractions, no wheezing or stridor, and minimal air entry. His oxygen saturation was 80% on room air. The infant was warm and well-perfused. A murmur was heard continuously throughout systole and diastole, and his abdomen was soft, with no organomegaly. The decision was made to intubate him because of his retractions and poor air entry. During the intubation procedure, laryngoscopy showed normal supraglottic structures and vocal cords. When a 3.0-mm endotracheal tube was passed through the vocal cords, an obstruction was encountered, but a 2.5-mm tube passed easily. The cause for the infant's current episode of respiratory failure is unclear, and a subspecialist is consulted to assist in his diagnosis and treatment.

Of the following, the MOST appropriate service to consult is

A. cardiology

B. general surgery

C. otolaryngology

D. pulmonology

Item 115

An 18-month-old boy is brought to the emergency department after his mother found him in her bathroom playing with an open bottle of iron-containing prenatal vitamins. She had purchased the bottle of 60 pills just 2 days earlier; she counts 25 pills remaining in the bottle. The boy is crying and fussy, but in no distress. He is afebrile and has a heart rate of 145 beats/min, respiratory rate of 24 breaths/min, and blood pressure of 90/50 mm Hg.

Of the following, the MOST appropriate next step is to

A. administer activated charcoal via nasogastric tube

B. administer intravenous deferoxamine

C. measure serum iron concentration

D. perform gastric lavage with bicarbonate

Item 116

A 16-year-old, previously healthy girl presents with a 1-week history of fever, sore throat, and severe fatigue. On physical examination, she is febrile (39.5°C), and has exudative pharyngitis; bilateral, tender, posterior cervical lymphadenopathy; and mild splenomegaly. A complete blood cell count shows leukocytosis of $16.0\times10^3/\mu L$ ($16.0\times10^9/L$), with 24% neutrophils, 20% monocytes, 42% lymphocytes, and 14% atypical lymphocytes. A rapid slide agglutination reaction test is positive for heterophile antibodies.

Of the following, the BEST next step in management for this girl is

A. acyclovir

B. corticosteroids

C. supportive care

D. valganciclovir

Item 117

A neonate with bilious emesis is being evaluated in the newborn nursery. Her mother is a 36-year-old gravida 3, para 1 woman with a history of a seizure disorder treated with levetiracetam. Prenatal laboratory results are significant for negative group B *Streptococcus* screening and rubella nonimmune status. The mother reports smoking half a pack of cigarettes daily during the pregnancy. The neonate was delivered vaginally with Apgar scores of 9 and 9 at 1 and 5 minutes, respectively.

Two hours after birth, the neonate had an episode of green emesis. On physical examination, her heart rate is 145 beats/min, blood pressure is 53/24 mm Hg, respiratory rate is 38 beats/min, and temperature is 36.3°C. She appears comfortable, with moderate abdominal distention and no tenderness on palpation. The remainder of her physical examination findings are unremarkable. A complete blood cell count shows a hemoglobin of 15 g/dL (150 g/L), platelet count of $279\times10^3/\mu L$ ($279\times10^9/L$), and white blood cell count of $10,200/\mu L$ ($10.2\times10^9/L$). An abdominal radiograph is obtained (Item Q117).

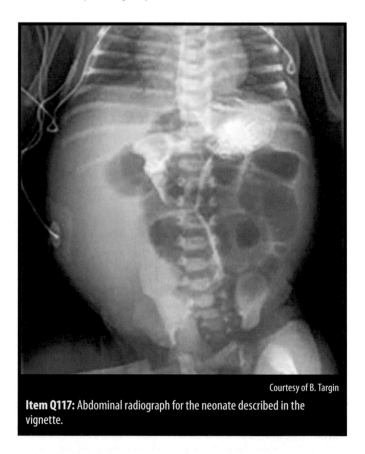

Courtesy of B. Targin

Item Q117: Abdominal radiograph for the neonate described in the vignette.

Of the following, this neonate's presentation is MOST likely due to

A. advanced maternal age

B. congenital rubella infection

C. exposure to levetiracetam

D. in utero cigarette exposure

Item 118

A 4 year old girl has rapid breathing. Her mother has counted her respiratory rate as 46 breaths/min. The girl has no signs of respiratory distress. She has not had fever, and there are no known ill contacts. She has an oxygen saturation of 99% in room air, a temperature of 37°C, and a respiratory rate of 48 breaths/min. She is irritable but comfortable and has no cough or wheeze. There is no increased breathing effort or use of accessory muscles. Breath sounds are clear, and the cardiac examination findings are normal. Pulses are equal and full. A chest radiograph is normal. Results of a urinalysis and a complete blood cell count and differential are normal.

Of the following, the historic information that is the MOST pertinent to this girl's presentation is

A. her maternal aunt has type 1 diabetes

B. an open bottle of chewable aspirin was found accessible in the home

C. respiratory syncytial virus has been reported in her day care center

D. she has recently been drinking more apple juice than usual

Item 119

A 3-year-old white boy is seen for concerns of leg bowing. His mother noticed that his legs appeared increasingly bowed over the past year. He eats a well-balanced diet and drinks at least 2 cups of milk per day. He is otherwise healthy. His weight is at the 25th percentile, and his height is at the 5th percentile. His legs appear bowed. His dentition is normal. The remainder of his physical examination findings are unremarkable. A right knee and lower leg radiograph is shown (Item Q119).

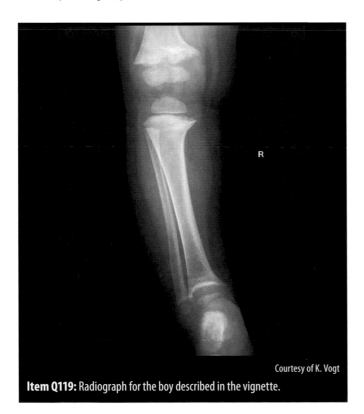

Courtesy of K. Vogt

Item Q119: Radiograph for the boy described in the vignette.

Laboratory data are shown:

Laboratory test	Result
Calcium	9.2 mg/dL (2.3 mmol/L)
Albumin	4.4 g/dL (44 g/L)
Phosphorus	1.8 mg/dL (0.6 mmol/L)
Alkaline phosphatase	640 U/L
Parathyroid hormone	40 pg/mL (40 ng/L) (Reference range, 10-65 pg/mL [10-65 ng/L])
25-hydroxyvitamin D	22 ng/mL (55 nmol/L)
1,25-dihydroxyvitamin D	20 pg/mL (52 pmol/L) (Reference range, 20-79 pg/mL [52-205 pmol/L])

Of the following, the BEST treatment for this boy is

A. calcium and calcitriol

B. calcium and cholecalciferol

C. phosphorus and calcitriol

D. phosphorus and calcium

Item 120

A 5-month-old male infant is being evaluated for growth failure, severe muscle weakness, delayed motor development, and global hypotonia. The mother reports a recent concern with his suck and swallow capabilities as well as 2 episodes of aspiration pneumonia. He was the product of a normal pregnancy and delivery. Development of symptoms, with progression, was noted after 2 months of age. Physical examination reveals a small, nondysmorphic infant with severe muscular weakness which spares the face. He is able to smile, laugh, and coo. He has mild contractures at the knees, postural tremor of the fingers, areflexia, and tongue fasciculations. He has normal male genitalia, with bilaterally descended testicles of normal size. Family history is unremarkable.

Of the following, the infant's MOST likely diagnosis is

A. Duchenne muscular dystrophy

B. Prader Willi syndrome

C. spinal muscular atrophy

D. Zellweger syndrome

Item 121

A 10-year-old boy has a 2-day history of throat pain and fever to 38.2°C. He has erythematous tonsils with petechiae on his soft palate. A rapid streptococcal antigen test result is positive. His mother states that he and his 3 siblings have had multiple throat infections over the past year, and these frequent infections are impairing her ability to keep her job. She requests a tonsillectomy to "get this taken care of once and for all." Over the past 3 years, the patient has had 7 visits for pharyngitis and 5 other positive rapid streptococcal antigen test results, including 2 performed during his siblings' visits while the patient was asymptomatic. He has an allergy to amoxicillin but no reaction to cephalosporins. Regarding sleep, his mother states that he has snoring only with upper respiratory infections, and there are no concerns about his behavior or school performance.

Of the following, the BEST next step in the care of this patient is

A. long-term prophylactic cephalosporin therapy

B. polysomnography

C. a referral to an otolaryngologist

D. watchful waiting

Item 122

A 13-year-old adolescent boy with cystic fibrosis is brought to the pulmonary clinic for follow up of *Mycobacterium abscessus* pulmonary infection. The treatment regimen includes amikacin via parenteral home antibiotic therapy, which he has been receiving for the last 4 weeks. His mother reports that he has been afebrile and has had resolution of cough. His respiratory status has returned to baseline. He has not had any medication-related adverse effects, including no concerns related to hearing.

Laboratory data obtained via his home health agency are shown:

Laboratory test	Result
Blood urea nitrogen	14 mg/dL (5.0 mmol/L)
Creatinine	0.6 mg/dL (53 μmol/L)

The last time an amikacin level was drawn was during the first week of therapy.

Of the following, the BEST description of the medical error in this patient is

A. commission

B. nonintercepted

C. preventable

D. sentinel

Item 123

During a 10-km run on a hot, humid day, a 16-year-old girl presents to the first-aid tent at the midpoint of the course. She reports being unable to continue running due to exhaustion and abdominal cramps. On physical examination, the girl has a heart rate of 148 beats/min, respiratory rate of 18 breaths/min, and a temperature of 38.8°C. She appears pale and sweaty.

Of the following, the girl's presentation is MOST consistent with

A. exercise-associated muscle cramps

B. exertional heat stroke

C. heat exhaustion

D. poor physical conditioning

Item 124

An 18-year-old girl is undergoing a health supervision visit and sports physical. Her parent denies any medical concerns, but states that the girl has become moodier and interacts with her family less than desired. During the confidential history, the girl states that she prefers to spend most of her time with her 20-year-old boyfriend. Physical examination shows bruising on the girl's upper arm which she claims is from playing volleyball. When it is noted that this bruise appears like someone grabbed her, she becomes tearful. She then discloses that her boyfriend sometimes yells at or pushes her. The girl's parents are not aware of this behavior, and she does not want them to be informed. The boyfriend always apologizes, so she forgives him and does not want to report him to the police. She assures you that she feels safe and is in no immediate danger. She is informed of her legal rights and resources, and an agreement is made to keep her confidence.

Of the following, the ethical principle that is BEST depicted by this decision is

A. autonomy

B. beneficence

C. justice

D. nonmaleficence

Item 125

A 14-year-old adolescent girl is brought to the emergency department for evaluation of right upper quadrant abdominal pain, fever, and vomiting. The symptoms began acutely 4 hours ago, shortly after eating pizza and ice cream. She is obese, but is otherwise healthy. She has a temperature of 39.5°C, heart rate of 130 beats/min, and blood pressure of 120/70 mm Hg. She appears uncomfortable and is trying to lie still. There is no scleral icterus. Cardiac examination reveals tachycardia. Respiratory examination findings are normal. Her abdomen is firm with involuntary guarding. She has pain with palpation in the right upper quadrant during deep inspiration.

Laboratory data are shown:

Laboratory test	Result
White blood cell count	$19.0 \times 10^3/\mu L$ ($19.0 \times 10^9/L$)
Total bilirubin	1.5 mg/dL (25.7 μmol/L)
Direct bilirubin	0.4 mg/dL (6.8 μmol/L)
Alanine aminotransferase	150 U/L
Aspartate aminotransferase	130 U/L
γ-Glutamyltransferase	120 U/L
Lipase	65 U/L

Of the following, the MOST appropriate next diagnostic test is

A. cholescintigraphy (HIDA scan)
B. computed tomography of the abdomen
C. ultrasonography of the abdomen
D. upper gastrointestinal series

Item 126

A 7-year-old boy is seen for difficulties in school. The boy's teacher has told his parents that he does not stay on task in class and lacks effort on his schoolwork. Their son has said that he is bored in class. The parents report that he is very curious and remembers everything. He is reading at the fourth grade level. Evaluation by a private psychologist indicates an IQ of 140. The boy's parents would like to know what to expect for his future.

Of the following, the BEST response to the parents' question is that their son will most likely

A. be advanced in all areas of development
B. benefit from grade advancement
C. need educational enrichment activities
D. require treatment with methylphenidate

Item 127

A 15-year-old girl develops right-sided facial weakness. She first noticed it when she woke up this morning when she was putting on eye makeup and could not close her right eye all the way. She then had difficulty drinking her usual protein shake because the fluid kept coming out of the right side of her mouth. The girl denies any recent illness or head injuries, but reports that her right ear was hurting yesterday and now seems overly sensitive to sounds. All of her vital signs are normal. Both tympanic membranes are pearly gray and there are no lesions in the external ear canals. When attempting to raise her eyebrows, the right side of her forehead does not move. Her right eye closure is weak and the right side of her mouth droops. Sensation on her face is normal, and she has full strength in all limbs.

Of the following, the management MOST likely to improve recovery is

A. amoxicillin
B. ophthalmology referral
C. prednisone
D. speech therapy referral

Item 128

A resident and supervising physician are seeing a 6-month-old infant for a health supervision visit. The infant's breastfeeding mother wonders when she can introduce cow milk to her infant. The resident asks about the differences between human milk and cow milk.

Of the following, the MOST accurate statement to include in the answer is that cow milk contains

A. less calcium
B. more fat
C. more protein
D. less sodium

Item 129

A 2-year-old boy scheduled for a ureteral reimplantation to correct severe ureteral reflux associated with recurrent urinary tract infections is seen for a preoperative evaluation. For the last 6 months, he has been receiving urinary tract infection prophylaxis with cefixime.

A preoperative laboratory evaluation is obtained. A complete blood cell count and the results of a metabolic panel (including liver function tests) are normal. The coagulation profile reveals:

Laboratory test	Result
Prothrombin time	14.7 s (reference range, 11-13.5 s)
Partial thromboplastin time	39 s (reference range, 25-35 s)

Of the following, the MOST likely cause of the abnormal laboratory values is

A. an acquired factor V deficiency
B. a congenital factor VIII deficiency
C. hypofibrinogenemia
D. a vitamin deficiency

Item 130

A 20-month-old previously healthy boy presents to the emergency department with a 0.5-cm simple laceration on the underside of his chin. He sustained this laceration 1 hour ago after tripping on a rug inside his home and hitting his chin on the corner of a table. He did not lose consciousness, and his behavior has been normal since he fell. The boy is very well-appearing with normal vital signs for his age. He has no allergies.

At the time of examination, the boy is playfully interacting with his mother and older sister. However, he becomes extremely anxious and screams loudly whenever approached by the physician. Despite the physician's gentle approach, reassurance, and multiple attempts to calm him using various distraction strategies, he screams and struggles to escape as he is examined and a topical anesthetic is applied to the laceration. It is determined that placement of 2 simple interrupted sutures, after thorough cleansing of the wound, will be required to appropriately repair the laceration. His mother asks if the physician could "please order something to keep him calm" during the anticipated procedure.

Of the following, the MOST appropriate medication option for this patient is

A. intramuscular morphine
B. intranasal midazolam
C. intravenous etomidate
D. intravenous propofol

 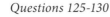

Item 131

A 15-year-old boy is being evaluated for blood in the urine of 1 day's duration. He describes the urine as bright red. He has no complaints of fever, frequency, painful urination, or flank pain. His vital signs are normal for his age, and his physical examination findings are normal. Urinalysis demonstrates a specific gravity of 1.015, pH of 6.0, 4+ blood, 4+ leukocyte esterase, and no protein or nitrites. Urine microscopy shows more than 100 red blood cells/high-power field (hpf), 10 to 50 white blood cells/hpf, and no crystals or bacteria.

Of the following, the MOST accurate statement regarding this boy's presentation is that

A. cystoscopy is routinely indicated for evaluation

B. there is usually a recognizable and apparent cause

C. urinary color reflects the degree of blood loss

D. urinary tract infection is a rare cause

Item 132

A 16-year-old adolescent girl is brought to the emergency department because of chest pain. The pain has been present for 1 day, and she describes it as sharp and severe and located in the inferior aspect of her sternum. She appears uncomfortable and states that she gets some relief from sitting up and leaning her elbows on her upper legs. She is afebrile, has a heart rate of 100 beats/min, respiratory rate of 25 breaths/min, blood pressure of 135/80 mm Hg, and oxygen saturation as measured by pulse oximetry of 100% on room air. Her physical examination findings are otherwise unremarkable. Electrocardiography is performed (Item Q132). Results from a basic metabolic panel and complete blood cell count are unremarkable. The C-reactive protein level is 3.5 mg/dL (33.3 nmol/L), and the troponin level is 5 ng/mL (5 µg/L). A chest radiograph has normal findings.

Of the following, the BEST next step in management is

A. activation of the cardiac catheterization team

B. administration of glucocorticoids

C. administration of intravenous immunoglobulin

D. administration of nonsteroidal anti-inflammatory drugs

Item 133

A 17-year-old adolescent boy is brought to the emergency department because of slurred speech. His mother reports that she tried to wake him at home and he was groggy with changes in his speech. In the emergency department, the patient is alert and oriented, and all of his vital signs are stable. When his mother is not in the room, he discloses that he had been drinking with his friends, and he does not want his mother to know. He and his friends drink daily after school (3 to 5 cans of beer), and sometimes he drives after he has been drinking. He reports that he has never gotten in a motor vehicle collision after he has been drinking, does not feel he has a problem, and knows he could stop drinking if he wanted to.

Of the following, the BEST next step in the management of this patient is to

A. break confidentiality and discuss the situation with his mother

B. make a safety contract with the patient that he will not drink and drive

C. order a blood alcohol level and urine toxicology screen

D. provide him with brochures on drug and alcohol rehabilitation programs for adolescents

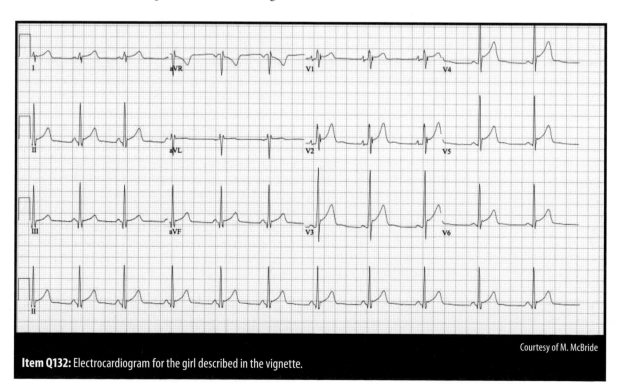

Courtesy of M. McBride

Item Q132: Electrocardiogram for the girl described in the vignette.

Item 134

An 8-year-old boy has been intubated and is receiving mechanical ventilation in the intensive care unit since he suffered a severe traumatic brain injury from a motor vehicle crash 5 days ago. He has had persistent intracranial hypertension despite a decompressive craniectomy, ventricular drainage, sedation, and mild hyperventilation. His sedation has been discontinued for 48 hours, and he is not receiving neuromuscular blockade. His electrolytes are normal. His vital signs are normal. On physical examination, the boy has flaccid tone and he is unresponsive to painful stimuli. His pupils are 5 mm and unreactive; corneal, cough, gag, oculovestibular, and oculocephalic reflexes are absent. No spontaneous respiratory effort was observed when the ventilator was disconnected for 5 minutes. Arterial blood gas partial pressure of carbon dioxide was 40 mm Hg before the ventilator was disconnected and 65 mm Hg at the end of the 5-minute period of apnea. Twelve hours later, the physical examination and apnea test were repeated, with the same results.

Of the following, the MOST appropriate next course of action in this case is to

A. declare death by neurologic criteria
B. recommend withdrawal of life-sustaining therapies
C. obtain radionuclide cerebral blood flow scan
D. recover organs for transplantation

Item 135

A 5-day-old male neonate is seen for his first health supervision visit. He was delivered at 39 weeks of gestation by a 28-year-old primiparous woman with an uncomplicated pregnancy. His postnatal course was complicated by breastfeeding difficulties and excessive weight loss. He did not pass the newborn hearing screen in either ear. The neonate's weight is 7% below his birth weight. His vital signs are normal for age. He has a flat midface, anteverted nares, micrognathia, and a bifid uvula. The remainder of his examination findings are normal.

Of the following, the MOST likely associated congenital anomaly is

A. atrial septal defect
B. corpus callosum agenesis
C. high myopia
D. hydronephrosis

Item 136

A 7-year-old girl with autism spectrum disorder is brought to the emergency department with decreased vision in her left eye. She has no other symptoms. There is no history of fever, vomiting, altered mental status, or weight loss. The family lives in rural Kentucky and has 2 puppies. There are no known tick or other animal exposures, including livestock. She has a history of occasionally eating dirt in her backyard. Her immunizations are up to date. The girl was born in the United States and has no history of international travel. She has not consumed raw or undercooked meats, has no sick contacts, and has not been taking any medications. On physical examination, she is alert and afebrile, with normal vital signs. Ophthalmologic examination reveals retinal abnormalities in the left eye (Item Q136).

The remainder of her physical examination findings are normal. Laboratory data are as follows.

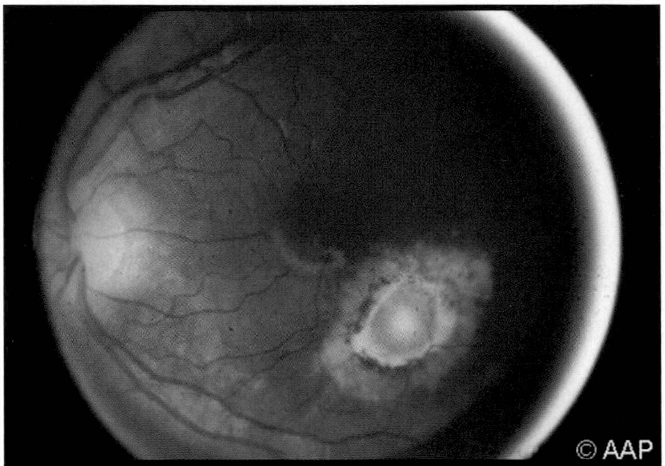

Reprinted with permission from H. Moffet and Kimberlin DW, et al, eds. *Red Book Online*. Itasca, IL: American Academy of Pediatrics; 2018.

Item Q136: Retinal abnormalities as described for the girl in the vignette.

Laboratory test	Result
White blood cell count	18,000/µL (18×10^9/L)
Platelet count	195×10^3/µL (195×10^9/L)
Neutrophils	45%
Eosinophil count	19%
Lymphocytes	36%
Hemoglobin	11.3 g/dL (113 g/L)

Of the following, the MOST likely cause of this girl's condition is

A. cysticercosis
B. toxocariasis
C. trichinosis
D. trichuriasis

Item 137

A 38-week-gestation neonate is brought to the nursery at 3 hours of age, after choking with an oral feeding. His mother is a 37-year-old woman with no significant medical history. On physical examination, the neonate is gagging with saliva in his mouth, and has a hypoplastic left thumb. The remainder of his examination findings are unremarkable. His chest radiographs are shown (Item Q137A and Item Q137B). An urgent cardiology consultation is conducted, and echocardiography reveals a patent foramen ovale.

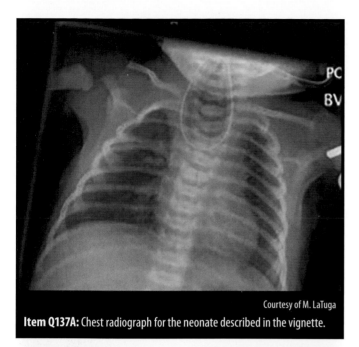

Courtesy of M. LaTuga

Item Q137A: Chest radiograph for the neonate described in the vignette.

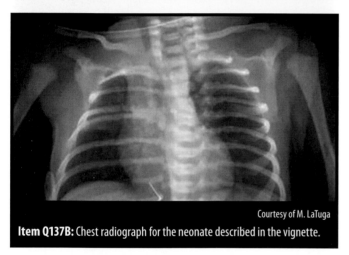

Courtesy of M. LaTuga

Item Q137B: Chest radiograph for the neonate described in the vignette.

Of the following, based on the neonate's clinical presentation, the MOST likely diagnosis is

A. CHARGE syndrome

B. Fanconi anemia

C. 22q11.2 syndrome

D. VACTERL association

Item 138

A 6-year-old boy is seen for a health supervision visit. His mother reports that he frequently coughs at night, he has to stop and rest when playing with friends, and he has excessive coughing when he has a viral respiratory infection. These symptoms have been present for several months following a severe viral illness, but they have not been severe enough that the mother felt the need for a sick visit. The family has a new dog in the house for about 1 year, and the maternal grandfather, who smokes, now lives with them. The boy's growth parameters are normal. He has an oxygen saturation of 99% on room air, a respiratory rate of 18 breaths/min, and a heart rate of 75 beats/min. He appears well and has no cough during the examination. His nasal mucosa is mildly boggy, and there is a small amount of clear mucus in the nasal antra. The posterior pharyngeal wall has a cobblestone appearance. Breath sounds are clear to auscultation, and cardiovascular examination findings are normal. The rest of the physical examination findings are unremarkable.

Office spirometry results are shown in Item Q138.

Item Q138. Spirometry results for the boy described in the vignette.

Result	Predicted	Best	% Predicted
FVC (L)	1.61	1.57	97%
FEV1 (L)	1.37	1.07	78%
FEV1/FVC	0.89	0.68	76%
FEF25-75% (L/s)	1.69	0.73	43%
PEFR (L/s)	3.18	2.37	74%
Vext %	—	1.91	—

FVC, Forced Vital Capacity (liters); FEV 1, Forced Expiratory Volume in 1 second (liters); FEF 25/75, Forced Expiratory Flow between 25% and 75% of FVC (liters/sec); PEFR, Peak Expiratory Flow Rate (liters/second); % pred, actual value as a percent of the predicted value for age and height

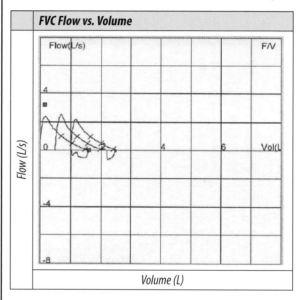

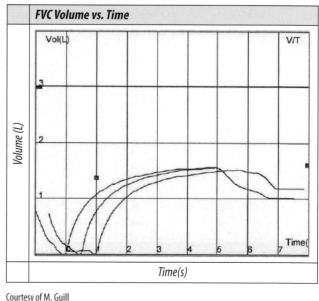

Courtesy of M. Guill

Of the following, the MOST effective approach to management in this child is

A. inhaled corticosteroid

B. oral albuterol

C. oral antihistamine

D. topical nasal corticosteroid

Item 139

A 13-year-old adolescent boy is seen for a routine health supervision visit. He and his mother have no concerns. He has a history of language delay and received speech therapy as a younger child. He has otherwise been healthy and takes no medication. His growth curve indicates tall stature (Item Q139). His adjusted mid-parental height is at the 50th percentile. His mother had menarche at 13 years of age, and his father had average timing of puberty. His legs appear disproportionately long, prompting measurement and calculation of an upper-to-lower segment ratio of 0.8. His sexual maturity rating is stage 3 for pubic hair. His testes are prepubertal in size. The remainder of his physical examination findings are normal.

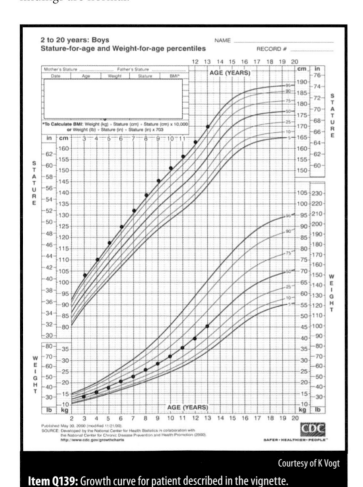

Item Q139: Growth curve for patient described in the vignette.

Courtesy of K Vogt

Of the following, the test that will MOST likely lead to the diagnosis is

A. echocardiography

B. an insulin-like growth factor-1 level

C. a karyotype

D. a serum homocysteine level

Item 140

A 3-year-old girl with a history of truncus arteriosus, submucosal cleft palate, mild hearing loss, and developmental delay presents for a new patient health supervision visit. Her mother reports a history of recurrent upper respiratory infections, including hospitalization at 6 months of age for respiratory syncytial virus. Chest radiography at that time revealed thymic hypoplasia. The girl also had feeding difficulties as a neonate, requiring nasogastric tube feeds for a short period.

Physical examination reveals hooding of the upper eyelids, ocular hypertelorism, overfolded helices, and a prominent nasal root with a nasal dimple/bifid nasal tip. Her height is at less than the 5th percentile.

Of the following, this girl is MOST likely to present with

A. hypercalcemia

B. hypocalcemia

C. pancytopenia

D. thrombocytopenia

Item 141

A 3-year-old girl has had fever for 6 days. Her father states that for the past 3 days her temperature has been at least 38.9°C, and it is not improving. He indicates that her eyes are red and she has a rash. He says she has been very cranky and that her appetite is decreased. He reports no vomiting, diarrhea, dysuria, cough, or trouble breathing. Her immunizations are up-to-date. The family was on vacation at a crowded amusement park for the first 3 days of her illness. She was seen at an urgent care center near the park where no etiology for her fever was found and no testing was done. Her temperature is now 38.9°C. She is irritable but interactive and cooperates with the examination. She has injected conjunctiva bilaterally without exudate, erythematous and cracked lips, and a polymorphous rash on her trunk and legs. The remainder of the physical examination findings are normal.

Of the following, the MOST appropriate next steps in the diagnostic approach for this child include

A. chest radiography, complete blood cell count with differential, blood culture, and urine culture

B. complete blood cell count with differential, comprehensive metabolic panel, C-reactive protein level, and urinalysis

C. nasopharyngeal swab for influenza A and B, rapid streptococcal antigen test, and heterophile antibody test

D. serum measles IgM antibody, complete blood cell count with differential, and nasopharyngeal swab for viral culture

Item 142

A 12-year-old boy is brought to the emergency department for evaluation of fever and right hip pain. He developed fever 7 days ago that has continued. Five days ago, he began to report pain over his right hip and developed a limp. He has not had any trauma. He has a temperature of 39.3°C, heart rate of 141 beats/min, respiratory rate of 24 breaths/min, and blood pressure of 125/69 mm Hg. He is distressed. Capillary refill time is 3 to 5 seconds with mild mottling. He has point tenderness over the proximal right femur but tolerates range of motion of the right hip.

Laboratory data are shown:

Laboratory test	Result
White blood cell count	5,960/μL (5.96 × 10⁹/L)
Neutrophils	73%
Lymphocytes	20%
Monocytes	7%
Hemoglobin	11.8 g/dL (118 g/L)
Platelet count	202 × 10³/μL (202 × 10⁹/L)
C-reactive protein	4.4 mg/dL (419.1 nmol/L)
Erythrocyte sedimentation rate	54 mm/h

Of the following, the BEST initial imaging study to obtain in this patient is

A. bone scan

B. computed tomography of the femur

C. radiography of the pelvis

D. ultrasonography of the hip

Item 143

A 15-year-old boy is being evaluated 1 day after his sister witnessed him having a seizure. The boy was in the bathroom getting ready for school when his sister heard a loud "thud." She opened the door to the bathroom and found her brother lying on the floor, unresponsive, with his arms and legs "jerking." The muscle movements lasted for less than 1 minute, after which her brother became alert and seemed "back to normal." The boy does not recall the episode. He reports feeling lightheaded for several minutes after the event. His medical history is otherwise unremarkable. His mother reports that she experienced similar episodes several years ago. The boy is currently asymptomatic and his physical examination findings are normal. He would like to return to basketball practice the following day.

Of the following, the MOST appropriate next steps in this boy's evaluation and management are

A. full clearance for sports with no further evaluation needed

B. rest from school and sports for 48 hours, followed by gradual return to activities if he remains asymptomatic

C. withhold clearance from sports, and perform a cardiac evaluation including electrocardiography

D. withhold clearance from sports, and perform a neurologic evaluation including magnetic resonance imaging of the brain

Item 144

A healthy 6-year-old girl is being evaluated at a new patient health supervision visit. Her parents ask about the girl's growth potential, because she has always been small for her age. She is currently at the 5th percentile for height and 25th percentile for weight. Her physical examination findings are unremarkable. No previous data are available to evaluate growth velocity. The father's height is 5'7" and the mother's height is 5'2". After calculating the midparental height using the population-based standard deviation of 1.67 inches (4.25 cm), the girl is suspected to have familial short stature.

Of the following, 95% of the time a girl with this history and physical examination is EXPECTED to have a final height that falls between

A. 4'11.5" and 5'9.5"

B. 5'1.2" and 5'7.8"

C. 4'10.7" and 5'5.3"

D. 5'2.8" and 5'6.2"

Item 145

An 11-year-old boy has had a cough for several weeks. He has also had a low-grade fever to 38.3°C associated with malaise that has waxed and waned. The cough was initially dry, but is now productive. His mother reports some wheezing. His immunizations are up-to-date, and he recently received his Tdap booster. He appears tired but nontoxic. He has a temperature of 37.7°C, oxygen saturation by pulse oximetry of 98%, and a respiratory rate of 20 breaths/min. There is no use of accessory muscles of respiration or retraction. Breath sounds are coarse, with diffuse rhonchi and crackles with scattered expiratory wheezes that do not fully resolve after inhalation of albuterol (2.5 mg) by wet nebulizer.

Of the following, the test MOST likely to be diagnostic for this patient is

A. nasal washing polymerase chain reaction for *Mycoplasma*

B. serology for Epstein-Barr virus antibodies

C. sputum for Gram stain and culture/sensitivity

D. throat swab for polymerase chain reaction for pertussis

The father of a 6-year-old girl is concerned about his daughter's learning. Although the child appears motivated at school, she has been unable to keep up with her peers. A psychoeducational evaluation has identified both cognitive and adaptive delays. The girl has qualified for an Individualized Education Program and will be placed in a special education classroom. Her father reports that the child's mother used various substances during her pregnancy and asks if any could have caused his daughter's disability. A picture of the girl is shown in Item Q146.

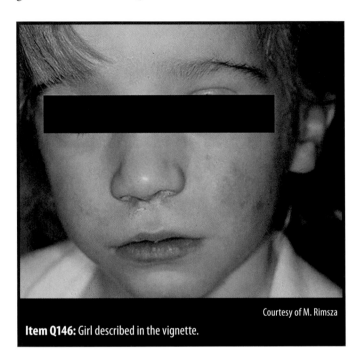

Courtesy of M. Rimsza

Item Q146: Girl described in the vignette.

Of the following, the substance MOST likely to have caused this child's difficulties is

A. cocaine

B. ethanol

C. marijuana

D. nicotine

A 9-month-old boy is being evaluated at a health supervision visit. He has just started sitting independently, but does not yet pull to stand. He can grab toys with each hand, but does not transfer them from hand to hand. He makes vowel sounds, but no consonants. His mother reports that about 1 month ago, the boy started having episodes during which he ducks his head down and his arms extend out. These happen in clusters, after which he cries. In response to your inquiries regarding family history, his mother reports that she previously had a raised, brown, leathery birthmark on her forehead for which she had laser treatment. Her sister's 2 children have autism and seizures. The boy's growth parameters are normal, and his general physical examination findings appear normal. He receives a detailed skin examination.

Of the following, the dermatologic findings MOST likely to be identified in this boy are

A. Item Q147A

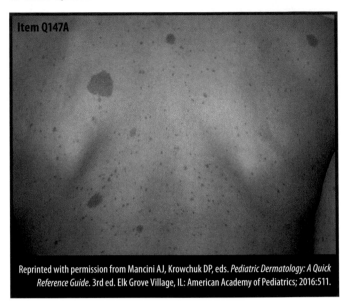

Reprinted with permission from Mancini AJ, Krowchuk DP, eds. *Pediatric Dermatology: A Quick Reference Guide.* 3rd ed. Elk Grove Village, IL: American Academy of Pediatrics; 2016:511.

B. Item Q147B

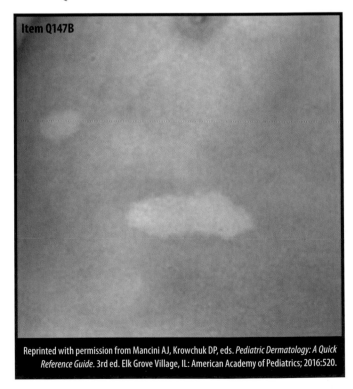

Reprinted with permission from Mancini AJ, Krowchuk DP, eds. *Pediatric Dermatology: A Quick Reference Guide.* 3rd ed. Elk Grove Village, IL: American Academy of Pediatrics; 2016:520.

C. Item Q147C

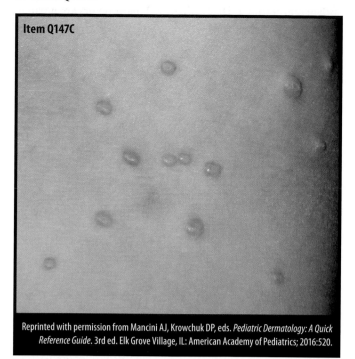

Item Q147C

Reprinted with permission from Mancini AJ, Krowchuk DP, eds. *Pediatric Dermatology: A Quick Reference Guide*. 3rd ed. Elk Grove Village, IL: American Academy of Pediatrics; 2016:520.

D. Item Q147D

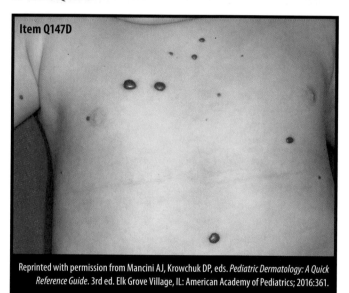

Item Q147D

Reprinted with permission from Mancini AJ, Krowchuk DP, eds. *Pediatric Dermatology: A Quick Reference Guide*. 3rd ed. Elk Grove Village, IL: American Academy of Pediatrics; 2016:361.

Item 148

A 15-year-old adolescent girl is brought to an urgent care center with right ear pain. A few days ago she was cleaning her right ear with a cotton-tipped applicator when she scraped the inside of her ear, which caused immediate pain and bloody drainage. Since then, her symptoms have worsened. Her temperature is 36.9°C. There is seropurulent fluid in the right external auditory canal with marked edema of the mucosa. The right tympanic membrane is perforated.

Of the following, the MOST appropriate topical treatment for this condition is

A. gentamicin

B. gentamicin with hydrocortisone

C. polymyxin B and bacitracin

D. polymyxin B and bacitracin with hydrocortisone

Item 149

An 18-month-old boy is seen for a health supervision visit. He has been well without significant illnesses since his last evaluation. He has had normal growth and development. His parents report that he still drinks from a bottle and estimate that he consumes 36 oz of cow milk per day.

He appears well but is pale. He is at the 35th percentile for height and the 30th percentile for weight (both decreased from the 40th percentile 6 months ago). He has a heart rate of 96 beats/min, blood pressure of 92/70 mmHg, respiratory rate of 22 breaths/min, and oxygen saturation of 99% on room air.

Laboratory data are shown:

Laboratory test	Result
White blood cell count	10,100/μL (10.1 × 10⁹/L)
Hemoglobin	7.9 g/dL (79 g/L)
Mean corpuscular volume	65 fL
Platelet count	510 × 10³/μL (510 × 10⁹/L)
Reticulocytes	0.9%

If left untreated, this patient is at an INCREASED risk for developing

A. acute lymphoblastic leukemia

B. milk protein allergy

C. neurocognitive changes

D. severe aplastic anemia

Item 150

A 17-year-old girl is brought to the emergency department (ED) by paramedics after her parents found her "passed out" in her room. The girl's parents state that she has been very upset over the past week, since her boyfriend of several months broke off their relationship. She has been crying frequently and having difficulty sleeping. One hour ago, the girl's mother found her lying on her bedroom floor and could not get her to wake up. The mother detected the scent of alcohol on her daughter and found an empty bottle of vodka in her closet.

On physical examination, the girl is lethargic and does not respond to verbal stimuli. She withdraws to pain and begins to cry as ED staff members place a peripheral intravenous catheter and begin to infuse normal saline. Her gag reflex is intact. Her temperature is 36°C, heart rate is 50 beats/min, respiratory rate is 12 breaths/min (with shallow respirations), and blood pressure is 92/60 mm Hg. The smell of alcohol is detected on the girl's breath and clothing. There are no signs of trauma. Her pupils are small (2 mm) and sluggishly reactive. Her skin is pale and clammy. The result of a bedside glucose test is normal, and a urine pregnancy test is negative. Her serum ethanol level is 50 mg/dL. Results of urine toxicology screening are pending. Electrocardiography reveals sinus bradycardia with no abnormalities.

Of the following, the BEST next management step for this girl is the administration of

A. activated charcoal, orally

B. dextrose, intravenously

C. fomepizole, intravenously

D. naloxone, intravenously

A 15-month-old girl presents to the emergency department (ED) for evaluation of fever for 2 days and decreased oral intake for 1 day. No other symptoms are reported. In the ED, her temperature is 39°C, heart rate is 120 beats/min, respiratory rate is 24 breaths/min, and blood pressure is 100/60 mm Hg. Her weight is 10 kg. The girl's physical examination findings are remarkable only for inflammation of the oropharynx. There are no signs of dehydration. After 3 hours of oral challenge, the girl has vomited twice and is refusing any oral fluids. Her initial laboratory values are as follows.

Laboratory test	Result
Sodium	139 mEq/L (139 mmol/L)
Potassium	4 mmol/L (4 mEq/L)
Chloride	105 mEq/L (105 mmol/L)
Blood urea nitrogen	14 mg/dL (5 mmol/L)
Serum creatinine	0.3 mg/dL (26.5 µmol/L)
Serum glucose	90 mg/dL (5 mmol/L)

The patient is admitted for intravenous antibiotics and fluids. Her daily sodium (Na) and potassium (K) requirements are estimated based on the Holliday Segar method.

Of the following, the MOST accurate estimate of this girl's daily requirement is

A. 10 mEq Na, 5 mEq K

B. 30 mEq Na, 20 mEq K

C. 30 mEq Na, 30 mEq K

D. 45 mEq Na, 30 mEq K

A 16-year-old adolescent girl is brought to the emergency department 45 minutes after passing out during her soccer game. She was running down the field with another player, going for the ball. She did not collide with another player or trip. She does not recall any pain or dizziness. She is otherwise healthy and very athletic. Her vital signs and physical examination findings are unremarkable.

Of the following, the test MOST likely to reveal the diagnosis is

A. electrocardiography

B. electroencephalography

C. orthostatic blood pressure measurements

D. plasma glucose level

A 17-year-old sexually active adolescent girl has had vaginal discharge for 2 weeks. She notices an odor when she urinates, and she worries that other people can smell it. She describes the discharge as thin and white with occasional itching. One week ago, she used an over-the-counter intravaginal miconazole preparation for 3 days with no symptom relief. She also tried a vaginal douche, which did not help. She reports no previous episodes of vaginal discharge, no dysuria, and no pain with sex. She has never been tested for sexually transmitted infections. She reports using condoms diligently for birth control.

Pelvic examination findings are significant only for a thin, grey, malodorous vaginal discharge. Wet mount microscopy of the discharge is performed (Item Q153).

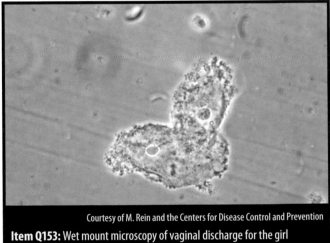

Courtesy of M. Rein and the Centers for Disease Control and Prevention

Item Q153: Wet mount microscopy of vaginal discharge for the girl described in the vignette.

Of the following, the MOST likely diagnosis is

A. bacterial vaginosis

B. *Candida albicans*

C. *Chlamydia trachomatis*

D. *Neisseria gonorrhoeae*

Item 154

A 15-year-old girl presents to an urgent care center with a 2-day history of vaginal itching, burning on urination, and a thick, white discharge. She is not sexually active. Her medical history is significant for rheumatic heart disease and subsequent mitral valve replacement with a prosthetic valve at age 12 years. She has no known drug allergies. Current medications include aspirin and warfarin. Physical examination is remarkable for a loud, mechanical S1 heart sound; vulvar and vaginal mucosal erythema; and a curd-like vaginal discharge. She was prescribed oral fluconazole for 3 days.

Of the following, the MOST likely adverse effect to be seen in this girl is

A. acute renal failure

B. bleeding

C. fulminant hepatic failure

D. thromboembolic stroke

Item 155

A 12-year-old boy is seen for a preparticipation sports physical evaluation. He has no concerns and is excited to play football in the upcoming fall season. His medical history is significant only for generalized joint hypermobility. He takes no medications and has no known allergies. His mother also has joint hypermobility; the family history is otherwise not significant.

Of the following, compared with his teammates, this boy is at INCREASED risk for

A. bone fracture

B. concussion

C. hyperthermia

D. joint dislocation

Item 156

A 2-hour-old neonate who was born at term by normal vaginal delivery to an 18-year-old gravida 2, para 1 woman with no pregnancy or delivery complications is being evaluated. At the time of delivery, the obstetrician noted an ulcerative lesion on her vaginal wall and sent a swab of the lesion for herpes simplex virus polymerase chain reaction testing. She has no known history of genital herpes. There is no history of premature or prolonged rupture of membranes, group B *Streptococcus* colonization, or positive screening for hepatitis B surface antigen, human immunodeficiency virus, or rapid plasma reagin. The neonate is well-appearing with normal physical examination findings. His complete blood cell count and alanine aminotransferase level are normal.

Of the following, the MOST appropriate next step in management for this neonate is (to)

A. at 6 hours of age, perform a diagnostic evaluation and start empiric intravenous acyclovir

B. at 24 hours of age, perform a diagnostic evaluation and start empiric intravenous acyclovir

C. immediately perform a diagnostic evaluation and start empiric intravenous acyclovir

D. observe closely with no empiric acyclovir therapy

Item 157

A resident research project is evaluating C-reactive protein (CRP) levels of 1 mg/dL or higher as a predictor of bacteremia in symptomatic term neonates transferred from the newborn nursery to the neonatal intensive care unit.

	Bacteremia	No bacteremia
CRP ≥1 mg/dL (95 nmol/L)	3	15
CRP <1 mg/dL (95 nmol/L)	3	79

Of the following, in this patient population, the calculated negative predictive value of a CRP less than 1 mg/dL is

A. 16%

B. 50%

C. 84%

D. 96%

Item 158

A 14-year-old adolescent boy is seen for a new concern about difficulty with exercise. His history is notable for seasonal allergic rhinitis with the recent development of perennial nasal symptoms. There is a strong family history of asthma, as well as a health and fitness orientation for the entire family. He has problems with cough and difficulty catching his breath after running more than a mile. He has been practicing for track competition season and running up to 5 miles at a time. His breathing problems start after 1 to 2 miles and persist for the rest of his run. He often has to stop running and walk for a while. One of his teammates has allowed him to use an albuterol inhaler before running, which has greatly improved his ability to run without discomfort. Results of pulmonary function testing are shown (Item Q158).

Item Q158. Spirometry results for the adolescent described in the vignette.

Result	Predicted	Best	% Predicted
FVC (L)	3.09	3.37	109%
FEV1 (L)	2.79	2.74	98%
FEV1/FVC	0.90	0.81	90%
FEF25-75% (L/s)	3.43	2.67	78%
PEFR (L/s)	---	4.83	---
Vext %	---	1.56	---

FVC, Forced Vital Capacity (liters); FEV 1, Forced Expiratory Volume in 1 second (liters); FEF 25/75, Forced Expiratory Flow between 25% and 75% of FVC (liters/sec);

PEFR, Peak Expiratory Flow Rate (liters/second); % pred, actual value as a percent of the predicted value for age and height

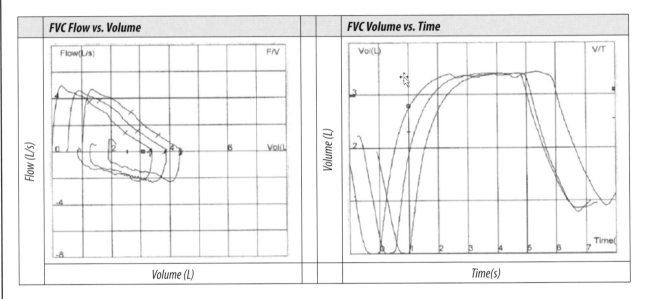

Courtesy of M. Guill

Of the following, the BEST approach to the management of this patient's problem is

A. daily inhaled corticosteroid

B. daily inhaled long-acting β-agonist

C. no medication

D. pre-exercise inhaled bronchodilator

Item 159

A 3-year-old boy is being evaluated for a 5-day history of a painful "diaper rash." His mother reports that he has pain with stooling or wiping. He is well in other respects and his medical history is unremarkable. The boy is afebrile and the only finding of note is the skin surrounding the anus (Item Q159).

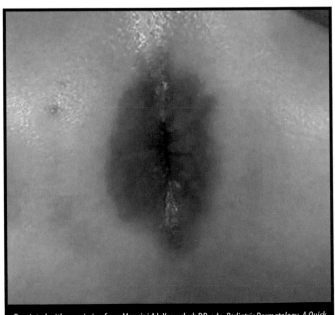

Reprinted with permission from Mancini AJ, Krowchuk DP, eds. *Pediatric Dermatology. A Quick Reference Guide.* 3rd ed. Elk Grove Village, IL: American Academy of Pediatrics; 2016. page 187

Item Q159: Findings as described for the boy in this vignette.

Of the following, the MOST appropriate treatment is

A. cephalexin orally

B. clotrimazole topically

C. hydrocortisone topically

D. nystatin orally

Item 160

A 3-year-old girl is brought to the emergency department after her parents had difficulty waking her this morning. She has been ill with an upper respiratory tract infection for the past 2 days, so has not been eating very well. She did not eat any of her dinner yesterday. Her past medical history is significant for short stature and slow weight gain. She is not on any medication. She is sleepy and difficult to arouse. The physical examination findings are otherwise unremarkable. A finger-stick glucose level is 36 mg/dL (2.0 mmol/L). Blood is drawn at the time of hypoglycemia. She is treated with 1 g/kg of intravenous dextrose, after which she becomes alert and talkative.

Laboratory results are shown:

Laboratory test	Result
Blood	
Glucose	32 mg/dL (1.8 mmol/L)
β-Hydroxybutyric acid	10 mg/dL (1720 μmol/L) (Reference range, fasting < 4.2 mg/dL [403 μmol/L])
Fatty acids (nonesterified)	80 mg/dL (2.8 mmol/L) (Reference range, 17-42 mg/dL [0.60-1.49 mmol/L])
Cortisol	28 μg/dL (772 nmol/L) (Reference range, AM 6.2-19.4 μg/dL [171-535 nmol/L])
Growth hormone	14 ng/mL (14 μg/L) (Reference range, > 10 ng/mL [10 μg/L] with stimulation)
Lactate	10.8 mg/dL (1.2 mmol/L) (Reference range, 4.5-20 mg/dL [0.5-2.2 mmol/L])
Blood alcohol content	0%
Urine	
Urinalysis	Large amount of ketones
Organic acids	Normal

Of the following, the MOST likely diagnosis is

A. fatty acid oxidation disorder

B. glycogen storage disease

C. hyperinsulinism

D. ketotic hypoglycemia

Item 161

A 10-year-old boy is at his health supervision visit. He has mild learning disabilities and speech delay. He is taller than most boys his age, while his parents are of average height. A karyotype reveals 47,XYY syndrome. You discuss the common features of this chromosomal abnormality with the parents.

Of the following, your discussion should include the STATEMENT that

A. macroorchidism develops during puberty

B. moderate to severe intellectual deficits are common

C. normal intelligence is expected

D. precocious puberty is typical

Item 162

A 4-year-old boy is seen for evaluation of food allergy. The boy was at a picnic 2 days ago and consumed a variety of food, including fried chicken, shrimp salad, deviled eggs, a gelatin salad containing multiple fruits, ice cream, and peanut butter cookies. Immediately after eating, he developed a macular nonpruritic rash on the right side of his mouth and chin that lasted about 30 minutes. Around the time the rash resolved, he became nauseated and vomited once. His mother reports no lip swelling, difficulty breathing, or urticaria. The boy takes cetirizine for seasonal allergies. His mother states that his paternal uncle has a history of food allergies, although she is not certain of the specific foods. His mother asks about food allergy testing.

Of the following, the MOST appropriate diagnostic approach for this child is to

A. defer allergy testing and reconsider if the boy has more severe reactions with continued exposure

B. order serum IgE testing to several common food allergens, with more specific testing if positive

C. refer to an allergist for skin-prick testing using only egg, shellfish, peanut, and milk

D. refer to an allergist for skin-prick testing using a panel of 20 common allergens

Item 163

A 2-week-old full-term male neonate has been hospitalized for 2 days after being brought to the emergency department for evaluation of fever. He was well until 1 day prior to admission when he developed fussiness and was noted to have a temperature of 38.5°C at home. In the emergency department, blood and urine specimens were obtained; however, his parents refused permission to perform a lumbar puncture. He has been receiving ampicillin 50 mg/kg/dose intravenously every 6 hours and gentamicin 4 mg/kg intravenously daily. He has had ongoing fever during the hospitalization, and his parents state that he continues to be fussy. He has a temperature of 38°C, heart rate of 153 beats/min, respiratory rate of 42 breaths/min, and blood pressure of 88/61 mm Hg. He is irritable, and there are scattered red macules with overlying pustules over the thorax. The remainder of the physical examination findings are normal.

Laboratory data are shown:

Laboratory test	Result
Blood culture	Pending
Urine culture	Escherichia coli

Escherichia coli susceptibilities are shown:

Laboratory test	Result
Ampicillin	≥ 32, resistant
Ceftriaxone	≥ 64, resistant
Ciprofloxacin	≤ 0.25, susceptible
Gentamicin	≤ 1, susceptible
Meropenem	≤ 0.25, susceptible
Nitrofurantoin	≤ 32, susceptible
Trimethoprim-sulfamethoxazole	≤ 20, susceptible

Of the following, the MOST appropriate antibiotic to use as monotherapy for this patient's infection is

A. gentamicin

B. meropenem

C. nitrofurantoin

D. trimethoprim-sulfamethoxazole

Item 164

A 4-year-old boy is being evaluated for leg pain and difficulty walking. His parents report that he woke up that morning and did not want to walk, refusing to take more than a few steps. He complains of pain in the back of both lower legs. His mother reports that the boy had a fever and "terrible cold," about 1 week ago, when he used an albuterol inhaler frequently. He has not had any rashes or joint swelling. There is no history of recent camping or travel. His family history is significant for a maternal grandmother with knee and hip arthritis. On physical examination, the boy has a temperature of 36.8°C. He has tenderness to palpation over the calf muscles bilaterally, and resists passive movement of the ankles. He will only take a few steps, and seems to shuffle his feet when he walks. His complete blood cell count and erythrocyte sedimentation rate are normal.

Of the following, the MOST likely cause of the boy's abnormal gait is

A. *Borrelia burgdorferi* infection

B. hypokalemia

C. influenza virus infection

D. juvenile idiopathic arthritis

Item 165

A 16-year-old girl is receiving a follow-up evaluation 4 weeks after she presented with dysuria and was diagnosed with chlamydia. She states that she took the single dose of azithromycin, 1 g orally, as prescribed. She denies dysuria, vaginal discharge, or recent sexual activity. Today the girl complains of heel pain and swelling for 1 week. On physical examination she is afebrile and well-appearing, with decreased range of motion of the left ankle with point tenderness to palpation and mild swelling at the insertion of the Achilles tendon on the calcaneus. The remainder of the physical examination findings are unremarkable. Laboratory tests show the following: white blood cells, 11,500/µL (11.5×10⁹/L) with normal differential; erythrocyte sedimentation rate, 25 mm/h; C-reactive protein, 2.0 mg/L (19 nmol/L); and negative urinalysis. The urine gonorrhea/chlamydia results are pending.

Of the following, the BEST initial management step for this girl is

A. doxycycline

B. ibuprofen

C. prednisone

D. physical therapy

Item 166

A 13-year-old adolescent girl is brought to an outpatient clinic with bilateral knee pain. Her symptoms began with right knee pain 6 months ago, followed by left knee pain 3 months ago. She experiences bilateral knee pain daily with morning stiffness. She recently developed right ankle pain and swelling. There is no history of injury or trauma. She reports that she has had intermittent fevers, fatigue, occasional oral ulcers, and a poor appetite. She has had an unintentional weight loss of 7 kg over the last 6 months. She reports intermittent abdominal pain, diarrhea, and nausea. She has a temperature of 36.1°C, heart rate of 99 beats/min, height of 160 cm (45th percentile), weight of 74.2 kg (95th percentile), and body mass index of 29.5 kg/m² (97th percentile). She is not distressed. Her abdomen is obese, soft, nontender, and without palpable masses. Rectal examination reveals an anal fissure, erythematous skin tags, and a small amount of exudate. She has swelling of the left knee and right ankle without significant erythema.

Laboratory data are shown:

Laboratory test	Result
White blood cell count	11,200/µL (11.2 × 10⁹/L)
Neutrophils	69%
Lymphocytes	25%
Monocytes	6%
Hemoglobin	7.1 g/dL (71 g/L)
Mean corpuscular volume	60 fL
Platelet count	658 × 10³/µL (658 × 10⁹/L)
Lactate dehydrogenase	340 U/L
Uric acid	4.7 mg/dL (280 µmol/L)
C-reactive protein	4.7 mg/dL (448 nmol/L)
Erythrocyte sedimentation rate	100 mm/h

Of the following, the test that is MOST likely to establish her diagnosis is

A. antinuclear antibody

B. bone marrow biopsy

C. colonoscopy

D. radiography of the right ankle and left knee

Item 167

An 8-year-old boy is evaluated because of his mother's concerns of challenging behaviors. She reports that he is unpleasant and refuses to do anything that is asked of him. He loses his temper easily and is argumentative. He deliberately annoys his siblings and blames them when he gets in trouble. He is disrespectful to his teacher and the staff at school.

Of the following, the BEST next step is to recommend a treatment program that teaches the parent to

A. apply consequences for challenging behaviors

B. delay response to unwanted behaviors

C. increase positive reinforcement of disruptive behaviors

D. vary response to undesired behaviors

Item 168

At a health supervision visit for a 2-month-old boy, the parents report that they have seen arm and leg twitching when he is asleep. This is usually a jerking of 1 arm, but it can move from 1 arm to the other and back again. It sometimes affects his legs. The jerking can last from 30 seconds up to 3 or 4 minutes. They have never seen it when he is awake and they have never seen jerking in his face. After it ends, he stays asleep. The parents are concerned, because the infant's father has a history of febrile seizures. The boy's physical examination findings are within normal parameters.

Of the following, the infant's MOST likely diagnosis is

A. benign infantile myoclonic epilepsy

B. benign sleep myoclonus of infancy

C. motor stereotypy

D. motor tics

Item 169

The parents of a 6-month-old infant being seen for a health supervision visit relate that his eyes have crossed since birth but lately it seems more frequent. His right eye crosses more than his left, but he shows no difficulty reaching for objects or recognizing his parents from across the room. The red reflex is symmetric bilaterally. On corneal reflex testing, the reflected image is revealed (Item Q169). Cover testing reveals no ocular deviation.

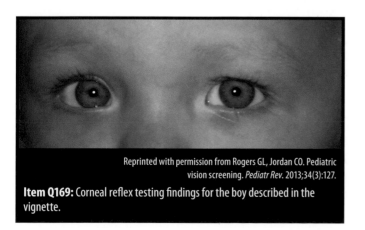

Reprinted with permission from Rogers GL, Jordan CO. Pediatric vision screening. *Pediatr Rev.* 2013;34(3):127.

Item Q169: Corneal reflex testing findings for the boy described in the vignette.

Of the following, the MOST appropriate diagnosis for this infant is right-sided

A. amblyopia

B. esotropia

C. exotropia

D. pseudostrabismus

Item 170

A 1-year-old boy was born with macrosomia, marked macroglossia, hypoglycemia, and an omphalocele.

Of the following, the MOST appropriate laboratory test(s) to include in a health screening plan for this patient is (are)

A. immunoglobulin levels

B. prothrombin time and partial thromboplastin time

C. serum α-fetoprotein

D. urine ketones

Item 171

A medical student has just assessed a healthy 2-year-old girl who placed a tiny plastic doll shoe in her left naris approximately 4 hours ago. Multiple attempts by the mother to dislodge the shoe by having the girl blow her nose have been unsuccessful. The student reports that the girl appears well and is in no distress. Her vital signs are normal for her age. The student visualized part of a plastic object lodged in the girl's left naris. There is some clear rhinorrhea from both nares, but no epistaxis.

Of the following, the MOST appropriate technique for the management of this patient is

A. application of topical neosynephrine to the left naris

B. insertion of a nasogastric tube into the left naris

C. irrigation of the left naris with sterile nasal saline spray

D. urgent referral to a pediatric otolaryngologist

Item 172

A 14-year-old boy presents for a health supervision visit. The boy is doing well at school, and his parents have no concerns. His vital signs include a temperature of 37.7°C, heart rate of 65 beats/min, respiratory rate of 14 breaths/min, and blood pressure of 120/74 mm Hg. His growth parameters and physical examination findings are normal. The boy's mother, age 38 years, was recently diagnosed with autosomal dominant polycystic kidney disease (ADPKD). His 55-year-old maternal grandfather has end-stage renal disease secondary to ADPKD, and is currently receiving dialysis.

Of the following, the extrarenal manifestation MOST likely to be seen with this disease is

A. biliary dysgenesis

B. cerebral aneurysm

C. lenticonus

D. portal fibrosis

Item 173

The mother of a 6-month-old female infant is concerned that the infant has caught an upper respiratory tract infection from her older siblings. She describes that the infant is not eating well and is breathing fast. The infant is tachypneic with intermittent grunting and an absence of nasal congestion. She is afebrile with a heart rate of 180 beats/min, blood pressure of 80/60 mm Hg, respiratory rate of 60 beats/min, and an oxygen saturation as measured by pulse oximetry of 94%. Her lungs have diffuse crackles. A gallop is noted on auscultation of the heart. Her liver is palpated 4 cm below the costal margin. She is sent to the emergency department for monitoring.

Of the following, the BEST next step in the management of this infant is to

A. administer hypertonic saline per nebulizer

B. administer normal saline (20 mL/kg)

C. perform abdominal ultrasonography

D. perform echocardiography

Item 174

A 15-year-old adolescent girl has pain with urination. For the past 3 days, she has a burning sensation every time she urinates. She has also noticed the need to urinate more frequently. She has been limiting the amount of fluid she drinks to try and reduce the number of times she needs to use the bathroom. She reports mild suprapubic pain but no back pain. She has no nausea, vomiting, diarrhea, or fever. She has a history of a urinary tract infection at 4 years of age. She reports that she has recently become sexually active, and has only had vaginal sex once.

Of the following, the MOST likely test(s) to establish the diagnosis is (are)

A. a complete blood cell count and blood culture

B. a nucleic acid amplification test for gonorrhea and chlamydia

C. potassium-hydroxide wet mount microscopy

D. a urine test strip analysis and culture

Item 175

A previously healthy 9-month-old girl is brought to the emergency department (ED) with fever, decreased oral intake, and difficulty breathing. The symptoms started 2 days ago with excessive fatigue and fussiness. Yesterday, she developed a fever of 38.3°C. Her mother took her to the pediatrician, who diagnosed her with bilateral acute suppurative otitis media and prescribed oral antibiotics along with acetaminophen and ibuprofen. Despite treatment, the fevers and fussiness persisted. She refused solid foods, took minimal fluids, and only made 1 wet diaper since being seen. The girl developed a diffuse, red macular rash. Last night, she was restless and inconsolable. On the day of admission, she became less active, her breathing became fast and labored, and she was grunting. On physical examination in the ED, she is lethargic and toxic-appearing. Her conjunctivae are injected. She has dry erythematous mucous membranes. The

girl is in moderate respiratory distress, breathing rapidly and shallowly with grunting. Crackles are heard throughout the chest. Her liver is palpable 4 cm below the costal margin. Her abdomen is soft, nontender, and moderately distended. Capillary refill time is 4 seconds.

Of the following, the MOST likely compensatory mechanism to improve cardiac output for this infant is

A. decreased afterload

B. decreased cardiac myocyte stretch

C. increased actin-myosin fiber interaction

D. increased heart rate

Item 176

A 14-year-old adolescent girl is brought to the emergency department for evaluation of severe sore throat. She has had a fever and throat pain for 1 day and reports difficulty opening her mouth because of pain. Her parents report that her voice sounds muffled. She appears ill. She has a temperature of 39.5°C, heart rate of 100 beats/min, and respiratory rate of 18 breaths/min. Her left tonsil is erythematous and enlarged, pushing her uvula to the right. She has tender anterior cervical lymphadenopathy. The remainder of her physical examination findings are normal.

Of the following, the MOST appropriate next step in management is

A. intravenous ampicillin-sulbactam

B. lateral neck radiography

C. magnetic resonance imaging of the neck

D. needle aspiration of left tonsil

Item 177

A 16-year-old black adolescent presents with a 5-week history of cough, headache, and fatigue. He was well until 5 weeks ago, when he developed fever, malaise, nonproductive cough, and headache. He received a 5-day course of azithromycin for presumed pneumonia. His fever resolved over several days, but the other symptoms persisted, along with weight loss, fatigue, and night sweats. During the past 2 weeks, his cough worsened, and he developed lower back pain. There are no sick contacts and no pets at home. The boy lives in California's San Joaquin Valley and has not travelled internationally. There is no known tuberculosis exposure. His immunizations are up to date. On physical examination, the boy is afebrile with a heart rate of 78 beats/min, respiratory rate of 16 breaths/min, and oxygen saturation of 92% on room air. He has diminished breath sounds in his left lower lung field and point tenderness over the lower thoracic spine. Chest radiography shows right lower lobe consolidation with marked paratracheal and hilar adenopathy. A radiograph of the spine shows a lytic bone lesion at T10.

Of the following, the best next test in this boy's evaluation is

A. biopsy of the bone lesion

B. computed tomography of the chest

C. serology

D. urine antigen assay

Item 178

A 15-hour-old neonate born at 39 weeks of gestation is being evaluated in the nursery. He was delivered vaginally with vacuum assistance. His mother has gestational diabetes that was controlled with metformin. His birth parameters were as follows: weight, 4.3 kg; length, 53 cm; and head circumference, 36 cm. On physical examination, the neonate's head circumference is 38 cm, heart rate is 170 beats/min, respiratory rate is 65 breaths/min, and blood pressure is 55/30 mm Hg. You note that he is pale, with normal work of breathing, mild forward displacement of the ears, and capillary refill of 3 to 4 seconds.

Of the following, the MOST likely explanation for this neonate's presentation is

A. hypoglycemia

B. pneumothorax

C. subgaleal hemorrhage

D. transient tachypnea of the newborn

Item 179

A 1-month-old female infant is brought to the emergency department by ambulance because her mother found her to be dusky and not breathing when asleep. She responded to stimulation by waking up and breathing but is now tachypneic and wheezing. There was no abnormal movement associated with the event, and her tone remained normal throughout the event. She was born at 36 weeks' gestation, had no problems in the newborn nursery, and went home with her mother. She has an oxygen saturation of 83% on room air, temperature of 37°C, respiratory rate of 60 breaths/min, and heart rate of 140 beats/min. The physical examination findings are notable only for tachypnea and diffuse expiratory wheezes with mild intercostal retraction. She is admitted to the hospital and placed on supplemental oxygen.

Of the following, the MOST appropriate next intervention for this infant is

A. barium swallow radiograph

B. intravenous ceftriaxone

C. nebulized albuterol solution

D. telemetric cardiorespiratory monitoring

Item 180

A 4-year-old boy is seen for a health supervision visit as a new patient. He was recently placed in foster care, and his prior medical records are not yet available. The child appears well and has normal vital signs and growth parameters. The physical examination findings are remarkable only for unique facial features (Item Q180A) and abnormal dentition (Item Q180B).

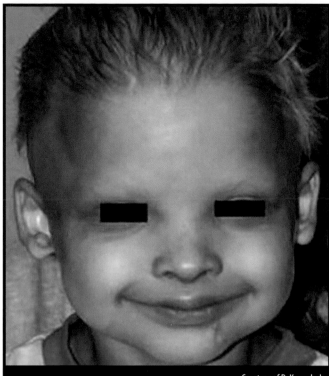

Courtesy of D. Krowchuk

Item Q180A: Facial features of the boy described in this vignette.

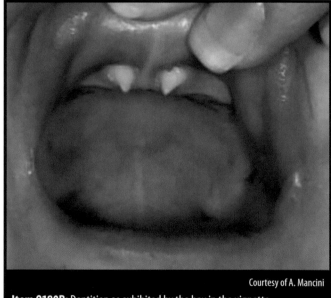

Courtesy of A. Mancini

Item Q180B: Dentition as exhibited by the boy in the vignette.

Of the following, the MOST likely diagnosis is

A. epidermolysis bullosa, recessive dystrophic type

B. hypohidrotic ectodermal dysplasia

C. incontinentia pigmenti

D. tuberous sclerosis complex

A pediatric residency program director has volunteered to score abstracts for his institution's annual research competition. The organizers sought volunteers among graduate medical education program directors because the majority of abstracts are submitted by graduate medical education trainees. One of the program director's assigned abstracts was submitted by one of his trainees. Although the program director is not listed as an author on the abstract, he assisted the trainee in finding a research mentor and provided advice on study design and data analysis.

Of the following, the BEST next step for this program director is to

A. ask a colleague to score the abstract for him

B. decline participation as an abstract scorer and ask the organizers to replace him

C. discuss the situation with the organizers and abstain from scoring this abstract

D. score the abstract using the rubric provided to ensure optimal objectivity

A 12-year-old girl is being evaluated for recurrent abdominal pain and pancreatitis. She has hepatosplenomegaly and crops of small yellow papules along her arms, legs, and buttocks (Item Q182). Laboratory evaluation reveals a triglyceride level of more than 2,000 mg/dL (22.6 mmol/L). The girl does not take any medications or supplements.

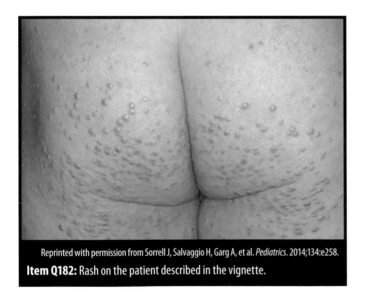

Reprinted with permission from Sorrell J, Salvaggio H, Garg A, et al. *Pediatrics*. 2014;134:e258.

Item Q182: Rash on the patient described in the vignette.

Of the following, the RECOMMENDED treatment for this disorder is

A. fish oil supplementation

B. glucocorticoids

C. restriction of dietary fat

D. restriction of dietary protein

A 3-month-old male infant is seen for evaluation of rhinorrhea and concern for an ear infection. His mother states that he has had no fever and no difficulty breathing, but he has been fussier than usual. His vital signs are normal for age. He is awake, smiling, and cooing. There is clear rhinorrhea and the tympanic membranes are grey and mobile. A 1-cm diameter circular bruise is seen on his left anterior chest wall. When asked about the bruise, his mother is unsure of the cause. She states that he tried to roll off of the changing table a few days ago, and she caught him at the edge of the table. She also states that his 2-year-old sibling "is sometimes rough with him." Four days ago, the infant's maternal uncle and grandmother started caring for him and his sibling during the evenings because his mother started a new job. She has no concerns for abuse and reports no family history of bleeding disorders.

Of the following, the next MOST appropriate step to investigate the etiology of this infant's skin finding is to

A. obtain a chest radiograph and, if an occult fracture is seen, refer the infant to the child protection clinic at a tertiary children's hospital

B. obtain a chest radiograph, complete blood cell count, and a prothrombin time, and refer the family to the state child welfare agency

C. obtain a complete skeletal survey and consult with a child protection specialist at the tertiary children's hospital by phone

D. place a photographic image in the infant's medical record and refer the infant to a dermatologist to estimate the age of the bruise

A 2,500-g male neonate was born at 35 weeks of gestation to a 32-year-old woman. She is from El Salvador and immigrated to the United States 6 weeks ago. During the first trimester, she developed a febrile illness that was characterized by rash and red eyes. She did not seek medical evaluation for this illness. The neonate is normocephalic with a head circumference of 33.5 cm (50th percentile). The remainder of the physical examination findings are normal. The mother expresses concern that her illness during the first trimester could have been caused by Zika virus.

Of the following, the BEST next step in the evaluation of this neonate is

A. head ultrasonography

B. ophthalmologic examination

C. standard pediatric care

D. Zika virus testing

Item 185

A 6-year-old boy is seen for evaluation of abdominal pain. He recently immigrated from El Salvador where he lived in a rural setting. This medical evaluation is his first in the United States. He has had intermittent abdominal pain for the last 8 months, which has been managed with over-the-counter medications. He has had occasional episodes of emesis. Yesterday, a worm was found in the emesis (Item Q185). He has a temperature of 37°C, heart rate of 105 beats/min, respiratory rate of 22 breaths/min, and blood pressure of 97/62 mm Hg. The physical examination findings are normal.

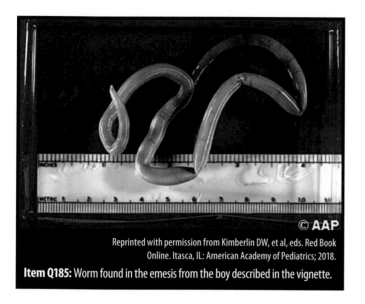

Reprinted with permission from Kimberlin DW, et al, eds. Red Book Online. Itasca, IL: American Academy of Pediatrics; 2018.

Item Q185: Worm found in the emesis from the boy described in the vignette.

Of the following, this infection was MOST likely to have been acquired via

A. contact with a contaminated fomite

B. ingestion of soil-contaminated food

C. ingestion of undercooked meat

D. larval dermal penetration

Item 186

A 16-year-old girl is being evaluated for right anterior thigh pain. She reports that 2 days ago she was hit in the front of the thigh by a hockey puck. She has been experiencing fairly severe pain in her thigh and still cannot fully bend her knee. On physical examination, the girl's right thigh girth is 2 cm more than the left. She has tenderness to palpation over the middle of the anterolateral thigh. Her knee flexion is 90 degrees on the right and 140 degrees on the left. Hip motion is full and symmetric.

Of the following, the MOST likely diagnosis for the girl in the vignette is

A. myositis ossificans

B. quadriceps contusion

C. quadriceps tendon rupture

D. stress fracture of the femur

Item 187

A 6-year-old girl is seen in April for evaluation of a persistent runny nose and cough. These symptoms have been present for several weeks, throughout the day and night. She reports frequent sneezing, itchy ears and throat, and cough. Her father hears her "sniff" frequently. The girl appears well and has no fever. Her vital signs are normal for age. Her nasal turbinates are pale and edematous, and she has cobblestoning of her posterior pharynx. Her lungs are clear and equal on auscultation bilaterally, with good air movement.

Of the following, the MOST appropriate treatment for her condition is

A. fluticasone nasal spray

B. oral diphenhydramine

C. oral prednisolone

D. phenylephrine nasal spray

Item 188

A 15-month-old boy is evaluated for ongoing concerns of poor weight gain. He has cystic fibrosis, which was diagnosed at birth, and exocrine pancreatic insufficiency. Although enzyme supplementation has been administered as directed and oral supplementation has been encouraged, he has been unable to gain weight. For several months, his weight-for-length percentile has decreased, and it is now at the eighth percentile. There is no history of regurgitation, vomiting, abdominal surgery, liver disease, or ascites. His pulmonary status is well controlled, and he has not required inpatient admission for pulmonary exacerbations. His cystic fibrosis team anticipates that additional long-term supplemental nutrition is needed. He has a weight of 8.8 kg (9th percentile) and length of 76.2 cm (15th percentile). He appears thin but in no distress. His examination findings are otherwise normal.

Of the following, the BEST option for improving this child's nutritional status is placement of a

A. central venous catheter

B. gastrostomy tube

C. jejunostomy tube

D. nasogastric tube

Item 189

A 2-year-old child is evaluated for concerns about his speech. He does not speak any understandable words and does not turn to his mother's voice when she calls his name. However, he smiles in response to social overtures, points to indicate interest in things, and plays appropriately with toys. He has no significant medical history. His physical examination findings are within normal limits. An audiology evaluation identifies hearing loss as the cause of his language delay. The boy's mother asks which communication approach will maximize the use of his residual hearing for the development of speech.

Of the following, the BEST response to the parent's question is

A. American sign language

B. the manual English method

C. the oral communication method

D. total language communication

Item 190

A 15-year-old boy is being evaluated for headaches. He feels the pain mostly in his forehead, and it is associated with nausea, vomiting, phonophobia, and photophobia. His vision becomes blurry, and sometimes everything turns gray for a few seconds. He reports ringing in his ears and dizziness during the headaches, but there are no dysesthesias. The headaches started 2 months ago and have increased in frequency and severity; they occur daily now. His current medications are doxycycline for acne, fluoxetine for anxiety, and an over-the-counter creatine supplement to build muscles. His mother and older brother get migraines, but the boy has never had severe headaches before. His vital signs show a blood pressure of 108/68 mm Hg, heart rate of 76 beats/min, and oxygen saturation by pulse oximetry of 99% on room air. His physical examination findings are within normal parameters, though his optic discs cannot be visualized because of his photophobia.

Of the following, the BEST next step in the evaluation and management of this boy is to

A. obtain brain imaging

B. perform a lumbar puncture

C. start a migraine prophylaxis medication

D. stop the creatine supplements

Item 191

A 12-year-old girl is evaluated for academic concerns. Her teachers describe her as inattentive and unfocused, although she behaves well otherwise. Her grades are below average, but recent statewide testing revealed above average scores in all subjects. At home, her parents worry that she does not listen and is sometimes irritable. She is a social girl who is active in team sports. A review of systems is notable for fitful sleep, snoring, and morning headaches. Her body mass index is at the 89th percentile. She has a hypernasal voice and breathes through her mouth. Her tonsils meet at the midline. The remainder of her physical examination findings are normal.

Of the following, the BEST test to confirm the diagnosis would be

A. attention-deficit/hyperactivity disorder–specific rating scale

B. an audiogram

C. polysomnography

D. psychoeducational testing

Item 192

A newborn is seen for a first health supervision visit. There is a family history of retinoblastoma, and his mother carries one wild-type *RB1* allele and one mutated *RB1* allele.

Of the following, this newborn's risk for developing retinoblastoma is

A. between 25% and 50%

B. between 75% and 100%

C. dependent on the father's genotype

D. no different than the general population

Item 193

A 4-year-old previously healthy girl is transported to the emergency department (ED) by Emergency Medical Services (EMS) after having a seizure. Earlier today the girl and her cousins were playing around the garage at her grandmother's house. About 1 hour ago, she suddenly seemed "drowsy and clumsy" and was noted to be "stumbling around like she was drunk." The girl then had 3 episodes of nonbilious vomiting. Soon after this, she began to "breathe funny" and had a generalized tonic-clonic seizure, leading her grandmother to call 911.

On arrival at the home, paramedics noted the girl to be obtunded and responsive only to painful stimuli. Her vital signs on arrival to the ED include a temperature of 36.4°C, heart rate of 80 beats/min, blood pressure of 78/50 mm Hg, respiratory rate of 40 breaths/min, and oxygen saturation of 90% on room air. The girl is obtunded, and responds inconsistently to painful stimuli. Her pupils are equal, round, and reactive to light. She has no signs of head trauma and no bruising of her skin. She is tachypneic with deep respirations, with clear lungs bilaterally. The tone in her extremities is decreased symmetrically. No other abnormalities are noted on neurologic examination, and the remainder of the girl's physical examination findings are unremarkable.

The girl's airway is secured via endotracheal intubation. Arterial blood gas reveals a pH of 7.05, partial pressure of carbon dioxide of 17 mm Hg, and serum bicarbonate of 7 mEq/L (7 mmol/L). Her other serum laboratory studies are pending. A urinalysis reveals the presence of blood, protein, and calcium oxalate crystals.

Of the following, the MOST likely cause of this girl's symptoms is

A. acute intracranial hemorrhage

B. carbon monoxide toxicity

C. ethylene glycol toxicity

D. hydrocarbon aspiration

Item 194

A 14-year-old-boy presents to the emergency department (ED) for evaluation of headaches. He has been having headaches off and on for the last few months, which are usually relieved by over-the-counter pain medications. He has no complaints of vomiting, blurring of vision, or waking up at night from these headaches. The family history is significant for hypertension in the father (diagnosed at age 25 years) and sister (diagnosed at age 18 years). In the ED, the boy's temperature is 37.6°C, heart rate is 66 beats/min, respiratory rate is 14 breaths/min, and blood pressure is 145/100 mm Hg. His physical examination findings and growth parameters are normal.

The results of the investigations performed due to concern about the boy's elevated blood pressure are as follows.

Laboratory Test	Patient Result
Sodium	139 mEq/L (139 mmol/L)
Potassium	2.9 mEq/L (2.9 mmol/L)
Chloride	100 mEq/L (100 mmol/L)
Bicarbonate	34 mEq/L (34 mmol/L)
Blood urea nitrogen	14 mg/dL (5 mmol/L)
Creatinine	0.7 mg/dL (61.8 μmol/L)
Glucose	98 mg/dL (5.4 mmol/L)
Calcium	9.6 mg/dL (2.4 mmol/L)
Phosphorus	5.2 mg/dL (1.6 mmol/L)
Urinalysis	Normal
Renal ultrasonography	Normal

Of the following, the MOST likely cause of the boy's hypertension is

A. Bartter syndrome
B. Gitelman syndrome
C. Gordon syndrome
D. Liddle syndrome

Item 195

A medical student rotating on the inpatient pediatric ward is learning about medical decision-making, including balancing risks and benefits and cost effective care. The roles of the physician's experiences, parental preferences, and study data in medical decision-making are discussed. The student asks how the risk-benefit ratio for treatment of any individual patient might be determined.

Of the following, the statistical concept that BEST addresses the student's question is

A. number needed to treat
B. paired t test
C. power
D. sample size

Item 196

A 16-year-old adolescent boy has been experiencing a burning sensation with urination for the past 5 days. He reports no hematuria, penile discharge, fever, vomiting, or diarrhea. He had a urinary tract infection at 24 months of age, but has otherwise been healthy. When his mother is not in the room, he discloses that he became sexually active 3 months ago and has had 2 female partners. He has not been using condoms consistently.

Of the following, the tests that are MOST likely to establish the diagnosis are

A. blood culture and complete blood cell count
B. comprehensive metabolic panel tests
C. nucleic acid amplification tests for gonorrhea and chlamydia
D. urinalysis and urine culture

Item 197

A 1-month-old boy is referred to the emergency department from his pediatrician's office because of failure to thrive. He was born at 36 weeks of gestation to a 20-year-old gravida 1, para 0 woman. She had appropriate prenatal care, and no complications were reported during the pregnancy or delivery. Perinatal testing results were unremarkable. The neonate's birthweight was 2.5 kg. He breastfed well in the nursery, passed meconium and urine within the first 24 hours, and was discharged from the hospital on day 2 after birth. His discharge weight was 2.32 kg. By his first health supervision visit, at age 10 days, he had regained his birthweight. Since then, the boy has had progressively increasing problems with feeding. He typically feeds for 10 minutes on each side, with a burping in between, and seems to adequately empty both breasts. For the last several days, he has had increasing vomiting with each burp, as well as after the feedings. The emesis is the color of milk, sometimes digested, and not projectile. It is more than would fill a teaspoon. The last 2 days before presentation, he has not been interested in feeding.

His current weight is 2.41 kg. His temperature is 37°C, heart rate is 120 beats/min, respiratory rate is 24 breaths/min, and blood pressure is 70/40 mm Hg. Physical examination reveals a poorly nourished infant who is sleeping comfortably. He is easily aroused, remains calm, and quickly falls back to sleep. Mucous membranes are dry, and his sclera are slightly icteric. He has skin tenting and muscle wasting. The infant is breathing comfortably, lungs are clear, and his heart has a regular rate and rhythm, with a soft, grade II/VI systolic crescendo-decrescendo murmur heard best in the right upper sternal border. His abdomen is scaphoid, soft, nontender, and nondistended, with no palpable masses. He has normal male genitalia. Laboratory results are as follows.

Laboratory Test	Result
Sodium	116 mEq/dL (116 mmol/L)
Potassium	3.0 mEq/dL (3.0 mmol/L)
Chloride	68 mEq/dL (68 mmol/L)
Bicarbonate	40 mEq/dL (40 mmol/L)
Glucose	62 mg/dL (3.4 mmol/L)

Of the following, the diagnostic test MOST likely to reveal the underlying cause of the infant's electrolyte disturbance is

A. abdominal ultrasonography
B. urine pH measurement
C. upper gastrointestinal radiographic series
D. plasma aldosterone/renin activity ratio

Item 198

A 5-year-old boy, who will be starting kindergarten in the fall, is seen for a health supervision visit. His medical history is not significant, but he has not been seen since he was 3 years old. The boy's mother has concerns about his coordination; he cannot skip, has difficulty balancing on 1 foot, and is slow when climbing stairs. He draws pictures of people and animals with at least 6 to 7 details and can use scissors. He tells stories and jokes, and will follow a 3- to 4-step command. The boy cannot read. The family history on his father's side is not significant. His mother's family history is unknown, because she was adopted as an infant. The boy's weight and height are at the 50th percentile. He appears well and has age-appropriate vital signs. He cannot skip, and when asked to stand from a seated position on the floor, he uses his arms to push himself up.

Of the following, the MOST appropriate next step in this boy's evaluation and management is to

A. evaluate his muscle weakness with a serum creatine kinase level

B. reassure his mother that the boy's development is normal

C. refer to early intervention for evaluation of global developmental delay

D. refer to physical therapy for evaluation of gross motor delay

Item 199

A community-based study was designed to investigate the burden of chronic fatigue and its related psychosocial exposures among young women in Nicaragua. Women aged 18 to 25 years were identified by random sampling of health records maintained at a primary health center over a period of 2 years. Consenting women were interviewed once using a structured questionnaire that elicited complaints of fatigue for at least 6 months (primary outcome measure) and associated psychosocial factors (such as mental health and gender inequality issues).

Of the women in the study, 10.1% (95% confidence interval 8.8%-11.4%) complained of chronic fatigue. Among the psychosocial factors assessed, intimate partner violence and anxiety were independently associated with chronic fatigue.

Of the following, the results of this study of chronic fatigue among women are MOST suggestive of its

A. etiology

B. incidence

C. prevalence

D. temporal trends

Item 200

A 3-day-old neonate born at 36 weeks' gestation is being evaluated. His mother had a history of gestational diabetes. He was born vaginally, with a birthweight of 3.5 kg. He has been breastfeeding every 2 to 3 hours since discharge from the hospital 24 hours after birth. On physical examination, his weight is 3.1 kg. He has jaundice, a high-pitched cry, weak suck, and mild generalized hypotonia.

Of the following, the test MOST likely to confirm this neonate's diagnosis is a

A. blood culture

B. serum ammonia level

C. serum bilirubin level

D. serum glucose level

Item 201

A 5-year-old boy is brought to the the emergency department by his mother who reports that he has had a cough that started the previous day. When he was picked up from day care he was noted to be coughing intermittently. The cough persisted throughout the night. There was no report of illness in his day care and no mention of any problem by the day care provider. He has not had fever, congestion, or other concerns. He is able to speak in sentences between coughing episodes and is not breathless or in distress. His mother has heard no stridor or audible wheeze.

He has an oxygen saturation of 98% on room air, heart rate of 115 beats/min, and respiratory rate of 25 breaths/min. Findings from an upper airway examination are normal. There is no increased work of breathing or intercostal retraction. On auscultation of the chest, there is a slight end expiratory wheeze in the lateral right middle lung field, but no other adventitious sounds. The remainder of the examination findings are unremarkable.

Of the following, the MOST important next step in his evaluation would be

A. a barium swallow radiograph with speech therapist

B. computed tomography of the chest with contrast

C. inspiratory and expiratory anterior-posterior chest radiographs

D. magnetic resonance imaging of the chest without contrast

Item 202

A 9-year-old boy with no significant medical history is seen for a routine health supervision visit. His mother asks if his thyroid function can be tested because both she and her sister have Hashimoto thyroiditis. The boy has no fatigue, constipation, temperature intolerance, or skin problems. He is growing normally with height at the 60th percentile and weight at the 40th percentile. He has a temperature of 37.1°C, heart rate of 72 beats/min, and blood pressure of 100/60 mm Hg. His thyroid is not enlarged. The remainder of the physical examination findings are normal.

Laboratory data are shown:

Laboratory Test	Result
Thyroid-stimulating hormone	1.5 mIU/L (Reference range, 0.3-4.2 mIU/L)
Thyroxine (total T$_4$)	4 µg/dL (51 nmol/L) (Reference range, 5.5-12.8 µg/dL [71-165 nmol/L])

Of the following, the MOST likely diagnosis is

A. central hypothyroidism
B. Hashimoto thyroiditis
C. iodine deficiency
D. thyroid-binding globulin deficiency

Item 203

Prenatal testing showed a neonate to have a complex congenital heart defect, holoprosencephaly, and symmetric intrauterine growth restriction. At delivery, physical examination reveals microcephaly, sloping forehead, cutis aplasia (Item Q203A), hypotelorism, microphthalmia, cleft palate, low-set ears with abnormal helices, bilateral cryptorchidism, and hypospadias. The infant had unusual feet and hands (Item Q203B). Echocardiography confirms a hypoplastic left heart.

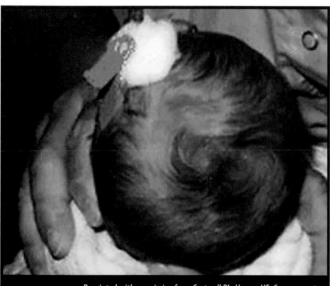

Reprinted with permission from Crotwell PL, Hoyme HE. Core concepts: chromosome aneuploidies. *NeoReviews*. 2012;13(1):e36.

Item Q203A: Cutis aplasia as seen in the neonate described in the vignette.

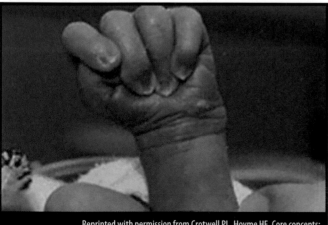

Reprinted with permission from Crotwell PL, Hoyme HE. Core concepts: chromosome aneuploidies. *NeoReviews*. 2012;13(1):e32.

Item Q203B: Hand anomaly as seen in the neonate described in the vignette.

Karyotype testing reveals the diagnosis.
Of the following, the neonate MOST likely has

A. 5p-deletion
B. 22q11.2 deletion
C. trisomy 13
D. trisomy 18

Item 204

An 8-year-old boy is seen as a new patient to establish primary care. He recently moved from another state. His father reports that his son is generally healthy, but has a history of asthma and egg allergy. His father reports that the egg allergy was diagnosed at 14 months of age after his son developed facial swelling and wheezing after eating scrambled eggs. He had seen an allergist at that time but has not seen one since. The father does not know if testing was done. He states that his son avoids eggs and egg-containing foods "as much as possible" and has not had any subsequent reactions. The Asthma Control Test is administered, and the boy has a score of 17, indicating suboptimal control. His father asks what should be done about the boy's asthma and egg allergy.

Of the following, the MOST accurate statement regarding the management of this child's allergy is

A. he has likely had inadvertent exposure to eggs; although he has not had any reactions, he should be referred for testing to confirm that he has outgrown the allergy
B. he has likely had inadvertent exposure to eggs, and more careful avoidance of eggs will likely improve his asthma symptoms
C. he has likely had inadvertent exposure to eggs; since he has had no reactions, he does not need further testing and can safely consume eggs
D. since it is unlikely he has outgrown his allergy, he should continue to avoid eggs and defer allergy testing until early adolescence

Item 205

A 6-month-old male infant who was born at 28 weeks' gestation is brought to the emergency department in November for difficulty breathing. He has had 3 days of rhinorrhea and a progressively worsening cough. Today, his parents noted that his breathing was rapid and labored. Since being discharged from the neonatal intensive care unit, he has been receiving palivizumab monthly. He has a temperature of 37.8°C, heart rate of 185 beats/min, respiratory rate of 70 breaths/min, blood pressure of 98/53 mm Hg, and oxygen saturation of 88% on room air. He is noted to have head bobbing, nasal flaring, and marked retractions. Auscultation of his lungs reveals coarse crackles diffusely.

Of the following, the diagnostic test that will MOST influence the management of this patient is

A. blood culture
B. chest radiography
C. urine culture
D. viral polymerase chain reaction assay

Item 206

An 8-year-old girl is being evaluated for a rash on her hand that developed 2 months ago. It began as a "bump" and has become larger, forming a ring. Her parents applied an over-the-counter antifungal cream without benefit. The physical examination findings are remarkable only for a skin-colored annulus with an elevated border overlying the 4th metacarpophalangeal joint of the left hand (Item Q206). The border is firm to palpation.

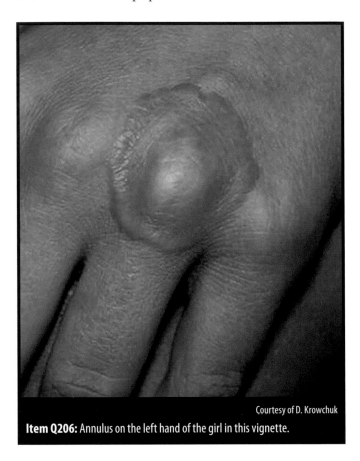

Courtesy of D. Krowchuk

Item Q206: Annulus on the left hand of the girl in this vignette.

Of the following, the MOST appropriate treatment is

A. clotrimazole topically
B. griseofulvin orally
C. hydrocortisone 1% topically
D. no intervention

Item 207

An 11-year-old boy is being evaluated for activity-related pain in his knees and ankles that began several years ago. He cannot recall any preceding injury or incident. His parents tell you that he does not like to participate in sports or other physical activity because of the joint pain. The boy and his family deny joint swelling, fevers, change in appetite or activity, rashes, and easy bruising. His maternal grandmother has knee arthritis. On physical examination, the boy has diffuse mild tenderness over the anterior aspect of both knees and the lateral and medial aspects of both ankles. He can extend both knees and both elbows to 15 degrees, and can touch his palms to the floor without bending his knees. The remainder of his physical examination findings are normal.

Of the following, the MOST appropriate next step in this boy's evaluation and management would be to

A. encourage physical activity and prescribe a physical therapy–directed home exercise program
B. order a complete blood cell count and C-reactive protein level
C. order bilateral radiography of the knees and ankles
D. write a note to exempt the boy from physical education and other sports activities

Item 208

During a health supervision visit, the parents of a healthy 4-year-old boy raise concerns about his behavior. A review of the medical record shows that the boy has had normal growth and development. The boy entered a preschool program this year. His teacher reports that he does not always share well or follow the rules, and sometimes he is aggressive toward other students to "get his way." The boy's parents deny behavior issues at home. He is their first child, so they have many questions about the most effective way to change his behavior.

Of the following, the BEST intervention to recommend to this boy's parents is to

A. discuss with him alternative acceptable means to "get his way"
B. initiate time-outs at home after bad conduct days
C. provide positive praise and rewards after good behavior days
D. take away a favorite toy or activity after bad conduct days

Item 209

A 9-year-old boy is brought to the emergency department for evaluation of abdominal pain associated with nonbilious, nonbloody emesis. His symptoms began acutely about 4 hours ago. The pain is epigastric and radiates to the back. The boy is on vacation with his family. His mother reports that similar symptoms have resulted in several hospitalizations since the age of 4 years. Aside from these episodes, he is otherwise healthy and growing normally. He does not take any prescribed or over-the-counter medications regularly. He is afebrile and has a heart rate of 120 beats/min, respiratory rate of 22 breaths/min, and blood pressure of 100/70 mm Hg. Growth parameters are normal for his age. He appears uncomfortable and in pain. His abdomen is firm and tender to palpation in the midepigastric region. There is no jaundice.

Laboratory data are shown:

Laboratory Test	Result
White blood cell count	12,000/µL (12.0 × 10⁹/L)
Neutrophils	63%
Lymphocytes	32%
Monocytes	5%
Hemoglobin	13.6 g/dL (136 g/L)
Platelet count	210 × 10³/µL (210 × 10⁹/L)
Lipase	954 U/L
Amylase	470 U/L
Total bilirubin	0.5 mg/dL (8.6 µmol/L)
Alanine aminotransferase	35 U/L
Aspartate aminotransferase	29 U/L

Abdominal ultrasonography demonstrates an edematous pancreas with calcifications.

Of the following, the MOST likely diagnosis is

A. gallstone pancreatitis

B. hemolytic-uremic syndrome

C. hereditary pancreatitis

D. viral pancreatitis

Item 210

An 8-year-old boy is seen for problems with learning. He reads slowly and has difficulty answering questions about what he has just read. He has problems spelling simple words. He can add single digit numbers but has difficulty identifying the value of coins and bills. He is pleasant and eager to please. He gets along well with his peers and likes to help out at school and at home. The boy's parents have requested an educational evaluation through his school for a possible learning disability. They state that the psychologist will be administering an IQ test and achievement tests. There is concern that the boy may have intellectual disability. A letter is written to the school psychologist to request additional standardized tests.

Of the following, the BEST test to address this concern is a measure of

A. adaptive function

B. long-term memory

C. processing speed

D. visual-motor integration

Item 211

A 16-year-old girl is being evaluated for headaches. The events start with severe pain behind her left eye and then spread to her whole forehead. She becomes sensitive to bright lights and noises, and feels nauseous. She denies numbness or tingling, tinnitus, or weakness and her vision does not change. The headache lasts until she throws up and then she falls asleep. The headaches started 7 months ago, at the beginning of the school year, and have steadily become more frequent. The girl is now having moderate headaches most days, and a severe headache 1 to 2 times a week. For the past 6 months, she has been using a topical retinoid for acne and takes ibuprofen as needed; she takes no other medications. Her father has similar headaches for which he takes hydrocodone. The girl has been taking ibuprofen 4 to 5 days a week, which is no longer effective. Her father is worried that ibuprofen is not working anymore and asks whether brain imaging would be appropriate. The girl's body mass index is 26 kg/m² (90th percentile); her pupils are equal, round, and reactive to light; on funduscopic examination the optic discs have crisp margins; and her eyes move equally in all directions. The remainder of her physical and neurologic examination findings are normal.

Of the following, the BEST next management step for this girl is to

A. order magnetic resonance imaging of the brain

B. order a lumbar puncture

C. start hydrocodone

D. stop ibuprofen

Item 212

A mother and father bring their infant to a routine health supervision visit. He responds to his own name, knows familiar faces, passes a toy from 1 hand to the other, and supports his weight with his legs and bounces.

Of the following, these developmental milestones are MOST typical for an infant whose age is

A. 4 months

B. 6 months

C. 9 months

D. 12 months

Item 213

A 14-year-old adolescent girl is seen for a follow-up evaluation of enlarged lymph nodes in her neck. She had been seen twice over the last 4 weeks for the same concern. At the first visit, reassurance was provided. At the second visit, she was given a prescription for high-dose amoxicillin. She states that she completed the antibiotics as prescribed, but that the lymph nodes have not changed. She reports no fevers, weight loss, or night sweats. She has not traveled outside the country during the last year and has no pets. Prior to the onset of the neck lymphadenopathy, she had been well with normal growth and development. She is up-to-date on all recommended immunizations.

She appears fatigued. She is at the 45th percentile for height and the 60th percentile for weight. She has a temperature of 37°C, heart rate of 82 beats/min, and blood pressure of 110/76 mm Hg. Her physical examination findings are remarkable only for palpable lymph nodes in the left posterior cervical chain. The largest is approximately 2 cm in diameter, firm, and nontender. There is no overlying erythema.

Laboratory data are shown:

Laboratory Test	Result
White blood cell count	12,500/μL (12.5 × 10⁹/L)
Hemoglobin	9.1 g/dL (91 g/L)
Mean corpuscular volume	88 fL
Platelet count	462 × 10³/μL (462 × 10⁹/L)
Erythrocyte sedimentation rate	82 mm/h

Of the following, the next MOST appropriate step in her management is to

A. obtain a chest radiograph

B. provide reassurance

C. treat her with a course of prednisone

D. treat her with high-dose amoxicillin/clavulanate

Item 214

A 15-year-old girl presents for follow-up of a nondisplaced fracture of the anterior wall of her right maxillary sinus. The girl was struck over her right cheek by a ball during a high school field hockey match last evening. She did not lose consciousness. Computed tomography of her facial bones, obtained in the emergency department, showed the fracture. No other injuries were identified.

Of the following, the MOST appropriate recommendation for ongoing management of this patient is

A. a 1-week course of oral amoxicillin-clavulanate

B. a 5-day course of oral prednisolone

C. follow-up with an otolaryngologist in 4 to 6 weeks

D. no medication or follow-up

Item 215

A full-term neonate who presented with respiratory distress immediately after delivery is being evaluated. He was born via normal vaginal delivery to a 30-year-old gravida 1, para 0 woman. The pregnancy was complicated by oligohydramnios. Prenatal ultrasonography performed at 19 weeks of gestation demonstrated bilateral hydronephrosis. The boy is currently receiving mechanical ventilation in the neonatal intensive care unit. His physical examination findings are otherwise unremarkable.

Laboratory tests show the following results.

Laboratory Test	Patient Result (SI Units)
Sodium	129 mEq/L (129 mmol/L)
Potassium	6.0 mEq/L (6.0 mmol/L)
Chloride	82 mEq/L (82 mmol/L)
Bicarbonate	15 mEq/L (15 mmol/L)
Blood urea nitrogen	45 mg/dL (16.0 mmol/L)
Creatinine	1.9 mg/dL (168 μmol/L)
Glucose	98 mg/dL (5.4 mmol/L)
Calcium	9.6 mg/dL (2.4 mmol/L)
Phosphorus	6.5 mg/dL (2.1 mmol/L)

Abdominal ultrasonography demonstrates bilateral hydronephrosis with renal cortical thinning and a thickened bladder wall.

Of the following, the MOST likely diagnosis in this neonate is

A. posterior urethral valves

B. ureteropelvic junction obstruction

C. ureterovesical junction obstruction

D. vesicoureteral reflux

Item 216

A 12-year-old girl is seen for evaluation of fatigue and left knee pain. For the past month, she has been taking naps in the middle of the day and has not been interested in participating in gym class, which she usually enjoys. She mentions that her right knee had been sore in the last week but that it seems much better now. She reports that she had an upper respiratory tract infection with a sore throat prior to the onset of fatigue. Her vital signs are normal for age. Her left knee is swollen, red, tender, and warm to the touch. Her right knee is without erythema or edema and is minimally tender to palpation. There is a grade 2/6 blowing systolic murmur over the left midclavicular line that was not noted on prior examinations. She has no rash or other skin findings. Her lungs are clear to auscultation bilaterally.

Of the following, the test MOST likely to reveal the diagnosis is

A. antistreptolysin O titer

B. C-reactive protein level

C. echocardiography

D. white blood cell count

Item 217

To determine how confident pediatric residents are at diagnosing eating disorders after completing their adolescent medicine rotation, a standardized pre- and post-test is given at the beginning and end of the rotation. Over the course of a year, 65 residents rotated on the service. The residents who took the rotation during the second half of the academic year tended to have more correct answers on the pre- and post-tests than the residents who did their rotation earlier in the year.

Of the following, the MOST likely explanation for this discrepancy is

A. the difference in scores is most likely due to systematic error

B. the pre- and post-tests are not reliable

C. the pre- and post-tests are not valid

D. the pre- and post-tests are reliable and valid

Item 218

A full-term female neonate is being evaluated in the well-child nursery. She was born to a 22-year-old gravida 1, para 0 woman via normal spontaneous vaginal delivery. Her Apgar scores were 8 and 9 at 1 and 5 minutes, respectively; birthweight was 2,700 g. The mother had adequate prenatal care, and there were no concerning findings on prenatal or perinatal screening tests. The neonate has been attempting to breastfeed, and she has not latched on successfully. At 48 hours after birth, her weight had decreased to 2,450 g. Physical examination findings were normal, with the exception of generalized jaundice. Her serum bilirubin level at that time was 16.2 mg/dL (277 μmol/L), and phototherapy was started. Today, 72 hours after birth, the infant appears less vigorous and is not interested in feeding. Her weight is 2,200 g, temperature is 37°C, heart rate is 170 beats/min, respiratory rate is 36 breaths/min, and blood pressure is 60/30 mm Hg. On physical examination today, the infant is sleepy and difficult to arouse; however, with noxious stimuli the infant cries normally. Her tone is normal, mucous membranes are dry, and she appears icteric. Her breathing is normal, and lungs are clear with good aeration. Heart sounds are regular, with a II/VI systolic ejection murmur. There is significant skin tenting and her extremities are cool, with 4-second capillary refill time.

Of the following, the BEST next step in management is to

A. administer a bolus of 0.9% normal saline, 20 mL/kg, intravenously
B. administer 0.2% normal saline at 16 mL/hour, intravenously
C. offer formula orally
D. perform a whole blood exchange transfusion

Item 219

An 8-year-old boy is seen for a health supervision visit. Neither he nor his parents have specific concerns or questions. His family history is significant for hypercholesterolemia, hypertension, and obesity in his father and obesity in his mother. The boy's height is 140 cm and his weight is 45 kg. His body mass index is 23 kg/m² (97th percentile for age) and has been in this range since 4 years of age. The family is counseled on evidence-based interventions to achieve a healthy body mass index.

Of the following, the intervention MOST likely to help this boy is

A. eliminating sugar-sweetened beverages from his diet
B. enrolling in a commercial weight-loss program
C. increasing dietary fiber in the form of whole grains
D. participating in an organized sport

Item 220

An 11-year-old girl presents with a 1-day history of nausea, abdominal cramping, watery diarrhea without blood or mucus, low-grade fever, malaise, and headache. Five days before presentation, she participated in a summer camp where she had contact with livestock, including preweaned calves, goats, and pigs. The campers also had access to a swimming pool and lake, and consumed meals prepared at a central kitchen. A garden provided lettuce and other produce for camp meals. Several other campers and staff members have become ill with diarrhea. The girl's temperature is 37°C, and her vital signs are normal. Her physical examination is only notable for evidence of mild dehydration.

Of the following, the MOST likely cause of this girl's illness is

A. *Bacillus cereus*
B. *Brucella melitensis*
C. *Cryptosporidium parvum*
D. enteropathogenic *Escherichia coli*

Item 221

A 4-month-old premature infant who was recently discharged from the neonatal intensive care unit is being evaluated. She was born at 26 weeks of gestation with a birthweight of 825 g. Her hospital course was remarkable for a spontaneous intestinal perforation on day 2 after birth, which was treated with an intra-abdominal drain. She also had a grade 2 right intraventricular hemorrhage. She remained intubated until 37 weeks of postconceptional age and was diagnosed with severe bronchopulmonary dysplasia. Physical examination reveals a healed scar in the left lower abdomen, mildly decreased central tone, and mild plagiocephaly. The mother wishes to know how prematurity will affect her daughter in her first year.

Of the following, the MOST likely complication to affect this girl will be

A. craniosynostosis
B. posthemorrhagic hydrocephalus
C. protein-losing enteropathy
D. pulmonary hypertension

Item 222

A 2-year-old boy has a history of wheezing with viral respiratory infections and uses daily inhaled corticosteroids plus albuterol by metered-dose inhaler or nebulizer when he is symptomatic. His mother calls after office hours because he has been sick for 2 days with fever to 38.9°C, cough, and wheezing. She has noticed rapid heart and respiratory rates when he is sleeping. She is using albuterol by metered-dose inhaler with spacer/mask combination, 2 puffs (90 μg each) twice daily, which has been effective for his wheezing in the past. She is concerned about increasing the frequency of dosing because of his rapid heart rate.

Of the following, the BEST advice to her is to

A. begin a course of oral corticosteroids
B. change from albuterol to a long-acting β-agonist inhaler
C. double the dose of inhaled corticosteroids with spacer/mask
D. use albuterol inhaler 2 to 4 puffs with spacer/mask every 3 to 4 hours

Item 223

A 14-year-old African American adolescent girl is seen for a preparticipation physical examination. She is concerned about her weight and would like to join the volleyball team to help her engage in regular physical activity. She has no significant medical history. A review of systems is remarkable for irregular menses since menarche at an age of 11 years. She estimates having 4 menstrual cycles per year.

Her last menstrual period was 2 weeks ago. Her mother has hypertension and had gestational diabetes. Her paternal grandfather had a myocardial infarction at 45 years of age. She has a blood pressure of 132/86 mm Hg and a heart rate of 96 beats/min. She has a height of 168 cm (88th percentile), weight of 82 kg (> 95th percentile), and body mass index of 29.3 kg/m^2 (> 95th percentile). She has acanthosis nigricans over the nape of her neck and mild hirsutism over her chin and lower abdomen. Physical examination findings are otherwise unremarkable. She had a normal fasting lipid profile a year ago.

Of the following, the BEST test to order is

A. a hemoglobin A$_{1c}$ level

B. an insulin level

C. a midnight salivary cortisol level

D. a thyroid-stimulating hormone level

Item 224

A 17-year-old boy develops tinnitus and hearing loss. He has played sports for years, and has recently noted a change in his balance. Magnetic resonance imaging of his brain reveals bilateral vestibular schwannomas. A hearing test, including brainstem auditory-evoked response analysis, reveals moderate sensorineural hearing loss bilaterally. The boy's mother has a history of persistent facial palsy, and a meningioma that warranted surgical removal in early adulthood.

Of the following, the MOST likely finding on this boy's eye examination is

A. coloboma

B. heterochromia

C. iris Lisch nodules

D. posterior subcapsular lens opacity

Item 225

A 4-year-old girl is seen for a health supervision visit. Her previous visit was at 36 months of age. She has had a gastrostomy tube since 10 months of age; it was placed because of poor weight gain and choking with oral feeds. Her mother reports that she has been in and out of the hospital for the past year for various problems, including recurrent febrile seizures, persistent vomiting and abdominal pain, gastrostomy site infections, and unexplained hypoglycemia, tachycardia, and hypoxia. She has undergone electroencephalography and abdominal ultrasonography multiple times, in addition to an endoscopy and colonoscopy; all results were normal. The results of a muscle biopsy to assess for mitochondrial abnormalities are pending. She is followed by 3 specialists at the local children's hospital. Her mother asks for referrals to a different children's hospital because her current specialists "can't figure her out." She also requests a referral to a surgeon for a central line placement because of previous difficulties securing an intravenous line and a wheelchair because of excessive falling and fatigue.

The girl is talkative and engaging. Her examination findings are normal, and she exhibits appropriate developmental skills. Her discharge summaries are reviewed. They state that the seizures, vomiting, and episodes of pain occurred prior to hospitalization and then resolved upon admission. There is no mention of abnormal serum glucose levels or abnormal vital signs.

Of the following, the next MOST appropriate step in managing this patient is to

A. contact the child protection team at the local children's hospital

B. grant the mother's request to replace her daughter's current specialists but not for the surgery evaluation or the wheelchair

C. refer the family to the state child welfare agency if the biopsy indicates no mitochondrial disorder

D. request that the mother find a primary care provider who is better equipped to handle complex patients

Item 226

A 9-year-old boy is brought to the emergency department for abdominal pain. The abdominal pain began 3 days ago and has been associated with fever. He has been using ibuprofen for pain control, which has provided some relief. This morning the pain woke him from sleep. There is no significant past medical history, and his immunizations are up-to-date. The boy was born in Mexico and moved to the United States 6 months ago. He has a temperature of 38.5°C, heart rate of 100 beats/min, respiratory rate of 22 breaths/min, and blood pressure of 109/65 mm Hg. He has abdominal tenderness over the right upper quadrant. Abdominal ultrasonography is attempted but cannot be completed because of his discomfort. Computed tomography of the abdomen reveals a hypoattenuating lesion in the liver (Item Q226).

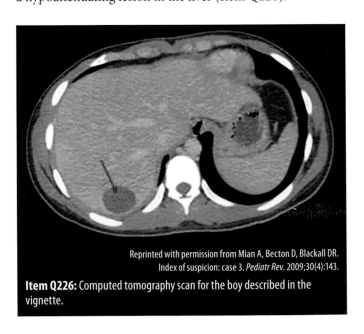

Reprinted with permission from Mian A, Becton D, Blackall DR. Index of suspicion: case 3. *Pediatr Rev.* 2009;30(4):143.

Item Q226: Computed tomography scan for the boy described in the vignette.

Of the following, the test MOST likely to determine the patient's diagnosis is

A. aspirate microscopy

B. serology

C. stool culture

D. stool microscopy

You are called to admit a 36-week-gestation male newborn to the nursery who was delivered vaginally to a 27-year-old gravida 3, para 1 woman. The mother's prenatal history is significant for an *Escherichia coli* urinary tract infection and positive group B *Streptococcus* (GBS) status. Rupture of membranes occurred 8 hours before delivery. The mother received 1 dose of intravenous penicillin 3 hours before delivery, for GBS prophylaxis. The neonate is rooming in with his mother and formula feeding well. The mother has a 4-year-old son at home, and requests that her newborn be discharged 24 hours after birth. You discuss with her the current guidelines for care of neonates born to GBS-positive mothers.

Of the following, the MOST appropriate management plan for this neonate would be

A. complete blood cell count, blood culture, and cefotaxime administration pending culture results

B. complete blood cell count and blood culture, with possible discharge at 24 hours of age

C. complete blood cell count and blood culture, with possible discharge at 48 hours of age

D. observation in the newborn nursery unit, with possible discharge at 24 hours of age

Item 228

A 14-year-old girl with type 1 diabetes mellitus is undergoing a sports preparticipation evaluation before the start of her first high school soccer season. Her parents ask your advice about managing her blood glucose levels, given the expected intensity of practice sessions. The girl has been successfully using an insulin pump for the past 6 months.

Of the following, the MOST appropriate statement to include when counseling the girl and her family is that

A. frequent snacking before exercise is the best way to mitigate her risk of hypoglycemia

B. she should avoid exercising early in the day, as that would increase her risk of hypoglycemia

C. she should decrease her basal infusion of insulin beginning 1 to 2 hours before exercise

D. the highest risk period for hypoglycemia is 30 minutes after she begins intense exercise

Item 229

At a routine health supervision visit, the parents of a 4-month-old girl raise a concern about her vomiting. The vomiting is described as nonbilious, nonbloody "spit up" that occurs a few minutes after nearly every feeding. The girl does not choke or cough with feedings. The emesis occurs effortlessly after feedings, often with burping. She is breastfed when her mother is home and given expressed breast milk by bottle when her mother is at work. She feeds on demand about every 4 hours and will readily take 6 to 8 ounces per bottle feeding. On occasion she has received cow milk formula as a supplement. The girl's parents believe she vomits slightly more volume after bottle feedings than breastfeedings. The type of milk does not seem to make a difference in the amount of vomiting. Her stools are soft and yellow. She is otherwise asymptomatic. The girl's growth curve is following the 25th percentile trajectory for length, weight, and fronto-occipital head circumference. Her parents want to discuss the prognosis for this condition.

Of the following outcomes, this condition is MOST likely to

A. improve with longer intervals between feedings

B. lead to other feeding/swallowing problems

C. resolve spontaneously by 12 months of age

D. result in poor weight gain and undernutrition

Item 230

A 16-year-old adolescent boy has concerns of weight loss and fatigue. His family believes he has lost 4.5 kg in the last 4 to 6 weeks. He also reports abdominal bloating and diarrhea. This week, a friend whom he had not seen for several months remarked that his eyes were yellow. He has no prior history of jaundice. His family is concerned about possible drug use because he has had difficulty walking steadily. He has a history of depression diagnosed at 13 years of age and treated with psychotherapy. There is no family history of liver disease, autoimmune diseases, or emphysema. He has normal vital signs for age. He has a weight of 47.7 kg (5th percentile), height of 167 cm (25th percentile), and body mass index of 17 kg/m² (5th percentile). He appears fatigued and jaundiced with scleral icterus. His abdomen is distended with a fluid wave. His liver edge is firm and at the right costal margin. His spleen is palpated 5 cm below the left costal margin. There is no edema. He has palmar erythema.

Laboratory data are shown:

Laboratory Test	Result
White blood cell count	6,000/µL (6.0 × 10⁹/L)
Hemoglobin	11.0 g/dL (110 g/L)
Platelet count	95 × 10³/µL (95 × 10⁹/L)
Conjugated bilirubin	4.5 mg/dL (77.0 µmol/L)
Alanine aminotransferase	245 U/L
Aspartate aminotransferase	215 U/L
Prothrombin time	18.0 s
International normalized ratio	1.6
Vitamin D, 25-hydroxy	9 ng/mL (22 nmol/L)
Urine toxicology screen	Negative

Of the following, the test that is MOST likely to establish the diagnosis is

A. α_1-antitrypsin level

B. ceruloplasmin

C. hepatitis C virus antibody

D. partial thromboplastin time

Item 231

A 15 year old adolescent boy is seen for a health supervision visit. His mother reports that his aunt was recently hospitalized for a suicide attempt. She describes her son as moody and sensitive like her sister. She is concerned about his risk for suicide completion.

Of the following, the factor MOST likely to increase his risk is

A. a diagnosis of attention-deficit/hyperactivity disorder

B. poor social communication skills

C. the presence of a firearm in the home

D. problems with academic achievement

Item 232

A 7-month-old boy is brought to the emergency department (ED) after he had a seizure at home. He had a runny nose and cough for 3 days and temperature of 38.3°C that morning. He was given acetaminophen and the fever resolved. Later that afternoon, he was playing on the floor when suddenly he fell over and his whole body started jerking. This lasted about 30 seconds and then stopped on its own, but he was sleepy afterwards. The Emergency Medical Service (EMS) was called. At the home, EMS found that the boy's blood glucose level was normal, and he was transported to the ED. In the ED, his temperature is 39.1°C, heart rate is 160 beats/min, and blood pressure is 90/60 mm Hg. He is sleepy, but wakes up readily during the examination. The remainder of his physical examination findings are normal. The boy's parents report that he has never had a seizure before, and he has no chronic medical problems. His development is age appropriate. His immunizations are up to date, with the most recent doses given at his 6-month health supervision visit 3 weeks ago. His cousin has autism and epilepsy.

Of the following, the MOST accurate statement you can make to this boy's parents is that

A. electroencephalography is indicated to determine his seizure recurrence risk

B. the immunizations may have triggered this seizure

C. the short duration of the seizure makes subsequent seizures less likely

D. the strongest risk factor for recurrent seizure is his age

Item 233

An otherwise healthy neonate in the newborn nursery has a well-developed rugated scrotum without palpable testes. The phallus is 2 cm in length with a urethral meatus at the base of the penile shaft just above the scrotum.

Of the following, the disorder MOST likely associated with this condition is

A. congenital adrenal hyperplasia

B. imperforate anus

C. renal agenesis

D. vesicoureteral reflux

Item 234

A 2-year-old girl is seen for a health supervision visit. She has been well with normal growth and development. She has had a normal appetite, although her parents report that she has been sleeping more than usual for the last few weeks. She is up-to-date on her vaccinations. She appears well but pale. She has a temperature of 37°C, heart rate of 130 beats/min, and blood pressure of 92/50 mm Hg. She is at the 45th percentile for both height and weight. The remainder of her physical examination findings are normal.

Laboratory data are shown:

Laboratory Test	Result
White blood cell count	5,500/µL (5.5 × 10⁹/L)
Neutrophils	55%
Lymphocytes	40%
Monocytes	5%
Hemoglobin	6.2 g/dL (62 g/L)
Mean corpuscular volume	75 fL
Platelet count	320 × 10³/µL (320 × 10⁹/L)
Reticulocytes	0.1%

Of the following, the test(s) MOST likely to confirm the diagnosis is (are)

A. flow cytometry of the peripheral blood

B. hemoglobin electrophoresis

C. serial hemoglobin and reticulocyte counts

D. a technetium-99m pertechnetate scan (Meckel scan)

Item 235

A 16-year-old boy presents to the emergency department (ED) for evaluation after a motor vehicle crash. Thirty minutes ago, the boy was driving on a rural highway, swerved to miss an animal in the road, and struck a tree. He was not wearing a seatbelt. His vehicle is an older pick-up truck that does not have airbags. He did not hit his head or lose consciousness, but did strike his chest on the steering wheel and has complained of severe chest pain since then.

On arrival at the ED, the boy is alert and fully oriented but appears anxious. His vital signs include a heart rate of 128 beats/min (regular rhythm), respiratory rate of 36 breaths/min, blood pressure of 110/70 mm Hg, and oxygen saturation of 90% on room air. He appears very uncomfortable, and is complaining of anterior chest wall pain. His airway is intact. There is significant bruising over his anterior chest wall, especially over the midsternal area. The boy is taking short, rapid breaths and reports that "it hurts to breathe." His breath sounds are clear and equal throughout, but his respirations are very shallow and you note intermittent paradoxical movement of a section of his right chest wall. His abdomen is soft and nontender. His cervical and thoracolumbar spine are nontender and without step-offs. His extremities are well-perfused, with normal pulses.

Chest radiography reveals a nondisplaced fracture of the sternum, as well as multiple anterior displaced fractures of the boy's right first, second, and third ribs and left second rib. The boy is placed on 100% oxygen via a nonrebreather face mask.

Of the following, the BEST next management step for this boy is

A. endotracheal intubation and mechanical ventilation
B. immediate operative management by a cardiothoracic surgeon
C. placement of an external splint device to stabilize the chest wall
D. placement of chest tubes bilaterally

Item 236

A 2-day-old neonate born to a 30-year-old primigravida by normal vaginal delivery is being evaluated. The neonate is feeding every 3 to 4 hours and has had 7 wet diapers in the last 24 hours. Prenatal ultrasonography at 19 weeks of gestation showed multiple cysts of different sizes in the right kidney. The neonate's vital signs include a weight of 3 kg, temperature of 37°C, heart rate of 140 beats/min, respiratory rate of 40 breaths/min, blood pressure of 80/44 mm Hg, and oxygen saturation of 97% with pulse oximetry on room air. Physical examination is significant for a mass in the right flank. Results of laboratory testing are as follows.

Laboratory Test	Patient Result (SI Units)
Sodium	138 mEq/L (138 mmol/L)
Potassium	4.5 mEq/L (4.5 mmol/L)
Chloride	100 mEq/L (100 mmol/L)
Bicarbonate	21 mEq/L (21 mmol/L)
Blood urea nitrogen	20 mg/dL (7.1 mmol/L)
Creatinine	0.8 mg/dL (70.7 μmol/L)
Calcium	9.6 mg/ dL (2.4 mmol/L)
Phosphorus	6.0 mg/dL (1.9 mmol/L)

Abdominal ultrasonography demonstrates multiple non-communicating cysts in the right kidney and a normal left kidney.

Of the following, the MOST likely diagnosis in this boy is

A. autosomal dominant polycystic kidney disease
B. autosomal recessive polycystic kidney disease
C. medullary cystic kidney disease
D. multicystic dysplastic kidney

Item 237

A 12-month-old girl who was born at 25 weeks' gestation is seen for follow-up in her primary care office. She was recently evaluated in a comprehensive neonatology follow-up clinic where she sees multiple specialists at a single visit. A medical student on rotation asks how the role as primary care provider within a medical home is different in a child with a complex medical history who is seen by multiple specialists compared to the role for a child who is otherwise healthy.

Of the following, the BEST response to the student is that this arrangement will

A. decrease communication between providers
B. decrease the quality of care provided by minimizing the role of the subspecialists
C. improve the overall quality of care
D. provide a set location for vaccinations and development checks only

Item 238

A 16-year-old adolescent girl is seen for a health supervision visit. She is healthy with no significant medical history. During a HEADSS (home and environment; education and eating; activities; drugs; sexuality; suicide, depression, and safety) assessment with her mother outside of the room, she reports that she identifies as being female but is attracted to both sexes. She has been dating a girl her age for the past 2 months and is feeling guilty because she does not believe her family will be accepting of this relationship. She becomes tearful and says that it has been difficult to lie to her parents about her feelings. She has never had sex of any type with a male or female partner.

Of the following, the BEST next step in management is to

A. advise her to stop dating the female partner
B. discuss birth control options and safe sex
C. recommend therapy to explore her feelings
D. start fluoxetine to address her depression

Item 239

A previously healthy, 4-month-old boy is admitted to the pediatric intensive care unit with acute hypoxic respiratory failure due to bronchiolitis. It is his third day of illness, and his second day on mechanical ventilation. His vital signs are as follows: temperature, 37°C; heart rate, 140 beats/min; respiratory rate, 30 breaths/min; and blood pressure, 80/40 mm Hg. His ventilator rate is set at 20 breaths/min, and he is receiving 50% oxygen. The infant appears comfortable on these settings. An attempt was made to decrease his ventilator settings several hours ago, but when the rate was decreased to 16 breaths/min, he started to breathe rapidly. The boy is sedated with a continuous infusion of morphine. He is generally sleepy, but spontaneously opens his eyes. He has occasional episodes of agitation, precipitated by noxious stimuli such as suctioning and phlebotomy, in which he cries and moves his head from side to side, but calms down with patting, rocking, or an extra dose of morphine intravenously.

Of the following, the MOST appropriate measure to prevent unplanned extubation in this patient would be to

A. administer continuous pharmacologic paralysis
B. apply continuous end-tidal carbon dioxide monitoring
C. ask the parents to hold the tube in place during episodes of agitation
D. ensure a 1:1 nurse-to-patient ratio

Item 240

During the confidential portion of his routine health supervision visit, a healthy 15-year-old boy inquires about testicular size. He has noticed that his left scrotum is larger than the right, so he is concerned that his right testicle is too small. He denies any acute changes in color, size, or pain in the scrotal area. He is not sexually active. On physical examination, the boy's sexual maturity rating is 4. You palpate a mass above the left testicle that feels like a bag of worms. This mass is most prominent when the patient is standing and decreases significantly when he is examined supine. The remainder of his physical examination findings are unremarkable.

Of the following, the MOST accurate statement about this condition is that

A. fertility problems will occur in 50% or more of adult men with this finding

B. it occurs in about one-third of adolescent boys

C. it needs no evaluation when asymptomatic

D. the larger the mass, the greater the risk for future testicular cancer

Item 241

A 6-year-old girl presents to the emergency department with a 16-day history of fever up to 38.3°C, malaise, headache, and fatigue. One week before this visit, she was evaluated by her pediatrician for these symptoms. A complete blood cell count and urinalysis at that time revealed normal values. Daily fevers and fatigue have persisted, and she has now developed right-sided abdominal pain. There are no sick contacts. The girl lives on a farm and has exposure to cats, dogs, horses, and cattle. She has not traveled internationally. There is no known tuberculosis exposure. Her immunizations are up to date.

On physical examination, the girl is afebrile with a heart rate of 78 beats/min, respiratory rate of 16 breaths/min, and oxygen saturation of 92% on room air. She has right upper quadrant tenderness and hepatosplenomegaly. The remainder of her physical examination findings are normal. Laboratory data show an elevated platelet count and an erythrocyte sedimentation rate of 75 mm/hour. Results are otherwise normal, including white blood cell count, hemoglobin, lactate dehydrogenase, uric acid, and liver and renal function tests. Blood and urine cultures are negative. A purified protein derivative skin test is negative and her chest radiograph is normal. Abdominal ultrasonography shows multiple hypoechoic lesions in the liver and spleen.

Of the following, the test MOST likely to establish this girl's diagnosis is

A. bone marrow biopsy

B. liver biopsy

C. serology

D. stool testing for ova and parasites

Item 242

A neonate is born at 35 weeks' gestation to a 19-year-old primigravida with limited prenatal care. Maternal history is significant for cigarette smoking during the pregnancy. Physical examination reveals the following (Item Q242).

The neonate is placed in a sterile plastic bag up to the axilla with the right side down, taking care to support the intestines.

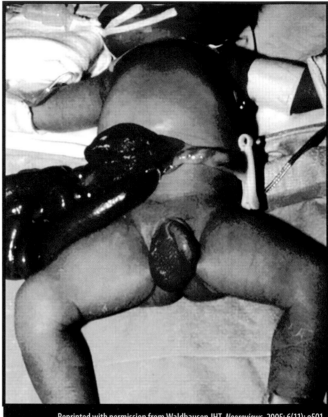

Reprinted with permission from Waldhausen JHT. *Neoreviews.* 2005; 6(11); e501

Item Q242: Findings for the neonate described in the vignette.

Of the following, the disorder MOST commonly associated with this congenital anomaly is

A. bladder exstrophy

B. hypoglycemia

C. necrotizing enterocolitis

D. Wilms tumor

Item 243

A 3-year-old girl has had recurrent respiratory infections. She has had chronic runny nose and nasal congestion since early infancy and has had 3 or 4 episodes of otitis media each year in addition to bronchiolitis at least once per year since birth. She is not in day care and stays at home with her mother. There is a family history of seasonal and perennial allergic rhinitis and a question of asthma. There are no pets in the house. The girl's mother smokes in a room with the door closed. She stopped smoking during pregnancy, but resumed smoking when the child was younger than 3 months.

The girl has normal growth parameters. Her oxygen saturation is 98% on room air, and she is afebrile. Tympanic membranes are dull and have a diffused light reflex. The nasal mucosa is swollen, and the airway is impaired but not obstructed; there is thin, clear mucus in the nares. Tonsils are grade 2+ and not inflamed. The girl has a wet cough and her breath sounds are coarse, with a few scattered rhonchi but no fine rales or wheezes.

Of the following, a discussion with the mother regarding potential ways to improve her child's health should focus on

A. the initiation of daily antihistamine therapy

B. keeping the windows open in the house for more fresh air

C. tobacco smoking cessation for the mother

D. the use of impermeable zippered covers on the child's mattress and pillows

Item 244

A 2-day-old male neonate is transferred to the neonatal intensive care unit for persistent hypoglycemia. He was born at 39 weeks' gestation by cesarean delivery due to breech position. The pregnancy was otherwise uncomplicated. Birth weight was 3,350 g. Due to jitteriness, a point-of-care blood glucose was measured with a result of 18 mg/dL (1.0 mmol/L). A confirmatory venous sample sent to the laboratory was 20 mg/dL (1.1 mmol/L). His glucose level has remained less than 50 mg/dL (2.8 mmol/L) despite frequent feeding. Upon arrival to the neonatal intensive care unit, a blood sample was obtained and intravenous dextrose-containing fluids were started. His physical examination findings are significant for a stretched phallic length of 1.8 cm. His right testicle is not palpable, and the left testicle is palpable high in the scrotum.

Of the following, the MOST likely cause of this neonate's hypoglycemia is

A. a fatty acid oxidation disorder

B. hyperinsulinism

C. hypopituitarism

D. transitional hypoglycemia

Item 245

A newborn with an unusual head shape and hand and foot abnormalities is being evaluated. The neonate's head is cone-shaped with occipital flattening (turribrachycephaly). Facial dysmorphology includes moderate midfacial hypoplasia, ocular hypertelorism, mandibular prognathism, beaked nose, and proptosis (Item Q245A). There is a "mitten-glove" deformity of the hands and feet, with varying degrees of syndactyly of the soft tissue and bones of the fingers and toes (Item Q245B). Echocardiography and renal ultrasonography results are normal. Computed tomography of the head confirms craniosynostosis of multiple skull bones (Item Q245C). Radiologic imaging of the extremities confirms soft tissue and bone syndactyly of the hands and feet (Item Q245D).

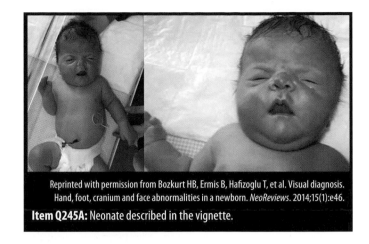

Reprinted with permission from Bozkurt HB, Ermis B, Hafizoglu T, et al. Visual diagnosis. Hand, foot, cranium and face abnormalities in a newborn. *NeoReviews.* 2014;15(1):e46.

Item Q245A: Neonate described in the vignette.

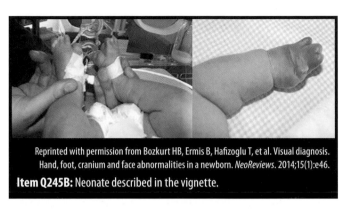

Reprinted with permission from Bozkurt HB, Ermis B, Hafizoglu T, et al. Visual diagnosis. Hand, foot, cranium and face abnormalities in a newborn. *NeoReviews.* 2014;15(1):e46.

Item Q245B: Neonate described in the vignette.

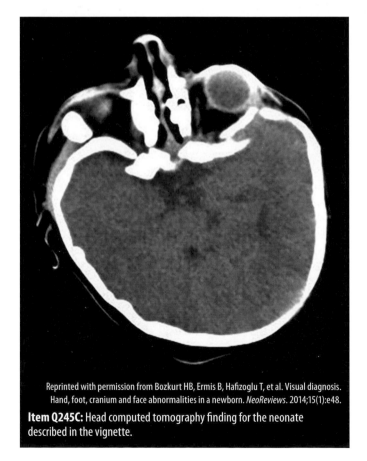

Reprinted with permission from Bozkurt HB, Ermis B, Hafizoglu T, et al. Visual diagnosis. Hand, foot, cranium and face abnormalities in a newborn. *NeoReviews.* 2014;15(1):e48.

Item Q245C: Head computed tomography finding for the neonate described in the vignette.

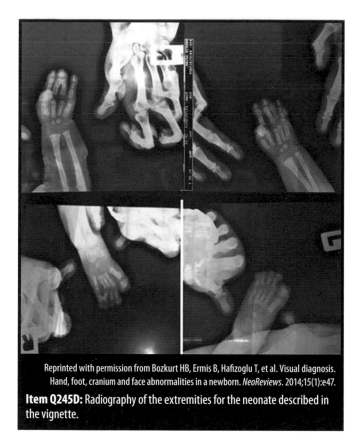

Reprinted with permission from Bozkurt HB, Ermis B, Hafizoglu T, et al. Visual diagnosis. Hand, foot, cranium and face abnormalities in a newborn. *NeoReviews*. 2014;15(1):e47.

Item Q245D: Radiography of the extremities for the neonate described in the vignette.

Of the following, the MOST likely diagnosis in this neonate is

A. amniotic band syndrome

B. Apert syndrome

C. Holt-Oram syndrome

D. Shprintzen-Goldberg syndrome

Item 246

A 6-year-old girl is seen for concerns about her balance. Over the past 3 days the girl has had 5 or 6 episodes where she states that the room is spinning and she has to grab onto something, such as a table or the edge of the sofa, to steady herself. She states that she feels like vomiting during these episodes, but has not vomited. The episodes last 1 minute or less. She recovers fully and acts normally in between episodes. She had 2 similar episodes 1 month ago, around the time a sibling was diagnosed with influenza. She had a tactile fever 2 weeks ago that lasted for a few hours and responded to ibuprofen. This episode was associated with cough and rhinorrhea that lasted a few days. The girl's father takes medication for migraines, a maternal aunt has multiple sclerosis, and her paternal grandfather died from a brain tumor.

She is sitting comfortably on the examination table and is engaged with her mother's smartphone. She talks about the game she is playing. The physical examination, including pneumotoscopy of the tympanic membranes and detailed neurologic examination, has normal findings.

Of the following, the BEST next step in management is to

A. obtain electroencephalography and magnetic resonance imaging of the brain

B. prescribe a 7-day course of oseltamivir and diazepam as needed to reduce symptoms

C. recommend watchful waiting and consult a neurologist if symptoms worsen

D. refer to physical therapy for nystagmus testing and canalith repositioning

Item 247

A 2-week-old full-term male neonate is seen for evaluation of eye drainage. Watery drainage along with mild eye swelling were first noted 3 days ago. He has had progressive worsening of these symptoms. He was born to a 21-year-old gravida 2, para 1 mother. The delivery was uneventful, and he went home with the mother at 2 days of age. He received topical erythromycin eye prophylaxis in the newborn nursery. His mother had intercourse with several partners during her pregnancy. Physical examination reveals abnormalities in the right eye (Item Q247).

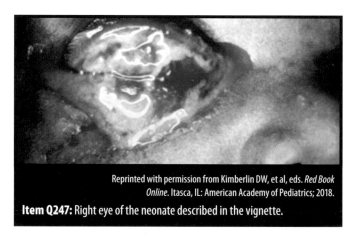

Reprinted with permission from Kimberlin DW, et al, eds. *Red Book Online*. Itasca, IL: American Academy of Pediatrics; 2018.

Item Q247: Right eye of the neonate described in the vignette.

Of the following, the MOST likely etiology for this neonate's illness is

A. adenovirus

B. *Chlamydia trachomatis*

C. herpes simplex virus

D. *Neisseria gonorrhoeae*

Item 248

A 9-month-old female infant with "spots" on her skin is being evaluated as a new patient. A few spots were present at birth but they have increased in number since. The girl is an only child. Her mother is unaware of family members with similar spots. Physical examination findings are remarkable only for the lesions shown in Item Q248A and Item Q248B.

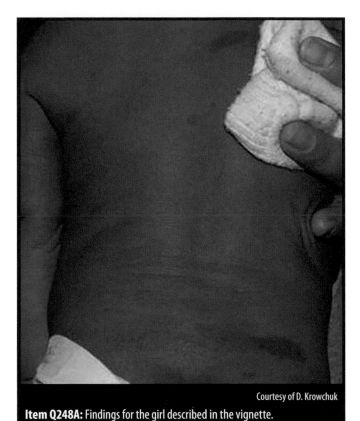

Item Q248A: Findings for the girl described in the vignette.

Courtesy of D. Krowchuk

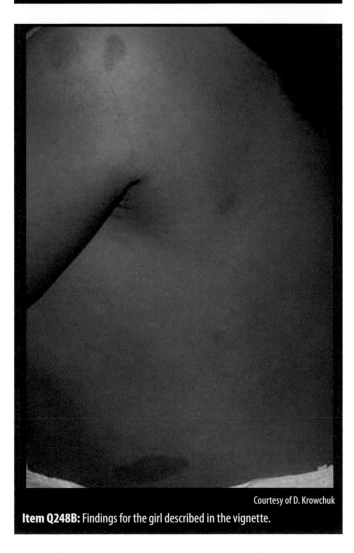

Item Q248B: Findings for the girl described in the vignette.

Courtesy of D. Krowchuk

Of the following, the BEST next step in management for this infant is

A. magnetic resonance imaging of the brain
B. no further evaluation
C. referral for developmental assessment
D. referral to an ophthalmologist

Item 249

A 10-year-old girl sustained an inversion injury to her left ankle at soccer practice. She was able to bear weight at the time of injury, but unable to continue playing soccer. On physical examination, mild-to-moderate swelling is noted over the lateral aspect of the left ankle. Her ankle motion is slightly limited in all directions due to pain. The ankle is tender to palpation over the anterior aspect of the distal tip of the fibula and the area just anterior and inferior to this bony landmark. She has no ligamentous laxity.

Of the following, the structure the girl is MOST likely to have injured is the

A. anterior talofibular ligament
B. deltoid ligament
C. distal fibula physis
D. peroneus brevis tendon

Item 250

The timing, sequence, and rationale behind the introduction of solid foods is an important topic at the routine 4-month health maintenance visit. An evidence-based discussion on infant nutrition should focus on the recommendations for infants at 4 months of age.

Of the following, the statement that MOST accurately reflects the latest recommendations is

A. adding a small amount of cereal in the bedtime bottle is not harmful and has been demonstrated to aid sleeping through the night, especially in large infants
B. between 6 and 11 months of age, 8 ounces of 100% fruit juice is recommended, in addition to complementary foods, to meet the daily requirements for vitamin C intake
C. delaying the introduction of solid foods beyond 4 to 6 months of age has not been shown to prevent the development of food allergies
D. the texture of complementary foods should be advanced strictly, following an age-based schedule, to help prevent future picky eaters

Item 251

A 7-year-old boy is being evaluated for "white spots" on his face that developed 6 weeks ago. He has no associated symptoms and has been in good health. The physical examination findings are notable only for the lesions shown in Item Q251.

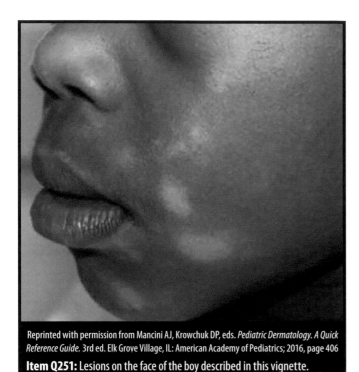

Reprinted with permission from Mancini AJ, Krowchuk DP, eds. *Pediatric Dermatology. A Quick Reference Guide.* 3rd ed. Elk Grove Village, IL: American Academy of Pediatrics; 2016, page 406

Item Q251: Lesions on the face of the boy described in this vignette.

Of the following, the MOST appropriate treatment is

A. clotrimazole topically

B. emollient topically

C. triamcinolone topically

D. ultraviolet B phototherapy

Item 252

A 15-year-old adolescent boy with a 5-day history of nausea, dark tarry stools, and dizziness is brought to the emergency department for a syncopal episode. He has previously had intermittent heartburn and mild abdominal pain, but not blood in his stools. He reports no recent use of nonsteroidal anti-inflammatory drugs or other over-the-counter medications. He also reports no alcohol or recreational drug use. He has a heart rate of 120 beats/min and blood pressure of 112/48 mm Hg. He is pale and fatigued. He has tachycardia and a grade 1/6 systolic murmur. His abdomen is soft and nontender without masses or hepatosplenomegaly. A digital rectal examination reveals purple, hemoccult-positive liquid stool.

A nasogastric tube is placed in the emergency department and reveals dark red blood. Two large-bore intravenous catheters are placed.

Laboratory results are shown:

Laboratory Test	Result
White blood cell count	8,000/µL (8.0 × 10⁹/L)
Hemoglobin	6.3 g/dL (63 g/L)
Mean corpuscular volume	91 fL
Platelet count	167 × 10³/µL (167 × 10⁹/L)
Prothrombin time	12.6 s
Partial thromboplastin time	35 s
Alanine aminotransferase	33 U/L
Aspartate aminotransferase	15 U/L
Total bilirubin	< 0.5 mg/dL (8.6 µmol/L)

Of the following, the BEST next step in management is to

A. administer packed red blood cells

B. perform abdominal ultrasonography with Doppler

C. perform endoscopy

D. perform a Meckel scan

Item 253

An 8-year-old boy is seen for concerns about his learning. His parents report that he is not performing at the level of his peers, especially in reading. He makes careless errors on his classwork and examinations. He is resistant to doing his homework, and it takes him much longer than it should to complete the work. He is described as distractible and forgetful. He has just been assessed through his school for a possible learning disability, and his parents are waiting for the results to be finalized. Attention-deficit/hyperactivity disorder is suspected, and the parents are asked to complete a standardized rating form and to give their son's teacher a teacher rating form. The results are reviewed, and a diagnosis of attention-deficit/hyperactivity disorder is made.

Of the following, the BEST next step in management is to recommend

A. classroom accommodations

B. cognitive behavioral therapy

C. extended school year services

D. re-evaluation by the school

Item 254

A previously healthy 7-year-old boy presents to the emergency department with cough and runny nose for 2 weeks, and fever and headache of 1 day's duration. On physical examination, his temperature is 39.4°C, heart rate is 122 beats/min, and blood pressure is 100/60 mm Hg. His physical examination shows erythematous nasal mucosa and clear nasal discharge; all other findings are within normal parameters. Soon after his initial evaluation he has a seizure. His mother reports that the seizure started in his left arm and leg and then his whole body started shaking. The seizure ends after 2 minutes, and the boy is lethargic. Over the next 10 minutes, he starts to wake up and move around, but his left arm and leg are weak.

Of the following, the BEST next step in this boy's evaluation and management is to

A. administer acetaminophen orally

B. administer lorazepam intravenously

C. perform brain imaging

D. perform a lumbar puncture

Item 255

The parents of a 3-month-old female infant with a history of severe eczema would like advice on introduction of peanuts into her diet. They have read that infants who have frequently occurring eczema that requires prescription-strength medications may benefit from early exposure to peanuts. The infant is referred to an allergy specialist, for which there is more than a month-long wait, and blood testing for peanut-specific IgE is performed. The result is 0.9 kU/L (normal < 0.35 kU/L).

Of the following, the parents are MOST likely to be advised that

A. peanuts should be avoided in the future

B. she undergo allergy testing for multiple foods

C. skin testing is not recommended because of her age

D. a supervised oral challenge of peanuts may be recommended

Item 256

A 2-year-old boy is seen by his pediatrician because his mother felt a "lump in his belly" while bathing him. Prior to this visit, the boy had been generally well, with normal growth and development. He has never been hospitalized or had surgery. His mother reports that he has seemed well and has had a normal activity level and appetite. He has had no weight loss, fevers, or vomiting.

The boy appears well and is in no distress. He has a temperature of 37°C, heart rate of 92 beats/min, and blood pressure of 96/68 mm Hg. He is at the 60th percentile for both height and weight. The remainder of his examination is only remarkable for a mass in the left flank, palpable at a level just above the umbilicus.

Urgent ultrasonography reveals a mass that appears to arise from the left kidney.

Of the following, this child's MOST likely diagnosis and prognosis is

A. adrenocortical carcinoma with less than 30% chance of being cured

B. neuroblastoma with a 50% chance of being cured

C. nephroblastoma with a greater than 70% chance of being cured

D. renal cell carcinoma with less than 30% chance of being cured

Item 257

A 14-month-old previously healthy boy is being evaluated for fussiness, refusal to eat, loose stools, and vomiting. His symptoms started last evening. The boy had fallen asleep at his usual bedtime; however, during the night he woke up frequently, crying. Each time, his mother could console him and soothe him back to sleep. This morning he has had episodes of crying every 20 to 30 minutes. Over the past 3 hours, he has had several episodes of vomiting and loose stools. He has refused to eat or drink since his symptoms began. The boy's mother reports that he seems much more sluggish than usual this morning, which she attributes to his poor sleep last night. He had cough and rhinorrhea last week, but has had no recent fevers. There is no history of recent trauma.

The boy's current vital signs are as follows: temperature, 37.8°C; heart rate, 165 beats/min; respiratory rate, 36 breaths/min; and oxygen saturation, 98% on room air. He appears lethargic, and is lying still in his mother's arms. He abruptly begins to cry loudly and "squirm around." This lasts for about 10 minutes before he falls asleep again.

On physical examination, there are no rashes or bruising. The boy's mucous membranes are dry. He is slightly tachypneic, but his lungs are clear with good air exchange. His abdomen is moderately distended. His extremities are cool with a capillary refill time of 2 seconds. He has no swelling of his joints. The remainder of his physical examination findings are unremarkable. The boy then passes an unformed soft stool that is positive for blood.

Of the following, the MOST likely diagnosis for this boy is

A. inguinal hernia

B. infectious enterocolitis

C. intussusception

D. Meckel diverticulum

Item 258

A 6-year-old boy presents to the emergency department (ED) for evaluation of recurrent facial swelling. He was evaluated by his pediatrician 1 week ago for a similar complaint, at which time he was treated with an antihistamine. Physical examination in the ED shows a healthy-appearing boy with normal growth parameters. He is afebrile with a respiratory rate of 18 breaths/min, heart rate of 84 beats/min, and blood pressure of 104/66 mm Hg. The only findings of significance on his examination are facial puffiness and periorbital edema. A urine test strip analysis demonstrates a specific gravity of 1.015, pH of 5.5, 3+ protein, and is negative for blood, leukocyte esterase, and nitrites.

Of the following, the MOST likely diagnosis in this boy is

A. focal segmental glomerulosclerosis

B. membranoproliferative glomerulonephritis

C. membranous glomerulonephritis

D. minimal change disease

Item 259

A 14-year-old adolescent boy is brought for a follow up visit. He went to an urgent care center last night with severe chest pain that occurred while playing soccer. He reports that he was running at full speed and had a sudden onset of sharp substernal pain that caused him to stop running to catch his breath. After resting for 10 minutes, he began to feel better. By the time he got to the urgent care center, the pain had resolved and he was told to follow up with his pediatrician. The boy has not felt this pain before. He is otherwise healthy. His vital signs are unremarkable. His lungs are clear, his abdomen is benign, and he has no reproducible chest wall tenderness. A grade 3/6 harsh systolic murmur is noted at the right upper sternal border.

Of the following, the BEST next step is to

A. order chest radiography without exercise restriction

B. order an exercise stress test with exercise restriction

C. order pulmonary function testing without exercise restriction

D. refer to a pediatric cardiologist with exercise restriction

Item 260

A 14-year-old adolescent girl is referred for evaluation of lower abdominal pain. She had menarche at 12 years of age. She initially had 1 period every 2 to 3 months, but for the past year she has had regular monthly periods accompanied by severe lower abdominal pain for the first 2 days that has had minimal response to ibuprofen. She misses 1 day of school monthly because of abdominal pain, nausea, and diarrhea. Her mother has a history of endometriosis. The girl has never been sexually active.

Of the following, the MOST likely diagnosis is

A. endometriosis

B. irritable bowel syndrome

C. ovarian cyst

D. primary dysmenorrhea

Item 261

A previously healthy 12-month-old boy is brought to the emergency department (ED) with a 2-day history of high fever, progressive irritability, poor feeding, and lethargy. His medical history is unremarkable. He was born at full term, has no drug allergies, and is fully immunized. On arrival in the ED, his vital signs are as follows: temperature, 40.5°C; heart rate, 180 beats/min; respiratory rate, 50 breaths/min; and blood pressure, 70/45 mm Hg. Pulse oximetry is 100% on room air. He has a generally toxic and lethargic appearance. With noxious stimulation, he opens his eyes, tries to move the examiner's hands away, and cries. Cough and gag reflexes are intact. His lungs are clear to auscultation, heart sounds are normal, and capillary refill time is 4 seconds. There are no rashes. A peripheral intravenous catheter is placed, and three 20 mL/kg boluses of normal saline are administered. Results of a lumbar puncture show 500 nucleated cells/µL, protein of 120 mg/dL, and glucose of 30 mg/dL (1.6 mmol/L).

Gram staining shows gram-positive cocci in pairs and chains. Serum electrolytes and renal function test results are normal. He is started on vancomycin 15 mg/kg intravenously every 6 hours and ceftriaxone 50 mg/kg intravenously every 12 hours. Vancomycin levels drawn immediately before and 1 hour after the second dose were 5.5 µg/mL and 15.6 µg/mL, respectively. The infectious disease service recommended steady state trough vancomycin levels in the 10- to 15-µg/mL range and peak levels in the 25- to 40-µg/mL range.

Of the following, the BEST next step in management of this boy's infection is to

A. administer dexamethasone 0.15 mg/kg intravenously every 6 hours

B. change the vancomycin interval to every 4 hours

C. continue the current antibiotic regimen

D. increase the vancomycin dose to 20 mg/kg

Item 262

A 5-year-old boy is being evaluated for right ear drainage that began 1 month ago. At that time, he was seen at an urgent care clinic and diagnosed with "swimmer's ear," for which he was treated with antibiotic otic drops 3 times daily for 7 days. The drainage has continued. He reports no pain, fever, or subjective hearing loss. He appears well and has age-appropriate vital signs. His right tympanic membrane is shown (Item Q262). The remainder of his examination findings are normal.

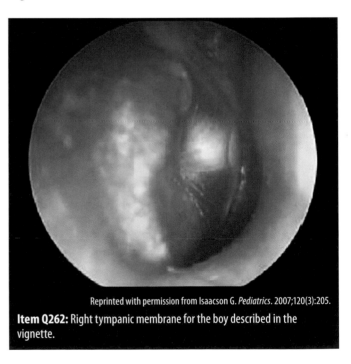

Reprinted with permission from Isaacson G. *Pediatrics*. 2007;120(3):205.

Item Q262: Right tympanic membrane for the boy described in the vignette.

Of the following, the MOST appropriate next step(s) is (are)

A. antibiotic-corticosteroid otic drops

B. oral antibiotics

C. reassurance and follow-up examination

D. referral to an otolaryngologist

Item 263

A 16-year-old adolescent with a history of acute myeloid leukemia was exposed to a cousin staying in the same household who developed a febrile illness and a varicella rash 1 day later. The exposure occurred 1 day before his cousin's illness. Six months ago, the patient received a matched, unrelated hematopoietic stem cell transplant. His posttransplant course was complicated by cutaneous chronic graft-vs-host disease treated with tacrolimus and corticosteroids, but he is currently not receiving any immunosuppressive therapy. Before transplantation, a serologic test for varicella zoster virus was negative, but he had received 2 doses of varicella vaccine at age 12 months and 5 years. The patient currently appears well and has normal physical examination findings.

Of the following, the MOST appropriate next management step for this patient is to administer

A. acyclovir

B. valacyclovir

C. varicella vaccine

D. varicella-zoster immune globulin

Item 264

A 10-year-old girl has new-onset wheezing. She has had both seasonal and perennial upper respiratory allergy symptoms since 6 years of age and wheezing with viral respiratory infections for the last 2 years. In the past, her wheezing has been easily controlled with inhaled albuterol. However, in the last 6 weeks she has had persistent wheezing with poor response to her albuterol inhaler. Her symptoms have been particularly bad at night, interrupting her sleep and waking her parents. Her mother reports that when they went away for a week to visit relatives, she had no wheezing, but the wheezing returned when they came home. She got a new cat about 2 months ago, but the cat does not go into the bedrooms. The girl has itchy, watery eyes and sneezing when she holds the cat.

She appears healthy and in no distress. Her vital signs are normal, and her growth parameters are at the 30th percentile. She has Dennie's lines and dark circles under her eyes in addition to a transverse nasal crease. The nasal mucosa is edematous, and the nasal airway is narrowed but not obstructed. She breathes primarily through her mouth. The oropharynx is clear. She has no increased work of breathing but scattered wheezes on forced expiration. The remainder of the physical examination findings are normal.

The MOST likely explanation for this girl's nocturnal wheezing is

A. delayed IgE-mediated response to cat dander

B. drying of respiratory mucosa from mouth breathing

C. immediate IgG-mediated response to house dust mites

D. rebound bronchoconstriction from albuterol inhaler overuse

Item 265

A 38-week-gestation female neonate is being evaluated in the full-term nursery. She was born 6 hours ago to a 36-year-old woman with a history of chronic hypertension. Her membranes ruptured 22 hours before delivery and she developed a fever of 39.5°C 2 hours before delivery. The mother's laboratory results are significant for group B *Streptococcus*–positive status and a white blood cell count of 16,000/μL (16.0×10⁹/L). She did not receive adequate intrapartum antibiotic prophylaxis. The neonate's weight is 2.2 kg, head circumference is 36 cm, and length is 45 cm. Her physical examination findings are unremarkable. She is comfortable in room air with normal work of breathing and normal perfusion.

Of the following, the STRONGEST predictor of this neonate's risk of early-onset infection is

A. birthweight less than 2.5 kg

B. gestational age

C. maternal fever

D. rupture of membranes longer than 18 hours

Item 266

A 9-year-old boy with type 1 diabetes recently had a health supervision visit. His tissue transglutaminase IgA antibody test result is positive. The test was done for screening purposes, given the increased prevalence of celiac disease in individuals with type 1 diabetes (5%). He has no signs or symptoms of celiac disease. Given a sensitivity of 96% and specificity of 97% of the tissue transglutaminase IgA antibody test, the likelihood ratio (sensitivity/[100-specificity]) for a positive test can be calculated as 32.

Based on this information, of the following you can BEST conclude that

A. the boy has celiac disease

B. the boy is now 32 times more likely to have celiac disease

C. the posttest probability of celiac disease can be determined by using the Fagan nomogram

D. the posttest probability of celiac disease would be the same if he did not have type 1 diabetes

Item 267

A 16-year-old boy has increasing episodes of anxiety, depression, apathy, irritability, mild cognitive decline, clumsiness, and jerking of his arms, legs, and face over the last year. His mother is concerned because the boy's father, who is currently 40 years old, had similar issues; his symptoms have now progressed to dystonia, severe writhing movements, unsteadiness, bradykinesia, rigidity, and moderate cognitive decline. The boy's paternal grandmother died after a similar progression of symptoms. She was ultimately confined to a wheelchair with an inability to speak or eat.

On physical examination, the boy is nondysmorphic. There is no hepatosplenomegaly. His examination is remarkable for slender extremities, with intermittent jerking movements, difficulty with extraocular movements, and poor balance on tandem gait analysis.

Of the following, given this boy's clinical symptoms and family history, his MOST likely diagnosis is

A. Duchenne muscular dystrophy

B. Huntington disease

C. Parkinson disease

D. spinal muscular atrophy

Item 268

A healthy 5-year-old girl is seen for a health supervision visit. Her mother is 38 weeks' pregnant and mentions that she is planning to deliver the new baby at home with a midwife. Her 5-year-old daughter was born full-term in a hospital and was observed in the neonatal intensive care unit for 2 days because of hypoglycemia. The mother has another child who was born at 32 weeks' gestation and spent 6 weeks in the neonatal intensive care unit. The mother has had one urinary tract infection during this pregnancy but reports no other pregnancy-related risk factors (eg, gestational diabetes, group B *Streptococcus* positivity). Her blood type is AB-positive. She inquires about post-birth follow-up care for the new baby.

Of the following, the MOST appropriate plan is to

A. arrange for a nurse visit to check the neonate's weight and a session with the lactation consultant between 24 and 48 hours after birth

B. arrange for serum glucose and bilirubin testing at 24 hours of age

C. instruct the mother to have the neonate seen by her pediatrician between 24 and 48 hours after birth to perform the newborn screen and screen for cyanotic congenital heart defects

D. instruct the mother to have the neonate seen by her pediatrician within 24 hours after birth to assess for dehydration, feeding problems, and hyperbilirubinemia

Item 269

A 2-month-old female infant is seen for a health supervision visit. She was diagnosed with sickle cell disease through newborn screening, followed by confirmatory testing by a hematologist at 3 weeks of age. Prophylactic penicillin was begun at the hematology visit. She is feeding and voiding well. Her mother does not have any concerns at today's visit. The infant has a temperature of 37.1°C, weight of 5.4 kg (75th percentile), length of 55 cm (25th percentile), and occipito-frontal circumference of 38.5 cm (50%). The spleen is not palpable. The remainder of the examination findings are unremarkable.

In addition to routine immunizations, the BEST plan for meningococcal vaccination in this patient is

A. conjugate vaccine at 11 years of age

B. conjugate vaccine today

C. serogroup B vaccine at 2 years of age

D. serogroup B vaccine today

Item 270

A 7-year-old girl sustained a tibia fracture during a family vacation. She was seen in an emergency department, placed in a hard splint, and instructed to use crutches to avoid weight bearing. She has a follow-up visit scheduled with an orthopaedic physician in 3 days. Over the past few hours, the girl has become very distressed. Her father calls the office stating that his daughter reports increased pain, despite taking the prescribed acetaminophen and hydrocodone suspension. The girl denies numbness or tingling in the foot. Her toes are visible, and the father states that they appear "normal."

Of the following, the MOST appropriate recommendation regarding this girl's care is to

A. add ibuprofen to the girl's current regimen of pain medications

B. apply ice packs to the foot over the splint

C. call the orthopaedic clinic and arrange for an outpatient visit in the next 24 hours

D. loosen the splint and take the girl to an emergency department immediately

Item 271

A neighborhood parent group is attending a presentation about general health, nutrition, and exercise for middle school-aged children. The school is located in a large urban area with few neighborhood parks. When it is suggested that bicycling together is a great form of family exercise, a concerned mother responds that she is afraid to allow her children to ride their bikes in the neighborhood due to the vehicular traffic. There is a lot of traffic on the residential streets, the intersections are very busy, there are no designated bike paths, and the sidewalks are heavily used by pedestrians. She asks for a recommendation about the safest way to ride bikes in this setting.

Of the following, the BEST recommendation in this setting is to ride

A. in the street against the vehicular traffic flow

B. in the street with the vehicular traffic flow

C. on the grass along the sidewalk

D. on the sidewalk

Item 272

A 17-year-old adolescent is seen for evaluation of a mildly pruritic rash on his chest and back that developed over the last 2 weeks. He is well in other respects and takes no medications. His temperature is 37°C, and other vital signs are normal. There are hypopigmented macules and patches on his chest and back (Item Q272).

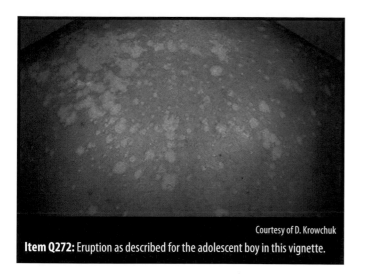

Courtesy of D. Krowchuk

Item Q272: Eruption as described for the adolescent boy in this vignette.

Of the following, the MOST appropriate initial treatment is

A. ammonium lactate topically
B. ketoconazole orally
C. minocycline orally
D. selenium sulfide topically

Item 273

A 3-month-old male infant is brought to the emergency department for vomiting that began 10 hours ago. Initially the emesis resembled formula, however over the last few hours his parents have noticed light-brown emesis. Although he has been more irritable than usual over the last day, he is now quiet and sleepy. His medical history is significant for heterotaxy syndrome, which was diagnosed prenatally, as well as gestational diabetes and maternal tobacco smoke exposure. He was born via spontaneous vaginal delivery at 39 weeks' gestation. His postnatal course was remarkable for diagnosis of a small ventricular septal defect, and he was discharged to home 5 days after birth. The infant currently appears lethargic. He has a temperature of 39.3°C and heart rate of 190 beats/min. His abdomen is distended and tender to touch. His extremities are warm, and he has a 7-mm hemangioma on his right arm. There is concern for bowel obstruction caused by midgut volvulus.

Of the following, the component of this infant's history that is MOST likely to be associated with his current condition is

A. gestational diabetes
B. heterotaxy syndrome
C. infantile hemangioma
D. maternal tobacco smoke exposure

Item 274

A 12-year-old boy is seen for a health supervision visit. His father is concerned about his poor grades in school and his lack of respect. When interviewed alone, the boy reports that his father is controlling and expects him to immediately obey his commands. He feels that he cannot do anything right and discloses that he has been using marijuana. There is concern regarding his risk for developing a substance use disorder.

Of the following, the factor from the boy's history MOST predictive of his developing this disorder is

A. academic failure
B. authoritarian parenting
C. early drug use
D. low self-esteem

Item 275

A 17-year-old adolescent girl is seen for a routine health supervision visit. She reports that she plans to attend a tanning salon prior to prom and summer vacation. Anticipatory guidance regarding tanning beds is provided.

Of the following, she is MOST likely to be counseled that this exposure

A. could provide sufficient vitamin D with brief exposure
B. may cause cataracts with long-term use
C. primarily emits ultraviolet B rays, which damage skin cells
D. would be acceptable if using sunscreen with a sun protection factor rating of at least 50

Item 276

A 4-month-old girl is being evaluated at a health supervision visit. She was born at term, and had no medical problems. Her parents report that the girl's head "wobbles" a lot, and she does not roll or push herself up when prone. She babbles, smiles at her parents, and tracks objects closely with her eyes. Her growth has been tracking along the 10th percentile in length, weight, and occipital frontal head circumference. Physical examination shows an alert infant who is lying on her back with a frog-leg posture. With inspiration her abdomen is distended. She smiles responsively, tracks faces, and her facial movements are symmetric and appear to be full strength. Her tongue has a trembling appearance. Her arms and legs are hypotonic, with a small amount of spontaneous movement. No deep tendon reflexes are elicited.

Of the following, the girl's MOST likely diagnosis is

A. cerebral palsy
B. congenital muscular dystrophy
C. infant botulism
D. spinal muscular atrophy

Item 277

A 2-year-old boy is brought to the emergency department because of refusal to bear weight on his right leg. His parents report that he began limping 4 days ago and that the limping has gotten progressively worse. His parents also report that he bruises very easily and that he had prolonged bleeding after circumcision as a newborn. There has been no known trauma to the leg. He has been afebrile.

He has a temperature of 36.7°C, heart rate of 130 beats/min, and blood pressure of 90/50 mm Hg. He appears pale. He refuses to bear weight on his right leg, and there is a fullness on palpation of the upper inner thigh. His right leg is flexed, and he experiences pain on flexion, extension, and external and internal rotation of the right hip. Ultrasonography of the right hip shows a large iliopsoas hematoma.

Of the following, the laboratory value MOST likely to be abnormal in this patient is

A. factor XIII level

B. partial thromboplastin time

C. platelet count

D. prothrombin time

Item 278

A 16-year-old girl is transported to the emergency department (ED) by Emergency Medical Services after her mother found her to be minimally responsive at home. The mother reports that the girl has been "devastated" over the past 2 weeks since a close friend died of suicide. When the patient did not come out of her room for breakfast this morning, the mother checked on her and could not get her daughter to awaken. She found a note in the girl's room expressing suicidal intent.

On arrival at the ED, the girl's vital signs include a temperature of 37.8°C, heart rate of 135 beats/min, respiratory rate of 14 breaths/min, blood pressure of 78/50 mm Hg, and oxygen saturation of 93% on room air. She does not respond to verbal stimuli, and responds only minimally as 2 peripheral intravenous catheters and a urinary catheter are placed. Her skin is dry and flushed. Her pupils are 4 mm in size with sluggish reactivity. You note no signs of traumatic injury. Electrocardiography reveals sinus tachycardia with broadening of the QRS complex (120 msec). On further questioning, the patient's mother states that many medications are accessible at home, because 2 elderly grandparents who take multiple medications live with the family.

Of the following, the MOST likely cause of this girl's presentation is

A. amitriptyline

B. clonidine

C. iron sulfate

D. metformin

Item 279

A 3-year-old girl is at a health supervision visit. The girl was diagnosed with bilateral grade IV vesicoureteral reflux after a urinary tract infection 6 months ago. The girl has been otherwise healthy, with normal growth parameters and development. She has been toilet trained since age 2 years. Her physical examination findings are normal. Urinalysis shows a specific gravity of 1.020, pH of 6.0, and no protein, blood, leukocyte esterase, or nitrites.

Of the following, it is MOST likely that in this disorder

A. antibiotic prophylaxis can be stopped after 1 year without urinary tract infection

B. bladder and bowel dysfunction is uncommon

C. the primary form is uncommon in children

D. spontaneous resolution is unlikely

Item 280

A 3-day-old neonate born at 28 weeks' gestation has a patent ductus arteriosus that was identified by echocardiography. The ductus is reported to have left-to-right (aorta-to-pulmonary artery) blood flow. The neonate is currently supported with continuous positive airway pressure of +5 on 21% FiO_2 and full enteral feeds. The neonate just completed a 48-hour course of antibiotics.

Of the following, the BEST management for this neonate at this time is to

A. administer indomethacin

B. monitor

C. refer for surgical ligation

D. repeat echocardiography in 48 hours

Item 281

A 17-year-old adolescent girl is seen for a health supervision visit. She was diagnosed with systemic lupus erythematosus 1 year ago after developing a rash on her chest. She has no kidney involvement. She is being treated with methotrexate, prednisone, and hydroxychloroquine. During a HEADSS (home and environment; education and eating; activities; drugs; sexuality; suicide, depression, and safety) examination, with her mother out of the room, she mentions that she takes her prednisone intermittently because she does not like that she has been gaining weight and thinks her face looks more round than usual. She has not discussed this issue with her rheumatologist. There is concern that her nonadherence with the prescribed medication regimen may cause a flare of her lupus.

Of the following, the BEST next step in the management of this patient is to

A. disclose to her mother that she is not being adherent with one of her medications

B. discuss the benefits of being adherent and that many medication adverse effects are temporary

C. refer her to a psychiatrist for evaluation of depression and start of antidepressant medication

D. use motivational interviewing to engage her in becoming more adherent with taking her medication

Item 282

A 15-year-old, previously healthy girl presents to the emergency department (ED) with altered mental status. She had gone to sleep the previous night within her usual routine, but did not wake up for school in the morning. Attempts by her mother to arouse her were unsuccessful, so she drove her to the ED. No fever, loss of appetite, exercise intolerance, fatigue, or mental health problems are reported. The girl is fully immunized, and has no known drug allergies. She does not take any medications, and her mother does not think there are any medications in the house. She is a straight A student who plays basketball, volleyball, and the violin. To her mother's knowledge, the girl does not go to parties, has not been dating, and is not sexually active. In the ED, her vital signs are as follows: temperature, 40.2°C; heart rate, 156 beats/minute; respiratory rate, 22 breaths/min; and blood pressure, 150/90 mm Hg. On physical examination, the girl is obtunded, with episodes of agitation including thrashing of the head and all extremities. With painful stimuli, she opens her eyes, moans, and stiffens her upper and lower extremities. Cough and gag reflexes are normal. Her pupils are 8 mm and minimally reactive. Mucous membranes are dry. There is neck stiffness and markedly increased tone of the upper and lower extremities. Deep tendon reflexes are 3/4 throughout. Her breathing is slightly rapid and deep, lungs are clear to auscultation, and her heart sounds are rapid with a grade II/VI systolic ejection murmur. Her abdomen is soft, nontender, and nondistended, extremities are warm with flash capillary refill, and her skin is diffusely erythematous with no rashes. You administer empiric antibiotic therapy.

Of the following, the BEST next step in management is intravenous

A. fomepizole

B. haloperidol

C. lorazepam

D. naloxone

Item 283

A 15-month-old black girl is evaluated for "bowing" of her legs. She was born at term and has been healthy. She was exclusively breastfed until 6 months of age, and since then continues to breastfeed and eat a variety of family foods. She has never taken any vitamins or medications. She is not yet walking alone, but is cruising. Her height and weight are in the 5th percentile for age, and her head circumference is in the 25th percentile for age. Her physical examination findings are remarkable only for bilateral, symmetric genu varum. A radiograph of her knees is shown (Item Q283). She has low levels of calcium, phosphorus, and 25-hydroxyvitamin D. She has elevated parathyroid hormone and alkaline phosphatase levels.

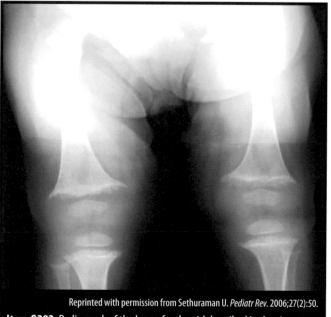

Reprinted with permission from Sethuraman U. *Pediatr Rev.* 2006;27(2):50.

Item Q283: Radiograph of the knees for the girl described in the vignette.

Of the following, the girl's MOST accurate diagnosis is

A. 1α-hydroxylase deficiency (vitamin D–dependent rickets type 1)

B. hereditary resistance to vitamin D (vitamin D–dependent rickets type 2)

C. hypophosphatemic rickets

D. vitamin D–deficient rickets

Item 284

A 4-year-old previously healthy, unimmunized Alaskan native girl is brought to the emergency department with a 1-day history of fever and a 4-hour history of drooling and respiratory distress. There are no sick contacts, no pets at home, and no recent travel. She has not received routine childhood vaccinations for philosophical reasons. She appears ill and has a temperature of 40°C, heart rate of 126 beats/min, and a respiratory rate of 32 breaths/min. Her blood pressure is normal. There is inspiratory stridor. The remainder of the physical examination findings are unremarkable. She is evaluated by an otolaryngologist and then undergoes urgent intubation in the operating room (Item Q284).

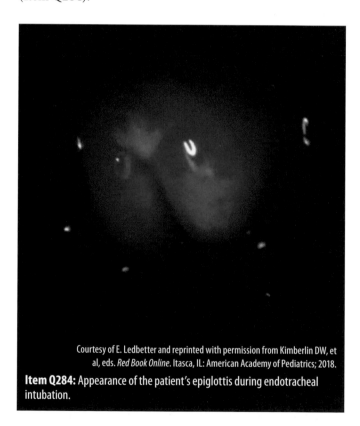

Courtesy of E. Ledbetter and reprinted with permission from Kimberlin DW, et al, eds. *Red Book Online.* Itasca, IL: American Academy of Pediatrics; 2018.

Item Q284: Appearance of the patient's epiglottis during endotracheal intubation.

Of the following, the BEST initial antimicrobial treatment is

A. ampicillin

B. ceftriaxone

C. clindamycin

D. vancomycin

Item 285

A 7-week-old premature female infant is currently admitted to the neonatal intensive care unit. She was born at 27 weeks' gestation because of placental abruption. Her early hospital course was notable for mild respiratory distress and anemia. By 6 weeks after birth, she was stable on room air and was tolerating 100% of caloric needs by enteral feeds of expressed breast milk, 70% delivered via nasogastric tube and 30% delivered by bottle. Yesterday, she developed fever, coffee-ground nasogastric output, and hypotension. Her abdominal examination showed distention. An abdominal radiograph demonstrated pneumatosis, and she was diagnosed with necrotizing enterocolitis. She was started on broad-spectrum antibiotics. Although her vital signs are now stable, a repeat abdominal radiograph today demonstrates persistent pneumatosis.

Of the following, the method of nutritional support that is MOST appropriate for this patient is

A. expressed breast milk via nasogastric tube
B. expressed breast milk via nasojejunal tube
C. peripheral parenteral nutrition
D. total parenteral nutrition

Item 286

An 8-day-old full-term neonate is being evaluated at an initial visit. She was delivered vaginally at home by her mother's friend, who is studying to be a midwife. Her 19-year-old mother has no significant medical history. She received limited prenatal care. The neonate has been breastfeeding well, with 2 to 3 wet diapers and multiple stools daily. Her mother says the girl's eyelashes on both eyes have been crusty. On physical examination, a clear discharge is noted from both eyes with mild conjunctival erythema.

Of the following, this neonate's MOST likely condition could have been prevented by

A. avoidance of perfumed baby shampoo
B. gentle massage of both nasal lacrimal ducts downward
C. ocular application of 0.5% erythromycin ointment
D. saline irrigation of the eyes

Item 287

A 15-year-old adolescent boy is seen for a sports pre-participation examination prior to starting cross-country track. He is concerned that his puberty is not progressing normally. His medical history is significant only for right orchidopexy at the age of 10 months. There is no family history of delayed puberty. A comprehensive review of systems is significant for the inability to smell strong odors. He runs an average of 10 miles per week. He has a blood pressure of 102/64 mm Hg and a heart rate of 68 beats/min. His weight is at the 25th percentile, height is at the 50th percentile, and body mass index is at the 20th percentile. His sexual maturity rating is grade 3 for pubic hair and grade 1 for genital development. He does not have axillary hair or facial hair. The remainder of his physical examination findings are unremarkable.

Of the following, the MOST likely diagnosis is

A. constitutional delay of puberty
B. functional hypogonadism
C. Kallmann syndrome
D. Klinefelter syndrome

Item 288

Newborn screening in a 4-day-old female neonate detects hyperphenylalaninemia. A pediatric metabolic specialist is consulted to obtain recommendations. The specialist recommends implementation of a phenylalanine-free diet and laboratory studies to include red blood cell dihydropteridine reductase assay and urine pterin analysis.

Of the following, ADDITIONAL supportive laboratory testing for the suspected diagnosis would include

A. serum amino acids
B. serum ammonia
C. urine succinylacetone
D. very-long-chain fatty acids

Item 289

An 18-month-old boy is seen for evaluation of a rash. He has a health supervision visit scheduled in 2 weeks. After the rash is evaluated, his mother asks if her son seems to be developing normally. She is especially worried because a friend's child the same age as her son was recently diagnosed with autism, and another friend's child recently started receiving therapy for a speech delay.

Of the following, the finding MOST concerning for a developmental delay in this child is if he does not

A. copy a circle
B. name objects pictured in a book
C. point to things that interest him
D. use 2-word phrases

Item 290

A 6-year-old boy is seen for a health supervision visit. His parents express concern that their son is not learning at the same pace as his classmates and that he prefers to play with the younger children on the playground. He occasionally flaps his hands when excited. He is flexible with changes in his routine and is generally eager to please his parents, teacher, and other adults. He eats well and does not become upset with loud noises. He requires assistance with dressing. The boy has a history of expressive and receptive language delay and is receiving speech therapy.

Of the following, the MOST appropriate next step in management is to

A. order electroencephalography and brain magnetic resonance imaging

B. provide the family with a prescription for applied behavioral analysis therapy

C. refer the boy and his family to start early intervention services

D. request a psychoeducational evaluation from the boy's school

Item 291

A previously healthy 13-year-old girl is brought to the emergency department because of altered mental status. She had been complaining of abdominal pain, nausea, and vomiting for 3 days before her presentation. For the past month, she has been drinking water and sports drinks excessively, and has been waking up in the middle of the night to urinate. During the day of admission, she became progressively somnolent, prompting her mother to bring her to the emergency department. On arrival, her temperature is 37.0°C; heart rate is 140 beats/min; respiratory rate is 50 breaths/min, and blood pressure is 100/60 mm Hg. Her oxygen saturation is 100% on room air. On physical examination, she responds to stimuli with moaning and withdrawal of extremities. She opens her eyes to command. Her pupils are 3 mm, equal, and reactive. Her eyes are sunken and her lips are cracked and dry. The girl's gag reflex is intact. Her extremities are cool, with a capillary refill of 3 seconds. Pulses are strong. Laboratory results are as follows:

Laboratory Test	Result
Sodium	124 mEq/L (124 mmol/L)
Potassium	7.0 mEq/L (7.0 mmol/L)
Chloride	100 mEq/L (100 mmol/L)
Bicarbonate	5 mEq/L (5 mmol/L)
Serum urea nitrogen	38 mg/dL (13.5 mmol/L)
Creatinine	1.4 mg/dL (124 μmol/L)
Glucose	1,350 mg/dL (74.9 mmol/L)
Capillary blood gas pH	6.95
Partial pressure of carbon dioxide	14 mmHg (1.8 kPa)
Base deficit	-25

Of the following, the best next management option for this girl is

A. 0.9% sodium chloride bolus, 10 mL/kg intravenously over 1 hour

B. 3% sodium chloride bolus, 5 mL/kg intravenously over 20 minutes

C. to administer intravenous insulin, 0.1 unit/kg

D. to perform rapid sequence endotracheal intubation

2019

PREP® Self-Assessment
Critiques, Images, and Answer Sheet

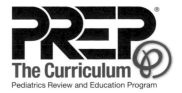

Item 1   Preferred Response: C

The boy in the vignette has diffuse low back pain that does not radiate. He denies systemic symptoms. Physical examination reveals tight hamstring muscles and tenderness over the paraspinal muscles. These features suggest mechanical low back pain. Physical therapy for core stabilization is the next best step in management.

Back pain is fairly common in school-aged children. The prevalence of back pain increases with age, approaching rates seen in adults by late adolescence. Although young people are more likely than adults to have an identifiable cause for their pain, most children with low back pain are diagnosed with mechanical (muscular) low back pain.

In children with a clear anatomic cause of back pain, spondylolysis is most common. Spondylolysis is a crack in the pars interarticularis, the posterior aspect of the vertebral ring. Individuals with spondylolysis typically report pain with extension of the lumbar spine and may experience some local radiation. Participation in sports with repetitive forward and back bending is thought to be a risk factor for the development of spondylolysis. When spondylolysis is bilateral (ie, 2 cracks occur in the same vertebral ring), the vertebral body may shift forward leading to spondylolisthesis.

Radiography is the preferred initial study for suspected spondylolysis. Posterior-anterior and lateral radiographs have a sensitivity of 50% to 60% for spondylolysis; oblique radiographs do not increase either sensitivity or specificity in most studies. Additional evaluation with magnetic resonance imaging (MRI) is indicated when there is a strong clinical suspicion for spondylolysis that is not seen on radiography. Historically, computed tomography (CT) and bone scintigraphy with single-photon emission CT (SPECT) were the preferred studies; however, due to the high radiation exposure with these tests, MRI is now preferred. The boy in the vignette does not have pain during activity or with lumbar extension, so additional evaluation for spondylolysis would not be the best next step.

Magnetic resonance imaging would be useful for identifying other structural conditions such as herniated nucleus pulposus, apophyseal ring fracture, osteoid osteoma, or bone cysts. However, these conditions are unusual causes of back pain in children, and this boy's history and physical examination point to a diagnosis of mechanical low back pain. Therefore, MRI to evaluate for other conditions would be reasonable if his symptoms do not improve with physical therapy. Exercise can be therapeutic for patients with muscular back pain and the boy in the vignette does not have pain during activity so rest from sports and gym class would not be the best treatment.

PREP Pearls

- Back pain is common in children and adolescents. Mechanical (muscular) low back pain is the most likely diagnosis.
- Children and adolescents with spondylolysis typically report back pain with extension.

American Board of Pediatrics Content Specification(s)/Content Area

- Plan the appropriate management of back pain
- Formulate a differential diagnosis of back pain in children of various ages
- Plan the appropriate evaluation of back pain

Suggested Readings

MacDonald J, Stuart E, Rodenberg R. Musculoskeletal low back pain in school-aged children: a review. *JAMA Pediatr.* 2017;171(3):280-287.

Sarwark JF, LaBella CR, ed *Pediatric Orthopaedics and Sports Injuries: A Quick Reference Guide.* 2nd ed. Elk Grove Village, IL: American Academy of Pediatrics; 2014.

Item 2   Preferred Response: A

The situation described in the vignette typifies the vulnerable child syndrome (VCS). The next best step in management is to discuss and address the mother's perception of the child's illness risk. Vulnerable child syndrome was first described in 1964 by Drs Green and Solnit who hypothesized that "parental reactions to an acute, life-threatening illness in a child may have long-term psychologically deleterious effects on both parents and children." The clinical hallmarks of VCS are parental over concern for minor health issues and excessive use of health services. A prior event that instigates parental anxiety, such as the history of hospitalization for bronchiolitis for the boy in this vignette, can often be identified. Parents are frequently perceived as demanding and overprotective, and they may inappropriately use medications. Secondary behavioral problems in the child are common and include separation anxiety, sleep disturbance, somatic complaints, academic underachievement, discipline issues, and aggression toward caregivers.

Families at greatest risk for VCS have predisposing risk factor(s) that may include:

- Environmental: Family stress, low levels of social support, low socioeconomic status, parents who rate their own health as poor
- Parental psychological conditions: Postpartum depression, obsessive-compulsive behavior, anxiety, unresolved grief over the death of a child or family member
- Complicated birth history: Maternal history of fertility problems or previous miscarriages, threatened abortion or health concerns of fetus, prematurity, hyperbilirubinemia, congenital anomalies
- Medical and family history: Preceding serious illness or injury to this child or a sibling, presence of a condition that is benign or resolved but considered serious to the parent (eg, functional heart murmur, colic), known familial or inheritable conditions

The best management approach to VCS is prevention. Clear and direct communication with parents explaining that their past experiences with illness can affect their perception of their child's health can be delivered in an empathetic manner. Clarification of the child's resolved health conditions and reassurance are key to the anticipatory guidance offered to prevent VCS. Regularly scheduled follow-up visits to discuss health concerns and behavioral issues are helpful in these cases. When new concerns arise, a thorough history and physical examination are primary. Extensive laboratory evaluation, radiologic studies, and referral to subspecialists should be avoided unless medically indicated. Based on this boy's medical history and physical examination findings, further laboratory tests to evaluate for an underlying immunodeficiency and referral to a pulmonary specialist for pulmonary function testing are not warranted. Providing an extended school excuse is not medically necessary and would indirectly reinforce the mother's concerns.

PREP Pearls

- Clear and direct communication with parents that past experiences with illness can affect their perception of their child's health is key to preventing vulnerable child syndrome.
- Families at greatest risk for vulnerable child syndrome have predisposing factors that may include environmental conditions, parental psychological conditions, complicated birth history, or a significant medical or family history.
- Secondary behavioral problems in the child and issues with parent-child interactions are common in vulnerable child syndrome.
- The hallmarks of vulnerable child syndrome are parental over concern for minor health issues and excessive use of health services.

American Board of Pediatrics Content Specification(s)/Content Area

- Understand factors predisposing to vulnerable child syndrome
- Provide anticipatory guidance to prevent vulnerable child syndrome

Suggested Readings

Green M, Solnit AJ. Reactions to the threatened loss of a child: a vulnerable child syndrome—pediatric management of the dying child, part III. *Pediatrics*. 1964;34(7):58-66.

Kokotos F. The vulnerable child syndrome. *Pediatr Rev*. 2009:30(5):193-194.

Pearson SR, Boyce WT. Consultation with the specialist: the vulnerable child syndrome. *Pediatr Rev*. 2004;25(10):345-349.

Item 3   Preferred Response: D

The boy in this vignette has exocrine pancreatic insufficiency (EPI) caused by Shwachman-Diamond syndrome, an autosomal recessive condition associated with skeletal abnormalities, neutropenia, and short stature. He has findings of neutropenia and multiple infections, anemia, thrombocytopenia, short stature, and low fecal pancreatic elastase level (indicative of EPI).

The pancreas is an integral organ for fat, carbohydrate, and protein digestion. The pancreas secretes digestive enzymes (lipase, amylase, and protease) in response to nutritional intake. Exocrine pancreatic insufficiency results when lipase secretion is less than 90% to 95% of the expected level and malabsorption occurs. Steatorrhea, excess fat in the stools, is often a presenting sign of EPI and is commonly accompanied by sequelae of fat malabsorption including weight loss, failure to thrive, and fat-soluble vitamin deficiency. In young children, severe and persistent diaper dermatitis may be a sign of fat malabsorption.

The most common cause of EPI in children is cystic fibrosis, which is caused by mutations in the cystic fibrosis transmembrane regulator protein, many of which can result in pancreatic insufficiency. Although EPI from cystic fibrosis can occur at any time in life, most children with EPI present at birth or shortly thereafter. Other causes of EPI include chronic pancreatitis, Johanson-Blizzard syndrome (a rare autosomal recessive disorder associated with hypothyroidism, developmental delay, and other congenital anomalies), and Pearson syndrome (a rare disorder associated with pancreatic fibrosis, severe anemia, and other multiorgan abnormalities).

Management of EPI is through oral pancreatic enzyme replacement therapy (PERT). The PERT dose is dependent on the weight of the child and the amount of fat ingested during a meal or snack. In the United States, the PERT dose is generally 2,000 lipase units/kg/meal and 1,000 lipase units/kg/snack. With PERT, fat absorption improves but is still not equivalent to normal pancreatic function. Fat-soluble vitamin status should be carefully monitored and supplemented appropriately, even if a child is adherent to PERT.

The boy in this vignette has no evidence of chronic pancreatitis; specifically there was no mention of recurrent episodes of abdominal pain and vomiting resulting in hospitalizations. Cystic fibrosis is unlikely given the bone marrow suppression and multiple extrapulmonary infections. A diagnosis of Fanconi anemia would not explain the EPI in this patient.

PREP Pearls

- Exocrine pancreatic insufficiency in children can present as steatorrhea, severe diaper rash, failure to thrive, and/or fat-soluble vitamin deficiency.
- Exocrine pancreatic insufficiency is managed with pancreatic enzyme replacement therapy and supplementation of fat-soluble vitamins.
- While cystic fibrosis is the most common cause of exocrine pancreatic insufficiency in children, other causes include chronic pancreatitis, Shwachman-Diamond syndrome, Pearson syndrome, and Johanson-Blizzard syndrome.

American Board of Pediatrics Content Specification(s)/Content Area

- Understand the etiology of pancreatic insufficiency
- Plan the appropriate management of pancreatic exocrine insufficiency
- Recognize the clinical features associated with pancreatic insufficiency

Suggested Readings

Bitton S, Pettei MJ. Exocrine pancreatic insufficiency. *Pediatr Rev*. 2016;27(2):85-87.

Uc A, Fishman DS. Pancreatic disorders. *Pediatr Clin N Am*. 2017;64(3):685-706.

Aggressive behaviors in children have been associated with prenatal exposure to substances including cocaine, alcohol, and tobacco. Of the answer choices offered, prenatal exposure to cocaine would be the most likely contributing factor for the boy in the vignette. Pediatric aggression may occur when a child who is biologically predisposed to aggression is subject to an environmental stressor. Epigenetic mechanisms are thought to be involved.

Biological factors contributing to the development and maintenance of aggression include the regulation of neurotransmitters and neural pathways. High levels of dopamine, low levels of serotonin, and low levels of GABA (γ-aminobutyric acid) are associated with aggression. Aggression is influenced by the interaction between the prefrontal cortex, which can inhibit actions, and the limbic system, where emotional arousal resides. Traumatic brain injury can result in aggression when the communication between these areas is disrupted. Hormones such as glucocorticoids and sex steroids also mediate aggression. Rapid and high release of cortisol and chronic low basal plasma cortisol levels have both been associated with aggressive behaviors. Rapid increase of testosterone in puberty can lead to behavioral disinhibition and aggression in boys.

Environmental factors contribute to aggressive behaviors. Exposure to violence is associated with aggressive behaviors in children. Harsh parental physical discipline and neighborhood violence portray aggression as an acceptable method for resolving conflicts. Maltreatment and trauma, particularly in the first 2 years of age, encompass negative social interactions that may lead to childhood and then adulthood aggression; these children may not develop appropriate emotional regulation or social skills. An *authoritarian* style of parenting, characterized by a high level of control and low level of warmth (eg, orders and commands given with expectations for obedience) is the parenting style most associated with aggression. Better psychosocial and mental health outcomes are seen with an *authoritative* parenting style, where a high level of control occurs in the setting of a high level of warmth (eg, expectations and rules clearly established with engaging and interactive parents). Indirect exposure to violence such as through media is also associated with aggressive behaviors in children. Additional environmental factors including low socioeconomic status, higher number of siblings, family discord or disruption, poor parental supervision, and peer rejection are related to aggression in children.

Aggression is more common in children with mental health conditions such as mood disorders (eg, posttraumatic stress disorder, depression, bipolar disorder) and disruptive behavior disorders (eg, oppositional defiant disorder, conduct disorder). Substance abuse (eg, alcohol, cocaine, methamphetamine) is associated with aggression. Children who have anxiety may demonstrate reactive aggression when their anxiety is triggered and the child is unable to cope. Children with an autism spectrum disorder may demonstrate aggression, particularly when unable to communicate and when feeling frustrated, anxious, or unwell. Impaired communication abilities as well as high impulsivity and low frustration tolerance can play a part in the high prevalence of aggression in children with genetic syndromes such as fragile X syndrome, Smith-Magenis syndrome, and Prader-Willi syndrome.

Risk factors for violence in children are listed in Item C4. An understanding of the contributors to childhood aggression can help pediatric practitioners to identify patients at highest risk for these behaviors and to address modifiable risk factors (eg, promoting positive parenting skills and interactions).

Item C4. Risk Factors for Pediatric Violence.

Individual	Family	Peer	Community/ Environment
History of aggression	Authoritarian parenting	Bullying	Low socioeconomic status
Mental illness	Inconsistent parenting	Ostracization	Poor school connection or involvement
Intellectual disabilities	Family violence	Gang involvement	Disorganized community
Learning disorders	Low parental involvement	Peer violence	Multiple placements or moves
Active substance abuse	Low parental education	Peer substance abuse	Access to guns
Brain trauma	Parent untreated mental illness or substance abuse		
Genetic syndromes	Criminal activity		
Temperament	Disrupted placement		
Prenatal illicit substance exposure	High family discord		
Early life trauma	Number of siblings		

Reprinted with permission from Austerman J. Violence and aggressive behavior. *Pediatr Rev.* 2017;38(2):74.

PREP Pearls

- Aggression is influenced by the interaction between the prefrontal cortex, which can inhibit actions, and the limbic system, where emotional arousal resides.
- Aggressive behaviors in children have been associated with prenatal exposure to substances including cocaine, alcohol, and tobacco.
- Children who have anxiety may demonstrate reactive aggression when their anxiety is triggered and the child is unable to cope.

American Board of Pediatrics Content Specification(s)/ Content Area

- Recognize the various environmental and biological contributors to the development and maintenance of aggressive behaviors

Suggested Readings

Austerman J. Violence and aggressive behavior. *Pediatr Rev.* 2017;38(2): 69-80.

Hawkins JD, Smith BH, Catalano RF. Delinquent behavior. *Pediatr Rev.* 2002;23(11):387-392.

Zarht DM, Melzer-Lange MD. Aggressive behavior in children and adolescents. *Pediatr Rev.* 2011;32(8):325-331.

Item 5   Preferred Response: B

The girl in the vignette has Guillain-Barré syndrome (GBS). The best next step is to perform a lumbar puncture to obtain a cerebrospinal fluid (CSF) specimen. Typically, the CSF results show cytoalbuminologic dissociation, with a high protein and normal white blood cell count. Early in the course of GBS, CSF studies may be normal.

Guillain-Barré syndrome often occurs after a respiratory or gastrointestinal illness, as described in the vignette. Other risk factors include back surgery, bone marrow transplantation, and trauma. There is a small association between GBS and influenza vaccine; for every million persons receiving the influenza vaccine between 1992 and 1994, there was 1 additional case of GBS. Symptoms of GBS include ascending paralysis, low back pain, and distal dysesthesias. The diagnosis is made clinically, with ancillary studies providing supporting evidence and ruling out other disorders. Cerebrospinal fluid white blood cells more than 50 per high-power field should prompt a search for concurrent infection. Magnetic resonance imaging of the lumbar spine with and without contrast may show nerve root enhancement, but can be normal in GBS. Electromyography and nerve conduction studies can confirm the presence of a neuropathy and determine whether there is demyelinating or axonal injury. Some or all of these tests can be performed when making a diagnosis of GBS, depending on the clinical situation and test availability. Treatment for pediatric GBS is typically intravenous immunoglobulin. Supportive care required for GBS includes close monitoring for progression of weakness, especially of the respiratory muscles, and monitoring for evidence of dysautonomia including cardiac arrhythmias, hypertension, bladder dysfunction, and ileus.

Creatine kinase is not recommended because the level would be elevated in a disorder of the muscles, such as influenza myositis, which can cause severe calf myalgias and distal weakness because of pain. Although the girl in the vignette had a prodromal respiratory illness and presents with distal lower extremity weakness, she does not have myalgias, and she has additional sensory symptoms that are more suggestive of a disorder of the nerves. Because the girl in the vignette most likely has GBS, she needs inpatient admission for treatment and clinical monitoring. Solely providing reassurance is not the best next step. Treatment for GBS is intravenous immunoglobulin; intravenous methylprednisolone is not indicated.

PREP Pearls

- Patients with Guillain-Barré syndrome should be monitored closely for progression of weakness, especially involving the muscles of respiration, and for dysautonomia.
- Risk factors for Guillain-Barré syndrome include antecedent respiratory or gastrointestinal infection, back surgery, and bone marrow transplantation. There is a very small association between influenza vaccine and Guillain-Barré syndrome.
- Treatment for Guillain-Barré syndrome is intravenous immunoglobulin.

American Board of Pediatrics Content Specification(s)/ Content Area

- Recognize risk factors associated with Guillain-Barré syndrome
- Plan the appropriate diagnostic evaluation of Guillain-Barré syndrome, and manage appropriately

Suggested Readings

Korinthenberg R, Schessl J, Kirschner J. Clinical presentation and course of childhood Guillain-Barré syndrome: a prospective multicentre study. *Neuropediatrics.* 2007;38(1):10-17.

Rosen BA. Guillain-Barré syndrome. *Pediatr Rev.* 2012;33(4):164-171.

Item 6   Preferred Response: C

The boy in this vignette has chronic urticaria, which is defined as the presence of hives, with or without angioedema, for 6 weeks or longer. The vignette describes hives with angioedema, defined as episodic submucosal swelling that affects nondependent parts of the body without pitting. Angioedema may develop within a period of minutes to hours. While acute urticaria and angioedema may result from IgE-mediated allergic reactions, no external allergic cause can be identified in 80% to 90% of children affected by chronic urticaria. In contrast, chronic urticaria is associated with various autoimmune disorders. Thyroid disease is the most common specific autoimmune disease associated with chronic urticaria. Additional symptoms related to a thyroid disorder may include weight changes or heat/cold intolerance.

While a specific etiology is rarely found for chronic urticaria, every effort should be made to determine a cause for these symptoms. A detailed history and physical examination form the basis of the initial evaluation. The history should focus on signs and symptoms associated with cutaneous lesions, including duration of lesions and associated angioedema. Chronic urticaria skin lesions are typically well-circumscribed, raised, erythematous papules/plaques, often with central pallor, transient (lasting a few hours to 24 hours), pruritic, and present for 6 weeks or longer.

Several practice parameters have been published for the diagnosis of chronic urticaria. While routine laboratory studies rarely reveal abnormalities if a history is not suggestive of an underlying etiology, initial recommended laboratory evaluation includes a complete blood cell count with differential, markers of inflammation (either erythrocyte sedimentation rate or C-reactive protein), and thyroid-stimulating hormone level. Standard treatment is aimed at supportive care as symptoms may last years, though chronic urticaria is typically self-limited and episodic. H1 antihistamines, sometimes in higher than usual doses, serve as first-line treatment in combination with H2 antihistamines and leukotriene modifiers. Systemic glucocorticoids in short courses may be needed to treat severe exacerbations.

To exclude specific etiologies, the evaluation should also focus on new drugs (eg, nonsteroidal anti-inflammatory drugs or antibiotics), recent travel, infections, atopic conditions, and a complete review of symptoms. Systemic symptoms such as fever, weight loss, or arthritis/arthralgias may be suggestive of systemic lupus erythematosus or another rheumatoid disorder, such as juvenile idiopathic arthritis, for which an evaluation might also include antinuclear antibodies, complement levels, and rheumatoid factor. Gastrointestinal symptoms, such as weight loss, recurrent abdominal pain, vomiting, persistent diarrhea, or chronic constipation should prompt consideration of celiac disease, for which evaluation would include tissue transglutaminase antibodies. While many patients with chronic urticaria perceive food-associated reactions, food allergies are rarely identified as an etiology, and allergy testing is not usually warranted.

PREP Pearls

- Chronic urticaria is defined as the presence of hives, with or without angioedema, for a period of 6 weeks or longer.
- Laboratory evaluation for the etiology of chronic urticaria should include an evaluation of the thyroid-stimulating hormone level.
- Thyroid disease is the most common specific autoimmune disease associated with chronic urticaria in children.

American Board of Pediatrics Content Specification(s)/Content Area

- Identify the etiologic agents that commonly cause urticaria, angioedema, and/or anaphylaxis
- Recognize the signs and symptoms of chronic urticaria, and manage appropriately

Suggested Readings

Confino-Cohen R, Chodick G, Shalev V, Leshno M, Kimhi O, Goldberg A. Chronic urticaria and autoimmunity: associations found in a large population study. *J Allergy Clin Immunol.* 2012;129(5):1307.

Joint Task Force on Practice Parameters. The diagnosis and management of urticaria: a practice parameter, part II: chronic urticaria/angioedema. *Ann Allergy Asthma Immunol.* 2000;85(6 pt 2):S521-S544.

Langley EW, Gigante J. Anaphylaxis, urticaria, and angioedema. *Pediatr Rev.* 2013;34(6):247-257.

Item 7 (PBLI) **Preferred Response: D**

The child in this vignette has symptomatic, severe anemia and a marked reticulocytosis. A schematic approach to developing a differential diagnosis for anemia is shown in Item C7. The reticulocytosis indicates that increased destruction of red cells (hemolysis) is the pathophysiologic cause of the anemia. Although the results of a direct antibody test are not reported in the vignette, factors in the child's history suggest that he is experiencing hemolysis caused by glucose-6-phosphate dehydrogenase (G6PD) deficiency, an X-linked red cell enzymopathy. These factors include his African American ethnicity, the acute onset of the illness, the association with trimethoprim-sulfamethoxazole, and the blister cells on the peripheral smear.

A mutation in *G6PD* on band Xq28 results in G6PD deficiency. Although there are more than 150 allelic mutations, 2 main variants are prevalent in the United States: G6PD A- and G6PD Mediterranean. The G6PD A- variant affects 10% of African American males, and the G6PD Mediterranean variant affects Americans of Middle Eastern descent. The G6PD enzyme is part of the pentose phosphate pathway. When there is inadequate cellular G6PD, there is reduced thiol glutathione and increased susceptibility to oxidative stress leading to hemolysis. While all cells in the body are affected in a G6PD-deficient state, the erythrocyte is particularly sensitive to oxidative stress.

The World Health Organization classifies G6PD deficiency based on severity of the enzyme deficiency and degree of hemolysis into classes I to V, with class I being the most severe. The G6PD A- variant is a class III variant, which most often presents with mild to moderate hemolysis only when the patient is exposed to certain triggers, including foods such as the fava bean and medications such as sulfa-based antibiotics and antimalarials. Blister cells and polychromatic macrocytes on a peripheral blood smear are hallmarks of G6PD deficiency–associated hemolysis.

Hemolysis associated with G6PD deficiency is managed symptomatically. There is no treatment, other than packed red blood cell support as needed for severe, life-threatening anemia and avoidance of substances that can trigger a hemolytic event. A critical part of the management of this child will be to educate his parents on foods and medications to avoid.

Although autoimmune hemolytic anemia, membranopathies, and hemoglobinopathies can lead to hemolysis and an elevated reticulocyte count, the history, physical examination findings, and peripheral blood smear findings described in this vignette are most consistent with G6PD deficiency.

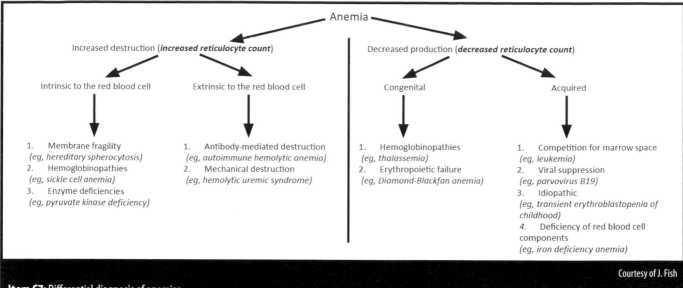

Item C7: Differential diagnosis of anemias.

Courtesy of J. Fish

PREP Pearls

- Although there are many variants of glucose-6-phosphate dehydrogenase deficiency, 2 variants are the most prevalent in the United States, with the A- variant affecting 10% of African American males.

- Glucose-6-phosphate dehydrogenase deficiency is an X-linked condition resulting in an ineffective response to intracellular oxidative stress. Erythrocytes are particularly sensitive and undergo hemolysis.

- Patients with glucose-6-phosphate deficiency should avoid specific medications and foods that induce increased oxidative stress.

American Board of Pediatrics Content Specification(s)/Content Area

- Recognize the inheritance pattern associated with G6PD deficiency
- Plan appropriate management of hemolysis in a patient with G6PD deficiency
- Recognize the clinical findings associated with G6PD deficiency in patients of differing ethnic backgrounds

Suggested Readings

Cappellini MD, Fiorelli G. Glucose-6-phosphate dehydrogenase deficiency. *Lancet.* 2008;371(9606):64-74.

Haley K. Congenital hemolytic anemia. *Med Clin North Am.* 2017;101(2):361-374.

Noronha SA. Acquired and congenital hemolytic anemia. *Pediatr Rev.* 2016;37(6):235-246.

Item 8   Preferred Response: A

The girl in the vignette has significant pain and distress secondary to a displaced femur fracture as well as numerous unsuccessful attempts to secure intravenous access. The best next step in management is to provide intranasal fentanyl for pain.

Acute pain affects many children, arising as a result of injury, illness, and/or necessary medical procedures. However, it is often inadequately assessed and treated. It is imperative that pediatric providers understand the appropriate use of pharmacologic and nonpharmacologic pain management modalities.

To provide guidance to practitioners, the American Academy of Pediatrics Committee on Pediatric Emergency Medicine and the Section on Anesthesiology and Pain Medicine published a clinical report on relieving pain and anxiety in pediatric patients in Emergency Medical Systems in 2012. This report emphasizes the importance of timely administration of analgesia to children with acute pain and anxiety, because this "affects the entire emergency medical experience and can have a lasting effect on a child's and family's reaction to current and future medical care" (Fein et al).

For children with severe pain who are seen in the emergency department and prehospital settings, optimal pain management requires rapid pain assessment and administration of a systemic opioid pain medication. Administration may occur through various routes, including transmucosal or intravenous. Intranasal fentanyl is a good option for relieving the severe pain experienced by the girl in the vignette. Studies have demonstrated that doses of fentanyl delivered via a transmucosal route have similar analgesic action to intravenous opioids. An advantage of transmucosal analgesics is the ability to provide rapid pain relief without the need for intravenous access.

Oral ibuprofen has been well-studied and shown to be effective in the management of mild to moderate pain for patients with no contraindications to receiving oral medications. However, this option would not be appropriate for the girl in the vignette because of the severity of her injury, high degree of pain and distress, and high likelihood that she will require procedural sedation and surgical intervention in the near future.

Oral sucrose solution has been found to decrease the response to painful stimuli, such as intravenous line insertion, heel stick, and lumbar puncture, in neonates and infants less than 6 months of age. While this option can be useful in reducing distress arising from procedure-related pain in neonates and young infants, it would not adequately address pain in a 2-year-old child with a displaced femur fracture.

Although the use of distraction techniques and other nonpharmacologic modalities can be an important component in helping to relieve anxiety in children and enabling them to better cope with acute pain, using distraction techniques alone would be inadequate for the girl in the vignette. Administration of an appropriate analgesic to this girl should not be delayed, given the severity of her pain and distress as well as the significant transport time anticipated.

PREP Pearls

- For children with severe pain seen in the emergency department and prehospital settings optimal pain management requires rapid pain assessment and administration of a systemic opioid pain medication.
- Timely administration of analgesia to children with acute pain and anxiety is critical, and can affect their reaction to future medical care.
- Transmucosal fentanyl has a similar analgesic action to intravenous opioids, providing rapid pain relief without the need for intravenous access.

American Board of Pediatrics Content Specification(s)/ Content Area

- Understand the appropriate use of pharmacologic pain management modalities
- Understand the appropriate use of nonpharmacologic pain management modalities
- Understand the risks associated with the use of narcotics for pain management

Suggested Readings

AAP Committee on Psychosocial Aspects of Child and Family Health and the Task Force on Pain in Infants, Children, and Adolescents. The assessment and management of acute pain in infants, children, and adolescents. *Pediatrics*. 2001;108(3):793-797.

Fein JA, Zempsky WT, Cravero JP; Committee on Pediatric Emergency Medicine and Section of Anesthesiology and Pain Medicine. Relief of pain and anxiety in pediatric patients in Emergency Medical Services. *Pediatrics*. 2012;130(5):1391-1405.

The most likely diagnosis for the boy in the vignette is hemolytic uremic syndrome (HUS), one of the most common causes of acute renal failure in children. A diagnosis of HUS should be considered in all children presenting with bloody diarrhea. A complete blood cell count (CBC) with review of the peripheral blood smear (PBS) is most likely to reveal the diagnosis for the boy in the vignette. Hemolytic uremic syndrome is characterized by the triad of microangiopathic hemolytic anemia, thrombocytopenia, and acute kidney injury. Enteric infection with organisms such as *Salmonella*, *Campylobacter*, *Yersinia*, amebiasis, or *Clostridium difficile* also present with abdominal pain and bloody diarrhea. Evaluation in such patients may reveal elevated serum creatinine and blood urea nitrogen levels, indicating acute renal failure (prerenal) secondary to dehydration. Patients with Henoch-Schönlein purpura (HSP) may also have similar symptoms in association with a palpable purpuric skin rash. The presence of thrombocytopenia and hemolytic anemia on the CBC and PBS showing schistocytes distinguishes these enteric infections and HSP from HUS.

Thrombocytopenia in HUS is due to consumptive coagulopathy secondary to platelet microthrombi formation triggered by the toxinemia. The presence of schistocytes (up to 10% of total red blood cells [RBC]) and helmet cells on PBS is indicative of mechanical hemolysis. Hemolysis in HUS is non–immune-mediated (direct antiglobulin test [Coombs test] is negative), and is due to RBC fragmentation from platelet microthrombi blocking the small blood vessels. In a patient with bloody diarrhea, the presence of schistocytes on the PBS is diagnostic of HUS.

Hemolytic uremic syndrome is categorized as diarrhea-positive (typical HUS) or diarrhea-negative based on the presence or absence of a diarrheal prodrome. The most common cause of diarrhea-positive HUS is Shiga toxin–producing *Escherichia coli* (STEC). Enterohemorrhagic *E coli* (EHEC) is the most common organism identified in STEC HUS; EHEC O157:H7 is the most common strain of EHEC associated with HUS in the United States. The most important reservoir for *E coli* O157:H7 is the gastrointestinal tract of cattle, sheep, and goats. The most frequent transmission route of EHEC is foodborne, via consumption of 1) uncooked contaminated meat (ground beef), 2) unpasteurized milk, or 3) fecal contamination of produce (fruits such as apples, unpasteurized apple cider, and vegetables such as spinach) and water. Secondary human-to-human contamination has been reported, and is especially a concern for affected children in daycare centers. *Shigella dysenteriae* type 1–associated HUS is usually more severe; this type occurs in the Indian subcontinent and southern Africa.

Patients with diarrhea-negative HUS are more likely to have an insidious or a relapsing clinical course, increased risk for end-stage renal failure, and an overall poorer prognosis. This form has been reported in association with malignancy, medications (cyclosporine, tacrolimus), systemic lupus erythematosus, pregnancy, and genetic mutations leading to uncontrolled activation of the alternate complement pathway.

Serum creatinine, electrolytes, and urinalysis are usually abnormal in patients with acute renal failure, but are not indicative of the underlying etiology. Evaluation for STEC infection includes stool testing for Shiga toxins (with an enzyme-linked immunosorbent assay) and cultures. However, the systemic manifestations of HUS usually develop nearly 7 days after diarrhea onset, whereas stool studies are more likely to be positive when performed within 6 days of onset.

PREP Pearls

- Hemolytic uremic syndrome is one of the most common causes of acute renal failure in children. It is characterized by the triad of microangiopathic hemolytic anemia, thrombocytopenia, and acute renal failure.
- The most common cause of diarrhea-positive HUS is Shiga toxin–producing *Escherichia coli*. Enterohemorrhagic *E coli*, especially *E coli* O157:H7, is the most commonly identified organism.
- The most frequent transmission route of enterohemorrhagic *E coli* is foodborne.

American Board of Pediatrics Content Specification(s)/Content Area

- Plan the appropriate initial management of hemolytic-uremic syndrome
- Recognize the clinical and laboratory findings associated with hemolytic-uremic syndrome

Suggested Readings

American Academy of Pediatrics. *Escherichia coli* diarrhea (including hemolytic-uremic syndrome). In: Kimberlin DW, Brady MT, Jackson MA, Long SS, eds. *Red Book: 2018 Report of the Committee on Infectious Diseases*. 31st ed. Itasca, IL: American Academy of Pediatrics; 2018:338-344.

Fiorino EK, Raffaelli RM. Hemolytic-uremic syndrome. *Pediatr Rev*. 2006; 27(10):398-399.

Van Why SK, Avner ED. Hemolytic-uremic syndrome. In: Kliegman RM, Stanton BF, St. Geme J, Schor NF, eds. *Nelson Textbook of Pediatrics*. 20th ed. Philadelphia, PA: Saunders; 2016:2507-2510.

Item 10   Preferred Response: D

The child in this vignette has elevated blood pressure in the right upper extremity and a delay in the right femoral pulse relative to the pulse in the right upper extremity. These findings are consistent with coarctation of the aorta, which requires surgical or transcatheter repair. Patients with coarctation of the aorta will have a lower systolic blood pressure in the extremities distal to the area of coarctation (ie, the legs), than is seen proximal to the narrowing (ie, the right arm). Some older patients may report leg claudication. Younger patients will typically present with a murmur. Neonates with a critical coarctation, (systemic blood flow is dependent on the presence of a patent ductus arteriosus) will present in shock if not prenatally diagnosed.

Secondary causes of hypertension include renovascular disease, some malignancies (eg, neuroblastoma or Wilms tumor), endocrine disorders (eg, hyperthyroidism), and certain medications. When hypertension is caused by an underlying or secondary cause, the treatment of choice is to fix the underlying cause, if possible. Essential hypertension is the

presence of hypertension without an underlying cause. In general, therapy for essential hypertension is initially focused on lifestyle modifications followed by pharmacologic interventions. Coarctation causing significant hypertension, as seen in the child in this vignette, requires repair by cardiac surgery or a transcatheter approach in the cardiac catheterization laboratory. Healthy diet and exercise, amlodipine, and enalapril are not beneficial next steps in the treatment of hypertension caused by coarctation of the aorta.

PREP Pearls

- Coarctation of the aorta can be suggested by an arm-leg blood pressure differential with a higher blood pressure in the right arm compared to the legs.
- Hypertension can be essential or secondary to another disease process.
- Treatment for hypertension associated with coarctation of the aorta is repair of the defect via surgery or cardiac catheterization.

American Board of Pediatrics Content Specification(s)/Content Area

- Plan the initial management of hypertension in a patient with coarctation of the aorta

Suggested Readings

Brady T. Hypertension. *Pediatr Rev*. 2012;33(12):541-552.

Dijkema EJ, Leiner T, Grotenhuis HB. Diagnosis, imaging and clinical management of aortic coarctation. *Heart*. 2017;103(15):1148-1155.

Nakamura K, Stefanescu Schmidt A. Treatment of hypertension in coarctation of the aorta. *Curr Treat Options Cardio Med*. 2016;18(6):40.

Torok RD, Campbell MJ, Fleming GA, Hill KD. Coarctation of the aorta: management from infancy to adulthood. *World J Cardiol*. 2015;7(11): 765-775.

Item 11   Preferred Response: B

The adolescent in this vignette has chronic health conditions, plans to go out of state for college, and will soon be responsible for managing his own care. Discussions regarding identifying and transferring to adult providers must start early in an effort to facilitate a smooth transition.

The Society of Adolescent Health and Medicine defines health care transition as "the purposeful, planned movement of adolescent and young adults with chronic physical and medical conditions from child-centered care to the adult-oriented health care system." An increasing number of youth with chronic medical conditions and special health care needs are living into adulthood. Approximately 500,000 youth transition into the the adult health care system annually. Chronic medical conditions include physical, behavioral, and emotional diseases. For the transition to be successful, it requires planning on the part of the patient, family, and health care providers. If proper planning is not done, transition to adult care is often a negative experience for adolescents and young adults that can lead to nonadherence with medication and follow-up appointments. This nonadherence ultimately affects their quality of life, disease outcome, and ability to complete their education, secure employment, and make a successful transition to adulthood.

There are several barriers in transition of care. First, many patients and their families have difficulty leaving the pediatric care setting and trusting a new provider. Second, in the adult care system, adolescents and young adults are expected to take responsibility for their health care and take a more active role in decision-making processes. Third, patients and their families need to be given anticipatory guidance regarding what will be expected of the adolescents and young adults in the adult care system, which can be difficult to navigate. It can also be difficult for parents to step back from the day-to-day management of their child's medical condition.

Health care transition is a process, and the earlier it is started the more likely it is to be successful. The American Academy of Pediatrics, American Academy of Family Physicians, and American College of Physicians recommend that discussions regarding transition begin at age 12 years, keeping in mind that transition planning must be focused on the cognitive and developmental stage of the patient.

Key elements of transition planning include the following:

- Start discussing transition early to better prepare patients, families, and health care providers.
- Transition planning has to be individualized. Coordination of care is a collaborative process discussed with the patient, family, pediatric specialist, adult specialist/provider, and primary care physician. The transferring and receiving physicians must be in communication.
- Assess the patient's readiness to start discussions around transition of care.
- Use written individualized transition plans, such as Got Transition (http://www.gottransition.org), and the University of North Carolina STARx. Got Transition includes 6 core elements of health care transition: transition policy, transition tracking and monitoring, transition readiness, transition planning, transfer of care, and transfer completion.
- Transfers of care should be during a time when the chronic condition is stable and not during acute medical crises.
- Some research supports the usefulness of transition coordinators as facilitators between the pediatric and adult health care systems.

For the patient in this vignette, discussing his medication with only his mother places the responsibility of compliance on the parent and does not make the patient an active participant in the management of his own health care. It is important to have adolescents involved in their health care visits and discuss their understanding of why they take certain medications, dosing schedules, and compliance. Inquiring about medication adverse effects and updating immunizations is an important aspect of any health supervision visit. However, if the transition planning process has not been started in an adolescent who has chronic medical conditions it would be imperative to begin open discussions in an effort to foster a smooth transition to the adult health care system.

American Board of Pediatrics Content Specification(s)/ Content Area

- Provide appropriate guidance to transition adolescents from pediatric to adult health care

Suggested Readings

Got Transition/Center for Health Care Transition Improvement. Six core elements of health care transition 2.0. http://www.gottransition.org/providers/index.cfm.

Mahan JD, Betz CL, Okumura MJ, Ferris ME. Self-management and transition to adult healthcare in adolescents and young adults: A team Process. *Pediatr Rev.* 2017;38(7):305-319.

Rosen DS, Blum RW, Britto M, Sawyer S, Siegel DM; Society of Adolescent Medicine. Transition to adult health care for adolescents and young adults with chronic conditions: a position paper of the Society of Adolescent Medicine. *J Adolesc Health.* 2003;33(4):309-311.

Sawyer S. Chronic health conditions in adolescents and young adults. *In: Neinstein LS, ed. Neinstein's Adolescent and Young Adult Health Care: A Practical Guide.* 6th ed. Philadelphia, PA: Wolters Kluwer; 2016:84-89.

Item 12   Preferred Response: D

The girl in this vignette, who has a severe traumatic brain injury, is oliguric and exhibiting signs of hypervolemia. The most likely cause of these findings is the syndrome of inappropriate antidiuretic hormone (SIADH), and the most common associated electrolyte disturbance is hyponatremia.

Syndrome of inappropriate antidiuretic hormone is most commonly caused by central nervous system pathology, including traumatic brain injury, hypoxic-ischemic encephalopathy, meningitis, encephalitis, intracranial hemorrhage, hydrocephalus, and stroke. Syndrome of inappropriate antidiuretic hormone from extracerebral antidiuretic hormone (ADH) release can also occur as a paraneoplastic syndrome, and with various pulmonary conditions, most frequently bronchiolitis, acute respiratory distress syndrome, and pneumonia.

Arginine vasopressin (AVP), also known as ADH, is a peptide hormone synthesized in the anterior hypothalamus and stored in the posterior pituitary gland. Release of AVP is induced by hyperosmolality detected by osmoreceptors in the hypothalamus and by low cardiac output detected by baroreceptors located in the carotid sinus, aortic arch, and left atrium. Vasopressin acts as a potent vasoconstrictor by binding to V1a receptors on vascular smooth muscle cells and increasing intracellular calcium via a phospholipase C–mediated mechanism. Vasopressin binding to V2 receptors, via a cyclic adenosine monophosphate mechanism, causes the insertion of aquaporin channels in the collecting duct of the distal nephron. Intraluminal water flows through the aquaporin channel back into the bloodstream, decreasing the excretion of water in the urine. This mechanism is important in maintaining the osmotic equilibrium of the serum. Failure of this process at the level of the pituitary or hypothalamus (central diabetes insipidus) or at the kidney (nephrogenic diabetes insipidus) results in excessive urine output, often up to 8 to 10 mL/kg per hour, dilute urine with specific gravity approaching 1.005, hypernatremia, and volume depletion.

In contrast, SIADH is marked by hyponatremia due to decreased water excretion, low urine output, high urine sodium for the degree of hyponatremia, and hypervolemia. Cerebral salt wasting, another cause of hyponatremia and high urine sodium, can also occur in severe traumatic brain injury. Although patients with cerebral salt wasting are more hypovolemic, it is often difficult to distinguish between the 2 conditions. Hypovolemic hyponatremia, another important cause of hyponatremia in critically ill patients, can be distinguished from SIADH by a low urine sodium (<20 mEq/L) and clinical signs of volume depletion. It should be noted that some or all of the findings of SIADH can occur due to a normal physiologic release of ADH from factors such as decreased cardiac output, thirst, and stress.

For the child in the vignette, hypocalcemia is not likely, because there is no indication of endocrine dysfunction or low dietary intake of calcium. Iatrogenic hyperchloremia can occur in traumatic brain injury from the administration of normal or hypertonic saline; however, urine output would be high. Hyperkalemia can occur in trauma, but usually when there is a concomitant crush injury or anuric renal failure.

PREP Pearls

- Arginine vasopressin decreases the excretion of water into the urine due to the insertion of aquaporin channels on the basolateral membrane of the collecting duct in the distal nephron.
- Arginine vasopressin, also referred to as antidiuretic hormone, is a peptide hormone secreted by the posterior pituitary gland.
- Syndrome of inappropriate antidiuretic hormone is marked by low urine output, hypervolemia, and high urine sodium and osmolality.

American Board of Pediatrics Content Specification(s)/ Content Area

- Recognize the role of head trauma in the development of SIADH

Suggested Readings

Ellison DH, Berl T. The syndrome of inappropriate antidiuresis. *N Engl J Med.* 2007;356:2064-2072.

Maesaka JK, Imbriano L, Mattana J, Gallagher D, Bade N, Sharif S. Differentiating SIADH from cerebral/renal salt wasting: failure of the volume approach and need for a new approach to hyponatremia. *J Clin Med.* 2014;3(4):1373-1385.

Reid-Adam J. Hyponatremia. *Pediatr Rev.* 2013;34;417-419.

The boy in this vignette has systemic juvenile idiopathic arthritis (JIA). Laboratory findings in this condition commonly include an elevated erythrocyte sedimentation rate and other signs of inflammation. Patients do not typically have leukopenia, elevated antinuclear antibody titer, or a positive rheumatoid factor.

The International League of Associations for Rheumatology recommends the division of JIA into 5 subsets: systemic arthritis, polyarthritis, oligoarthritis, enthesitis-related arthritis, and psoriatic arthritis. Epidemiology, clinical features, and associated laboratory findings for these subsets are shown in Item C13. Some children with JIA have symptoms that do not fill diagnostic criteria for a single subset, and some children may change categories over time as their disease evolves.

PREP Pearls

- Juvenile idiopathic arthritis can be divided into 5 subsets: systemic arthritis, polyarthritis, oligoarthritis, enthesitis-related arthritis, and psoriatic arthritis.
- Systemic juvenile idiopathic arthritis typically presents with high, daily fever for at least 2 weeks, rash, lymphadenopathy, hepatosplenomegaly, serositis, and arthritis in 1 or more joints. Inflammatory laboratory markers will be elevated, but patients typically have a normal antinuclear antibody titer and a negative rheumatoid factor.

American Board of Pediatrics Content Specification(s)/ Content Area

- Recognize the laboratory findings associated with juvenile rheumatoid (idiopathic) arthritis and its complications
- Recognize the clinical findings associated with the various types of juvenile rheumatoid (idiopathic) arthritis

Suggested Readings

Espinosa M, Gottlieb BS. Juvenile idiopathic arthritis. *Pediatr Rev.* 2012;33(7):303-313.

Prakken B, Albani S, Martini A. Juvenile idiopathic arthritis. *Lancet.* 2011;377(9783):2138-2149.

Item C13. Characteristics of Subsets of Juvenile Idiopathic Arthritis.

JIA Subset	Age at Onset	Sex Ratio	Symptoms	Laboratory Findings
Systemic arthritis	Childhood	F = M	• Arthritis in ≥ 1 joints • Fever • Rash • Lymphadenopathy • Hepatosplenomegaly • Serositis • > 50% of arthritis is destructive	↑↑ ESR ↑↑ WBC ↑↑ Ferritin ↓↓ Hgb Normal ANA titer Negative RF
Polyarthritis	Biphasic peaks (2-4 and 10-14 years)	F >> M	• Arthritis in ≥ 5 joints in first 6 months of illness • > 50% of arthritis is destructive	↑ ESR Normal WBC ↑ Ferritin ↓ Hgb Low ANA titer +/− RF
Oligoarthritis	Toddlers	F >>> M	• Arthritis in < 5 joints • Large joints commonly affected (rarely hip) • +/− uveitis/iritis • Destructive arthritis is rare	↑ or Normal ESR Normal WBC Normal Ferritin Normal Hgb Low ANA titer Negative RF

Enthesitis-related arthritis	Pre-adolescents, adolescents	M >> F	• Arthritis and enthesitis
			• May develop:
			  • iritis
			  • ankylosing spondylitis
			  • reactive arthritis
			  • inflammatory bowel disease−associated arthritis
				↑ or Normal ESR
				↑ or Normal WBC
				↑ or Normal ferritin
				↓ or Normal Hgb
				Normal ANA titer
				Negative RF
				HLA-B27 positive

Psoriatic arthritis	Biphasic peaks (2-4 and 9-11 years)	F > M	• Arthritis and psoriatic rash, or
			• Arthritis and at least 2 of following:
			  • 1st degree relative with psoriasis
			  • dactylitis
			  • nail pitting
			  • +/− iritis
				↑ or Normal ESR
				↑ or Normal WBC
				↑ or Normal ferritin
				↓ or Normal Hgb
				Elevated ANA titer
				Negative RF

Abbreviations: ANA, antinuclear antibody; ESR, erythrocyte sedimentation rate; Hgb, hemoglobin; RF, rheumatoid factor; WBC, white blood cells.

Courtesy of I. Larson.

Item 14　　　　　　　　　　　**Preferred Response: B**

Adults (≥18 years of age) who have been immunized against polio by completion of routine vaccine series of oral polio vaccine (OPV) or inactivated polio vaccine (IPV) are considered immune for life, but the precise duration of immunity is unknown. Fully immunized adults who intend to travel to, and remain in, a polio-endemic country for more than 4 weeks are at increased risk of exposure to wild poliovirus (WPV) or vaccine-derived poliovirus (VDPV), and should receive a dose of IPV before departure. Based on current data, no additional booster dose with IPV is recommended for adults. Unimmunized, incompletely immunized, or adult travelers with an unknown polio immunization status should receive 3 doses of IPV following the accelerated schedule and minimum intervals recommended by the Advisory Committee on Immunization Practices.

Remarkable progress has been made in global polio eradication, with an over 99% estimated reduction in the number of polio cases since 1988, translating to more than 16 million people saved from paralytic disease. An estimated 350,000 cases occurred in more than 125 endemic countries in 1988 compared with 37 reported cases in 2016. Of the 3 serotypes of WPV (type 1, type 2, and type 3), type 1 poliovirus accounts for all recent polio cases caused by WPV. Eradication of WPV type 2 was certified in 1999 and the last case of WPV type 3 was reported from Nigeria in November 2012.

In the United States, the last case of indigenous acquisition of naturally occurring WPV was reported in 1979. All other cases of polio since 1986 have been vaccine-associated paralytic poliomyelitis (VAPP) in OPV recipients or their contacts. Introduction of IPV as a part of the immunization series in 1997 resulted in a steep decline in VAPP cases; in 2000, an all IPV-vaccine series was routinely implemented in the United States. There have been no reports of circulating WPV in the United States for many decades. In addition, with the recent success of the global polio eradication program, there is a very low risk of contact with imported wild-type polioviruses except in the setting of foreign travel to polio-endemic countries, such as Nigeria, Afghanistan, and Pakistan.

In the United States, a total of 4 doses of IPV at ages 2, 4, 6 to 18 months, and 4 to 6 years is currently recommended for all infants and children as part of a routine immunization series. The minimum recommended interval between IPV doses 1 and 2 and between doses 2 and 3 is 4 weeks, and the minimum interval between doses 3 and 4 is 6 months. The minimum age for dose 1 of IPV is 6 weeks. In situations of high-risk exposure, such as travel to a polio-endemic country, the minimum age and intervals should be used for administration of IPV. The fourth IPV dose should be given after age 4 years, irrespective of the previous number of doses administered, and at least 6 months after receiving the previous vaccine dose. Incompletely immunized children and adolescents should receive the complete schedule of IPV doses following the accelerated schedule and minimum intervals recommended by the American Academy of Pediatrics Committee on Infectious Diseases (https://redbook.solutions.aap.org/selfserve/ssPage.aspx?SelfServeContentId=Immunization_Schedules).

The following children and adolescents should receive an additional dose of IPV: (1) those who are up to date with their polio immunization or have completed the routine IPV series but traveling to a polio-endemic country and staying for more than 4 weeks, and (2) those who received their last IPV dose more than 12 months before the date they will be departing the country to which they are traveling. Children who receive this additional 4th IPV dose between 18 months through 4 years will still need an IPV booster dose at age 4 years or later.

In 2014, the World Health Organization (WHO) declared the international spread of WPV as a public health emergency of international concern. The risk of international spread is highest from countries with ongoing endemic circulation of WPV or VDPV, a polio outbreak, or evidence from an environmental source (eg, sewage) of WPV or VDPV circulation. In May 2017, the WHO issued updated guidance regarding the administration of polio vaccine. The Centers for Disease Control Travelers' Health website (www.cdc.gov/travel) and the Global Polio Eradication Initiative website (www.polioeradication.org/Dataandmonitoring/Poliothisweek.aspx) are good resources for up-to-date information regarding reported WPV and VDPV cases, travel notices, and vaccine recommendations. Clinicians should document all polio vaccinations on an International Certificate of Vaccination or Prophylaxis for long-term travelers and residents. The polio vaccine must be received between 4 weeks and 12 months before the date of departure from the polio-infected country to meet the departure requirement (wwwnc.cdc.gov/travel/news-announcements/polio-guidance-new-requirements).

PREP Pearls

- Adults who received a complete polio immunization series in childhood and intend to travel to and stay for more than 4 weeks in a polio-affected country should receive a single lifetime booster dose of IPV before departure.

- Before traveling to polio-endemic areas, travelers should ensure that they have received the recommended age-appropriate polio immunization series.

- In the United States, a total of 4 doses of inactivated polio vaccine at ages 2, 4, and 6 to 18 months and 4 to 6 years is currently recommended for all infants and children.

American Board of Pediatrics Content Specification(s)/Content Area

- Understand the efficacy and safety of the poliovirus vaccine
- Know the indications, contraindications, and schedules for the poliovirus vaccine, including under special circumstances (eg, unimmunized adult contacts)

Suggested Readings

American Academy of Pediatrics. Poliovirus infections. In: Kimberlin DW, Brady MT, Jackson MA, Long SS, eds. *Red Book: 2018 Report of the Committee on Infectious Diseases.* 31st ed. Itasca, IL: American Academy of Pediatrics; 2018:657-664

Orenstein WA; Committee on Infectious Diseases. Eradicating polio: how the world's pediatricians can help stop this crippling illness forever. *Pediatrics.* 2015;135(1):196-202.

World Health Organization. Polio vaccines: WHO position paper, March 2016-recommendations. Vaccine. 2017;35(9):1197-1199.

Item 15	Preferred Response: C

The neonate in the vignette with trisomy 21 has polycythemia, but is clinically asymptomatic. The most appropriate management choice is close observation.

Polycythemia is defined by a hematocrit (Hct) greater than 65% on a sample obtained from a vein or central vessel. Samples obtained by heel stick often have a falsely elevated Hct. The incidence of polycythemia is approximately 1% to 2% among term neonates, occurring because of either increased red blood cell production or passive transfusion of red blood cells. During gestation, erythropoietin production is stimulated by hypoxemia. Therefore, maternal conditions that result in a relative hypoxic environment may result in elevated red blood cell production and polycythemia. Risk factors for polycythemia among neonates include delivery in high-elevation areas; gestational age of more than 40 weeks; small size for gestational age; maternal diabetes; maternal hypertension; maternal history of cigarette smoking; trisomy 13, 18, or 21; neonatal Graves disease; congenital adrenal hyperplasia; cyanotic congenital heart disease; and neonatal hypothyroidism. Passive transfusion of red blood cells may occur with delayed cord clamping or twin-to-twin transfusion syndrome.

Most neonates with polycythemia are asymptomatic. They often have a ruddy appearance. Clinical signs and symptoms of polycythemia may include irritability, tachypnea, hypoglycemia, lethargy, thrombocytopenia, pulmonary hypertension, stroke, necrotizing enterocolitis, renal vein thrombosis, and seizure. Clinical findings are due to hyperviscosity, not the elevated red blood cell count. Neonatal red blood cells are more likely than those of older children to become deformed and clump, increasing the risk of hyperviscosity. However, because viscosity cannot be measured with bedside testing, clinicians must use hematocrit as a proxy when deciding whether or not to treat polycythemia.

Neonates should be treated with partial exchange transfusion if they are symptomatic with a Hct greater than 60% or have a Hct greater than 70%, whether symptomatic or not. Treating polycythemia may not improve outcomes. Among neonates with asymptomatic polycythemia, a randomized trial comparing partial exchange transfusion with conservative management with observation did not show a decrease in long-term complications with partial exchange transfusion. The long-term complications of polycythemia may be related to the effects of hypoxia during gestation, rather than the polycythemia itself.

For the neonate in the vignette, there is no evidence of hypotension, hypoperfusion, or dehydration that would warrant a bolus of normal saline. A platelet transfusion is not indicated for a platelet count greater than $100 \times 10^3/\mu L$ $(100 \times 10^9/L)$.

PREP Pearls

- Neonates with polycythemia and hematocrit (Hct) values of 65% to 69% who are clinically asymptomatic should be closely observed.
- Polycythemia with Hct greater than 70% should be treated with partial exchange transfusion.
- Risk factors for neonatal polycythemia include delivery in high-elevation areas; gestational age of >40 weeks; small size for gestational age; maternal diabetes, hypertension, and history of cigarette smoking; trisomy 13, 18, or 21; neonatal Graves disease and hypothyroidism; congenital adrenal hyperplasia; cyanotic congenital heart disease.

American Board of Pediatrics Content Specification(s)/ Content Area

- Recognize the risks associated with polycythemia in newborn infants, and manage appropriately

Suggested Readings

Kates EH, Kates JS. Anemia and polycythemia in the newborn. *Pediatr Rev.* 2007;28:33.

Maheshwari A, Carlo WA. Plethora in the newborn infant (polycythemia) In: Kliegman RM, Stanton BF, St Geme JW, Schor NF, eds. *Nelson Textbook of Pediatrics.* 20th ed. Philadelphia, PA: Saunders Elsevier; 2016:880-889

The boy in this vignette most likely has persistent asthma, based on symptoms of chronic cough, frequent night cough, and exercise intolerance. The normal physical examination findings do not rule out asthma, and the most common cause of cough in conjunction with exercise intolerance for children is asthma. Asthma is one of the most misdiagnosed conditions in pediatric medicine, both by underdiagnosis and overdiagnosis. The most appropriate initial diagnostic test for asthma in patients of school age or older is spirometry. Some might argue that obtaining pulse oximetry would be appropriate before spirometry, and that, indeed, is often a part of routine vital signs. But of the choices available, spirometry is the most appropriate next step. If there is sign of obstruction, repeating spirometry 15 to 20 minutes after administration of inhaled bronchodilator could establish reversible airflow obstruction.

Chest radiography is an imprecise tool for the evaluation of asthma. In young children who cannot perform spirometry, radiography may be helpful if there is evidence of hyperinflation or air trapping. But, most often any changes will be nonspecific.

Methacholine challenge is rarely needed in children. Most often, children with persistent cough or significant daily symptoms will show obstruction on spirometry with demonstration of reversibility; in that case, there is no need for methacholine challenge as a diagnostic tool. In the presence of cough without wheeze and normal spirometry, it might be appropriate to do a methacholine challenge if no other etiology can be found for the cough. But, for most children with cough or shortness of breath related to exercise, an exercise challenge with lung function monitoring is a better diagnostic test.

Despite the family history of cystic fibrosis, and in the age of newborn screening, cystic fibrosis is unlikely in the context of normal growth parameters and lack of gastrointestinal symptoms. If there were nonreversible obstruction on spirometry, then a chest radiograph and possibly sweat chloride test would be indicated as secondary evaluation tools despite his normal growth.

PREP Pearls

- If there is sign of airway obstruction on spirometry, repeating spirometry 15 to 20 minutes after administration of inhaled bronchodilator could establish reversible airflow obstruction, indicating the diagnosis of asthma.
- Spirometry provides objective information about airway obstruction that may be missed from history or physical examination alone.

American Board of Pediatrics Content Specification(s)/ Content Area

- Understand the basic terminology and purpose of various pulmonary function tests

Suggested Readings

Kaslovsky R, Sadof M. Spirometry for the primary care physician. *Pediatr Rev.* 2014;35(11):465-475.

Looijmans-van den Akker I, van Luijn, K, Verheij T. Overdiagnosis of asthma in children in primary care: a retrospective analysis. *Br J Gen Pract.* 2016;66 (644):e152-e157.

Wood PR, Hill VL. Practical management of asthma. *Pediatr Rev.* 2009; 30(10):375-384.

Item 17 Preferred Response: D

The adolescent boy in this vignette has an enlarging red nodule adjacent to a hyperpigmented plaque (Item C17A). These findings are concerning for melanoma (the nodule represents an amelanotic lesion) and, accordingly, prompt referral to a dermatologist for excision is indicated. For a lesion that is not exhibiting a benign course (ie, is "EFG": elevated, firm, and growing progressively for > 1 month), providing reassurance that the lesion will resolve without intervention, applying a topical antibiotic, or cauterizing with silver nitrate would not be appropriate.

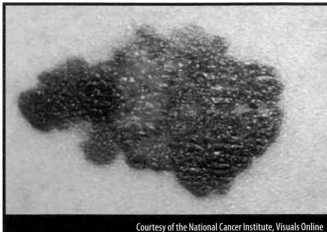

Courtesy of the National Cancer Institute, Visuals Online

Item C17B: Malignant melanoma exhibiting asymmetry, border irregularity, and color variegation.

- A = Amelanotic: Lesions lack visible pigment (Item C17A). Most amelanotic melanomas (70%) will appear pink or red (and may mimic a pyogenic granuloma, Item C17C), but some may be skin colored and resemble warts.
- B = Bleeding, bump: Lesions often are papules or nodules that may ulcerate or bleed, not flat lesions.
- C = Color uniformity
- D = De novo, any diameter: lesions often do not arise in preexisting melanocytic nevi and may measure 6 mm or more in diameter.

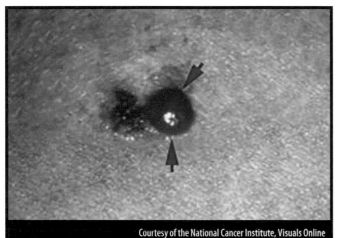

Courtesy of the National Cancer Institute, Visuals Online

Item C17A: Erythematous nodule (arrows) representing an amelanotic melanoma. To the left of nodule is an area of irregular pigmentation that is the early radial growth phase of superficial spreading melanoma.

Only 0.5% of new cases of malignant melanoma occur in patients younger than 20 years. Several studies have documented that melanomas in children and adolescents may not meet the conventional ABCD criteria (asymmetry, border irregularity, color variegation, diameter > 6 mm) (Item C17B shows a melanoma that meets these conventional criteria). In a 2013 retrospective study by Cordoro et al, 60% of patients 0 to 10 years of age and 40% of patients 11 to 19 years of age with malignant melanoma did not exhibit these criteria. In addition, most melanomas (67%) appeared de novo, not in a preexisting congenital or acquired melanocytic nevus. In both children and adolescents, recent evolution (the "E" dded to the ABCDs) was reported for nearly all lesions. Based on these data, the authors proposed additional criteria to assist in the diagnosis of melanoma in children and adolescents:

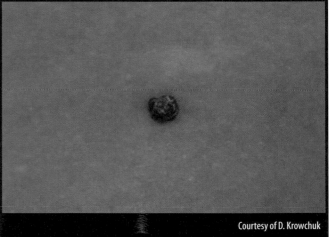

Courtesy of D. Krowchuk

Item C17C: A pyogenic granuloma is a red to purple papule that usually is pedunculated and often has a collarette of scale at its base.

The physical findings most often exhibited by children and adolescents with melanoma are summarized in Item C17D.

Item C17D. Prevalence of Physical Findings in Pediatric Melanoma.*

Physical Finding	Age 0-10 y	Age 11-19 y
Amelanosis	77%	23%
Bump (raised lesion)	100%	87%
Bleeding	53%	22%
Consistent color	87%	48%
Denovo appearance	67%	63%
Diameter ≤ 6 mm	73%	53%

* Percentages represent approximations.

Adapted and reprinted with permission from Cordoro KM, Gupta D, Frieden IJ, McCalmont T, Kashani-Sabet M. Pediatric melanoma: results of a large cohort study and proposal for modified ABCD detection criteria for children. *J Am Acad Dermatol*. 2013;68(6):918.

PREP Pearls

- If a lesion is "EFG" (elevated, firm, and growing progressively for > 1 month), consider the possibility of an amelanotic or nodular melanoma.
- Melanomas in children often do not exhibit the conventional ABCD detection criteria (asymmetry, border irregularity, color variegation, diameter > 6 mm).
- Pediatric melanomas often are pink or red, papular or nodular, and have uniform color and smooth borders.

American Board of Pediatrics Content Specification(s)/Content Area

- Recognize the clinical findings associated with melanoma

Suggested Readings

Cordoro KM, Gupta D, Frieden IJ, McCalmont T, Kashani-Sabet M. Pediatric melanoma: results of a large cohort study and proposal for modified ABCD detection criteria for children. *J Am Acad Dermatol*. 2013;68(6):913-925.

National Cancer Institute, Surveillance, Epidemiology, and End Results Program. Cancer stat facts: melanoma of the skin. http://seer.cancer.gov/statfacts/html/melan.html.

Slade AD, Austin MT. Childhood melanoma: an increasingly important health problem in the USA. *Curr Opin Pediatr* 2014;26(3):356-361.

Item 18   Preferred Response: D

The patient in this vignette has recurrent diabetic ketoacidosis (DKA) with 3 episodes in the past year. The most common cause of recurrent DKA is insulin omission. Adolescent girls are a higher risk group for recurrent DKA. Often, recurrent DKA is a symptom of an underlying psychosocial problem. Examples include intentional insulin omission for weight loss ("diabulimia"), depression, poor coping skills, or a mechanism of escape from an undesirable social situation. Thus, recurrent DKA should prompt a behavioral health evaluation. An interdisciplinary approach to the management of recurrent DKA includes diabetes education, psychosocial evaluation, medical treatment, and appropriate adult supervision.

The most common cause of DKA in individuals whose diabetes is managed with an insulin pump is interruption of insulin delivery, usually caused by a compromised infusion site. Insulin pumps deliver only rapid-acting insulin, so when interrupted, DKA occurs more quickly than in individuals receiving a long-acting basal insulin injection. Education is critical for the prevention of DKA in individuals on an insulin pump. Ketones should be monitored at home during times of significant hyperglycemia and on sick days. Additional insulin and oral fluid are needed if ketones are present, and the additional insulin should be administered by injection. Families should also have 24-hour access to medical advice by telephone.

Infection is a rare cause of recurrent DKA. Proper education on sick-day management is essential for preventing DKA. Sick-day management includes close monitoring of blood glucose and ketone levels, as well as 24-hour telephone access to medical advice. Extra insulin is often needed because of the stress of illness. Abdominal pain and vomiting are symptoms of DKA that are often confused with gastroenteritis and resolve with treatment of the DKA. An elevated white blood cell count, as seen in the patient in this vignette, is associated with DKA due to the stress response. It should not be interpreted as a sign of infection without other indications of infection.

Excessive carbohydrate intake does not cause DKA. Insulin deficiency to the extent that the body's basic fuel requirements are not met causes DKA. Excessive carbohydrate intake without adequate bolus insulin coverage causes hyperglycemia but not DKA as long as there is enough insulin to deliver enough glucose to meet the body's basic fuel requirements.

Inadequate basal insulin dose is not the cause of recurrent DKA for the patient in this vignette. She is prescribed 0.5 units/kg/day of long-acting basal insulin glargine, which is a typical dose for her age. Even if her prescribed dose is not keeping her blood glucose levels in the target range, it is enough to prevent DKA.

PREP Pearls

- Diabetes education on sick-day management and insulin pump malfunction is critical for diabetic ketoacidosis prevention.
- Recurrent diabetic ketoacidosis is often a symptom of an underlying psychosocial problem.
- The most common cause of recurrent diabetic ketoacidosis is insulin omission.

American Board of Pediatrics Content Specification(s)/Content Area

- Recognize the clinical and laboratory manifestations of adrenal insufficiency
- Differentiate the clinical and laboratory findings associated with adrenal insufficiency from those of the inappropriate secretion of antidiuretic hormone

Suggested Readings

Jefferies CA, Nakhla M, Derraik JG, Gunn AJ, Daneman D, Cutfield WS. Preventing diabetic ketoacidosis. *Pediatr Clin North Am.* 2015;62(4): 857-871.

Wolfsdorf JI, Allgrove J, Craig ME, et al; International Society for Pediatric and Adolescent Diabetes. ISPAD Clinical Practice Consensus Guidelines 2014. Diabetic ketoacidosis and hyperglycemic hyperosmolar state. *Pediatr Diabetes.* 2014;15 Suppl 20:154-179.

Item 19   **Preferred Response: C**

The neonate in the vignette has classic CHARGE syndrome, an autosomal dominant disorder. CHARGE is a mnemonic for *c*oloboma, *h*eart defects, choanal *a*tresia, *r*etarded growth and development, *g*enital abnormalities, and *e*ar anomalies. Neonates with this condition can present with multiple life-threatening conditions. If CHARGE syndrome is suspected, the neonate should undergo urgent evaluation of the heart, airway, feeding, and genitourinary tract. Hearing should also be evaluated.

The diagnosis of CHARGE syndrome is based on clinical findings and imaging. The only known gene to be associated with CHARGE syndrome is the *CHD7* gene, and mutations are detectable in 65% to 70% of persons presenting with the clinical syndrome. Genetic testing is available.

The diagnostic criteria for CHARGE (Item C19) syndrome are:

- Definite CHARGE syndrome: 4 major characteristics or 3 major and 3 minor characteristics
- Probable CHARGE syndrome: 1 or 2 major characteristics and several minor characteristics

The girl in the vignette had all 4 major criteria and several minor criteria.

Item C19. Diagnositic Criteria for CHARGE Syndrome.

Major diagnostic criteria
• Ocular colobomas
• Choanal atresia
• Cranial nerve dysfunction or anomaly (eg, anosmia, facial palsy, auditory nerve hypoplasia, or swallowing problems)
• External ear anomalies, middle ear defects, Mondini defect, temporal bone abnormalities
Minor diagnostic criteria
• Genital hypoplasia
• Developmental delay
• Cardiovascular anomalies
• Growth deficiency
• Cleft lip and/or palate
• Tracheoesophageal fistula or esophageal atresia
• Facial dysmorphology (square face with prominent forehead, flat midface, broad nasal root)

Adapted and reprinted with permission from Lalani SR, Hefner MA, Belmont JW, Davenport SLH. Charge syndrome. *GeneReviews*.

In the case of this neonate, *CHD7* gene mutation analysis would be an appropriate method to confirm the presence of this disorder. This type of diagnostic genetic testing involves postnatal single gene analysis, and would be a cost-effective method that avoids testing of genes that do not fit the infant's clinical presentation. The type of genetic testing indicated is based on a child's specific clinical presentation, and could include a karyotype, fluorescent in situ hybridization analysis, microarray, multigene panel testing, or whole exome sequencing. Multigene panel testing is indicated when one wants to examine many genes simultaneously, which could be implicative for a clinical presentation, such as hypertrophic cardiomyopathy or Noonan syndrome. A microarray or karyotype is appropriate to evaluate patients presenting with intellectual disability, autism, or multiple congenital anomalies as a baseline genetic test. Single gene analysis may be ordered if a specific syndrome is highly suspected. Whole exome sequencing can be used to identify the underlying molecular basis of a genetic disorder in an individual who has undergone prior extensive genetic testing with no unifying etiology identified.

22q11.2 deletion syndrome presents with congenital heart disease, palatal abnormalities, characteristic facial features, learning problems, hypocalcemia, immune deficiency, kidney abnormalities, and hearing loss. These children do not have colobomas or choanal atresia.

Branchio-oto-renal syndrome (BOR) is characterized by deafness, external ear deformities, lateral semicircular canal hypoplasia, branchial arch anomalies, and renal malformations. The lack of other major criteria of CHARGE syndrome makes them easily distinguishable. BOR is caused by mutations of *EYA1* and *SIX1*.

Treacher Collins syndrome is characterized by mandibular and zygomatic hypoplasia, coloboma of the lower eyelids, absent lower eyelashes, external ear abnormalities, and pre-auricular hair displacement onto the cheekbones. Diagnosis is made via clinical and radiographic findings. Genetic testing is available for the 3 genes known to cause this disorder: *TCOF1*, *POLR1C*, and *POLR1D*.

PREP Pearls

- CHARGE syndrome defines a constellation of clinical findings including coloboma, heart defects, choanal atresia, retarded growth and development, genital abnormalities, and ear anomalies.

- In postnatal single gene analysis, a single gene is analyzed based on a child's clinical presentation, which is highly suspect for a specific syndrome or diagnosis. It is a cost-effective method that avoids unnecessary testing of genes that do not fit the clinical situation.

- Neonates with CHARGE syndrome can present with multiple life-threatening conditions. Urgent evaluation of the heart, airway, gastrointestinal tract, and genitourinary tract, improves morbidity and mortality and optimizes outcome. Hearing should also be evaluated.

Suggested Readings

Lalani SR, Hefner MA, Belmont JW, Davenport SLH. CHARGE syndrome. *GeneReviews*. http://www.ncbi.nlm.nih.gov/books/NBK1117/.

National Human Genome Research Institute. https://www.genome.gov/19516567/faq-about-genetic-testing/.

Zentner GE, Layman WS, Martin DM, Scacheri PC. Molecular and phenotypic aspects of CHD7 mutation in CHARGE syndrome. *Am J Med Genet A*. 2010;152A:674-686.

Item 20   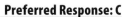   **Preferred Response: C**

The mother of the child in this vignette should be reported to the state child welfare agency for suspected neglect. While involvement of a practice's social worker or care coordinator is an appropriate intervention for cases of episodic or mild neglect, that resource has been exhausted in this case. Additional assistance from the care coordinator or bargaining with or threatening to report the mother as a means to prompt obtaining a single episode of recommended care is unlikely to adequately address the common root causes of neglect, including poverty, lack of social support, family and neighborhood stress, domestic violence, and a caregiver's mental health and substance abuse problems. Furthermore, the mother's neglect has been longstanding; this chronic neglect is particularly detrimental to a child's development and often requires intense, ongoing involvement with community-based caseworkers.

Approximately three-quarters of child maltreatment cases involve neglect. Neglect is legally defined at the federal level as a caregiver's act, or failure to act, which results in or places a child at risk for harm, abuse, or exploitation. At the state level, it is often further defined as failure to provide food, clothing, shelter, medical care, education, or supervision, such that the child's well-being is compromised. The diagnosis of medical neglect, which typically stems from failing to seek care when a child is obviously seriously ill or failing to carry through on recommendations for care, requires that the following criteria be met:

- A child is harmed or at risk of harm because of lack of health care.
- The recommended care would benefit the child.
- The benefit of care significantly outweighs the risk.
- The family has access to care but has not used it.
- The caregiver understands the clinician's recommendations.

The physical and psychological effects of neglect are serious. Neglect, particularly chronic neglect, can result in aggression and conduct problems; negative self-esteem; anxiety; cognitive and language delays; poor growth; and social-emotional impairment. As with physical and sexual abuse, chronic neglect can result in posttraumatic stress disorder. In addition to environmental and family factors, a caregiver's unemployment, young age, inability to cope with stress, and mental health/substance abuse problems are risk factors for neglect. Protective factors include a nurturing relationship between caregiver and child, social connections, and a caregiver's understanding of child development. Developmental delays and other chronic conditions place a child at risk for neglect; a child's emotional and social competence are protective.

When a report to the state child welfare agency is made, the clinician should disclose this to the caregiver. Rather than blaming the caregiver, the clinician should explain his or her desire to support the caregiver to best care for his or her child and alleviate some of the stress or barriers the caregiver is experiencing. Emphasizing a caregiver's strengths and being empathetic can help a clinician build rapport with the caregiver. Because most caregivers reported for suspicion of neglect retain custody of their children, the clinician in this vignette will likely continue caring for the girl and should maintain a positive, collaborative relationship with her mother, to the degree possible.

PREP Pearls

- Because chronic neglect benefits most from intensive, long-term involvement with community-level caseworkers, a referral to the state child welfare agency is often warranted.
- Neglect, particularly chronic neglect, disrupts the typical development of caregiver-child attachment and can result in behavior and emotional problems, especially for younger children.

Suggested Readings

Child Welfare Information Gateway. Acts of omission: an overview of child neglect. http://www.childwelfare.gov/pubs/focus/acts/index.cfm.

Child Welfare Information Gateway. Chronic childhood neglect. https://www.childwelfare.gov/pubs/chronic_neglect.cfm.

Dubowitz H. Neglect in children. *Pediatr Ann*. 2013;42(4):73-77.

Jenny C; Committee on Child Abuse and Neglect, American Academy of Pediatrics Recognizing and responding to medical neglect. *Pediatrics*. 2007;120(6):1385-1389.

Naughton AM, Maguire SA, Mann MK, et al. Emotional, behavioral, and developmental features indicative of neglect or emotional abuse in preschool children: a systematic review. *JAMA Pediatr*. 2013;167(8):769-775.

The clinical and laboratory findings for the boy in this vignette best support a diagnosis of pyogenic arthritis. In a child with acute onset of limp associated with fever, ill appearance, and marked limitation in range of motion, infection should be at the forefront of the differential diagnosis.

In patients with pyogenic arthritis, fever and limited range of motion of the affected joint are almost always present. External signs of inflammation may not always be present, depending on the site of disease. Septic arthritis of the hip is more difficult to diagnose than septic arthritis of the knee or ankle because external signs (erythema, swelling) tend to be absent as a result of the internal location of the joint. However, localizing the affected site should not be difficult because limitation in range of motion would be expected.

If there is concern for infection in the setting of arthritis or a joint effusion, laboratory tests including a complete blood cell count, C-reactive protein level, erythrocyte sedimentation rate, and blood culture are obtained. Radiographs are helpful as an initial diagnostic study to rule out a fracture. A sizeable effusion can sometimes be appreciated in traditional radiographs, although they are not the most sensitive study for an effusion. Ultrasonography can also be considered to assess for the presence of an effusion, especially for the hip. Joint aspiration is the best test for confirming the diagnosis. Joint fluid analysis in pyogenic arthritis typically yields a white blood cell count of $50,000/\mu L$ ($50 \times 10^9/L$) or greater that is predominantly neutrophilic. Magnetic resonance imaging can be pursued as a second-line test, particularly if there is concern for concurrent osteomyelitis.

Empiric treatment of pyogenic arthritis in children should include an antimicrobial expected to have activity against *Staphylococcus aureus* and streptococcal species. Considerations should be given to providing empiric coverage for methicillin-resistant *S aureus*, especially if there is a high rate of these infections in the community. In children of preschool age and younger, *Kingella kingae* can be an important cause of pyogenic arthritis, and antimicrobials should be adjusted to cover *K kingae* in addition to the other common bacterial pathogens.

The clinical illness for the boy in this vignette had acute onset and thus would not be consistent with a diagnosis of juvenile idiopathic arthritis, which can be made only after persistent symptomatology (joint pain, swelling, stiffness) for 6 weeks.

Transient synovitis of the hip often occurs after viral infections. The patient in this vignette had a viral upper respiratory tract infection preceding the current illness, which could invoke consideration of transient synovitis. It can be difficult to distinguish between transient synovitis and pyogenic arthritis, particularly in the case of more indolent infections. However, the patient in this vignette has high fever, leukocytosis, a very elevated C-reactive protein level, and marked limitation in range of motion, which is more suggestive of pyogenic arthritis. In general, the acuity of symptoms and elevation of inflammatory marker levels is milder in transient synovitis than would be expected in pyogenic arthritis. The modified Kocher criteria can be used to help discern the 2 clinical entities (Item C21). Each criteria fulfilled by a patient gives stronger weight to a diagnosis of pyogenic arthritis over transient synovitis. In transient synovitis, imaging typically reveals small effusions, and joint fluid analysis would be expected to yield a white blood cell count between $5,000/\mu L$ and $15,000/\mu L$ (5-$15 \times 10^9/L$).

Item C21. Kocher Criteria for Septic Arthritis of the Hip.

Temperature > 38.5°C
White blood cell count >12,000/µL (12×10⁹/L)
Erythrocyte sedimentation rate >40 mm/h
Inability to ambulate
C-reactive protein >2.5 mg/L (23.8 nmol/L)*

* C-reactive protein not part of the original Kocher criteria.

Reprinted with permission from Herman MJ, Martinek M. The limping child. *Pediatr Rev.* 2015;36(5):190.

A traumatic effusion could be considered in this patient, especially given the history of a fall. However, fever and elevated levels of inflammatory markers are strongly suggestive of an infection, which could have been seeded by a primary traumatic process.

PREP Pearls

- Empiric treatment of pyogenic arthritis in children should include an antimicrobial expected to have activity against *Staphylococcus aureus* and streptococcal species, and in young children, *Kingella kingae* should also be covered.

- High fever, leukocytosis, elevated inflammatory marker levels, and inability to ambulate help distinguish pyogenic arthritis from transient synovitis.

- In the setting of pyogenic arthritis, fever and limited range of motion are almost always present, but external signs (erythema, swelling) vary depending on the site of disease.

American Board of Pediatrics Content Specification(s)/Content Area

- Plan the appropriate antimicrobial management of pyogenic arthritis
- Plan the appropriate diagnostic evaluation of pyogenic arthritis in patients of various ages
- Recognize the clinical findings of pyogenic arthritis or arthritis associated with rheumatic fever in patients of various ages

Suggested Readings

Arnold JC, Bradley JS. Osteoarticular infections in children. *Infect Dis Clin North Am.* 2015; 29(3):557-574.

Herman MJ, Martinek M. The limping child. *Pediatr Rev.* 2015; 36(5): 184-195.

The adolescent boy in the vignette has *corrected* vision of worse than 20/40 in 1 eye. Thus, he is considered a functionally 1-eyed athlete. If he were to sustain an eye injury resulting in vision loss in his better-seeing eye, this could result in significant disability. Baseball, basketball, hockey, lacrosse, and racket sports are among the activities typically considered high risk for eye injury, and the boy would require protective eyewear for participation in these sports.

Wrestling has historically been considered a sport with a low risk of eye injury. However, a recent study examining high school and college injury databases demonstrated that wrestling had the 4th highest rate of eye injury (after women's basketball, women's field hockey, and men's basketball). There is no commercially available protective eyewear for wrestling. Although custom-made eye protection may be available, the use of eye protection is typically not feasible for competitive wrestlers. Therefore, the boy in the vignette should not participate in wrestling.

The American Academy of Pediatrics (AAP) policy statement *Protective Eyewear for Young Athletes* outlines recommendations for eye protection for each sport. Eye injuries account for a relatively small percentage of the total number of sports injuries overall and only a small fraction of these result in severe dysfunction. However, because protective eyewear is easy to use and very effective at preventing eye injuries, protective eyewear is recommended for essentially all sports with a risk of eye injury. Eyewear used by athletes should conform to the American Society for Testing Materials (ASTM) standards for a particular sport as outlined in the AAP statement.

PREP Pearls

- Athletes are considered functionally 1-eyed if they have corrected vision of worse than 20/40 in 1 eye.
- Baseball, basketball, hockey, lacrosse, and racket sports are considered high risk for eye injury.
- Eyewear used by athletes should conform to the American Society for Testing Materials standards for a particular sport as outlined in the American Academy of Pediatrics policy statement *Protective Eyewear for Young Athletes*.

American Board of Pediatrics Content Specification(s)/Content Area

- Recognize the indications for the use of eye goggles during sports activities

Suggested Readings

American Academy of Pediatrics Committee on Sports Medicine and Fitness. Protective eyewear for young athletes. *Pediatrics*. 2004;113 (3 Pt 1):619-622.

Boden BP, Pierpoint LA, Boden RG, Comstock RD, Kerr ZY. Eye injuries in high school and collegiate athletes. *Sports Health*. 2017;9(5):444-449.

The type of measuring device used to administer liquid medications and the units marked on the device influence parents' ability to deliver an accurate dose. A syringe labeled in 0.5-mL increments is the best dosing device to provide this parent to ensure 2.5 mL of amoxicillin will be correctly administered. Although medication cups may be more accessible and perceived as more acceptable to parents, evidence shows there is an increased likelihood of dosing errors when liquid medications are given by cup compared with syringe. This occurs across health literacy and language groups, and is especially true for smaller amounts of medication. Medication errors by parents are more likely when teaspoon or tablespoon units are used compared with milliliter units. Also the use of dosing tools that are labeled with both milliliter and teaspoon units leads to more errors.

Parents commonly administer the incorrect dose of medication to their children. The ability of parents to understand medication dosing is related to their literacy and numeracy skills. The dose, formulation, and frequency of prescribed medications must be clearly explained. Provision of dosing tools closely matched to the prescribed dose volume is an important strategy to help reduce medication dosing errors. Prescribing easy-to-dose volumes when selecting the formulation of medications is another strategy. Pictographic depiction of dosage is also an effective means to ensure understanding and reduce medical errors at home. The use of household spoons as measuring devices should always be discouraged because of inaccuracy and inconsistency in volume. Over-the-counter products should provide clear directions and a concordant measuring device for parents to use.

Pediatric health care providers need to understand the impact of product packaging on medication safety, plus the role medical device design plays in the prevention of medical errors. Several medical organizations have issued statements that recognize the importance of clarity and precision for dosing orally administered liquid medications.

The American Academy of Pediatrics Committee on Drugs policy statement from April 2015 includes the following recommendations:

- Metric-based dosing with milliliters should be used exclusively.
- Medications should be dosed to the nearest 0.1, 0.5, or 1 mL.
- The concentration of the medication and the frequency of administration should be clearly noted on prescriptions.
- Appropriate-volume milliliter-based dosing devices should be distributed with the medication.
- Syringes are the preferred dosing device. Measuring cups and spoons calibrated and marked in milliliters are acceptable alternatives.
- Advanced counseling strategies to ensure parental understanding and adequate health literacy and numeracy should be offered.

American Board of Pediatrics Content Specification(s)/ Content Area

- Understand the role of medical device design in prevention of medical error
- Understand the impact of product naming and packaging on medication safety

Suggested Readings

Committee on Drugs. Metric units and the preferred dosing of orally administered liquid medications. *Pediatrics*. 2015;135(4);784-787.

Leonard MS. Patient safety and quality improvement: reducing risk of harm. *Pediatr Rev*. 2015;36;448-458.

Shonna Yin H, Parker RM, Sanders LM, et al. Liquid medication errors and dosing tools: a randomized controlled experiment. *Pediatrics*. 2016;138(4)e20160357.

Shonna Yin H, Parker RM, Sanders LM, et al. Pictograms, units and dosing tools, and parent medication errors: a randomized study. *Pediatrics*. 2017;140(1):e20163237.

Item 24   Preferred Response: C

The patient in this vignette has primary lactase deficiency. She has symptoms concerning for carbohydrate malabsorption (bloating, flatulence, and diarrhea), which are worse with lactose intake. Primary lactase deficiency occurs most commonly in adolescents and adults, although it can also occur in early childhood or infancy. Certain ethnic and racial populations, including African Americans, Native Americans, and Asian Americans, are at the highest risk for developing primary lactase deficiency. Lactase deficiency can also occur as a secondary phenomenon, for example following infectious enteropathy. This patient's symptoms, in the context of her age and ethnicity, are consistent with primary lactase deficiency. Diagnosis may be made clinically by removal of dietary lactose. If symptoms improve, referral to a gastrointestinal specialist may not be necessary. Lactose breath hydrogen testing is available as an objective measure of lactose malabsorption.

Lactase, an enzyme in the intestinal brush border, digests lactose (a disaccharide) to galactose and glucose (monosaccharides). The digestion of disaccharides to monosaccharides allows the intestine to absorb carbohydrates. When brush border enzymes are not present, undigested carbohydrates reach the colon where bacterial metabolism of carbohydrates produces gases. Symptoms include bloating, flatulence, abdominal cramping, and diarrhea.

Lactose intolerance/lactase deficiency is the most common disorder of carbohydrate malabsorption. Fructose malabsorption and sucrase-isomaltase deficiency are other key carbohydrate malabsorptive disorders. Fructose malabsorption is dependent on the amount of fructose ingested and is more common with large volumes of high-fructose–containing foods. Sucrase-isomaltase deficiency is a congenital deficiency of both sucrase and isomaltase enzymes, resulting in severe infantile diarrhea, failure to thrive, vomiting, and dehydration after starch/sugars are introduced into the diet. This deficiency is more common in native Greenlanders and Alaskans.

Galactosemia is an inborn error of metabolism, presenting early in infancy with feeding difficulties, liver damage, cataracts, and shock or liver failure, symptoms not seen in the patient in this vignette. Hereditary fructose intolerance, not to be confused with fructose malabsorption, is an inborn error of metabolism, presenting with hypoglycemia, liver disease/liver failure, and poor growth once infants are exposed to fructose (formula or solid foods). Sucrase-isomaltase deficiency would also present in infancy and is therefore not consistent with this case.

American Board of Pediatrics Content Specification(s)/ Content Area

- Recognize the clinical features associated with a carbohydrate malabsorption disorder
- Recognize the ethnic differences in the development of lactase and sucrase maltase deficiency

Suggested Readings

CaJacob NJ, Cohen MB. Update on diarrhea. *Pediatr Rev*. 2016;37(8): 313-322.

Hammer HF, Hammer J. Diarrhea caused by carbohydrate malabsorption. *Gastroenter Clin N Am*. 2012;41(3):611-627.

Item 25   Preferred Response: B

The boy in this vignette is demonstrating irritability, grandiosity, increased goal-driven activity, and decreased need for sleep. Because he also has a close relative with behaviors consistent with bipolar disorder, this boy is most likely to have bipolar disorder. While there is overlap with the symptom profiles for attention-deficit/hyperactivity disorder (eg, hyperactivity, impulsivity, distractibility), depression (eg, irritability), disruptive dysregulation mood disorder (eg, chronic irritability, angry outbursts, aggression), and oppositional defiant disorder (eg, irritability, anger), the episodic nature, grandiosity, and decreased need for sleep distinguish bipolar disorder from these other conditions. Disruptive dysregulation mood disorder is a new diagnosis introduced in the fifth edition of the *Diagnostic and Statistical Manual of Mental Disorders* that encompasses a persistently irritable mood with severe temper outbursts occurring on average 3 or more times per week.

Bipolar disorder has a prevalence of 1% to 3% in children and adolescents. The course of the condition is variable and mood tends to fluctuate rapidly. Bipolar disorder I is diagnosed when there is at least 1 episode of mania (elevated or irritable mood and energy or goal-directed activity for at least 7 days, causing severe impairment or warranting hospitalization). Bipolar II disorder is diagnosed when there is at least 1 episode of major depression and at least 1 episode of hypomania (elevated or irritable mood and energy or goal-directed activity for at least 4 days, not enough to cause severe impairment or to warrant hospitalization). The episodes of mania or hypomania are accompanied by 3 or more symptoms of grandiose ideation, decreased need for sleep, rapid speech, distractibility, flight of ideas, increased goal-directed activity, or over-involvement in activities with high risk for adverse consequences. When present, episodes of major depression can alternate with the mania (bipolar I) or hypomania (bipolar II) or may co-occur with mania or hypomania (mixed state). The child's moods exceed what is expected for the child's developmental age and are inappropriate for the context in which they occur. Pediatric bipolar disorder is more likely in children who exhibit excessive activity or silliness, significantly decreased need for sleep, and/or inappropriate sexual behaviors (without exposure to sexual activity or abuse). Bipolar disorder is also more likely when psychosis is present (eg, hallucinations). While mid- or older adolescent patients may present similarly to adults with bipolar disorder (eg, clear-cut mood episodes), younger children are more likely to have rapid or short mood episodes, or to present with mixed states, severe irritability, or disruptive behaviors. Attention-deficit/hyperactivity disorder, oppositional defiant disorder, and anxiety disorders commonly coexist with bipolar disorder in children.

Both biological and environmental factors contribute to the development of bipolar disorder in children and adolescents. A significant risk factor for bipolar disorder is a family history of the condition. Genetic studies on bipolar disorder indicate a heritability of greater than 80%. Parents with bipolar disorder are much more likely to have children with bipolar disorder than parents without bipolar disorder. First-degree relatives of children with bipolar disorder have an increased risk of bipolar disorder. Twin and adoption studies also support a genetic predisposition. Neuroimaging studies indicate involvement of several areas of the brain (limbic, frontotemporal, frontostriatal). Environmental contributors to poor prognosis include low socioeconomic status, family dysfunction or conflict, and trauma (eg, physical, sexual, emotional).

PREP Pearls

- A significant risk factor for bipolar disorder is a family history of the condition.
- Disruptive dysregulation mood disorder is a new diagnosis introduced in the fifth edition of the *Diagnostic and Statistical Manual of Mental Disorders* that encompasses a persistently irritable mood with severe temper outbursts occurring on average 3 or more times per week.
- In bipolar disorder, the child has episodes of elevated or irritable mood and energy or goal-directed activity (mania with at least 7 days of symptoms or hypomania with 4-6 days of symptoms). This activity may be accompanied by grandiose ideation, decreased need for sleep, rapid speech, distractibility, and flight of ideas.
- While mid- or older adolescent patients may present similarly to adults with bipolar disorder (eg, clear-cut mood episodes), younger children are more likely to have rapid or short mood episodes, or to present with mixed states, severe irritability, or disruptive behaviors.

American Board of Pediatrics Content Specification(s)/ Content Area

- Recognize the various environmental and biological contributors to the development of bipolar disorder in children and adolescents
- Recognize the clinical findings associated with bipolar disorder in children and adolescents

Suggested Readings

Lee T. Pediatric bipolar disorder. *Pediatr Ann.* 2016;45(10):e362-e366.

Tang MH, Pinsky EG. Mood and affect disorders. *Pediatr Rev.* 2015;36(2):52-61.

Wozniak J, Biederman J. Bipolar disorder in children. In: Augustyn M, Zuckerman B, Caronna EB, eds. *The Zuckerman Parker Handbook of Developmental and Behavioral Pediatrics for Primary Care.* 3rd ed. Philadelphia, PA: Wolters Kluwer; 2011:151-154

Item 26	Preferred Response: A

The boy in the vignette had an unwitnessed event that caused an acute loss of consciousness. The differential diagnosis for this includes head injury, intoxication, infection (meningitis or encephalitis), cardiogenic syncope, vasovagal syncope, and seizure. His evaluation in the emergency department is not suggestive of other underlying causes, therefore, seizure is a possibility. In children with new-onset seizure, electroencephalography can identify an epilepsy syndrome in about 50% of cases.

Lumbar puncture would be indicated if the boy had signs of meningitis or encephalitis, such as fever, meningismus, or purpuric rash. Without these signs, lumbar puncture is not likely to reveal any abnormalities. Magnetic resonance imaging of the brain is unlikely to show a cause for his altered level of consciousness, especially because computed tomography scan of the head was normal and his neurologic examination does not show any focal abnormalities. Diffuse, symmetric hyperreflexia, sometimes with upgoing toes on plantar stroking, can be seen after a generalized tonic-clonic seizure, and does not necessarily imply a structural brain abnormality. Hyperammonemia can cause altered consciousness, but would not cause hyperreflexia and there are no signs of hepatic dysfunction so this test is unlikely to identify any abnormality.

American Board of Pediatrics Content Specification(s)/ Content Area

- Identify the various etiologies of an altered level of consciousness
- Plan the appropriate initial evaluation of an altered level of consciousness

Suggested Readings

Camfield P, Camfield C. Special considerations for a first seizure in childhood and adolescence. *Epilepsia*. 2008;49(suppl 1):40-44.

Sadleir LG, Scheffer IE. Optimizing electroencephalographic studies for epilepsy diagnosis in children with new-onset seizures. *Arch Neurol*. 2010; 67(11):1345-1349.

Item 27   **Preferred Response: B**

The neonate in this vignette has findings characteristic of galactosemia, a metabolic disease caused by deficiency of enzyme activity or impairment of liver function resulting in elevated blood galactose concentration. Classic galactosemia of infancy presents within the first few days after birth and the initiation of cow milk–based formula or breastfeeding with signs and symptoms as described in the vignette. Abnormal laboratory results include liver dysfunction (hyperbilirubinemia, abnormal liver function test results, and coagulopathy), metabolic acidosis, galactosuria (indicated by the presence of reducing substances in the urine), and hemolytic anemia. Among infants with galactosemia, sepsis is most often caused by *Escherichia coli*. Cataracts associated with galactosemia may resolve if a lactose-free formula is initiated shortly after birth.

A cataract is a lens opacity that may occur at any age. It is a common yet preventable cause of blindness in children. Early recognition is critical for a good visual prognosis. Approximately 50% of congenital cataracts are idiopathic and 25% are genetic; the remainder are caused by infection, metabolic disease, and acquired causes. Galactosemia, as described in the vignette, is one of the most common metabolic causes of congenital cataracts. Additional associated metabolic diseases include hypoparathyroidism, hypoglycemia, and diabetes mellitus. Intrauterine infections, such as TORCH infections (toxoplasmosis, other [syphilis, varicella zoster], rubella, cytomegalovirus, herpes simplex) are commonly associated with congenital cataracts. Genetic etiologies include chromosomal abnormalities, such as trisomies 13, 18, and 21, and other syndromes. Risk factors for developing cataracts include prematurity, low birthweight, exposure to maternal diabetes, ocular trauma, toxins such as glucocorticoids or ionizing radiation, and familial forms. Hereditary forms of pediatric cataracts, which are inherited most commonly in an autosomal dominant fashion, may be present at birth or develop over time. Any offspring or siblings of a patient with childhood-onset cataracts should be referred to an ophthalmologist.

Prompt recognition and management of congenital cataracts is crucial for prevention of blindness. Therefore, every newborn should be evaluated for a red reflex in a darkened room with an ophthalmoscope. First, each eye should be examined individually from a distance of 1 to 2 feet, followed by the Bruckner reflex, during which both eyes are examined simultaneously from 2 to 3 feet. Immediate referral to an ophthalmologist is needed for findings such as an asymmetric, absent, dulled, or opaque red reflex; dark spots in the red reflex; or leukocoria (white reflex). After 3 months of age, poor tracking, lack of fixation, nystagmus, or squinting would warrant a referral. The American Academy of Pediatrics recommends assessment of visual acuity with instrument-based screening beginning at 1 year of age through 5 years of age or until visual acuity can be assessed reliably using an eye chart, usually at about 6 years of age.

Aniridia is the absence of an iris and is most commonly associated with WAGR syndrome (*W*ilms tumor, *a*niridia, *g*enital abnormalities, *r*etardation). Coloboma is a developmental defect of the eye in which one or more ocular structures are missing tissue. Colobomas are often associated with syndromes, such as CHARGE syndrome (*c*oloboma, *h*eart defects, choanal *a*tresia, growth *r*etardation, *g*enital abnormalities, *e*ar abnormalities). Glaucoma is a type of optic neuropathy that may be associated with elevated intraocular pressure. Primary congenital, infantile, and juvenile glaucoma are rare, but secondary glaucoma may develop in the setting of conditions including Sturge-Weber syndrome, aniridia, and retinopathy of prematurity and as a consequence of cataract surgery, tumors, trauma, or exposure to steroids.

American Board of Pediatrics Content Specification(s)/ Content Area

- Recognize the clinical findings associated with congenital cataracts
- Identify risk factors associated with the development of cataracts in patients of various ages
- Recognize the various disorders that may be associated with congenital cataracts

Suggested Readings

American Academy of Pediatrics, Committee on Practice and Ambulatory Medicine, Section on Ophthalmology, American Association of Certified Orthoptists, American Association for Pediatrics Ophthalmology and Strabismus, American Academy of Ophthalmology. Visual system assessment in infants, children, and young adults by pediatricians. *Pediatrics*. 2016;137(1):1-3.

Davenport KM, Patel AA. Cataracts. *Pediatr Rev*. 2011;32(2):82-83.

Grady NEG, Millard D. Congenital galactosemia. *NeoReviews*. 2017;18(4): e228-e233.

Item 28	Preferred Response: D

The patient in this vignette has symptoms of superior vena cava syndrome, which occurs when there is external compression of the superior vena cava, resulting in reduced blood return from the upper body and head to the heart. This leads to venous congestion in the face and arms as well as increased intracranial pressure. Over 90% of cases of superior vena cava syndrome are caused by cancer, and the chest radiograph for this patient shows a mediastinal mass. In children and adolescents, the most common cause of superior vena cava syndrome is a mediastinal mass.

Given the location of the mass on the radiograph, there should be concern not just for compression of the superior vena cava, but also of the right atrium. Should the mass completely compress the right atrium, there would be no blood return to the heart, and cardiac arrest would ensue. The factors helping to maintain the patency of the right atrium are gravity and negative intrathoracic pressure. Thus, lying the patient down on his back would worsen the compression of the right atrium, as would sedating the patient. The best management option for the patient's respiratory distress is to maintain him awake, sitting up, and with positive pressure.

The patient is a very poor candidate for general anesthesia as this would result in the loss of the negative intrathoracic pressure, increasing the risk of right atrial collapse. Consulting a surgeon for a biopsy would thus not be the next best step in management. Obtaining chest computed tomography would necessitate lying the patient supine on his back, thereby increasing the risk for right atrial collapse from the mass. As the compression in the chest is occurring distal to the larynx, the endotracheal tube would not bypass the obstruction and the sedation could potentially lead to cardiac arrest.

PREP Pearls

- For patients with mediastinal masses, there should be concern for maintaining the patency of the right atrium. Factors contributing to the risk for collapse of the right atrium include gravity and negative intrathoracic pressure; thus, these patients should not be lying flat supine, and sedation should be avoided.
- Signs and symptoms of superior vena cava syndrome often include edema of the face and arms, headache, and cough.
- Superior vena cava syndrome is caused by compression of the superior vena cava, most often by cancer.

American Board of Pediatrics Content Specification(s)/ Content Area

- Recognize the clinical findings associated with a chest mass
- Recognize the need for immediate evaluation of a child with a chest mass who is at risk of acute respiratory failure

Suggested Readings

Buhtoiarov IN. Pediatric lymphoma. *Pediatr Rev*. 2017;38(9):410-423.

Pearson JK, Tan GM. Pediatric anterior mediastinal mass: a review article. *Semin Cardiothorac Vasc Anesth*. 2015;19(3):248-54.

Prusakowski MK, Cannone D. Pediatric oncologic emergencies. *Emerg Med Clin North Am*. 2014;32(3):527-548.

Item 29	Preferred Response: D

The 4-year-old unimmunized boy in the vignette has signs, symptoms, and radiographic findings that are highly suggestive of acute epiglottitis. The best next step in management for this boy is administration of 100% humidified oxygen, along with obtaining expert consultation to secure his airway.

Epiglottitis, an infection or inflammatory process involving the epiglottis and surrounding supraglottic structures, is a relatively rare but life-threatening cause of acute stridor and respiratory difficulty in children. Historically, infection with *Haemophilus influenzae* type B (HIB) was most often responsible for causing epiglottitis. The epidemiology of the disease has changed because of routine vaccination against HIB, which has drastically decreased the incidence of epiglottitis. Other organisms that may cause epiglottitis include *Streptococcus pneumoniae*, *Staphylococcus aureus*, β-hemolytic streptococci, other types of *H influenzae* (A, F, and nontypeable), *H parainfluenzae*, *Klebsiella*, *Pseudomonas*, and multiple viruses. Epiglottitis may also arise from direct trauma or thermal injury to supraglottic structures.

Children with epiglottitis are typically febrile and toxic-appearing with drooling. Symptoms may include severe sore throat, dysphagia, and pain/tenderness over the anterior neck. Intermittent stridor (without cough), respiratory distress, anxiety, and a "tripod" position (leaning forward on outstretched hands with the neck extended and mouth open) are characteristic signs. These signs should raise providers' suspicion of upper airway compromise and warrant immediate intervention to stabilize the patient's airway. Caution should be used during the physical examination in children with suspected epiglottitis; they should not be forced out of a position of comfort or agitated, because it could worsen their airway obstruction.

The diagnosis of epiglottitis is largely clinical. Plain radiographs of the neck can help differentiate epiglottitis from other causes of stridor and respiratory distress (such as croup and upper airway foreign body), but they are not required or recommended if clinical suspicion of epiglottitis is high. A classic radiographic finding in patients with epiglottitis is the "thumbprint sign" (Item C29) seen on lateral neck radiography, which is created by a swollen, rounded epiglottis projecting into the hypopharynx. Neck radiographs (and any other studies) should *not* be obtained if doing so would cause a child to become agitated (which could potentially cause worsening airway compromise) or delay definitive management of a tenuous airway.

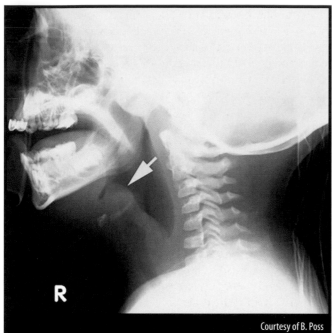

Item C29: Lateral radiograph of the neck in epiglottitis. There is enlargement of the epiglottis (arrow) giving the "thumb" sign.

Courtesy of B. Poss

In children with suspected epiglottitis, the most urgent priority in management is maintenance and stabilization of the airway. A provider with experience in airway evaluation and management (such as an otolaryngologist and/or anesthesiologist) should be immediately consulted. Patients should be allowed to remain in a position of comfort until the epiglottis can be visualized and a definitive airway can be established in a controlled setting, such as the operating room. Attempts to visualize the epiglottis should not be made in a setting (or by personnel) unequipped to manage an obstructed airway. Because of their smaller-diameter airways and the potential for rapid disease progression, many experts agree that younger children (<5 years) with epiglottitis should undergo intubation in a controlled setting, regardless of whether they have respiratory distress.

Nebulized albuterol would not be helpful in the management of epiglottitis, because this disease involves inflammation of the upper airway structures and not reversible constriction of the lower airways. In addition, administration of albuterol to the boy in the vignette could potentially agitate him, worsening his respiratory distress.

Although ceftriaxone and vancomycin would be appropriate parenteral antibiotics to treat the bacterial pathogens that could cause epiglottitis, placing an intravenous line and initiating antibiotics would be contraindicated at this point in this boy's care. He should be kept calm and in his position of comfort until a definitive airway can be secured. Intravenous antibiotic therapy can be initiated after control of his airway is established.

Intramuscular dexamethasone would not be the recommended first step in this boy's management. The role of corticosteroids in the treatment of epiglottitis has not been clearly established, as retrospective studies have not supported their efficacy in improving outcomes, and data from randomized clinical trials are not available. Administering an intramuscular injection to this child could agitate him and should be delayed until his airway is secured.

PREP Pearls

- Children with epiglottitis are typically febrile and toxic-appearing with drooling, severe sore throat, dysphagia, and pain/tenderness over the anterior neck, intermittent stridor without cough, respiratory distress, anxiety, and a "tripod" position.
- Epiglottitis is a relatively rare but life-threatening cause of acute stridor and respiratory difficulty in children.
- In children with suspected epiglottitis, the most immediate priority in management should be stabilization of the airway.

American Board of Pediatrics Content Specification(s)/Content Area

- Plan the appropriate clinical and laboratory evaluation of epiglottitis
- Plan the appropriate management of epiglottitis

Suggested Readings

Hopper EC, Perry H. Stridor. In: Shaw K, Bachur R, eds. *Fleisher and Ludwig's Textbook of Pediatric Emergency Medicine.* 7th ed. Philadelphia, PA: Lippincott Williams & Wilkins; 2015;chap 70.

Virbales J, Smith L. Upper airway obstruction. *Pediatr Rev.* 2015;36(2): 62-73.

Item 30   **Preferred Response: A**

The boy in the vignette has persistent microscopic hematuria (2 urine samples positive for blood over a 1-year period), proteinuria, and family history of renal failure and deafness (maternal uncle). This is suggestive of Alport syndrome (AS), an inherited disorder of basement membrane collagen characterized by involvement of the kidneys (always), ears (often), and eyes (occasionally).

Hematuria is the earliest manifestation and universal symptom in patients with AS. It is usually detected in childhood or even at birth. Seventy-four percent of patients present with hematuria by age 6 years. Patients with AS may present with gross/macroscopic hematuria or asymptomatic microscopic hematuria. Male patients fare poorly, with progression to renal failure by age 20 years (juvenile type) or 40 years or later (nonprogressive or adult type). Progressive renal failure associated with AS is characterized by increasing proteinuria, elevated serum creatinine, and the development of hypertension and anemia. Important extrarenal manifestations of AS include hearing loss and lenticonus. Bilateral sensorineural hearing loss (initially high frequency and progressively involving lower frequencies) develops over the first decade, with boys being more severely affected.

Hematuria may present as visible blood in the urine or microscopic hematuria. Microscopic hematuria is defined as more than 5 red blood cells (RBCs) per high-power field (hpf). In children, a single urinalysis will be positive for microscopic hematuria in up to 4% of samples. This incidence decreases to less than or equal to 1% for 2 or more urine samples. One-third of children with 2 or more urinalysis results positive for hematuria will have persistent microscopic hematuria (positive result on repeat test after a 6-month interval).

Asymptomatic isolated microscopic hematuria, frequently seen in children, is usually transient and benign in etiology. Persistent microscopic hematuria, hematuria with proteinuria, presence of RBC casts, dysmorphic RBCs on urine microscopy, or microscopic hematuria with associated symptoms suggest an underlying etiology requiring further evaluation, including referral to a subspecialist (Item C30). In the case of gross hematuria, a detailed history, physical examination, and urinalysis usually provide clues to the underlying cause.

In X-linked dominant AS, the most common mode of inheritance, males are affected and females are asymptomatic carriers. Gene defects of the α chain of collagen type IV lead to abnormal protein assembly, causing the characteristic abnormalities of AS. Genes encoding for these chains have been identified most commonly on chromosome Xq22 (COL4A5, COL4A6). COL4A3 or COL4A4 mutations lead to autosomal recessive or dominant AS, respectively, with similar disease severity in male and female patients.

Children with myoglobinuria will present with myalgia and muscle weakness, along with dark urine associated with muscle breakdown (rhabdomyolysis). This most often occurs with viral myositis, trauma associated with extensive muscle injury, excessive exertion, drug overdose, seizures, or metabolic disorders (hypokalemia increases the risk of rhabdomyolysis). Laboratory evaluation of myoglobinuria will demonstrate a urine dipstick test positive for blood and the absence of RBCs on microscopy, unlike the boy in the vignette. The urine in myoglobinuria has a clear sediment (lack of RBC) with a supernatant that is red because of the myoglobin pigment.

Glomerular hematuria (eg, nephritis) is usually described as cola, tea, or brown colored. In patients with glomerular or lower urinary tract bleeding, the supernatant is clear, while the sediment is red (presence of RBCs). Glomerulonephritis (GN) refers to immune-mediated (noninfectious) inflammation of the renal parenchyma. Depending on the severity of renal failure, serum chemistries may show azotemia and dyselectrolytemia. Further characterization of acute GN requires complement evaluation and, if clinically indicated, serologic evaluation for underlying vasculitis. Children with AS or immunoglobulin A nephritis may present with asymptomatic persistent microscopic hematuria, recurrent episodes of gross hematuria, or acute GN within just days of a viral infection.

Systemic lupus erythematosus (SLE) is a chronic inflammatory disease with multisystem involvement that may include skin, joints, kidneys, lungs, nervous system, serosal membranes, or other organs. Children with SLE may present with renal involvement alone, with hematuria and proteinuria on routine examination, nephrotic syndrome (proteinuria, edema, and hypoalbuminemia), or acute nephritis (acute renal failure, hematuria, and hypertension).

PREP Pearls

- Alport syndrome is an inherited disorder of basement membrane collagen characterized by involvement of the kidneys (always), ears (often), and eyes (occasionally). Hematuria is the earliest manifestation and a universal symptom in patients with Alport syndrome.

- Asymptomatic isolated microscopic hematuria frequently seen in children, is usually transient and benign in etiology.

- Persistent microscopic hematuria, hematuria along with proteinuria, presence of red blood cell casts, dysmorphic red blood cells on urine microscopy, or microscopic hematuria with associated symptoms suggests an underlying etiology requiring further evaluation.

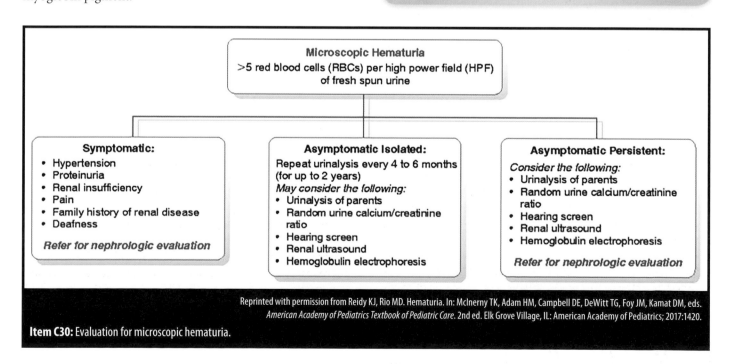

Reprinted with permission from Reidy KJ, Rio MD. Hematuria. In: McInerny TK, Adam HM, Campbell DE, DeWitt TG, Foy JM, Kamat DM, eds. *American Academy of Pediatrics Textbook of Pediatric Care.* 2nd ed. Elk Grove Village, IL: American Academy of Pediatrics; 2017:1420.

Item C30: Evaluation for microscopic hematuria.

American Board of Pediatrics Content Specification(s)/ Content Area

- Formulate a differential diagnosis of persistent microscopic hematuria with and without persistent proteinuria
- Plan the appropriate clinical and laboratory evaluation of microscopic hematuria

Suggested Readings

Massengill SF. Hematuria. *Pediatr Rev.* 2008;29:342-348.

Reidy KJ, Rio MD. Hematuria. In: McInerny TK, Adam HM, Campbell DE, DeWitt TG, Foy JM, Kamat DM, eds, American Academy of Pediatrics, Elk Grove Village, IL, 2017: 1420.

Item 31   Preferred Response: D

The neonate in this vignette is found on pulse oximetry screen to have an oxygen saturation of 88% in the right hand and 99% in the right foot. The presence of a patent ductus arteriosus (PDA) can result in different pulse oximetry findings in different extremities. Typically, the resistance in the pulmonary vascular bed is lower than the resistance of the systemic vascular bed, resulting in blood flow through a PDA from the aorta to the pulmonary artery, or left-to-right flow. This scenario would not result in differential pulse oximetry values for the right hand and lower extremity. The presence of pulmonary hypertension or an aortic obstruction (coarctation of aorta or interrupted aortic arch) with a PDA can result in differential cyanosis, which is characterized by a pulse oximetry reading that is higher in the right hand relative to a lower extremity. The neonate in this vignette, however, has a higher oxygen saturation in the right foot, which is called reverse differential cyanosis. Reverse differential cyanosis is seen in D-transposition of the great arteries when either pulmonary hypertension or aortic arch obstruction is also present. Given the findings of reverse differential cyanosis in this neonate, transposition of the great arteries is the most likely cardiac defect. The pulse oximetry screen with these findings should dictate prompt transfer to a pediatric facility with a congenital heart disease team.

Dextro-transposition of the great arteries is a congenital heart lesion in which the great arteries are switched from their typical location, resulting in parallel circulations instead of in-series circulations. "Blue" blood from the vena cava flows to the right atrium, into the right ventricle, out the aorta, and back around to the vena cava. "Red" blood flows from the pulmonary veins to the left atrium, the left ventricle, and then out the pulmonary arteries to return to the left atrium via the pulmonary veins. For a neonate to survive, there needs to be mixing of these 2 circulations, which ideally occurs at a nonrestrictive (big enough so that pressures on either side are equal) atrial level shunt. Although less mixing can take place across a PDA, its presence can be sufficient. Initiation of prostaglandin infusion to maintain an open ductus arteriosus can be life saving. Even in the presence of a PDA, neonates with no atrial level shunt or an atrial level shunt that is restrictive will be cyanotic (sometimes dramatically so) until a balloon atrial septostomy is performed. The neonate will require an arterial switch operation soon after birth.

Given the potential morbidity and mortality for newborns with critical congenital heart disease, most states have enacted a mandatory critical congenital heart disease (CCHD) screening prior to discharge from the newborn nursery. This screening assesses for the presence of a pulse oximetry reading of 95% or less or a difference of greater than 3% between the right hand and foot. Further details are available on the Centers for Disease Control and Prevention website (https://www.cdc.gov/ncbddd/heartdefects/hcp.html).

Ebstein's anomaly can present with varying degrees of cyanosis, depending on the degree of severity of the lesion, but will not present with reverse differential cyanosis. Hypoplastic left heart syndrome may result in cyanosis and may also present with differential cyanosis, but not reverse differential cyanosis. Pulmonary atresia will result in cyanosis but not reverse differential cyanosis.

PREP Pearls

- Differential cyanosis is the result of pulmonary hypertension or aortic obstruction, and reverse differential cyanosis is the result of pulmonary hypertension or aortic obstruction and D-transposition of the great arteries.

- D-transposition of the great arteries results in 2 parallel circulations, and mixing of the circulations is necessary for oxygen delivery. While a patent ductus arteriosus can help with that, an atrial level shunt is ideal.

- Most states require critical congenital heart disease (CCHD) screening prior to discharge from the newborn nursery. Oxygen saturations should be greater than 95%, with no more than a 3% difference between preductal and postductal oxygen saturations.

American Board of Pediatrics Content Specification(s)/ Content Area

- Recognize the clinical findings of transposition of the great arteries

Suggested Readings

Division of Birth Defects and Developmental Disabilities, Centers for Disease Control and Prevention. Congenital heart defects (CHDs): information for healthcare providers. https://www.cdc.gov/ncbddd/heartdefects/hcp.html.

Mahle WT, Newburger JW, Matherne GP, et al. Role of pulse oximetry in examining newborns for congenital heart disease. A scientific statement from the American Heart Association and American Academy of Pediatrics. *Circulation.* 2009;120(5):447-458.

Roth P. Pulse oximetry and the neonate. *Pediatr Rev.* 2016; 37(9):402-405.

Silberbach M, Hannon D. Presentation of congenital heart disease in the neonate and young infant. *Pediatr Rev.* 2007;28(4):123-131.

Item 32   Preferred Response: D

Self-esteem is defined as confidence in one's abilities and self-worth. Low self-esteem can influence an adolescent's psychological and physical development. The adolescent girl in this vignette is displaying signs of low self-esteem in that she is bullied about her appearance, does not have a support network at school, and has failing grades and evidence of nonsuicidal self-injury (NSSI) via cutting. She would benefit from counseling to address her thoughts about herself, identify areas that can be modified to improve her outlook, and develop coping skills to deal with comments from her peers at school.

Poor self-esteem has been associated with anxiety, depression, and suicide. According to the fifth edition of the *Diagnostic and Statistical Manual of Mental Disorders*, major depressive episodes in adolescents usually last between 4 to 9 months and often go unrecognized. The key features of depression in adolescents are a depressed or irritable mood for the majority of the day, sadness, and lack of interest in activities. Other diagnostic criteria include changes in weight (> 5% loss or gain), insomnia or hypersomnia, fatigue or loss of energy, psychomotor agitation or slowing, feelings of worthlessness or guilt, poor concentration, and suicidal thoughts or attempts. The diagnosis requires 5 of the 9 criteria to be present for at least 2 weeks and must include a depressed or irritable mood and lack of interest in activities.

Children who are overweight and obese are more likely to be bullied. Bullying includes verbal commentary, physical threats, spreading rumors, and social isolation. Children who are bullied often have low self-esteem and higher rates of depression and other mental health disorders, are more prone to substance abuse, and may have limited opportunities because of dropping out of school. Schools that use anti-bullying interventions tend to have less violence overall. However, many schools do not get involved and leave it up to the child and their parents to identify solutions. Schools that do not provide a safe learning environment and fail to enforce no-bullying policies are conveying a message for students to tolerate and accept abusive behavior.

Nonsuicidal self-injury is inflicting harm to one's own body without intent of committing suicide. It may include cutting, burning, biting, or punching. There is an 18% lifetime prevalence of NSSI amongst adolescents. Adolescents that repeatedly engage in self-injurious behaviors have a greater risk of committing suicide. Individuals who self-injure often report engaging in these behaviors for short-term relief of stress, to punish themselves, to deal with feelings of emptiness, and to communicate their feelings to others. Pediatricians and other primary care providers are often the first to identify that an adolescent is engaging in NSSI. The SOARS (suicidal ideation, onset, aftercare, reasons, and stage of change) model can be used to screen for NSSI and determine the appropriate type of brief intervention.

The adolescent in this vignette is morbidly obese with acanthosis nigricans. She should be screened for type 2 diabetes mellitus with a hemoglobin A_{1C} test and fasting plasma glucose test. She would also benefit from nutrition counseling by a dietitian and a discussion regarding adolescent weight loss programs in an effort to prevent long-term consequences such as cardiovascular disease, type 2 diabetes mellitus, hyperlipidemia, and nonalcoholic fatty liver disease. However, if her thoughts about herself and mood are not addressed first with therapy, it is unlikely she will be motivated to make other types of positive lifestyle changes toward improving her health.

PREP Pearls

- Adolescents should be asked about factors that may influence their self-esteem, such as support networks at home and school, bullying, and self-injury.
- Psychotherapy can be used to help adolescents process their feelings and develop healthy coping mechanisms to address negative interactions with peers.

American Board of Pediatrics Content Specification(s)/ Content Area

- Identify outcomes and plan the management of a poor self-image in adolescence

Suggested Readings

Glew GM, Frey KS, Walker WO. Bullying update: are we making any progress? *Pediatr Rev.* 2010;31(9):e68-e74.

Trzesniewski KH, Donnellan MB, Moffitt TE, Robins RW, Poulton R, Caspi A. Low self-esteem during adolescence predicts poor health, criminal behavior, and limited economic prospects during adulthood. *Dev Psychol.* 2006;42(2):381-390.

Westers NJ, Muehlenkamp JJ, Lau M. SOARS model: risk assessment of nonsuicidal self-injury. *Contemp Pediatr.* 2016;33(7):25-31.

Item 33   Preferred Response: B

The child in the vignette has suffered an asphyxial brain injury due to an unsafe sleeping environment. Although he has not suffered a cardiac arrest, he is breathing slowly and irregularly. His hypoxia is manageable with the administration of supplemental oxygen, but his ventilation is inadequate. Therefore, the most appropriate next management step is positive pressure ventilation.

Asphyxia is a condition of inadequate arterial oxygen content resulting in end-organ damage. The etiology of asphyxia varies significantly with age. Perinatal asphyxia can be caused by nuchal cord, placental abnormalities, chorioamnionitis, sepsis, airway and breathing derangements, meconium aspiration, preeclampsia, and prematurity. In infants, such as the child in this vignette, the most common cause of asphyxia is accidental suffocation. Asphyxia can also result from intentional suffocation, abusive head trauma/shaken baby syndrome, preexisting airway or breathing problems, or accidents such as drowning or foreign body airway obstruction. In cases of sudden unexplained infant death, an unsafe sleeping environment is often discovered, such as cosleeping, excessive bedding, soft surfaces, prone positioning, or the presence of loose objects. Prevention, via anticipatory guidance and an ongoing public campaign over the last few decades regarding safe infant sleeping practices, has greatly reduced the incidence of sudden infant death syndrome.

Asphyxia in children results in death in many cases. In contrast to adults, in whom cardiac arrests are generally cardiac in origin, the most common causes of pediatric cardiac arrests are respiratory. Therefore, if reversed, timely intervention can prevent death. Unlike sudden cardiac arrest from causes such as arrhythmia and coronary ischemia, asphyxial cardiac arrest occurs gradually. When hypoxia starts to occur, arterial oxygen content decreases, but cardiac output is maintained. Oxygen delivery falls, but the process of oxygen extraction by end-organ tissues maintains homeostasis for a period that can vary, depending on the suddenness of the breathing derangement. As hypoxia and reduced oxygen delivery worsen, cardiac output decreases, leading to end-organ ischemia. Cardiac arrest can occur due to myocardial ischemia.

Other than death, the most important consequence of asphyxia in children is hypoxic-ischemic encephalopathy. Thus, the most important therapeutic considerations include restoration of airway and breathing function, and supportive care of the brain. The child in the vignette suffered asphyxia in an unsafe sleeping environment, but was discovered before cardiac arrest. His hypoxia was corrected with supplemental oxygen, but ventilation remained inadequate, as evidenced by respiratory acidosis on blood gas analysis. Thus, positive pressure ventilation is the best next step in management.

Hypercapnia can lead to vasodilation of the cerebral vasculature, and subsequent elevation in cerebral blood flow, cerebral blood volume, and intracranial pressure. Early in the course of brain injury, this can worsen cerebral edema and lead to derangements in local tissue oxygen delivery. In severe cases, brain herniation can occur. In contrast, hyperventilation causes cerebral vasoconstriction. While this could temporarily prevent herniation in severe cases, decreased cerebral blood flow can cause tissue ischemia. Hyperventilation in pediatric neurointensive care has been extensively studied and has not been shown to improve outcome; instead, ventilation strategies to achieve a normal PCO_2 are recommended. Although therapeutic hypothermia has been shown to improve outcome after perinatal asphyxia and in adults following cardiac arrest, a National Institutes of Health–funded, multicenter, randomized trial on therapeutic hypothermia after pediatric cardiac arrest (THAPCA trial) did not show any benefit for hypothermia. Although the child in the vignette is acidotic, improving the ventilation would be more beneficial in this case than administering sodium bicarbonate.

PREP Pearls

- In cases of asphyxia in children, the most important therapeutic considerations include restoration of airway and breathing function and supportive care of the brain.
- In cases of sudden unexplained infant deaths, an unsafe sleeping environment is often discovered, such as cosleeping, excessive bedding, soft surfaces, prone positioning, or the presence of loose objects.
- In pediatric neurointensive care, ventilation strategies to achieve a normal PCO_2 are recommended.

American Board of Pediatrics Content Specification(s)/Content Area

- Recognize the clinical findings associated with cerebral edema in an asphyxiated patient

Suggested Readings

Moler FW, Silverstein FS, Holubkov R, et al. Therapeutic hypothermia after in-hospital cardiac arrest in children. *N Engl J Med.* 2017;376(4):318-329.

Moon RY, Fu L. Sudden infant death syndrome: an update. *Pediatr Rev.* 2012;33(7):314-320.

Shapiro-Mendoza CK, Parks SE, et al. Variations in cause-of-death determination for sudden unexpected infant deaths. *Pediatrics.* 2017; 140(1). pii: e20170087.

Item 34	Preferred Response: B

The infant in this vignette should be referred to an ophthalmologist for evaluation of strabismus. Although it is normal for infants to have a disconjugate gaze in the first 2 to 4 months after birth, eye movements should be conjugate by 6 months. Even in young infants, disconjugate gaze should be random; the report of 1 eye that consistently moves in a specific direction (eg, the right eye turning inward, as the parents in this vignette report) warrants careful examination. It would not be appropriate to consider referral for this patient only if she has a family history of childhood visual impairment. Because of the time-sensitive nature of treatment, delaying referral until after repeat examination at the next health supervision visit would not be indicated.

Visual impairment can arise from pathology at any point along the visual pathway, including problems in the visual media (cornea, anterior chamber, lens, and vitreous), retina, or along the neurovisual pathway (optic nerve, optic chiasm, retrochiasmal pathway, and cortex). Amblyopia, or reduced visual acuity because of abnormal visual development early in life, is the most common cause of visual impairment in children, affecting 1% to 4% of pediatric patients. Amblyopia can be classified based on its cause:
- Strabismic amblyopia: abnormal alignment of the eyes
- Refractive amblyopia: significantly different refractive error in the 2 eyes
- Deprivational amblyopia: interruption of the visual axis

Early detection and treatment of amblyopia improves outcomes. Treatment is most effective when initiated before age 7 years.

Children with visual impairment can present with various findings or may be asymptomatic. Parents may note abnormal eye movements or behavioral changes (eg, squinting, holding reading materials at unusual distances, or difficulties with tasks requiring clear vision). Older children may report headache, blurred vision, or double vision. Because many children with visual impairment are asymptomatic, the US Preventive Services Task Force and the American Academy of Pediatrics recommend screening all children during routine health supervision visits. Screening recommendations are shown in Item C34.

Item C34. Vision Screening Recommendations.

Age	Evaluation	Indications for Referral
Newborn (0–1 mo)	Examine outer structures of the eye and red reflex before the neonate leaves the newborn nursery	Abnormal red reflex requires urgent consultation
		History of retinoblastoma in parent or sibling
1 mo - 3 y	History	Poor tracking by 3 months
	Vision assessment; fix and follow	Abnormal red reflex
	External examination	Chronic tearing or discharge
	Ocular motility	
	Pupil examination	
	Red reflex evaluation	
3 - 5 y	History	Strabismus
	Vision assessment: LEA and Allen figures, HOTV letters, tumbling Es, Snellen chart	Chronic tearing or discharge
	External examination	Fail vision screen (cannot read 20/40 with one or both eyes or two-line difference between eyes) or photoscreening
	Ocular motility	Uncooperative after 2 attempts
	Pupil examination	
	Red reflex evaluation (photoscreening)	
	Ophthalmoscopy	
≥ 5 y	History	Strabismus
	Visual acuity	Cannot read at least 20/30 with one or both eyes or 2-line difference between eyes
	External examination	Fail photoscreening
	Ocular motility	Not reading at grade level
	Pupil examination	
	Red reflex evaluation (photoscreening)	
	Opthalmoscopy	
At-risk children of any age	History	Retinopathy of prematurity
	Visual acuity	Family history of retinoblastoma, congenital glaucoma or congenital cataracts
	External examination	Systemic diseases with associated retinal dystrophies/degenerations
	Ocular motility	Nystagmus
	Pupil examination	Neurodevelopmental delays
	Red reflex	
	Opthalmoscopy	

Adapted and reprinted with permission from the American Association for Pediatric Ophthalmology and Strabismus.

American Board of Pediatrics Content Specification(s)/ Content Area

- Recognize the clinical findings associated with visual impairment
- Identify the various causes of visual impairment

Suggested Readings

Jefferis JM, Connor AJ, Clarke MP. Amblyopia. *BMJ*. 2015;351:h5811.

Rogers GL, Jordan CO. Pediatric vision screening. *Pediatr Rev*. 2013;34(3): 126-133.

Item 35   Preferred Response: A

The outbreak of severe conjunctivitis among preterm infants in the neonatal intensive care unit (NICU), described in the vignette, is highly characteristic of adenovirus-associated epidemic keratoconjunctivitis (EKC). Adenovirus is a double-stranded, nonenveloped DNA virus that is viable for prolonged periods on environmental surfaces and fomites and is refractory to many forms of disinfection. Adenovirus serotypes 8, 19, and 37 are the most frequent causes of EKC. The disease is very contagious, causing outbreaks in the hospital and community.

Epidemic keratoconjunctivitis is characterized by severe follicular conjunctivitis with associated corneal inflammation (keratitis). Symptoms include significant pain, purulent discharge, photophobia, and blurry vision. Preauricular lymphadenopathy and subconjunctival hemorrhage may be noted. Adenovirus can be detected from eye secretions with culture or antigen testing; however, polymerase chain reaction is being increasingly used for rapid diagnosis because of its sensitivity and availability.

Adenovirus-associated EKC outbreaks have been reported worldwide and are associated with significant morbidity. Epidemic keratoconjunctivitis can result from direct or close contact with infected health care workers (HCWs) or contaminated equipment during ophthalmologic examinations. Outbreaks have been identified in various hospital settings including ophthalmology clinics, NICUs (following eye examinations for retinopathy of prematurity), as well as day-care centers with subsequent spread of infection to local hospitals. Simultaneous community transmission has also been reported.

Outbreaks of EKC are often difficult to control given the resistance of adenovirus to desiccation; prolonged viral shedding, ranging from days to weeks after symptom resolu-tion; high level of contagion; and large number of individuals affected. Adenovirus can survive in ophthalmic solutions and on equipment and other surfaces for more than 1 week. In addition to EKC, health care outbreaks of adenovirus-associated respiratory tract and enteric infections have been reported in hospitals and long-term care facilities. Outbreaks of adenovirus-associated pharyngoconjunctival fever can occur after exposure to contaminated water from swimming pools and shared towels.

To prevent EKC transmission, stringent infection control measures are required in all settings where ophthalmologic services are provided. Health care workers must be aware of adenovirus-associated EKC, adhere to basic infection control measures, and report suspected outbreaks or clusters of EKC infections to the local or state health department. In the case of an outbreak, enhanced control measures must be instituted in a timely fashion to prevent prolonged adenovirus transmission. Contact precautions are recommended for the duration of the illness for hospitalized patients with adenovirus conjunctivitis.

During EKC outbreaks, HCWs are the most frequently implicated sources of transmission. Recommended infection control measures in health care settings include (1) strict compliance with hand hygiene; (2) use of disposable gloves for any potential exposure to ocular discharge; (3) single-use disposable eye devices when feasible, and prompt disinfection of multiuse equipment after each use; (4) cohorting of suspected cases, and (5) furloughing of HCWs and staff with EKC. Other interventions include increased frequency of environmental surface disinfection and sterilization of instruments.

Chlamydia trachomatis is an important cause of neonatal conjunctivitis, but infection is not known to be communicable. Conjunctivitis or keratitis following primary herpes simplex virus (HSV) infection can occur as part of skin, eye, and mouth disease in the newborn. Spread of HSV in the NICU from infected HCWs has been infrequently reported, but does not result in EKC. Respiratory syncytial virus is known to cause health care–associated respiratory outbreaks in neonates and immunocompromised hosts, but does not typically result in EKC.

American Board of Pediatrics Content Specification(s)/ Content Area

- Recognize the clinical features associated with adenovirus infection
- Understand the epidemiology of adenovirus

Suggested Readings

Binder AM, Biggs HM, Haynes AK, et al. Human adenovirus surveillance - United States, 2003-2016. *MMWR Morb Mortal Wkly Rep.* 2017;66(39): 1039-1042.

Centers for Disease Control and Prevention (CDC). Adenovirus-associated epidemic keratoconjunctivitis outbreaks—four states, 2008-2010. *MMWR Morb Mortal Wkly Rep.* 2013;62(32):637-641.

Gordon YJ, Gordon RY, Romanowski E, Araullo-Cruz TP. Prolonged recovery of desiccated adenoviral serotypes 5, 8, and 19 from plastic and metal surfaces in vitro. *Ophthalmology.* 1993;100(12):1835-1840.

Item 36 — Preferred Response: C

Based on the maternal history and neonate's physical findings, oligohydramnios sequence is the most likely diagnosis. Mothers may develop oligohydramnios because of premature rupture of membranes or impaired fetal urine production. Because fetal lung development is dependent on sufficient exposure to amniotic fluid, neonates born to mothers with oligohydramnios often have poorly developed lung tissue. However, the degree of lung hypoplasia is not proportional to the amount of amniotic fluid present in the uterus. Therefore, it is difficult to predict the degree of respiratory distress until delivery. These neonates are also at risk for pulmonary hypertension and abnormal muscle growth and development. Neonates born to a mother with oligohydramnios may have facial features that appear compressed. They may also present with contractures such as the ankle contracture noted in the neonate in the vignette.

Oligohydramnios sequence is a series of findings resulting from oligohydramnios. In contrast, amniotic band sequence is a disruption of normal limb development typically caused by either constricting bands of amniotic tissue or a vascular insult. These neonates will often present with normal proximal limb development and distal abnormalities. The neonate in the vignette does not have a distal limb abnormality.

Maternal urinary tract infection may be associated with early-onset neonatal sepsis. However, it does not impair development. For neonates born prematurely before 37 weeks of gestation, normal development is interrupted but resumes postnatally. While postnatal organ development may not be normal, premature birth is not associated with physical malformations.

In 1946, obstetrician Dr Edith Potter described the characteristic facial features of neonates with renal agenesis. Potter syndrome specifically refers to oligohydramnios sequence resulting from bilateral renal agenesis. However, in practice, clinicians often refer to this set of physical findings as Potter syndrome irrespective of the cause of oligohydramnios.

PREP Pearls

- Neonates with pulmonary hypoplasia also may have pulmonary hypertension.
- Oligohydramnios sequence describes pulmonary hypoplasia, growth restriction, compressed facies, and abnormal positioning of the hands and feet in neonates born to mothers with low amniotic fluid levels.
- The extent of pulmonary hypoplasia is not proportional to amniotic fluid levels in utero.

American Board of Pediatrics Content Specification(s)/Content Area

- Identify the features associated with the oligohydramnios tetrad (Potter syndrome), and manage appropriately

Suggested Readings

Curry CJ, Jensen K, Holland J, et al. The Potter sequence: a clinical analysis of 80 cases. *Am J Med Genet.* 1984;19(4):679-702.

Elder JS. Congenital anomalies and dysgenesis of the kidneys. In: Kliegman RM, Stanton BF, St Geme JW, Schor NF, eds. *Nelson Textbook of Pediatrics.* 20th ed. Philadelphia, PA: Saunders Elsevier; 2016:2554-2556.

Joyce E, Ellis D, Miyashita Y. Nephrology. In: Zitelli BJ, McIntire SC, Nowalk AJ, eds. *Zitelli and Davis' Atlas of Pediatric Physical Diagnosis.* 7th ed. Philadelphia, PA: Elsevier; 2018: 510-539.

Item 37 — Preferred Response: D

The patient in this vignette has exercise-induced vocal cord dysfunction (VCD) or paradoxical vocal cord motion. Failure to develop objective signs of airway obstruction on formal exercise testing, combined with the characteristic flattened inspiratory arm of the flow-volume loop when she is symptomatic, are the findings most consistent with this diagnosis as opposed to exercise-induced asthma. Hints from the history include sensation of tightness in the upper chest and feeling that she cannot take in a good breath. Symptoms of VCD often begin early in the exercise session and are associated with the intensity of exercise. The sensation of the inability to breath worsens as exercise intensity peaks and airflow increases across the relatively narrow vocal cords.

Often patients with VCD will have tried inhaled bronchodilator and found no benefit. It is important to ask more specifically about the symptom of wheezing. Patients with paradoxical vocal cord motion will usually have an inspiratory "wheeze," which is actually the adventitial noise made when pulling air inward over a narrowed upper airway and not the fine expiratory wheeze characteristic of small airway obstruction in asthma. Item C37 illustrates an upper airway endoscopy from a patient with vocal cord dysfunction.

Vocal cord dysfunction is often mistaken for asthma, and it is not uncommon to have coexistent asthma and VCD in the same patient. In cases where the history is suggestive of exercise-induced asthma but there is not a good response to pretreatment with albuterol, the next most likely diagnoses are VCD and anxiety, which manifest similar symptoms.

A multimedia element is available for this critique on PREP® SA Online at www.pedialink.org.

Courtesy of M Guill

Item C37: Upper airway endoscopy from a patient with vocal cord dysfunction. Listen carefully over the background noise as the speech therapist coaches the patient to breathe in and out, and see the paradoxical vocal cord motion (closure on inspiration and opening on expiration). Then listen to the therapist coach the patient in short, sniffing breaths with long nasal exhalation to produce normal vocal cord function within the respiratory cycle.

It is unlikely that this patient would have severe enough anemia from menorrhagia to interfere with her ability to exercise, and the anemia would not cause "wheezing" or difficulty taking in a deep breath. Cardiomyopathy is a possible diagnosis, but the lack of cardiac findings on physical examination and the presence of objective information pointing to another diagnosis make this unlikely. Another possible diagnosis would be deconditioning as a cause for exercise-related dyspnea. But, deconditioning is generally not associated with wheezing or stridor/stertor.

PREP Pearls

- A patient's description of "wheezing" may not always represent the same pathophysiology that the physician considers to be wheezing.
- If a patient has atypical symptoms of exercise-induced asthma or does not respond to inhaled bronchodilator, another diagnosis should be considered.
- Vocal cord dysfunction can mimic asthma and often be mistaken for asthma.

American Board of Pediatrics Content Specification(s)/ Content Area

- Formulate a differential diagnosis for exercise intolerance

Suggested Readings

Abu-Hasan M, Tannous B, Weinberger M. Exercise-induced dyspnea in children and adolescents: if not asthma then what? *Ann Allergy Asthma Immunol.* 2005;94(3):366-371.

Boulet L-P, O'Byrne PM. Asthma and exercise-induced bronchoconstriction in athletes. *N Engl J Med.* 2015;372(7):641-648.

Tilles SA. Exercise-induced respiratory symptoms: an epidemic among adolescents. *Ann Allergy Asthma Immunol.* 2010;104(5):361-367.

Item 38	Preferred Response: A

A congenital, skin-colored, subcutaneous nodule that is firm to palpation and located on the lateral forehead or lateral orbital ridge likely represents a dermoid cyst. Entities that may mimic a dermoid cyst and features that differentiate them include:

- Epidermal cyst: Usually not present at birth (typically occur in adolescents and adults), may exhibit a central punctum (Item C38A)
- Infantile hemangioma: Usually not present at birth, compressible, not firm
- Juvenile xanthogranulomas: Usually not present at birth, appear as a dome-shaped orange papule or nodule (Item C38B)

Dermoid cysts are the result of entrapment of ectodermal tissues along lines of embryonic fusion. They are present at birth but may go unnoticed until they become larger (Item C38C), infected, or inflamed. Dermoid cysts are firm, noncompressible, nonpulsatile nodules that do not transilluminate. Most often they occur near the eyes, especially the lateral eyebrow, but they may be located on the nose, scalp (overlying the anterior fontanelle or midline occiput), or spine. Lesions involving the nose or midline scalp may be associated with intracranial extension, and lesions over the

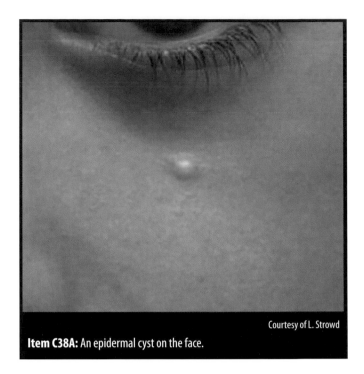

Courtesy of L. Strowd

Item C38A: An epidermal cyst on the face.

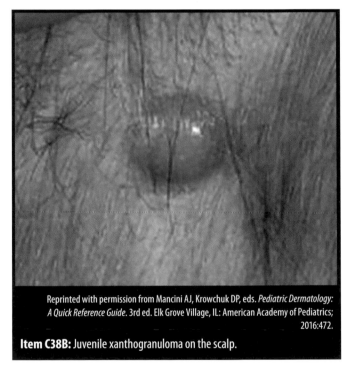

Reprinted with permission from Mancini AJ, Krowchuk DP, eds. *Pediatric Dermatology: A Quick Reference Guide.* 3rd ed. Elk Grove Village, IL: American Academy of Pediatrics; 2016:472.

Item C38B: Juvenile xanthogranuloma on the scalp.

spine may be associated with spinal dysraphism. A dermal sinus tract may also occur. This appears as a pit, sometimes with a tuft of protruding hair or keratinous drainage. Sinuses involving the midline craniospinal axis, including the nasal bridge, occiput, and midline back, raise concern for connection with the underlying central nervous system and risk of meningitis. All patients who have midline dermoid cysts or sinuses should undergo imaging (typically magnetic resonance imaging but occasionally computed tomography) to evaluate for possible intracranial extension. This evaluation is especially important if excision is planned. Lesions located near the eyebrow or on the lateral forehead do not require imaging before excision.

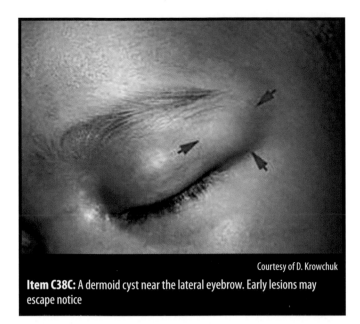

Item C38C: A dermoid cyst near the lateral eyebrow. Early lesions may escape notice

Courtesy of D. Krowchuk

PREP Pearls

- Dermoid cysts are firm, noncompressible, slowly growing nodules located most often on or near the lateral eyebrow.
- Lesions located in the midline (glabella, occipital scalp, midline back) or midline dermal sinuses require imaging to assess for central nervous system extension.

American Board of Pediatrics Content Specification(s)/Content Area

- Recognize the clinical findings associated with a dermoid

Suggested Readings

American Academy of Pediatrics Section on Dermatology. Dermoid cysts. In: Mancini AJ, Krowchuk DP, eds. *Pediatric Dermatology: A Quick Reference Guide*. 3rd ed. Elk Grove Village, IL; American Academy of Pediatrics: 2016:459-462.

Sewell MJ, Chiu YE, Drolet BA. Neural tube dysraphism: review of cutaneous markers and imaging. *Pediatr Dermatol*. 2015;32(2):161-170.

Item 39   Preferred Response: C

The patient in this vignette has an incidentally found thyroid nodule measuring 1.5 cm in greatest diameter. Her thyroid function test results are normal. According to current guidelines, a fine needle aspiration (FNA) biopsy with ultrasonography guidance is indicated to evaluate for thyroid cancer.

Indications for ultrasonography-guided FNA include a nodule of at least 1 cm in diameter or risk factors for malignancy on history, physical examination, or ultrasonography. Risk factors include a history of prior radiation to the head and neck, most commonly in cancer survivors, or a family history of thyroid cancer, especially medullary thyroid cancer. Medullary thyroid cancer is associated with the *RET* proto-oncogene and inherited in an autosomal dominant manner. Nodules that are firm, irregular, or fixed or that show microcalcifications or irregular margins on ultrasonography confer increased risk for malignancy. Abnormal cervical lymph nodes on palpation or by ultrasonography suggest regional metastases to the neck.

Thyroid function test results for the patient in this vignette are normal, indicating that the nodule is not hyperfunctioning. If the thyroid-stimulating hormone (TSH) level was suppressed, nuclear thyroid scintigraphy would be indicated to determine if the nodule is hyperfunctioning. Treatment for hyperfunctioning thyroid nodules is surgical, and preoperative FNA is not needed. Hyperfunctioning nodules are rarely malignant. For the patient in this vignette, obtaining nuclear thyroid scintigraphy would be indicated only if her TSH level was suppressed.

Thyroid cancer occurs in about 25% of thyroid nodules in children and adolescents, vs about 5% in adults. Papillary thyroid carcinoma, the most common thyroid cancer type in both children and adults, is more aggressive in childhood than adulthood but survival is better. Follicular thyroid carcinoma and medullary thyroid carcinoma are rare in pediatric patients. Medullary thyroid carcinoma has 100% penetrance in individuals with multiple endocrine neoplasia type 2A and 2B, which are inherited in an autosomal dominant manner. Pheochromocytoma and hyperparathyroidism are other components of type 2, in addition to a marfanoid body habitus and mucosal neuromas in type 2B.

Ultrasonography is the preferred imaging modality for thyroid nodules. For suspicious nodules, neck ultrasonography should also be performed to evaluate for abnormal cervical lymph nodes. Further evaluation should include a TSH level and referral to a subspecialist experienced in the evaluation and management of pediatric thyroid nodules.

For the patient in this vignette, reassuring her that no additional testing is indicated is not the best answer given the size of her nodule. Similarly, recommending repeat thyroid ultrasonography in 6 months is not the best answer because FNA is indicated.

PREP Pearls

- Evaluation of thyroid nodules includes a thyroid-stimulating hormone level, thyroid ultrasonography, and referral to a subspecialist experienced in the evaluation and management of pediatric thyroid nodules.
- Thyroid cancer occurs in about 25% of pediatric thyroid nodules, vs about 5% in adults.
- Thyroid nodules of 1 cm or greater warrant ultrasonography-guided fine needle aspiration.

American Board of Pediatrics Content Specification(s)/Content Area

- Plan the appropriate evaluation and management of a thyroid mass/nodule
- Recognize the clinical features associated with a thyroid cyst/tumor

Suggested Readings

Francis GL, Waguespack SG, Bauer AJ, et al; American Thyroid Association Guidelines Task Force. Management guidelines for children with thyroid nodules and differentiated thyroid cancer. *Thyroid*. 2015; 25(7):716-759.

Geddes G, Butterly MM, Patel SM, Marra S. Pediatric neck masses. *Pediatr Rev*. 2013;34(3):115-124.

Osipoff JN, Wilson TA. Consultation with the specialist: thyroid nodules. *Pediatr Rev*. 2012;33(2):75-81.

The boy in the vignette has Marfan syndrome, which is an autosomal dominant connective tissue disorder with a great degree of variability in clinical presentation even among members of the same family. Classic manifestations include ocular, cardiovascular, and skeletal involvement. Cardiac involvement includes dilation of the aorta, mitral valve prolapse, tricuspid valve prolapse, and proximal pulmonary artery enlargement. Children with this syndrome are at risk for aortic rupture; therefore, yearly echocardiographic monitoring for increased aortic root diameter is recommended, with intermittent surveillance of the entire aorta with computed tomography or magnetic resonance angiography beginning in young adulthood. The most common ocular manifestation is myopia; however, upward dislocation of the lens (ectopia lentis), retinal detachment, glaucoma, and early cataract formation are also frequently noted. Annual ophthalmologic slit-lamp examination is recommended. Skeletal findings include tall stature, scoliosis, pectus excavatum, pectus carinatum, arachnodactyly, and disproportionately long extremities. Facial features consist of a long and narrow face with deep-set eyes, downslanting palpebral fissures, malar hypoplasia, and micrognathia/retrognathia.

Marfan syndrome, caused by mutations in the *FBN1* gene, is typically diagnosed based on family history and characteristic systemic findings. Ectopia lentis and aortic aneurysm have high specificity and clinical significance for a diagnostic consideration of Marfan syndrome. Seventy-five percent of individuals have an affected parent, while 25% of probands have a sporadic de novo pathogenic mutation.

Ehlers Danlos syndrome is a group of disorders with a common feature of joint hypermobility. There are multiple subtypes, including classic, kyphoscoliotic, and vascular. Clinical findings include skin hyperextensibility, abnormal wound healing, easy bruising, and atrophic scarring.

Loeys Dietz syndrome is an autosomal dominant disorder that shares many features with Marfan syndrome including the pectus deformity, scoliosis, and aortic root aneurysm; however, several findings are not seen in Marfan syndrome, including hypertelorism, bifid uvula, craniosynostosis, cleft palate, and generalized arterial tortuosity along with dissections throughout the entire arterial tree.

Sotos syndrome is an autosomal dominant overgrowth syndrome characterized by a distinctive facial appearance with a broad forehead, sparse frontotemporal hair, downslanting palpebral fissures, long and narrow face, and malar flushing. Height and/or head circumference are greater than 2 standard deviations above the mean. Learning disability is common, varying from early developmental delay to mild, moderate, or severe intellectual deficit.

PREP Pearls

- In patients with Marfan syndrome, surveillance consists of an annual comprehensive physical and an ophthalmologic (including slit-lamp) examination, and echocardiography
- Marfan syndrome is an autosomal dominant connective tissue disorder with variable expression among members of the same family. Classic manifestations include ocular, cardiovascular, and skeletal involvement.
- Marfan syndrome, caused by mutations in the *FBN1* gene, is clinically diagnosed based on family history and characteristic systemic findings.

American Board of Pediatrics Content Specification(s)/ Content Area

- Recognize the clinical and laboratory findings associated with Marfan syndrome

Suggested Readings

Dietz H. Marfan syndrome. *GeneReviews.* https://www.ncbi.nlm.nih.gov/books/NBK1335/.

Goyal A, Keramati AR, Czarny MJ, Resar JR, Mani A. The genetics of aortopathies in clinical cardiology. *Clin Med Insights Cardiol.* 2017;11: 1179546817709787.

Tinkle BT, Saal HM, the Committee on Genetics. Health supervision for children with Marfan syndrome. *Pediatrics.* 2013;132(4):1059-1072.

The first-line therapy for sleep problems for the child in this vignette is to educate his caregivers on behavioral interventions to improve his sleep hygiene. While many children with neurodevelopmental conditions may benefit from medication for sleep, medication should be used only after behavioral interventions have been instituted.

One quarter to one-half of typically developing preschoolers and up to 80% of children with neurodevelopmental conditions have ongoing sleep problems. Screening tools such as questions based on the BEARS mnemonic (bedtime problems, excessive daytime sleepiness, awakening at night, regularity and duration of sleep, snoring) can help identify sleep disorders in primary care. For children aged 2 to 5 years, 11 to 12 hours of sleep per night is desired. School-aged children should sleep slightly less, 10 to 11 hours per night. Children with neurodevelopmental disorders may need even less sleep.

Behavioral insomnia of childhood (BIC) is diagnosed in children who have difficulty falling and/or staying asleep related to a behavioral problem. Sleep-onset association type BIC is diagnosed when the child depends on a certain stimulus to fall asleep and/or return to sleep after awakening at night. Limit-setting type BIC is diagnosed when the child stalls or refuses to go to sleep.

Proper sleep hygiene is the first-line therapy for most sleep disorders and is similar for children with and without neurodevelopmental conditions. The bedroom should be cool, dark, and quiet. Bedtime routines should be short, predictable, and soothing. Books and songs can be soothing; videos are not recommended. The routine should start at a consistent time and take ideally 15 to 30 minutes and no longer than one hour. Daytime naps should have a similar consistency in timing, length, and routine.

Teaching a child to fall asleep alone is an important skill to facilitate sleep onset and return to sleep after waking at night. The child should be guided to bed (ie, "tucked in") when he or she is drowsy but not asleep. Caregivers who lie in bed while children fall asleep can extinguish this behavior over time by gradually moving further from the bed over a few weeks until they are outside the bedroom. Children waking during the night and then coming into a caregiver's room should be promptly and consistently returned to their own bed. Positive rewards can be used to promote remaining in one's own bed all night.

Other sleep problems include night terrors, nightmares, and sleepwalking. Night terrors occur in about 3% of children aged 4 to 12 years and typically in the first few hours of sleep. Children appear frightened, sit up in bed, but are unresponsive; vocalizations are common. This problem is self-limited in most cases and requires no specific treatment. Nightmares tend to occur in the latter half of the night. Good sleep hygiene, a night light, and security objects can be helpful. Sleepwalking occurs in 3% to 5% of children, typically between 4 and 8 years of age. Management is generally focused on keeping children out of harm's way. Most cases remit by puberty. Medical conditions, such as persistent asthma and obstructive sleep apnea, as well as stress and anxiety, can affect sleep in children. Stimulants and corticosteroids can also negatively affect sleep.

There are few studies to guide the use of medications for sleep in children with neurodevelopmental conditions. In children with iron deficiency, iron supplementation may help improve the quality of sleep. Melatonin, a pineal gland hormone that regulates sleep, is often used for children with neurodevelopmental conditions. Initial dosing is 1 to 3 mg given 30 to 60 minutes prior to bedtime. The dose can be increased by 1 to 3 mg every 1 to 2 weeks up to a maximum dose of 10 mg. If there is no response after titrating to 6 mg per night, higher doses are unlikely to be helpful. Clonidine, an α_2-adrenergic agonist, can be prescribed if melatonin is not effective. It is particularly helpful in children with concurrent behavior problems. Clonidine should also be started at a low dose and titrated over time. Caution is warranted in children taking other central nervous system depressant medications. Trazodone, a sedating antidepressant, and gabapentin, a GABA (γ-aminobutyric acid) precursor often used for chronic pain, can be prescribed if other alternatives fail, but studies to guide their use in sleep disorders are limited.

Polysomnography involves gathering cardiorespiratory data with or without electroencephalography during sleep. It is typically performed in a sleep laboratory and is used to diagnose sleep-related breathing disorders (eg, obstructive sleep apnea), periodic limb movement disorder, sleep-related seizures, narcolepsy, and other sleep-wake disorders. Due to a lack of symptoms such as snoring or respiratory pauses in this patient, a sleep study would not be indicated.

PREP Pearls

- Improving sleep hygiene is the first-line therapy for sleep disorders with a behavioral component.
- Medications (eg, melatonin) can be a useful adjunct to good sleep hygiene in children with neurodevelopmental conditions and sleep disorders.

American Board of Pediatrics Content Specification(s)/Content Area

- Counsel parents regarding appropriate bedtime routines for their children
- Understand the effects of various medications on sleep

Suggested Readings

Bhargava S. Diagnosis and management of common sleep problems in children. *Pediatr Rev.* 2011;32(3):91-99.

Blackmer AB, Feinstein JA. Management of sleep disorders in children with neurodevelopmental disorders: a review. *Pharmacotherapy.* 2016; 36(1):84-98.

| Item 42 | Preferred Response: D |

The additional vaccine that is most appropriate for the girl in this vignette is Tdap. Infection with *Bordetella pertussis* provides only short-term protection against future pertussis infection. Thus, a documented infection should not alter the standard immunization schedule. Therefore, the patient in the vignette should receive a pertussis-containing vaccine as is routinely recommended at the 11- to 12-year-old visit.

In childhood, a total of 6 doses of pertussis-containing vaccine are recommended. Children younger than 7 years receive DTaP in a 5-dose series, typically at ages 2, 4, 6, and 15 to 18 months as well as 4 to 6 years. Individuals 7 years of age or older receive Tdap, which has reduced concentrations of pertussis antigens. One dose of Tdap is given at 11 to 12 years of age. Any person 19 years of age or older who has not previously received a dose of Tdap should receive one. It is important that health care workers receive one dose of Tdap if they have not previously received this vaccination. The only group for which more than one dose of Tdap is recommended is pregnant women. The vaccine should be administered with each pregnancy between 27 and 36 weeks' gestation as the best means of protecting young infants from pertussis.

Reactions to pertussis-containing vaccine include local-site reactions (redness, tenderness, localized swelling) and potentially systemic symptoms including crying, anorexia, vomiting, and moderate fever. A small percentage of patients can experience swelling of the entire extremity where the vaccine was administered. Entire-limb swelling typically occurs after the fourth or fifth dose of DTaP, resolves spontaneously, and is not a contraindication to future vaccination.

The whole-cell pertussis vaccine was plagued by issues of reactogenicity. The occurrence of seizures, typically febrile seizures, with whole-cell pertussis vaccine was estimated to be 1 in 1,750 doses. Postlicensure studies of the acellular vaccine did not reveal an increased risk for seizures. Similarly, hypotonic-hyporesponsive episodes occurred after whole-cell pertussis vaccine with the same frequency. While acellular pertussis vaccines are considered to be safer than whole-cell pertussis vaccines, the long-term efficacy of acellular vaccines is inferior to the whole-cell vaccines.

Contraindications to pertussis vaccine include anaphylaxis following a previous vaccination or development of encephalopathy that cannot be ascribed to another reason in the 7-day period following pertussis vaccination. That said, there is no evidence that links pertussis vaccination with any acute-onset neurologic illness.

Waning immunity is felt to be largely responsible for the resurgence in cases of pertussis in the United States in the last few decades. Immunity to pertussis wanes over a period of 7 to 20 years after vaccination. Several epidemics in the United States have revealed high attack rates in the 7- to 10-year-old and 10- to 14-year-old age groups, coinciding with the expected timeframe for waning from the last dose of DTaP in the childhood series (4 to 6 years). In 2005, it was recommended that the Tdap booster be given at 11 to 12 years to help overcome waning immunity in older children and adolescents.

The girl in this vignette should receive a pertussis-containing vaccine at this visit; therefore, DT and Td would not be appropriate. She should not receive DTaP because it is only licensed for children younger than 7 years.

PREP Pearls

- A documented pertussis infection should not alter the standard immunization schedule.
- In childhood, a total of 6 doses of pertussis-containing vaccine are recommended: DTaP in a 5-dose series, typically at ages 2, 4, 6, and 15 to 18 months as well as 4 to 6 years, and 1 dose of Tdap at 11 to 12 years.
- Waning immunity is felt to be largely responsible for the resurgence in cases of pertussis seen in the United States in the last few decades.

American Board of Pediatrics Content Specification(s)/Content Area

- Know the indications, contraindications, schedules, and possible complications associated with pertussis vaccine
- Recognize the effects of waning immunity to pertussis in contacts of infected patients
- Understand the difference between the whole-cell and acellular pertussis vaccines

Suggested Readings

American Academy of Pediatrics. Pertussis (whooping cough). In: Kimberlin DW, Brady MT, Jackson MA, Long SS, eds. *Red Book: 2018 Report of the Committee on Infectious Diseases.* 31st ed. Itasca, IL: American Academy of Pediatrics; 2018:620-633.

Jakinovich A, Sood S. Pertussis: still a cause of death, seven decades into vaccination. *Curr Opin Pediatr.* 2014;26(5):597-604.

Robinson CL, Romero JR, Kempe A, Pellegrini C, Szilagyi P. Advisory Committee on Immunization Practices recommended immunization schedule for children and adolescents aged 18 years or younger–United States, 2018. *MMWR Morb Mortal Wkly Rep.* 2018;67(5):156-157.

The knee radiographs of the girl in the vignette demonstrate a small, well-defined radiolucent cortical lesion with a surrounding rim of sclerosis; this appearance is consistent with a nonossifying fibroma (NOF; also referred to as a "fibrous cortical defect"). Nonossifying fibromas, very commonly seen in children, are typically discovered incidentally. Nonossifying fibromas larger than 50% of a bone's diameter carry a risk of pathologic fracture and should be followed every 6 to 12 months with radiographs. Small NOFs resolve spontaneously, and do not require follow-up.

Nonossifying fibromas can have a similar appearance to fibrous dysplasia. Fibrous dysplasia lesions, while benign, tend to enlarge with growth and have a significant risk of pathologic fracture. Unlike NOFs, fibrous dysplasia lesions are found in the medullary canal and cause thinning of the adjacent bony cortex.

Unicameral, or 'simple' bone cysts (UBCs), are fluid-filled cysts surrounded by a thin rim of bone. They most commonly originate in the proximal humerus (Item C43) or proximal femur. Although most UBCs are found incidentally, some cases are discovered after a pathologic fracture occurs. Children with UBCs in locations where a fracture is likely to lead to surgery, such as the femoral neck, should be referred to an orthopaedic surgeon for treatment with either corticosteroid injection or operative management.

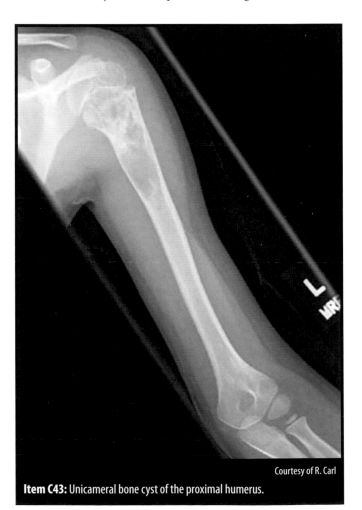

Courtesy of R. Carl

Item C43: Unicameral bone cyst of the proximal humerus.

Aneurysmal bone cysts (ABCs) are blood-filled loculated cysts. Aneurysmal bone cysts can be distinguished from UBCs based on their loculated appearance and tendency to have an eccentric location. They may be discovered incidentally or after pathologic fracture. Some children with ABCs experience pain even without fracture. All children with ABCs should be referred to orthopaedic surgery for operative treatment.

When evaluating radiolucent lesions, sclerosis or thickening of the bone surrounding a defect is indicative of a stable, benign lesion. Lesions that expand beyond the cortex and do not have distinct margins are more concerning for malignancy, and would merit evaluation by oncology or orthopaedic surgery.

PREP Pearls

- Bone lesions that expand beyond the cortex, and do not have distinct margins, are concerning for malignancy and warrant referral to oncology or orthopaedic surgery.
- Sclerosis of the bone surrounding a radiolucent defect is indicative of a stable, benign lesion.

American Board of Pediatrics Content Specification(s)/ Content Area

- Formulate a differential diagnosis of a bone cyst
- Understand the natural history of a bone cyst

Suggested Readings

Canavese F, Wright JG, Cole WG, Hopyan S. Unicameral bone cysts: comparison of percutaneous curettage, steroid, and autologous bone marrow injections. *J Pediatr Orthop.* 2011;31(1):50-55.

Donaldson S, Wright JG. Simple bone cysts: better with age? *J Pediatr Orthop.* 2015;35(1):108-114.

Sarwark JF, LaBella CR, eds. *Pediatric Orthopaedics and Sports Injuries: A Quick Reference Guide.* 2nd ed. Elk Grove Village, IL: American Academy of Pediatrics; 2014.

Item 44   **Preferred Response: B**

Sexual abuse of children is a common problem. Pediatric health care providers are in a position to be the first to identify cases and must be prepared to provide ongoing emotional support to the victims and their parents or caregivers. Of the psychosocial and environmental factors listed, the greatest risk for child sexual abuse is living in a single parent family (family structure). There is no association between child sexual abuse and ethnicity or socioeconomic status. Most perpetrators are male and known to the child; they may be family members, relatives, friends, teachers, coaches, babysitters, or other trusted authority figures. Adolescents are at risk for intimate partner violence, date rape, or less commonly, forceful sexual assault by a stranger.

Teenagers and young adults have the highest rates of being sexually assaulted. The majority of victims are female. Alcohol remains the most common date rape drug. Individuals with intellectual or physical disabilities are at an increased risk for sexual assault and acquaintance rape. Child victims are physically or emotionally vulnerable and may be victimized because they are eager for attention and affection. Children whose families have other psychosocial stressors, such as parental conflict, addiction, or mental health issues are also at greater risk.

Sexual abuse can lead to profound adverse behavioral and emotional consequences; these reactions may occur immediately or present at a later time, and may persist for years. Child and adolescent survivors of sexual abuse may present with various behavioral concerns. They may be withdrawn, angry, depressed, anxious, inattentive, or aggressive. They may have nonspecific complaints, such as sleep disturbance, academic problems, recurrent pain, or somatization. Young children may exhibit sexualized behavior, including imitation of adult sexual acts, that is inappropriate for their age and developmental stage. Adolescents may have early-onset and high-risk sexual behavior or sexual dysfunction. Low self-esteem, eating disorders, self-mutilation, and substance abuse are common consequences. Mental health problems may include suicidal ideation and attempts. The impact on the survivor varies depending on the age at onset, severity, frequency, and duration of the abuse. An important mitigating factor is the presence of a supportive protective parent or adult caregiver who believes the disclosure of abuse. Mental health interventions and other community resources should be offered to the patient and caregivers.

PREP Pearls

- Most perpetrators of sexual abuse are male and known to the victim.
- Sexual abuse can lead to profound adverse behavioral and emotional consequences; these reactions may occur immediately or at a later time, and may persist for years.
- There is no association between child sexual abuse and ethnicity or socioeconomic status.

American Board of Pediatrics Content Specification(s)/ Content Area

- Understand the epidemiology of and the psychosocial and environmental risk factors for sexual abuse
- Understand the behavioral and emotional consequences of child sexual abuse

Suggested Readings

Chiena A, Goldson E. Child sexual abuse. *Pediatr Rev.* 2017;38(3):105-118.

Crawford-Jakubiak JE, Alderman EM, Leventhal JM. AAP Committee on Child Abuse and Neglect, AAP Committee on Adolescence. Care of the adolescent after an acute sexual assault. *Pediatrics.* 2017;139(3):e20164243.

Fortin K, Jenny C. Sexual abuse. *Pediatr Rev.* 2012;33(1):19-32.

Item 45 — Preferred Response: B

The patient in this vignette has giardiasis (also known as *Giardia intestinalis*, *Giardia lamblia*, or *Giardia duodenalis*) with evidence of acute diarrhea and steatorrhea after a recent camping trip. Giardiasis causes an enteropathy or inflammation of the small intestine; if significant enough, this can lead to malabsorption (as seen in this patient with steatorrhea), weight loss, and failure to thrive. Anemia may be caused by poor iron absorption. Hematochezia or hemoccult-positive stools are not expected features of giardiasis.

Giardia is a flagellated protozoan pathogen and is the most common intestinal parasitic infestation in the world. Transmission can occur from person-to-person contact or after ingestion of contaminated water or food. The incubation period typically lasts 1 to 3 weeks. A person with giardiasis can continue to excrete cysts while untreated for weeks to months (and will remain infectious during this time).

Diagnosis of giardiasis is most frequently made with stool testing. Even with a high index of clinical suspicion, stool testing should be performed to confirm the diagnosis of giardiasis. Direct microscopic examination of a diarrheal stool (ova and parasite examination) has a sensitivity of 75% to 95%. Specific enzyme immunoassay has a sensitivity of 95% and specificity of 98% to 100%. Endoscopy is not required for diagnosis; however, if performed, duodenal fluid may be aspirated and evaluated for direct microscopic examination and/or enzyme immunoassay, and duodenal biopsies can demonstrate active *Giardia* infestation. Treatment options for *Giardia* in children include metronidazole, nitazoxanide, and tinidazole. Because giardiasis results in an enteropathy, transient lactose intolerance may occur; thus, a low-lactose diet may be temporarily helpful for symptom control.

Clostridium difficile infection would typically manifest as profuse bloody diarrhea, which was not present in this case. The pancreatic elastase level would be abnormal with pancreatic insufficiency; in this patient, the steatorrhea is the result of an enteropathy, not pancreatic insufficiency. Stool culture or polymerase chain reaction would test for bacterial causes of colitis.

PREP Pearls

- Giardiasis should be suspected in patients with malabsorptive diarrhea.
- Giardiasis is the most common intestinal parasitic infection worldwide and is transmitted by person-to-person contact or by ingesting contaminated water or food.
- Diagnosis of giardiasis is confirmed with direct microscopic evaluation and/or *Giardia*-specific enzyme immunoassay of stool samples.

American Board of Pediatrics Content Specification(s)/Content Area

- Plan the appropriate diagnostic evaluation when *Giardia lamblia* infestation is suspected
- Understand the epidemiology of *Giardia lamblia*
- Recognize the clinical features associated with *Giardia lamblia* infestation, and manage appropriately

Suggested Readings

American Academy of Pediatrics. *Giardia intestinalis* (formerly *Giardia lamblia* and *Giardia duodenalis*) infections (giardiasis). In: Kimberlin DW, Brady MT, Jackson MA, Long SS, eds. *Red Book: 2018 Report of the Committee on Infectious Diseases. 31st ed.* Itasca, IL: American Academy of Pediatrics; 2018:352-355.

Mmbaga BT, Houpt ER. *Cryptosporidium* and *Giardia* infections in children: a review. *Pediatr Clin North Am.* 2017;64(4):837-850.

Item 46 — Preferred Response: D

The girl in this vignette is demonstrating symptoms of posttraumatic stress disorder (PTSD). Her symptoms of poor concentration, withdrawal, startling easily, and sleep disturbance began after she and her family experienced a threat of harm from wildfires. The primary treatment of children with PTSD is evidence-based trauma-focused psychotherapy. In trauma-focused cognitive-behavioral therapy, a therapist works with both parent and child. The therapist assists the child in discussing and processing the trauma. The therapist works with the child to restructure troubling thoughts and to learn coping strategies and skills. The therapist teaches the parent skills to manage the child's symptoms and to communicate with their child about the trauma.

Posttraumatic stress disorder can develop in children and adolescents after experiencing actual or threatened harm to themselves or to others. These traumatic events may include interpersonal violence (eg, physical, sexual, domestic), natural disasters, accidents (eg, motor vehicle collisions), war, or serious injury. Approximately 16% of children exposed to a traumatic event develop PTSD. Children who are exposed to interpersonal violence, sexual abuse, a high threat to life, or war are more likely to develop PTSD.

Posttraumatic stress disorder is diagnosed when symptoms are present for at least a month and result in impaired functioning. Intrusive and uncontrollable thoughts and hyperarousal (eg, difficulty falling or staying asleep) are characteristic. Children actively avoid and are distressed with reminders of the trauma (eg, memories, places, people, smells, sounds, sights). Children may have physical symptoms (eg, abdominal pain) and may be fearful, agitated, or angry. Hypervigilance can cause these children to startle easily, be irritable, and be fearful of strangers. They feel unsafe and may have difficulty concentrating.

In young children (ie, up to 5 years of age), PTSD may present as aggression, temper tantrums, withdrawal, sleep disturbance with recurrent nightmares or fear of sleeping by themselves, difficulty separating from parents, and repetitive play about the traumatic event. These young children may withdraw and be less interested in exploring their environment to avoid cues of their previous trauma. School-age children may demonstrate aggression, anger, and withdrawal. They may feel helpless and overwhelmed. Adolescents may be preoccupied with the meaning of the event and feelings of guilt (eg, survivor's guilt). They may take more risks than previously or may fear an early death.

While medications such as selective serotonin reuptake inhibitors are sometimes considered for treatment of PTSD, they are usually not indicated unless a coexisting disorder such as anxiety or depression is also present. α-Adrenergic agents have been proposed to decrease hyperarousal symptoms or address sleep problems but current evidence is not sufficient to recommend their use for treatment of PTSD. Parent-child interaction therapy is a parent behavioral training treatment program that teaches parents positive engagement and communication with their children and effective strategies for managing difficult behaviors (eg, aggression, defiance). It is typically used for parents with young children with disruptive behaviors.

PREP Pearls

- Children who are exposed to interpersonal violence, sexual abuse, a high threat to life, or war are more likely to develop posttraumatic stress disorder.
- In young children (ie, up to 5 years of age), posttraumatic stress disorder may present as aggression, temper tantrums, withdrawal, sleep disturbance with recurrent nightmares or fear of sleeping by themselves, difficulty separating from parents, and repetitive play about the traumatic event.
- Posttraumatic stress disorder is diagnosed in children and adolescents who have experienced actual or threatened harm to themselves or others and who manifest symptoms of intrusive and uncontrollable thoughts, avoidance and distress with reminders of the trauma, and altered cognitions and mood for at least a month with resultant impairment in functioning.
- The primary treatment of children with posttraumatic stress disorder is evidence-based trauma-focused psychotherapy, which involves a therapist working with both parent and child.

American Board of Pediatrics Content Specification(s)/ Content Area

- Recognize the clinical findings associated with post-traumatic stress disorder in patients of various ages, and manage appropriately

Suggested Readings

Copeland-Linder N. Posttraumatic stress disorder. *Pediatr Rev.* 2008;29(3):103-104.

Kelly P. Posttraumatic stress disorder. *Pediatr Rev.* 2012;33(8):382-383.

Saxe G. Posttraumtic stress disorder in children. In: Augustyn M, Zuckerman B, Caronna EB, eds. *The Zuckerman Parker Handbook of Developmental and Behavioral Pediatrics for Primary Care.* 3rd ed. Philadelphia, PA: Wolters Kluwer; 2011:302-304.

Item 47 **Preferred Response: D**

The Langley Model for Improvement, often called the Model for Improvement, is a framework used to create improvement in many systems, including healthcare. It starts with 3 questions that generate corresponding statements:

Question	Statement
What are we trying to accomplish?	Aim
How will we know that a change is an improvement?	Measurement
What changes can we make that will lead to an improvement?	Changes that may lead to an improvement

Once these statements are defined, the changes are tested in a Plan-Do-Study-Act (PDSA) cycle (Item C47). The results of the PDSA cycle may or may not demonstrate whether the aim was achieved, and may be used to generate new changes, which are then followed by a new PDSA cycle. In the project in the vignette, the first PDSA cycle was completed but the results showed that the average time actually increased instead of decreasing. Discussion among the team members revealed a possible reason for this result. Of the response choices, the best next step is to do another PDSA cycle, for instance, in the same season as the baseline data are gathered.

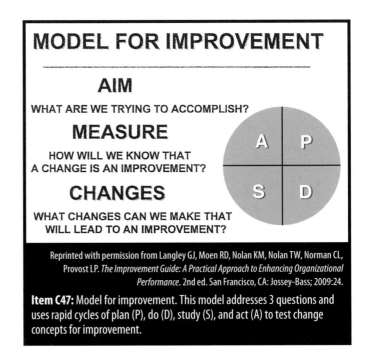

Item C47: Model for improvement. This model addresses 3 questions and uses rapid cycles of plan (P), do (D), study (S), and act (A) to test change concepts for improvement.

Changing the Aim statement would only be helpful if the goal for improvement has changed. Unexpected PDSA results should prompt changes in the improvement plan and additional PDSA cycles, not a change in the Aim.

Correct interpretation of PDSA cycle results is important to achieving the Aim. In the vignette, the time the patient was ready-to-be-seen actually increased after the changes were implemented, but a reason for this increase was found to be unrelated to the change. It would be incorrect to assume that the changes were ineffective after this 1 PDSA cycle. Quality improvement requires looking at data or processes (ie, trends) over time.

The scale of the project does not necessarily correlate to the achievement of quality improvement. Smaller scale projects can often be completed more quickly than larger scale projects. An advantage of the Langley Model for Improvement framework is that it allows for multiple, rapid PDSA cycles that can ultimately lead to quality improvement in a relatively brief time.

American Board of Pediatrics Content Specification(s)/ Content Area

- Identify the components of the Langley Model for Improvement
- Recognize that quality improvement requires looking at data or processes (ie, trends) over time
- Recognize that analysis of variation in data is critical in quality improvement to understand whether the variation is actually improvement

Suggested Readings

EQIPP. eqipp.aap.org.

Horbar JD, Plsek PE, Leahy K, NIC/Q 2000. Establishing habits for improvement in neonatal intensive care units. *Pediatrics*. 2003;111 (suppl E1):e397-e410. http://pediatrics.aappublications.org/content/111/ Supplement_E1/e397.

Institute for Healthcare Improvement. www.ihi.org/resources/Pages/ HowtoImprove.

Langley GJ. *The Improvement Guide: A Practical Approach to Enhancing Organizational Performance*. 2nd ed. San Francisco, CA: Jossey-Bass; 2009.

Item 48	Preferred Response: D

The adolescent in this vignette has zinc deficiency after undergoing bariatric surgery 2 years ago. The most common type of bariatric surgery is the Roux-en-Y gastric bypass, during which the surgeon creates a small gastric pouch (about 1 ounce in size). The small intestine is then divided into 2 portions. The Roux limb, which connects the small gastric pouch to the jejunum, is then attached to the bottom portion of the duodenum, creating the Y connection (Item C48). Food passes directly from the small gastric pouch to the jejunum bypassing the remaining stomach, which continues to produce gastric juices that flow through the duodenum and Y connection. Patients who receive gastric bypass surgery require ongoing vitamin supplementation to prevent deficiencies of micronutrients, including zinc.

Symptoms of mild zinc deficiency include taste and smell impairment, night blindness, and depressed immunity. Severe zinc deficiency is associated with alopecia, bullous pustular dermatitis, diarrhea, and frequent infections due to a depressed immune system. Conditions associated with zinc deficiency are varied. Acrodermatitis enteropathica is an autosomal recessive defect in intestinal zinc absorption that presents with bullous acral dermatitis, growth failure, diarrhea, and infections. Various diseases result in zinc deficiency, such as Crohn disease, renal disease, liver disease, cystic fibrosis, and sickle cell disease. Exclusive breastfeeding in mothers with low zinc levels in breast milk and dietary

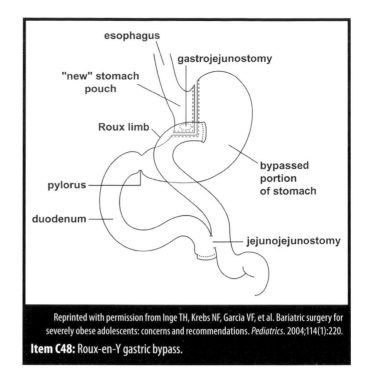

Reprinted with permission from Inge TH, Krebs NF, Garcia VF, et al. Bariatric surgery for severely obese adolescents: concerns and recommendations. *Pediatrics*. 2004;114(1):220.

Item C48: Roux-en-Y gastric bypass.

zinc depletion in developing parts of the world are also causes of zinc deficiency. Treatment of zinc deficiency is 1 to 3 mg/kg/day orally of elemental zinc.

Chromium deficiency is uncommon and generally presents in hospitalized patients in the setting of malnutrition with increased metabolic demands or increased catabolism. Other at-risk patients include individuals with short bowel syndrome, burns, or traumatic injuries and individuals who receive parenteral nutrition. Manifestations of chromium deficiency may include impaired glucose tolerance, although studies are conflicting. The recommended daily allowance of chromium for children is 11 to 15 µg/day.

The presentation of copper deficiency in children includes fragile or kinky hair, depigmented skin, myeloneuropathy (muscle weakness), edema, hepatosplenomegaly, and osteoporosis. Neurologic symptoms may also be present, such as ataxia, neuropathy, and cognitive deficits. Hematologic manifestations include microcytic hypochromic anemia and neutropenia. Risk factors for developing copper deficiency include gastrointestinal surgery (including bariatric surgery), chronic diarrhea or other malabsorptive disorders (including celiac disease), excessive zinc ingestion, or overtreatment of Wilson disease. Menkes disease, or "kinky hair syndrome," is an X-linked genetic disorder resulting from a mutation in the transport protein facilitating copper uptake from the intestine; symptoms of copper deficiency in Menkes disease develop in infancy. The recommended daily allowance for copper intake in children is 340 µg/day.

Magnesium deficiency manifests clinically in a variety of manners:

- Neuromuscular: tremor, tetany, muscle spasms/cramps, involuntary movements (athetoid or choreiform), convulsions, apathy, weakness, delirium, and coma
- Cardiovascular: widening of the QRS complex and peaking of T waves, widening of PR interval, and atrial and ventricular arrhythmias

- Calcium metabolism: hypocalcemia, hypoparathyroidism, and parathyroid hormone resistance
- Potassium metabolism: hypokalemia

Primary intestinal hypomagnesemia is an X-linked recessive genetic defect in magnesium absorption that presents in the neonatal period with secondary hypocalcemia. Gitelman syndrome is caused by a recessive genetic mutation resulting in renal magnesium wasting that presents with hypokalemic metabolic alkalosis and hypocalciuria. Familial hypomagnesemia with hypercalciuria and nephrocalcinosis is caused by an autosomal recessive genetic defect resulting in renal magnesium wasting that presents in childhood or adolescence with symptomatic hypocalcemia. Additionally, patients at risk for magnesium deficiency include those with gastrointestinal illness (acute/chronic diarrhea, malabsorption, steatorrhea, acute pancreatitis) or gastrointestinal surgery, including gastric bypass. Volume expansion, untreated diabetes mellitus, alcoholism, hypercalcemia, and acquired tubular renal dysfunction are also associated with magnesium deficiency. Medications associated with magnesium deficiency include proton pump inhibitors, diuretics, antibiotics (aminoglycosides, amphotericin, and pentamidine), calcineurin inhibitors, cisplatin, and antibodies targeting epidermal growth factor. Repletion of magnesium deficiency is dependent on whether the patient is symptomatic and whether renal function is decreased.

PREP Pearls

- Micronutrient deficiencies can occur from rare genetic defects as well as secondarily from an array of acquired disorders including gastrointestinal surgeries.
- Without appropriate supplementation, one of the long-term adverse effects of bariatric surgery is micronutrient/trace mineral deficiency.

American Board of Pediatrics Content Specification(s)/ Content Area

- Identify the conditions that are associated with a deficiency of various trace minerals (eg, zinc, copper, magnesium, chromium)

Suggested Readings

American Academy of Pediatrics, Committee on Nutrition. Trace elements. In: Kleinman RE, Greer FR, eds. *Pediatric Nutrition*. 7th ed. Elk Grove Village, IL: American Academy of Pediatrics; 2014:467-568.

Inge TH, Krebs NF, Garcia VF, et al. Bariatric surgery for severely obese adolescents: Concerns and recommendations. *Pediatrics*. 2004;114(1):217-223.

Salle A, Demarsy D, Poirier AL, et al. Zinc deficiency: a frequent and underestimated complication after bariatric surgery. *Obes Surg*. 2010;20(12):1660-1670.

Shankar P, Doylan M, Sriram K. *Micronutrient deficiencies after bariatric surgery. J Nutr*. 2010;26(12):1031-1037.

The radiograph in this vignette reveals an absent radius. This congenital anomaly is most often associated with thrombocytopenia with absent radius (TAR) syndrome, which is a genetic disorder inherited in a complex, compound manner. It is associated with a deletion at band 1q21.1 and also requires 1 of 2 polymorphisms at *RBM8A*.

Thrombocytopenia with absent radius presents with bilateral absent radii with shortened forearms with flexion at the elbow, resulting in an appearance of clubbed arms, but with sparing of the thumb. The normal thumb helps to distinguish this disorder from Fanconi anemia. Other defects of the upper extremities, cardiac defects, a persistently elevated white blood cell count, and anemia can be present with TAR. The thrombocytopenia tends to improve with time in most cases, and the platelet count can be normal after the first year of age. The thrombocytopenia in the first year of age can be life-threatening, but severe bleeding can be prevented through the use of prophylactic transfusions of single-donor platelets when the platelet count drops below a predetermined, age-dependent threshold.

The absent radii are a hallmark of TAR that distinguishes it from other congenital thrombocytopenias. While there are many rare congenital thrombocytopenia syndromes, some of the more common syndromes include:

- Bernard-Soulier syndrome: an autosomal recessive disorder causing the absence of functional platelet glycoprotein Ib and a resultant absence of the platelet Ib/IX complex. This absence results in an inability to bind von Willebrand factor. Bernard-Soulier syndrome is a giant platelet disorder, with platelets often exceeding the size of the red blood cell.
- Wiskott-Aldrich syndrome: an X-linked disorder that presents with thrombocytopenia with very small platelets, eczema, and an immune deficiency.
- MYH9 (myosin heavy chain 9) disorders: varied diseases that result from disruption of *MYH9*. These diseases include May-Hegglin anomaly and Sebastien, Fechtner, Epstein, and Alport syndromes.

Although TAR can present with cardiac defects, these do not commonly require extracorporeal membrane oxygenation. Some patients with TAR require packed red blood cell transfusions, but many more require single-donor platelet transfusions. Kidney failure is not associated with TAR.

PREP Pearls

- Severe bleeding in patients with thrombocytopenia with absent radius syndrome can be prevented through the use of single-donor platelet transfusions when the platelet count falls below a predetermined minimum threshold.
- The thrombocytopenia in thrombocytopenia with absent radius syndrome tends to improve with time and may be resolved after the first year of age.
- Thrombocytopenia with absent radius syndrome is a compound genetic disorder that presents with absent radii and severe thrombocytopenia in the neonatal period.

- Recognize the laboratory findings associated with thrombocytopenia
- Plan appropriate management of thrombocytopenia associated with TAR syndrome
- Recognize the clinical findings associated with Wiskott-Aldrich syndrome

Suggested Readings

Cremer M, Sallmon H, Kling PJ, Bührer C, Dame C. Thrombocytopenia and platelet transfusion in the neonate. *Semin Fetal Neonatal Med.* 2016; 21(1):10-18.

de Ybarrondo L, Barratt MS. Thrombocytopenia absent radius syndrome. *Pediatr Rev.* 2011;32(9):399-400.

Sillers L, Van Slambrouck C, Lapping-Carr G. Neonatal thrombocytopenia: etiology and diagnosis. *Pediatr Ann.* 2015;44(7):e175-80.

Item 50 　　　　　　　　Preferred Response: A

The 3-year-old girl in the vignette sustained extensive esophageal burns and later developed esophageal strictures by ingesting a household cleaning substance. She most likely ingested an alkaline product, such as drain cleaner.

Most caustic ingestions in young children occur in their homes, where both toxic alkaline and acidic products are often readily available. These products may cause significant toxicity if ingested. Caustics—also known as corrosives— are concentrated acidic, alkaline, or oxidizing agents. Many are found in common household products including drain cleaners, toilet bowl cleaners, laundry detergents, stain and mildew removers, floor cleaners, oven cleaners, swimming pool cleaners, rust removers, phenol-based disinfectants, swimming pool products, and batteries.

All household chemical products should be stored in their original labeled containers and kept out of the reach of children at all times to prevent accidental exposure. The US Centers for Disease Control and Prevention estimate that more than a half million children are treated emergently each year for acute poisoning with corrosives. Ingestion of even small amounts of a corrosive alkaline substance, such as drain cleaners, toilet bowl cleaners, or rust remover, can result in serious penetrating injuries to mucosal and skin surfaces by liquefaction necrosis. Acidic substances tend to cause injury via coagulation necrosis; acids carry a relatively lower risk of esophageal perforation, but are still capable of producing serious injury.

Patients ingesting corrosive substances typically present with odynophagia, dysphagia, drooling, intraoral injury, and esophageal burns and/or ulcerations. There is a significant potential for later development of strictures. Additional signs and symptoms may include vomiting with hematemesis, respiratory difficulty with stridor or wheezing, hoarseness, retrosternal chest pain, dyspnea, and burns on the face, hands, or chest. Significant burns to the eyes may occur with any ocular exposure. Because the primary mode of injury is direct tissue corrosion, systemic symptoms are rare. Apart from distress caused by pain, mental status is usually normal in affected children.

The most pressing clinical concern after a caustic ingestion is the potential for airway and/or esophageal injury. The presence or absence of intraoral injuries does not always correlate with the presence of injury to the lower airway or esophagus. Early airway visualization and protection are indicated in any child presenting with a suspected caustic ingestion and stridor or respiratory distress. Evaluation of the esophagus with upper endoscopy is indicated in children with a history strongly suggesting ingestion of a corrosive product and in those with intraoral burns or other symptoms related to the ingestion.

The ingestion of household bleach, insecticide, or lamp oil would not typically cause the esophageal injury seen in this child.

Although household bleach (sodium hypochlorite) is a substance with an alkaline pH (pH ~12), retrospective studies of children ingesting liquid household bleach have found that accidental ingestion is typically associated with a benign clinical course and does not require hospitalization or pharmacologic interventions.

Ingestion of an insecticide could result in organophosphate toxicity, characterized by clinical signs and symptoms related to the overactivation of cholinergic receptors by excess acetylcholine. The classic features of cholinergic toxicity can be recalled with the mnemonic SLUDGE: salivation, lacrimation, urination, defecation/diarrhea, gastrointestinal upset, and emesis. Although tachypnea, bradycardia, and pupillary constriction are among the expected abnormalities resulting from insecticide ingestion, this ingestion would not typically result in esophageal injury.

Lamp oil is a hydrocarbon-based product, and ingestion would primarily cause respiratory distress due to pulmonary aspiration. In acute situations, patients who ingest/aspirate a hydrocarbon present with coughing, gagging and choking. Physical examination findings may include fever, tachypnea, cyanosis, and abnormal lung sounds which may include crackles and wheezing. Direct central nervous system effects of the hydrocarbon may lead to lethargy, seizures, or even coma.

PREP Pearls

- All household chemical products should be stored in their original labeled containers and kept out of the reach of children at all times to prevent accidental exposure.
- Ingestion of even small amounts of a corrosive alkaline substance can result in serious penetrating injuries to mucosal and skin surfaces due to liquefaction necrosis. The most pressing clinical concern is the potential for airway and/or esophageal injury.
- Most caustic ingestions in young children occur in their homes. Common products include: drain, toilet bowl, floor, and oven cleaners; laundry detergents; stain, mildew, and rust removers; phenol-based disinfectants; swimming pool products; and batteries.

American Board of Pediatrics Content Specification(s)/
Content Area

- Recognize the signs and symptoms of ingestion of a caustic substance, and manage appropriately
- Know the common household sources of acids and alkali

Suggested Readings

Harley EH, Collins MD. Liquid household bleach ingestion in children: a retrospective review. *Laryngoscope*. 1997;107(1):122-125.

Kay M, Wyllie R. Caustic ingestions in children. *Curr Opin Pediatr* 2009; 21(5):651-654.

Turner A, Robinson P. Respiratory and gastrointestinal complications of caustic ingestion in children. *Emerg Med J*. 2005;22:359-361.

Item 51	Preferred Response: A

Flank pain radiating to the groin, hematuria (gross or microscopic), and difficulty on urination are indicative of kidney stones. An underlying risk factor for renal stone formation, such as a urinary metabolic abnormality, urinary tract infection, and/or structural abnormality of the genitourinary tract, is identified in nearly 80% of children with renal stones. Urinary metabolic abnormality, reported in 40% to 50% of children with recurrent stones, is the most commonly identified risk factor for renal stones. Therefore, the current recommendation is to evaluate all children with renal stones for urinary metabolic disorders. Of the metabolic abnormalities listed in the vignette, hypercalciuria is the most commonly identified. High urinary concentrations of calcium, cystine, oxalate, and uric acid, due to increased renal excretion and/or low urine volume, are associated with crystal formation leading to the development of renal stones. Increased urinary excretion of citrate (most important), magnesium, and pyrophosphate is associated with a decreased risk of renal stone formation, and a low level of these inhibitors is associated with an increased risk for nephrolithiasis in children and adults.

The urinary metabolic evaluation requires a 24-hour urine collection, which is analyzed for the presence of solutes associated with increased risk for stone formation and for decreased excretion of inhibitors of renal stone formation. The 24-hour urine collection should be performed after hospital discharge, when the patient is at home doing normal activities, consuming a regular diet, free of infection, and without intravenous fluid therapy. Evaluation for an underlying metabolic abnormality in children with suspected renal stones is indicated irrespective of the imaging results. Patients and parents should be instructed on the collection of urinary stones, and to bring in any stones passed in the urine, so that they can be sent for chemical analysis.

PREP Pearls

- High urinary concentrations of calcium, cystine, oxalate, and uric acid are associated with crystal formation leading to renal stone formation. Hypercalciuria is the most commonly identified metabolic cause of renal stones.
- Increased urinary excretion of citrate (most important), magnesium, and pyrophosphate is associated with decreased risk for renal stone formation, and a low level of these inhibitors is associated with an increased risk for nephrolithiasis in children and adults.
- Urinary metabolic abnormality is the most commonly identified risk factor for renal stones.

American Board of Pediatrics Content Specification(s)/ Content Area

- Recognize factors contributing to the development of urinary tract stones
- Plan the appropriate management of urinary tract stones

Suggested Readings

Gearhart JP, Herzberg GZ, Jeffs RD. Childhood urolithiasis: experiences and advances. *Pediatrics*. 1991;87(4):445.

McKay CP. Renal stone disease. *Pediatr Rev*. 2010;31:179-188.

Item 52	Preferred Response: D

Coronary heart disease is an important contributor to morbidity and mortality. About 20% of patients discharged from the hospital for acute coronary artery disease are younger than 55 years. This disease process begins during childhood, making screening for and treating hypercholesterolemia an important public health concern and focus for pediatric providers.

As outlined in 2011 by the Expert Panel on Integrated Guidelines for Cardiovascular Health and Risk Reduction in Children and Adolescents (sponsored by the National Institutes of Health and the National Heart, Lung, and Blood Institute), for children between the ages of 2 years and 8 years who have a parent with a total cholesterol of 240 mg/dL (6.22 mmol/L) or greater, a fasting lipid profile should be obtained and then repeated after 2 weeks to 3 months, regardless of the result, because the average of these results should be used to dictate therapy, as outlined in the guideline. While it would be appropriate to counsel on diet and exercise, the recommended evaluation as outlined by the guidelines should be completed first. Additionally, it would be premature to recommend pharmacologic intervention.

After the screening process is complete, any necessary intervention or therapy is dictated by age and the specific lipid abnormality (ie, is the low-density lipoprotein cholesterol level or the triglyceride level primarily elevated?). Counseling on diet and exercise are of paramount importance in the management of these patients. However, some children will need pharmacologic intervention. See Item C52 for more detailed recommendations.

PREP Pearls

- For children between the ages of 2 years and 8 years who have a parent with a total cholesterol of 240 mg/dL (6.22 mmol/L) or greater, a fasting lipid profile should be obtained and then repeated after 2 weeks to 3 months.
- In 2011, the Expert Panel on Integrated Guidelines for Cardiovascular Health and Risk Reduction in Children and Adolescents (sponsored by the National Institutes of Health and the National Heart, Lung, and Blood Institute) outlined guidelines for screening and treatment of pediatric patients at risk.

Item C52. Evidence-Based Recommendations for Dietary Management of Elevated LDL Cholesterol, Non-HDL Cholesterol, and Triglyceride Levels for ages 2-21 years.

Elevated LDL cholesterol: CHILD-2–LDL	Strength of Evidence
Refer to a registered dietitian for family medical nutrition therapy	Grade B strongly recommend
25%-30% of calories from fat, ≤7% from saturated fat, ~10% from monounsaturated fat; <200 mg/d of cholesterol; avoid trans fats as much as possible	Grade A recommend
Supportive actions:	
Plant sterol esters and/or plant stanol esters[a] up to 2 g/d as replacement for usual fat sources can be used after 2 y of age in children with familial hypercholesterolemia	
Plant stanol esters as part of a regular diet are marketed directly to the public; short-term studies have found no harmful effects in healthy children	
The water-soluble fiber psyllium can be added to a low-fat, low-saturated-fat diet as cereal enriched with psyllium at a dose of 6 g/d for children 2–12 y of age and 12 g/d for those ≥12 y of age	
As for all children, 1 h/d of moderate-to-vigorous physical activity and <2 h/d of sedentary screen time are recommended.	
Elevated triglycerides or non-HDL cholesterol: CHILD-2–TG	
Refer to a registered dietitian for family medical nutrition therapy[b]	Grade B strongly recommend
25%–30% of calories from fat, ≤7% from saturated fat, ~10% from monounsaturated fat; <200 mg/d of cholesterol; avoid trans fats as much as possible	Grade A recommend
Decrease sugar intake	Grade B recommend
Replace simple with complex carbohydrates	
No sugar-sweetened beverages	
Increase dietary fish to increase ω-3 fatty acids[c]	Grade D recommend

• **Grades** reflect the findings of the evidence review; **recommendation levels** reflect the consensus opinion of the expert panel; and **supportive actions** represent expert consensus suggestions from the expert panel provided to support implementation of the recommendations (they are not graded). Values given are in mg/dL. To convert to SI units, divide the results for TC, LDL cholesterol, HDL cholesterol, and non-HDL cholesterol by 38.6; for triglycerides, divide by 88.6.

[a] Can be found added to some foods, such as some margarines.

[b] If the child is obese, nutrition therapy should include calorie restriction, and increased activity (beyond that recommended for all children) should be prescribed. See "Overweight and Obesity" for additional age-specific recommendations.

[c] The FDA and the Environmental Protection Agency advise women of childbearing age who may become pregnant, pregnant women, nursing mothers, and young children to avoid some types of fish and shellfish and eat fish and shellfish that are low in mercury. For more information, call the FDA's food information line toll-free at 1-888-SAFEFOOD or visit **www.cfsan.fda.gov/~dms/admehg3.html**.

Reprinted with permission from Expert Panel on Integrated Guidelines for Cardiovascular Health and Risk Reduction in Children and Adolescents; National Heart, Lung, and Blood Institute. Expert panel on integrated guidelines for cardiovascular health and risk reduction in children and adolescents: summary report. *Pediatrics*. 2011;128(S5):S2.

American Board of Pediatrics Content Specification(s)/ Content Area

- Understand the importance of cholesterol/lipid screening examinations
- Understand the recommendations of the National Cholesterol Education Program for Children

Suggested Readings

Belay B, Belamarich P, Racine AD. Pediatric precursors of adult atherosclerosis. *Pediatr Rev.* 2004;25(1):4-16.

Expert Panel on Integrated Guidelines for Cardiovascular Health and Risk Reduction in Children and Adolescents; National Heart, Lung, and Blood Institute. Expert panel on integrated guidelines for cardiovascular health and risk reduction in children and adolescents: summary report. *Pediatrics.* 2011;128(S5):S213-S255.

Kavey RW, Daniels SR, Lauer RM, Atkins DL, Hayman LL, Taubert K. American Heart Association guidelines for primary prevention of atherosclerotic cardiovascular disease beginning in childhood. *Circulation.* 2003;107(11):1562-1566.

Item 53 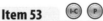 **Preferred Response: A**

Adolescence is a time of physical, psychological, and social maturity as individuals transition from childhood to adulthood. Neuroimaging studies have demonstrated dramatic development of the brain during adolescence and into young adulthood, with the development of higher cognitive functioning such as decision making, organization, hypothetical thought, and reasoning skills occuring later. Throughout adolescence there is progression from concrete thought to abstract thought. Individuals who engage in concrete thought tend to focus on physical objects and literal meanings, whereas individuals who engage in abstract thought can think about experiences they have not had or think through potential consequences of behavior. Not everyone has a smooth transition from concrete to abstract thought, and many adults remain concrete in their thought processes. This transition period can often be difficult for the adolescent as well as parents, teachers, and health care providers.

The developmental phases of adolescence are divided into the early stage (10-13 years of age), middle stage (14-17 years of age), and late stage (18-21 years of age). There are psychosocial processes associated with each stage. Young adulthood is defined as 18 to 25 years of age.

Early adolescence (10-13 years of age) is characterized by the initiation of puberty, self-absorption, impulsivity, and concrete thought. Children in this stage are trying to establish independence from their parents and are less interested in family related activities. They start to rely on their friendships for support. These youth are adjusting to their new bodies. They can be preoccupied with themselves and may develop dissatisfaction with how they look. This is a time when adolescents may start to diet, compare themselves to others, and develop eating disorders. Youth in early adolescence often think that everyone else is looking at or thinking about them (ie, "the imaginary audience"). They also start to develop emotional feelings and may have opposite- or same-sex attractions. Youth in this stage often have a need for privacy. They might start writing in a diary or closing the door to their room. They will also test the limits of their parents and other authority figures to see what they can get away with. Because they can also be impulsive, they are prone to taking more risks. As providers, it is important that we consider what we say to youth in this stage of development because our recommendations, comments, and advice may be misconstrued with these concrete thinkers.

Middle adolescence (14-17 years of age) is characterized by the peer group becoming even more important, greater independence, development of personal identity, and movement from concrete to abstract thought. School becomes more academically challenging and encourages these youth to develop better organizational skills and think more abstractly. This is often the most trying period of time for parents. Peer groups or "cliques" become a primary focus, with a great need for youth to conform in terms of thoughts, values, and clothing. Peer pressure often becomes an issue. Romantic relationships develop, and during this stage teenagers often experiment and become sexually active. There is also planning for the future in regard to career goals. This stage of development is known for the "personal fable." For example, a youth may believe someone else can get pregnant if they have unprotected sex, but it would not be an issue for themself. Adolescents in this stage often feel invincible and will engage in high-risk behaviors, such as drug and alcohol use, risky sexual behavior, and dangerous driving. The leading cause of death for individuals 15 to 19 years of age are accidents (unintentional injuries). Adolescents between 15 and 19 years of age also have the highest incidence rates of sexually transmitted infections (STIs). Youth in this stage are also able to appreciate and learn from their own experiences.

Late adolescence (18-21 years of age) is characterized by more intense planning for the future, the ability to think abstractly, comfort with one's identity and self, and taking on more responsibility and functioning independently of one's parents. During this stage, pubertal changes are complete, but youth may still be focused on improving how their body looks by diet and exercise. There is often more focus on individual relationships rather than peer group interactions. One's values and beliefs are more clearly defined. Youth in this stage will often start to appreciate that their parents do have valuable advice to share and are knowledgeable.

The adolescent girl in this vignette is an example of a youth in middle adolescence. She is aware she does not want to become pregnant but is engaging in high-risk sexual behaviors by having unprotected sex. This alludes to the personal fable. She is hesitant to start a birth control method based of the experiences of her friends. It would not be useful to discredit her friends, as their opinions carry weight. But as her provider, you can provide information (risks, benefits, and side effects) on all of the available methods so that she can make an independent and informed decision on her own. It would be helpful to assess her readiness to incorporate this information into her decision-making process via motivational interviewing techniques.

The provision of condoms and STI screening need to be addressed, but are not the best way to reduce this teenager's risk for pregnancy. For a sexually active teenager, STI screening should be done at a minimum of once per year. Offering condoms and encouraging use is a fundamental component of safe sex counseling. Waiting 3 months to let this adolescent contemplate if she would like a birth control method increases her chance of pregnancy.

PREP Pearls

- Adolescence is a time of biopsychosocial development, and there are significant cognitive shifts from concrete to abstract thought.
- Consider what stage of development an adolescent is in when deciding the best way to counsel about a medical-related issue.
- The goal of moving through adolescence is to become an independent and productive individual in society.

American Board of Pediatrics Content Specification(s)/Content Area

- Understand the timing of and factors influencing the development of concrete thinking and abstract reasoning in adolescents, and provide health advice accordingly

Suggested Readings

Hazen E, Schlozman S, Beresin E. Adolescent psychological development: a review. *Pediatr Rev.* 2008;29(5):161-168.

Sanders RA. Adolescent psychosocial, social, and cognitive development. *Pediatr Rev.* 2013;34(8):354-359.

Sherer S, Radzik M. Psychosocial development in normal adolescents and young adults. In: Neinstein LS, Katzman DK, Callahan ST, Gordon CM, Joffe A, Rickert VI, eds. *Neinstein's Adolescent and Young Adult Health Care: a Practical Guide.* 6th ed. Philadelphia, PA: Wolters Kluwer; 2016: 38-43.

The girl in the vignette has cardiogenic shock, and is receiving several therapies to improve cardiac output. Of the choices, the best site from which to obtain a blood sample for blood gas analysis would be an internal jugular venous catheter.

Cardiogenic shock is a condition of inadequate oxygen delivery to end organs as a result of low cardiac output. Understanding several mathematical equations is essential to understanding the relationships among cardiac output, oxygen delivery, and oxygen consumption in cardiogenic shock.

- Oxygen delivery = Arterial oxygen content × Cardiac output
- Cardiac output = Stroke volume × Heart rate
- Oxygen content = (1.34 × hemoglobin concentration × % oxygen saturation) + 0.003 × PO_2
- Oxygen consumption = Cardiac output × (arterial oxygen content − mixed venous oxygen content)

Equation 1 demonstrates that improvement in oxygen delivery requires that arterial oxygen content and cardiac output be optimized. Equation 2 shows that cardiac output can be increased by increasing the heart rate and/or by improving stroke volume (which in turn depends on preload, afterload, and contractility). Equation 3 expresses the oxygen content of blood as the amount bound to hemoglobin plus the amount dissolved in blood. Equation 4 shows that the body's oxygen consumption is equal to cardiac output multiplied by the difference between the arterial oxygen content (amount of oxygen supplied to the end-organs) minus the mixed venous oxygen content (blood returned after consumption of oxygen by end-organs, ie, pulmonary arterial).

Cardiac output can be quantitatively measured using pulmonary arterial catheters and indirect calorimetry, but this practice is uncommon in pediatrics. One can assume that because the patient with shock is not exercising, oxygen consumption is relatively constant during therapy. Thus, cardiac output can be qualitatively determined by measuring the difference in oxygen content between arterial and mixed venous blood. Because arterial and venous hemoglobin concentrations are equal, and the amount of oxygen dissolved in the blood is mathematically negligible, as shown in equation 3, a simplified approach is to calculate the arteriovenous oxygen saturation difference. The arterial oxygen saturation can be measured with either pulse oximetry or a radial artery catheter. Pulmonary arterial catheters are rarely placed in children, therefore, an internal jugular catheter with the tip in the junction between the superior vena cava and right atrium can be used to closely approximate mixed venous blood. Generally, an arteriovenous oxygen saturation difference of 20% to 30% indicates normal cardiac output, whereas greater than 40% indicates shock.

It is important to understand that for these relationships to hold, the venous blood sample must be obtained from a central venous source to represent the entire body. Antecubital venous blood reflects the oxygen delivery-consumption relationships of the lower arm, but not the rest of the body. The same concept holds for fingerstick capillary blood, which may contain some arterial blood as well. Blood from a radial arterial catheter would accurately reflect arterial oxygen content, but without a measurement of central venous blood saturation, arteriovenous oxygen saturation difference cannot be calculated.

It should be noted that many point-of-care blood gas machines can also measure lactic acid levels, bicarbonate concentration, and base deficit, all of which can be useful information in the treatment of patients with shock. Although blood samples obtained from any of the sites listed can measure these parameters, acid-base disturbance from lactic acidosis is a late finding in shock and not as sensitive a measure as arteriovenous oxygen difference.

PREP Pearls

- Acid-base disturbance from lactic acidosis is a late finding in shock and not as sensitive a measure as arteriovenous oxygen difference.
- An arteriovenous oxygen saturation difference of 20% to 30% indicates normal cardiac output, whereas greater than 40% indicates shock (the venous sample must be from a central venous source).
- Cardiogenic shock is a condition of inadequate oxygen delivery to end organs as a result of low cardiac output.

American Board of Pediatrics Content Specification(s)/Content Area

- Understand the limitations of capillary blood gas analysis

Suggested Readings

Mtaweh H, Trakas EV, Su E, Carcillo JA, Aneja RA. Advances in monitoring and management of shock. *Pediatr Clin North Am.* 2013; 60(3):641-654.

Subramaniam S, Rutman M. Cardiogenic shock. *Pediatr Rev.* 2015;36;225.

Turner DA, Cheifetz IM. Shock. In: Kliegman RM, Stanton BF, Schor NF, St. Geme JW, Behrman RE, eds. *Nelson's Textbook of Pediatrics.* 19th ed. Philadelphia, PA. Elsevier-Saunders; 2011:309-310.

Item 55   **Preferred Response: D**

The girl in this vignette has Stevens-Johnson syndrome (SJS). Treatment is supportive, although it is essential that potentially causative medications be discontinued immediately. Studies have not shown conclusive benefit from intravenous immunoglobulin or corticosteroid administration. Although secondary bacterial infections are common, prophylactic antibiotics are not indicated and have been associated with increased mortality.

Stevens-Johnson syndrome and toxic epidermal necrolysis (TEN) are manifestations of the same pathologic process of cell-mediated epidermal and mucosal necrosis. The 2 conditions differ in the extent of skin involvement, with less than 10% of a patient's body surface area affected in SJS, 10% to 30% affected in SJS/TEN overlap, and more than 30% of the body surface area affected in TEN. Medications are believed to be the most common trigger of SJS and TEN in children, and many other cases are associated with infection. Common triggers include nonsteroidal anti-inflammatory medications, sulfa-containing antibiotics, phenobarbital, carbamazepine, and lamotrigine, as well as infections with *Mycoplasma pneumoniae*, cytomegalovirus, herpes simplex virus, and hepatitis A virus.

Patients with SJS/TEN typically present with fever, myalgias, malaise, and other flu-like symptoms. Several days later, patients develop macules with purpuric centers that evolve into vesicles and bullae, as well as mucosal lesions. Large areas of skin may detach. Ocular signs and symptoms can include eye pain, photophobia, purulent conjunctivitis, keratitis, and endophthalmitis. Mucosal symptoms may include stomatitis, vaginitis, and urethritis. Extensive skin involvement can cause fluid and protein loss, pain, and hypothermia, and in severe cases, can lead to hypovolemic shock and multiorgan failure. Secondary bacterial infections and sepsis are the leading causes of mortality in patients with SJS/TEN.

Morbidity and mortality are reduced with early diagnosis and early discontinuation of causative medications. Treatment is supportive, with careful attention to pain management, fluid and electrolyte balance, and wound care. Patients may require transfer to a burn center for comprehensive wound care.

It is important to distinguish SJS/TEN from erythema multiforme (EM). Patients with EM do not have systemic symptoms of fever and malaise. Skin lesions in EM are targetoid without epidermal detachment, and patients have either little or no mucosal involvement (Item C55).

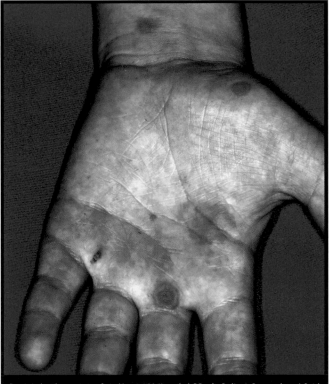

Reprinted with permission from Mancini AJ, Krowchuk DP, eds. *Pediatric Dermatology: A Quick Reference Guide.* 3rd ed. Elk Grove Village, IL: American Academy of Pediatrics; 2016:608.

Item C55: Targetoid skin lesions seen in a patient with erythema multiforme.

PREP Pearls

- In children, Stevens-Johnson syndrome/toxic epidermal necrolysis is commonly triggered by medications (eg, nonsteroidal anti-inflammatory drugs, sulfa-containing antibiotics, and antiepileptic medications) or infections (eg, *Mycoplasma pneumoniae*, cytomegalovirus, herpes simplex virus, and hepatitis A virus).
- Patients with Stevens-Johnson syndrome/toxic epidermal necrolysis present with fever and flu-like symptoms followed by macules with purpuric centers that develop into vesicles and bullae. Patients typically have mucosal involvement (conjunctivitis, stomatitis, urethritis, and/or vaginitis).
- Stevens-Johnson syndrome and toxic epidermal necrolysis are presentations along a spectrum of disease severity.
- Treatment for Stevens-Johnson syndrome/toxic epidermal necrolysis requires the prompt removal of any potentially causative medications and supportive care, with attention to pain management, fluid and electrolyte status, and wound care.

American Board of Pediatrics Content Specification(s)/Content Area

- Recognize the clinical features of Stevens-Johnson syndrome and manage appropriately
- Recognize the clinical spectrum of erythema multiforme

Suggested Readings

Alerhand S, Cassella C, Koyfman A. Stevens-Johnson syndrome and toxic epidermal necrolysis in the pediatric population: a review. *Pediatr Emerg Care.* 2016;32(7):472-476.

Ferrandiz-Pulido C, Garcia-Patos V. A review of causes of Stevens-Johnson syndrome and toxic epidermal necrolysis in children. *Arch Dis Child.* 2013; 98(12):998-1003.

Powers S, Carter-Beard G. Rash, eye pain, lesions in an adolescent. *Pediatr Rev.* 2010;31(12):e86-e90.

Item 56	Preferred Response: D

Recreational water–associated illnesses result from exposure to microorganisms or chemicals in locations that may be treated (eg, pools and hot tubs) or untreated (eg, lakes and oceans). Swimmers are a key source of the infectious pathogens that contaminate recreational water. Ingestion of contaminated water can result in infection, despite adequate chlorination. In the vignette, the outbreak of diarrheal illness among adults and school-age children in the community after visiting a wading pool is highly characteristic of *Shigella* infection. Swimming-related *Shigella* outbreaks have been well described in the United States due to inadequately disinfected pools and use of the pools by individuals with diarrhea. Inadvertent swallowing of even a small amount of infected water can cause infection because the inoculum dose for *Shigella* is very low; fewer than 10 organisms can result in transmission. The organisms can survive for up to 6 months in water and 1 month in food.

Shigella sonnei is a well-recognized cause of gastroenteritis in children. Transmission of *Shigella* bacteria typically occurs via the fecal-oral route by direct human-to-human contact in households. Contaminated water, food, or fomites, or sexual contact are other modes of transmission. Risk factors for *Shigella* infection include age less than or equal to 5 years, daycare center attendance, crowded residential settings (eg, military recruits, dormitories), men who have sex with men, and travel to endemic low and middle-income countries where sanitation is poor. Single cases of *Shigella* can spread to the community. Children in diapers cared for at daycare centers are recognized as a common source for spread of *Shigella* infection.

Shigella are gram-negative bacilli that include 4 species (*Shigella dysenteriae*, *S sonnei*, *Shigella flexneri,* and *Shigella boydii*). In the United States, *Shigella* is estimated to cause approximately half a million diarrheal illnesses each year, with more than 5,400 hospitalizations and 38 deaths. In 2011, in the United States, *S sonnei* accounted for the majority of infections.

The typical incubation period of shigellosis is 1 to 3 days. The large intestine is often infected, causing an illness characterized by watery or mucoid stools and/or dysentery, nausea, emesis, abdominal pain, and tenesmus. Infants with *Shigellosis* can develop high fever, severe dehydration, and self-limited seizures. In some cases, the illness may be severe, resulting in hospitalization. *Shigella* species can be isolated from stool culture, but more sensitive molecular detection with multiplex polymerase chain reaction platforms is frequently used for rapid diagnosis of *Shigella* and other bacterial, viral, and parasitic pathogens.

S sonnei infection is self-limited in most cases. While mild cases do not require antimicrobial therapy, treatment is recommended for immunocompromised individuals or those with severe illness. Given high rates of resistance of *Shigella* isolates in the United States to ampicillin (25%) and trimethoprim-sulfamethoxazole (43%), empiric antimicrobial treatment options for severe disease in children include azithromycin or ceftriaxone and ciprofloxacin in adults. Outbreaks of multidrug-resistant *S sonnei* gastroenteritis in daycare centers has been reported. *Shigella* strains with reduced susceptibility to azithromycin are a major concern among adults, especially men who have sex with men.

Other frequently reported pathogens causing recreational water–associated outbreaks include *Cryptosporidium*, *Giardia*, norovirus, and *Escherichia coli* O157:H7.

Prevention of recreational water–associated illness requires epidemiologic surveillance and outbreak detection, environmental hygiene maintenance, appropriate disinfection, and water quality controls. The public and venue staff must be educated on healthy swimming behaviors to prevent the spread of recreational water–associated illness, including 1) avoidance of swimming during diarrheal illness; 2) not swallowing pool water, and 3) adherence to strict hygiene measures (https://www.cdc.gov/healthywater/swimming/swimmers/steps-healthy-swimming.html).

Bacillus cereus is an important toxin-mediated foodborne illness, but it is not transmissible from person-to-person. *Campylobacter* species are a leading bacterial cause of foodborne gastroenteritis in children, often causing bloody diarrhea; infection rate is lower compared with infections caused by *Shigella* species. Enterotoxigenic *E coli* causes watery diarrhea among infants living in low- and middle-income countries, and is a common cause of traveler's diarrhea in all age groups. It has also been implicated in outbreaks of acute gastroenteritis on cruise ships.

PREP Pearls

- Common pathogens causing recreational water–associated outbreaks of acute gastroenteritis include *Cryptosporidium*, *Shigella*, *Giardia*, norovirus, and *Escherichia coli* O157:H7.
- The public and venue staff must be educated on healthy swimming behaviors to prevent the spread of recreational water–associated illness.
- Transmission of *Shigella* typically occurs via the fecal-oral route. Contaminated water, food or fomite exposure, or sexual contact can result in transmission.

American Board of Pediatrics Content Specification(s)/Content Area

- Plan appropriate management for a patient with *Shigella* infection
- Recognize the clinical features associated with *Shigella* infection
- Understand the epidemiology of *Shigella* species

Suggested Readings

American Academy of Pediatrics. *Shigella* infections. In: Kimberlin DW, Brady MT, Jackson MA, Long SS, eds. *Red Book: 2018 Report of the Committee on Infectious Diseases*. 31st ed. Itasca, IL: American Academy of Pediatrics; 2018:723-727.

Centers for Disease Control and Prevention (CDC). Shigellosis outbreak associated with an unchlorinated fill-and-drain wading pool—Iowa, 2001. *MMWR Morb Mortal Wkly Rep*. 2001;50(37):797-800.

Hlavsa MC, Roberts VA, Kahler AM, et al; Centers for Disease Control and Prevention (CDC). Outbreaks of illness associated with recreational water—United States, 2011-2012. *MMWR Morb Mortal Wkly Rep*. 2015; 64(24):668-672.

Item 57	Preferred Response: D

The girl in this vignette has altered chest wall mechanics due to her rotoscoliosis and neuromuscular dysfunction. These altered mechanics lead to ineffective cough and poor airway clearance. Inadequate airway clearance is the underlying mechanism of poor recovery from what should be minor respiratory infections. With severe scoliosis, the musculoskeletal mechanics of cough are impaired, and it is difficult to generate enough power from the diaphragm for an effective cough and to clear secretions.

Although viral respiratory infections are triggers for wheezing in predisposed children, there is nothing in the history or examination findings to suggest wheezing or airway hyperreactivity. Poor airway clearance and ineffective cough can lead to bronchiectasis from repeated infections, but the girl's chest radiograph does not suggest bronchiectasis, and the most proximate cause of her symptoms is poor airway mechanics rather than its long-term outcome.

Hypogammaglobulinemia is associated with recurrent sinopulmonary infections, however they are usually bacterial rather than viral infections. The girl's history of 3 episodes of pneumonia is concerning, but she has not had infections in other sites to raise a major concern for hypogammaglobulinemia.

Chest wall deformities due to neuromuscular dysfunction or skeletal dysplasias can impair the integrity of cough and adequate airway clearance, leading to a cycle of ongoing cough and retained secretions. The mechanism is a decrease in the bellows function of the chest wall, leading to a relatively restrictive pulmonary process from musculoskeletal cause rather than from intrinsic restrictive lung disease. Poor clearance of secretions, particularly in the context of even mild respiratory illness, produces a local environment conducive to secondary infection. Children with these conditions often have escalating cycles of cough and infection until the bellows function is improved by correction of the skeletal deformity or until measures are taken to improve airway clearance independently of the bellows function of the chest wall and diaphragm.

PREP Pearls

- Chest wall deformities that lead to decreased ability to cough and clear the airway may also underlie chronic respiratory symptoms.
- Neuromuscular dysfunction is often responsible for poor airway mechanics and ineffective airway clearance, potentiating recurrent respiratory illnesses.

American Board of Pediatrics Content Specification(s)/ Content Area

- Recognize the association of thoracic deformities with restrictive pulmonary disease

Suggested Readings

Ellis DG. Chest wall deformities. *Pediatr Rev.* 1989;11(5):147-151.

Panitch HB. The pathophysiology of respiratory impairment in pediatric neuromuscular diseases. *Pediatrics.* 2009;123(suppl 4):S215-S218.

Item 58	Preferred Response: B

The girl in this vignette has growth failure secondary to a craniopharyngioma. Brain magnetic resonance imaging (MRI) is the test most likely to reveal the diagnosis. Poor linear growth, headaches, and vision problems are common presenting symptoms of craniopharyngioma. Growth hormone deficiency is the most common anterior pituitary hormone deficiency at the time of diagnosis, manifesting as growth problems. Other pituitary hormone deficiencies may also be present and can contribute to abnormal growth. The other symptoms of craniopharyngioma are caused by increased intracranial pressure and mass effect on the optic chiasm.

Craniopharyngioma is the most common suprasellar tumor in childhood. These tumors originate from the remnants of Rathke's pouch and are benign, but they can cause significant problems because of their location and mass effect. The peak incidence in childhood is between 5 and 14 years of age. The standard imaging modality is MRI with and without contrast. Craniopharyngioma appears as a cystic mass on MRI (Item C58). Characteristic intratumoral calcifications can be seen on computed tomography. Treatment is associated with significant morbidity, specifically panhypopituitarism, diabetes insipidus, hypothalamic obesity, and vision loss.

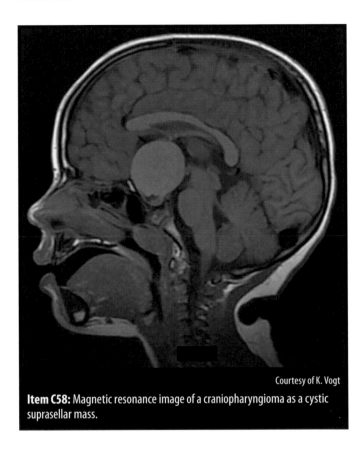

Courtesy of K. Vogt

Item C58: Magnetic resonance image of a craniopharyngioma as a cystic suprasellar mass.

Bone age radiography is often obtained as part of a growth evaluation but would not reveal the diagnosis. A karyotype is obtained in a growth evaluation to rule out Turner syndrome. The presentation of the girl in this vignette is not consistent with Turner syndrome. A thyroid-stimulating hormone level is indicated but would not reveal the diagnosis in this case.

The growth curve for the girl in this vignette shows declining height percentiles. After age 3 years and outside of the peripubertal period, crossing height percentiles is never normal and should be evaluated. When height velocity is decreased with relative preservation of weight, an endocrine or genetic disorder should be suspected. These endocrine disorders include growth hormone deficiency, hypothyroidism, and glucocorticoid excess (Cushing syndrome). In addition to declining growth velocity, Cushing syndrome is usually also associated with marked weight gain. Common genetic disorders associated with declining growth velocity include Turner syndrome and Noonan syndrome.

Familial short stature and constitutional delay of growth and puberty are considered normal variants and are associated with normal childhood growth velocity. Familial short stature is associated with normal growth velocity along a percentile consistent with an individual's genetic potential (target height percentile based on the parents' heights). Target height (adjusted midparental height) can be calculated as follows:

For girls: [mother's height + father's height − 5 inches (13 cm)]/2

For boys: [mother's height + father's height + 5 inches (13 cm)]/2

The final height of most individuals is within 2 inches (1 standard deviation) on either side of this calculated target height.

Familial short stature is associated with a bone age concordant with chronologic age and normal pubertal onset and progression. Final adult height is consistent with target height.

Constitutional delay of growth and puberty is associated with normal childhood growth velocity at a percentile below that expected based on target height. Length may cross percentiles prior to age 3 years due to "channelling" into their childhood growth percentile. Bone age is delayed and pubertal onset is later than average. Children with constitutional delay may cross height percentiles around the typical time of the pubertal growth spurt as they continue to grow at a normal prepubertal growth rate while their peers are experiencing increased pubertal growth velocity. These individuals grow for a longer period of time, have a later pubertal growth spurt, and end up at a normal final adult height. Usually there is a family history of constitutional delay of growth and puberty, commonly referred to as a "late bloomer."

PREP Pearls

- After age 3 years and outside of the peripubertal period, crossing height percentiles is never normal and should be evaluated.
- When height velocity is decreased with relative preservation of weight, an endocrine or genetic disorder should be suspected.

American Board of Pediatrics Content Specification(s)/ Content Area

- Understand the natural history of genetic (familial) short stature
- Plan the evaluation of a child with short stature or whose height percentiles have decreased
- Distinguish among constitutional short stature, genetic (familial) short stature, and growth hormone or thyroid deficiencies by growth chart evaluation
- Understand the natural history of constitutional growth delay

Suggested Readings

Braun LR, Marino R. Disorders of growth and stature. *Pediatr Rev.* 2017; 38(7):293-304.

Rogol AD, Hayden GF. Etiologies and early diagnosis of short stature and growth failure in children and adolescents. *J Pediatr.* 2014;164(5 suppl): S1-S14.e6.

Rose SR, Vogiatzi MG, Copeland KC. A general pediatric approach to evaluating a short child. *Pediatr Rev.* 2005;26(11):410-420.

Item 59 — Preferred Response: B

The girl in the vignette has classic fetal alcohol syndrome (FAS). To diagnose FAS, a physician should identify 3 cardinal features: abnormal facial features, growth deficiency, and central nervous system problems. The possibility of prenatal alcohol exposure is not required to clinically make the diagnosis, but should be discussed with the child's parents. In cases of adoption or foster care, the maternal history may be unknown. Classic facial features include midfacial hypoplasia, smooth philtrum, thin upper lip, micrognathia, short palpebral fissures, epicanthal folds, small jaw, and microcephaly. Prenatal growth deficiency is typical, as are continued postnatal growth problems. Height and weight are typically less than the 10th percentile. Central nervous system findings include attention/hyperactivity problems, hypotonia, decreased impulse control, poor coordination and memory, learning disabilities (especially in math), speech and language delays, intellectual disability, impaired executive function, and sleep problems. Heart defects may occur; ventricular septal defects and atrial septal defects are most commonly seen.

No specific laboratory test is available to confirm a diagnosis of FAS; it is a clinical diagnosis. There is no reported "safe" level of alcohol use during pregnancy. Any form of alcohol exposure during any trimester poses a similar risk. The neurocognitive impacts are lifelong and are completely preventable if a woman abstains from alcohol use during pregnancy.

Some children exposed to alcohol in utero develop alcohol-related neurodevelopmental disorder or neurobehavioral disorder associated with prenatal alcohol exposure. These children lack the physical stigmata commonly seen with FAS, but have the associated intellectual disabilities and problems with behavior and learning. Abnormalities may be noted on brain imaging. These children typically require an individualized education plan in school; speech, occupational, and physical therapy; specialized math tutoring; executive function training; and parenting and behavior management training. They often require referral to a child psychiatrist to manage the behavioral problems.

Angelman syndrome is associated with intellectual disability, gait ataxia, microcephaly, severe speech delay, and a characteristic happy demeanor with inappropriate laughter and excitability. Developmental delay becomes evident at around 6 months of age; many of the characteristic features do not become apparent until after 1 year of age. Developmental regression is not a common feature of this disorder; however, seizures are quite common. Facial features can include a wide mouth with wide-spaced teeth, prognathism, and a protruding tongue.

Noonan syndrome presents with characteristic facial features, short stature, varying degrees of developmental delay, and congenital heart defects. Facial features include low-set ears with fleshy helices, broad or webbed neck, and wide-spaced, downslanting eyes with epicanthal folds. Common congenital heart defects include pulmonary valve stenosis, atrial septal defect, and hypertrophic cardiomyopathy. Wide-spaced nipples and an unusual chest shape with superior pectus carinatum/inferior pectus excavatum are typical. Microcephaly is not a common feature. Multigene panel testing is available for Noonan syndrome.

Rett syndrome, caused by a *MECP2* gene mutation, is an X-linked neurodevelopmental disorder that predominantly affects girls. Affected girls typically have normal early growth and development (6-18 months) followed by a characteristic slowing of development, loss of purposeful hand movements, distinctive hand wringing, decreased brain growth (acquired microcephaly), loss of coordination, gait abnormalities, developmental regression, autistic-like behaviors, seizures, and intellectual disability. Apraxia and breathing difficulties while awake are quite common. Diagnosis commonly is made at 2 to 3 years of age.

PREP Pearls

- Neurologic problems in fetal alcohol syndrome include attention-deficit/hyperactivity problems, decreased impulse control, poor coordination and memory, learning disabilities (especially in math), speech and language delays, intellectual disability, impaired executive function, and sleep problems.

- The classic phenotype for fetal alcohol syndrome includes growth deficiency, midfacial hypoplasia, smooth philtrum, thin upper lip, micrognathia, short palpebral fissures, epicanthal folds, small jaw, and microcephaly.

- There is no reported "safe" level of alcohol use during pregnancy; a fetus can be affected during any trimester.

American Board of Pediatrics Content Specification(s)/Content Area

- Recognize the clinical and laboratory features associated with fetal alcohol syndrome, and manage appropriately

Suggested Readings

American Academy of Pediatrics. Fetal alcohol spectrum disorders program. https://www.aap.org/en-us/advocacy-and-policy/aap-health-initiatives/fetal-alcohol-spectrum-disorders-toolkit/Pages/default.aspx.

Centers for Disease Control and Prevention. Fetal alcohol syndrome disorders. https://www.cdc.gov/ncbddd/fasd/index.html.

Hagan JF Jr, Balachova T, Bertrand J, et al; on behalf of Neurobehavioral Disorder Associated With Prenatal Alcohol Exposure Workgroup, American Academy of Pediatrics. Neurobehavioral disorder associated with prenatal alcohol exposure. *Pediatrics.* 2016;138(4):pii: e20151553.

Williams JF, Smith VC, the Committee on Substance Abuse. Fetal alcohol spectrum disorders. *Pediatrics.* 2015;136(5):e1395-1406.

The newborn in this vignette has an isolated preauricular ear pit. For newborns with an isolated, unilateral preauricular pit or skin tag and no other risk factors, the risk of renal anomalies is, at most, slightly higher than in the general population. It is reasonable to forego renal ultrasonography in such newborns. In newborns with external ear anomalies who have other congenital anomalies or dysmorphic features, a family history of deafness, ear, or renal anomalies, or a maternal history of gestational diabetes, the likelihood of clinically significant structural renal anomalies is higher, and renal ultrasonography is warranted. Outer and middle ear anomalies include microtia, protruding ears, external auditory canal atresia, and malformations of the ossicles in the middle ear. In newborns with external ear abnormalities, 5% to 40% will have congenital anomalies involving other organs. Ear and/or renal anomalies are associated with several genetic syndromes. Thus, diligence is required when looking for other congenital malformations on examination when an ear anomaly is noted. Such conditions include CHARGE syndrome (coloboma, heart defects, atresia choanae, poor growth and/or intellectual disability, urogenital anomalies, and ear anomalies), DiGeorge syndrome (22q11.2 deletion), and branchio-oto-renal syndrome.

About 0.5% to 1% of all newborns have preauricular skin tags or pits; most are isolated findings and not part of a genetic syndrome. Several studies have addressed the question of which newborns with ear anomalies should undergo screening for renal anomalies; however, these studies are often limited by small sample size and geographic isolation. In one chart review study of 42 patients with ear anomalies undergoing renal ultrasonography in one medical center, 12 (29%) had renal anomalies. Of these 12, only 1 infant (11%) had no other congenital anomalies or risk factors, such as a family history of deafness, ear, or renal anomalies, or a maternal history of gestational diabetes. Other studies have reported similar results, suggesting that the risk of renal anomalies in children with isolated preauricular skin tags or pits is similar to or slightly higher than the 1% to 3% risk in the general population. Furthermore, many renal anomalies found are of indeterminate clinical significance or often resolve without treatment (eg, hydronephrosis). Thus, renal ultrasonography is not warranted based on the isolated presence of preauricular skin tags or pits.

Hearing screening is recommended for all newborns. However, it is important to also note that the risk of permanent hearing impairment is 5-fold higher in newborns with preauricular skin tags or pits, compared to newborns without these anomalies. Similar to renal anomalies, the highest risk of hearing impairment was found in newborns with external ear anomalies in the setting of other congenital anomalies, particularly craniofacial syndromes.

American Board of Pediatrics Content Specification(s)/ Content Area

- Recognize disorders commonly associated with malformed external and middle ears
- Know the significance of preauricular sinuses and pits

Suggested Readings

Arora RS, Pryce R. Is ultrasonography required to rule out renal malformations in babies with isolated preauricular tags? *Arch Dis Child.* 2004;89(5):492-493.

Roth DA, Hildesheimer M, Bardenstein S, et al. Preauricular skin tags and ear pits are associated with permanent hearing impairment in newborns. *Pediatrics.* 2008;122(4):e884-e890.

Wang RY, Earl DL, Ruder RO, Graham JM Jr. Syndromic ear anomalies and renal ultrasounds. *Pediatrics.* 2001;108(2):e32.

Item 61	Preferred Response: D

The antimicrobial that would best treat the boy in this vignette is doxycycline. The clinical triad of fever, rash, and headache in a patient that has travelled to an area endemic to Rocky Mountain spotted fever (RMSF) should raise concern for a rickettsial infection for which doxycycline is the optimal therapeutic agent.

Rocky Mountain spotted fever results from infection with *Rickettsia rickettsii* and is a tick-borne infection. Incubation ranges from 2 to 14 days. Humans, who are accidental hosts, can become infected as an infected tick feeds and releases the organism via its salivary glands or if a tick is crushed upon attempted removal. Cases are reported throughout the United States, although a high concentration comes from the south-central and mid-Atlantic states in a strip stretching from Oklahoma to North Carolina. Corresponding with expected tick activity, most cases occur during summer months. The incidence of RMSF is increasing in the United States. In 2008, a total of 2,563 cases were reported to the Centers for Disease Control and Prevention, which was a 4-fold increase over the number of cases reported in 2000. Infections caused by *R rickettsii* also occur in Central and South America.

The clinical spectrum of RMSF varies from a gradual or self-limited illness to an abrupt life-threatening illness. Most children experience high fever and rash, and a large portion have the triad of fever, rash, and headache. The rash evolves from a macular exanthem early in the illness to a maculopapular then petechial and purpuric rash several days into illness. The rash also tends to spread from the distal extremities centripetally. Lymphadenopathy, hepatosplenomegaly, peripheral edema, and meningismus can occur with relative frequency.

The principal histopathologic feature of infection with *R rickettsii* is endothelial injury and vascular permeability. The petechial rash results from focal vasculitis in the epidermis. Vascular fluid leakage into organ tissue can lead to characteristic symptoms, such as headache caused by increased intracranial pressure.

Laboratory aberrations, including thrombocytopenia, hyponatremia, and elevated levels of hepatic transaminases, occur in over half of the cases of RMSF and result from endothelial injury and capillary leak.

It is critical to start antimicrobial therapy as soon as RMSF is suspected instead of waiting for confirmation of the infection. Delay in treatment can result in adverse outcomes. The preferred treatment in children of all ages, including children younger than 8 years, is doxycycline. Patients should be treated for 3 days after fever resolves, usually between 5 to 10 days total.

Although RMSF can have symptomatic overlap with other life-threatening infections, the constellation of findings in a patient with travel to an endemic region must raise concern for a rickettsial infection. Ampicillin is fairly narrow in coverage, although it has a role is several infections, including infections caused by ampicillin-susceptible *Streptococcus* species, *Enterococcus* species, and *Listeria monocytogenes*. Amoxicillins have a role in treatment of another tick-borne infection, Lyme disease, but not in the treatment of RMSF. In children, azithromycin is typically used for the treatment of intracellular infections caused by *Mycoplasma pneumoniae*, *Bartonella henselae*, and nontuberculous mycobacteria. Ceftriaxone would be an appropriate empiric choice if targeting *Neisseria meningitidis*, which can have a clinical presentation similar to RMSF. Neither macrolides nor β-lactam antibiotics are effective for the treatment of RMSF.

American Board of Pediatrics Content Specification(s)/ Content Area

- Recognize the clinical features associated with Rocky Mountain spotted fever
- Plan the appropriate management of suspected or confirmed Rocky Mountain spotted fever
- Understand the epidemiology of Rocky Mountain spotted fever

Suggested Readings

American Academy of Pediatrics. Rocky Mountain spotted fever. In: Kimberlin DW, Brady MT, Jackson MA, Long SS, eds. *Red Book: 2018 Report of the Committee on Infectious Diseases*. 31st ed. Itasca, IL: American Academy of Pediatrics; 2018:697-699.

Razzaq S, Schutze G. Rocky Mountain spotted fever: a physician's challenge. *Pediatr Rev*. 2005;26(4):125-129.

Woods C. Rocky mountain spotted fever in children. *Pediatr Clin N Am*. 2013;60(2):455-470.

Item 62   Preferred Response: C

The infant in the vignette has congenital talipes equinovarus (TEV) or clubfoot. The widely accepted treatment for TEV is known as the Ponseti method. Treatment involves 3 stages: serial long leg casting, surgery to cut the Achilles tendon (for most infants), and long-term bracing to maintain the corrected position. Most orthopaedic providers recommend beginning treatment in the first few weeks after birth, provided the child is healthy without more pressing medical issues. The boy in the vignette should be referred immediately to an orthopaedic provider to initiate casting.

Talipes equinovarus deformity is the most common congenital foot deformity that requires treatment. Features include a high arch, adducted position of the forefoot, hindfoot varus, and plantar flexion contracture. Talipes equinovarus develops by 16 weeks of gestation, and can often be detected on prenatal ultrasonography. Most children treated with the Ponseti method have excellent foot appearance and function later in life.

Metatarsus adductus, a flexible, adducted positioning of the forefoot, is a common foot deformity that results from intrauterine positioning. Children with metatarsus adductus have a curved appearance of the lateral edge of the foot. This diagnosis can be distinguished from TEV on physical examination; infants with metatarsus adductus have normal ankle motion, while those with TEV are fixed in a plantarflexed position. Some providers recommend stretching exercises to promote resolution of metatarsus adductus. Casting and splinting may be useful for infants with metatarsus adductus that persists beyond age 6 months, though this condition almost always resolves spontaneously by the age of 3 to 4 years. Metatarsus varus is a term used to denote a rigid adducted position of the forefoot (ie, the foot cannot be stretched into a normal position). Infants with metatarsus varus should be referred to an orthopaedic physician for treatment with casting and/or splinting.

Home stretching and reverse last shoes (shoes designed to pull the forefoot into an abducted position) are not indicated for the treatment of TEV. Surgical reconstruction of the foot was historically the treatment of choice for TEV. However, multiple studies have shown that children treated with the Ponseti method have better functional outcomes than those treated with surgery, so this technique is now considered the 'gold standard'.

PREP Pearls

- Talipes equinovarus (clubfoot) is the most common congenital foot deformity that requires treatment.
- The 'gold standard' technique for the treatment of talipes equinovarus is the Ponseti method which includes serial casting, surgery to cut the Achilles tendon, and bracing.
- The features of talipes equinovarus include a high arch, adducted position of the forefoot, hindfoot varus, and plantar flexion contracture.

American Board of Pediatrics Content Specification(s)/Content Area

- Recognize the clinical findings associated with clubfoot and the need for prompt referral

Suggested Readings

Mosca V. The foot. In: Weinstein SL, Flynn HM, eds. *Lovell & Winter's Pediatric Orthopaedics*. 7th ed. Philadelphia: Lippincott Williams & Wilkins; 2013;chap 29:1389-1525.

Item 63   Preferred Response: C

The classic electrolyte and acid-base imbalance associated with infantile hypertrophic pyloric stenosis is hypochloremic, hypokalemic metabolic alkalosis. The duration of vomiting is directly related to the severity of this abnormality. The initial goals of management are to assess hydration status, evaluate for electrolyte abnormalities, and institute appropriate intravenous fluid therapy to correct the disturbances before surgical intervention.

The infant in the vignette demonstrates many of the clinical features commonly associated with infantile hypertrophic pyloric stenosis, which include:

- progressive nonbilious nonbloody vomiting that is clearly different from any baseline spitting up
- male sex
- age at onset 2 to 8 weeks
- previously healthy with good weight gain and growth parameters
- no fever, diarrhea, or other symptoms concerning for an underlying infection
- not in acute distress
- appears hungry
- abdomen is soft; a palpable mass ("olive") may be noted in the right upper quadrant and/or intestinal peristalsis may be visible on physical examination
- history of normal newborn screen
- degree of dehydration and malnutrition is related to the duration of the illness

The incidence of pyloric stenosis is 1 to 3 per 1,000 live births. Boys are affected 4 times more frequently than girls. The incidence is higher in white infants. Premature infants may present at an older chronologic age and with less forceful vomiting and hunger. The etiology is likely multifactorial, including genetic predisposition and environmental factors (maternal smoking, bottle feeding, macrolide exposure).

American Board of Pediatrics Content Specification(s)/ Content Area

- Recognize the clinical features associated with pyloric stenosis, and manage appropriately
- Recognize the acid-base changes associated with pyloric stenosis, and manage appropriately

Suggested Readings

Dinkevich E, Ozuah PO. Pyloric stenosis. *Pediatr Rev.* 2000;21(7)249-250.

Hsu BS, Lakhani SA, Wilhelm M. Acid-base disorders. *Pediatr Rev.* 2016; 37(9):361-369.

Reddy S, Kamat DM. Pyloric stenosis. In: McInerny TK, Adam HM, Campbell DE, DeWitt TG, Foy JM, Kamat DM, eds. *American Academy of Pediatrics Textbook of Pediatric Care*. 2nd ed. Elk Grove Village, IL: American Academy of Pediatrics; 2017:2551-2554.

Item 64   Preferred Response: A

The boy in this vignette likely has juvenile polyposis syndrome (JPS). Although the polyps removed are classified as juvenile polyps, the presence of 5 or more polyps suggests a diagnosis of JPS. Children with a suspected polyposis syndrome should be referred for genetic testing to confirm the diagnosis and follow surveillance guidelines.

Juvenile polyps are the most common type of colonic polyp in children. Typically manifesting as painless causes of rectal bleeding in young children, they are benign. Polypectomy during colonoscopy is indicated for confirmation of diagnosis and resolution of symptoms. Most commonly, simple juvenile polyps are present in the rectosigmoid colon. If less than 5 juvenile polyps are present, the diagnosis is likely simple juvenile polyps, and routine follow-up colonoscopy is not recommended. However, if symptoms recur, repeat colonoscopy is indicated.

Polyposis syndromes should be suspected in children with 5 or more juvenile polyps, adenomatous polyps, and/or a family history of polyposis or early colorectal cancer. Children or adults with 5 or more juvenile polyps may have JPS. Most commonly, patients describe painless rectal bleeding; however, some patients may experience diarrhea, abdominal pain, or bowel obstruction from intussusception. Mutations in *SMAD4*, *BMPR1A*, and *ENG* are associated with JPS. Patients with JPS have an increased risk of colorectal and gastric cancer, and surveillance with endoscopy and colonoscopy is recommended annually if polyps are present and every 3 years if no polyps are found. Patients with *SMAD4* mutations are also at increased risk for vascular malformations.

Other polyposis syndromes include Peutz-Jeghers syndrome, which is caused by *STK11/LKB1* mutations and characterized by mucocutaneous macules and polyps throughout the gastrointestinal tract that can result in intussusception, and familial adenomatous polyposis (FAP) syndrome, which is caused by *APC* mutations and characterized by numerous adenomatous polyps and significant risk for colorectal cancer. Both syndromes have increased risk for extraintestinal malignancies and have specific screening guidelines.

If a polyposis syndrome is suspected, genetic testing is recommended. Referral to a colorectal surgeon may be appropriate in cases with severe polyposis and increased risk of colorectal cancer (particularly in young adults with FAP syndrome), but it is not appropriate for the boy in this vignette because the diagnosis has not been established. Because the boy has 5 or more polyps, a polyposis syndrome is very likely; thus, surveillance colonoscopy would be indicated every 1 to 3 years as appropriate. Thyroid ultrasonography is indicated in children with FAP because of the increased risk of papillary thyroid cancer. However, the boy is this vignette did not have adenomatous polyps, thus he does not have FAP.

American Board of Pediatrics Content Specification(s)/ Content Area

- Recognize the clinical features associated with juvenile polyposis
- Recognize the significance of a solitary juvenile polyp

Suggested Readings

Haidle JL, Howe JR. Juvenile polyposis syndrome. *GeneReviews*. https://www.ncbi.nlm.nih.gov/books/NBK1469.

Iglesias IM, Fernandez A, Smith-Singares E, Soyemi K, Arcia R. Abdominal pain, nausea, and vomiting in a 12-year-old girl. *Pediatr Rev.* 2016;37(2):83-85.

Kay M, Eng K, Wyllie R. Colonic polyps and polyposis syndromes in pediatric patients. *Curr Opin Pediatr.* 2015;27(5):634-641.

The boy in the vignette has localized back pain, leg weakness, and urinary retention. A neurologic examination shows numbness in a dermatomal distribution in his middle back, where the back pain is, right lower extremity proximal weakness, brisk lower extremity reflexes, and a right upgoing toe. Together, this suggests a lesion of the spinal cord, most likely at or slightly above the level of the back pain and numbness. The best diagnostic test in this case is magnetic resonance imaging of the spinal cord with and without contrast. A brain lesion could cause most of his symptoms and signs, except the sensory loss over the area in his back. The sensory loss is due to involvement of the exiting dorsal roots and sensory nerves, and localizes the lesion to the spinal cord. Magnetic resonance imaging of the brain may eventually be recommended, especially if the boy is found to have a tumor, but it is not the best initial diagnostic test. Electromyography and nerve conduction study could confirm dysfunction of peripheral nerves, but the upper motor neuron signs of hyperreflexia and a right upgoing toe suggest a central nervous system lesion, so this would not be the best next test. Similarly, urodynamic studies may confirm bladder dysfunction, but would not be the best next test.

The boy in this vignette most likely has a spinal cord tumor, such as the schwannoma seen on T1 sagittal view of a magnetic resonance image with contrast of the thoracic spine (Item C65). Localized back pain and lower extremity weakness are common presenting signs of spinal cord tumors; bowel and bladder dysfunction can also occur. Untreated bladder dysfunction can result in recurrent urinary tract infections, vesicoureteral reflux, and autonomic dysreflexia which can be life-threatening. Clinicians should always assess for bowel and bladder dysfunction in patients with spinal cord disorders.

PREP Pearls

- Spinal cord tumors commonly present with localized back pain and lower extremity weakness. Bowel and bladder dysfunction can also occur.
- Untreated bladder dysfunction can result in recurrent urinary tract infections, vesicoureteral reflux, and autonomic dysreflexia which can be life-threatening.

American Board of Pediatrics Content Specification(s)/ Content Area

- Recognize the significance of bladder and bowel dysfunction in spinal cord disease
- Plan the initial neurodiagnostic evaluation of acute spinal cord dysfunction

Suggested Readings

Kliegman RM, Stanton BF, St Geme JW, Schor NF. *Spinal cord disorders. In: Nelson Textbook of Pediatrics*. 20th ed. Philadelphia, PA: Elsevier; 2016;chap 606:2952-2959.

Wilson PE, Oleszek JL, Clayton GH. Pediatric spinal cord tumors and masses. *J Spinal Cord Med*. 2007;30(suppl 1):S15.

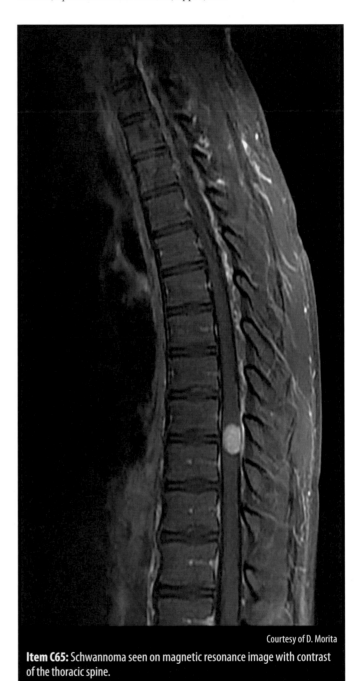

Courtesy of D. Morita

Item C65: Schwannoma seen on magnetic resonance image with contrast of the thoracic spine.

Despite significant improvements in blood lead levels (BLLs) in children over the last few decades due to banning or eliminating lead-based substances, increased awareness, and widespread screening, lead toxicity remains a significant public health dilemma. There is no safe blood lead concentration. In 2012, the Centers for Disease Control and Prevention (CDC) recommended a lower threshold for acceptable BLLs of less than 5 µg/dL (0.2 µmol/L), which the American Academy of Pediatrics (AAP) adopted. The AAP Recommendations for Preventive Pediatric Healthcare, consistent with the CDC, recommend universal screening for lead toxicity at 12 months and 24 months for children who are eligible for Medicaid, receive government assistance, or live in high-risk environments. Expanded targeted screenings may be recommended by local and state health departments depending on risk factors. Immigrant and refugee children are also a high-risk population and should be screened upon entering the country. While a fingerstick lead level is an acceptable first step for screening, a confirmatory venous BLL must be obtained for fingerstick levels of 5 µg/dL (0.2 µmol/L) or greater because of the increased hand-to-mouth behaviors of young children and possible contamination of exposed skin.

Environmental lead is ubiquitous. It exists in the air, soil, dust, and water. However, most causes of lead exposure result from contaminated manmade sources. Lead-based paint, banned in the 1970s, continues to exist in many homes built before the 1950s and is a major source of lead toxicity. Home renovations, repair, construction, abatement, or decay may also lead to lead-laden dust. Soil contaminated with gasoline, prior to the elimination of lead in the 1980s, or from former mine or smelter communities is another cause of lead toxicity. Tap water stagnant in old or corroded lead-based pipes is another contributing source. Additional exposures include nutritional supplements, folk medicines, ceramic dishware, imported foods or candies, and cosmetics.

Lead toxicity can occur at any BLL and affects different organ systems, although the vast majority of affected children are asymptomatic. Manifestations include abdominal pain, constipation, growth failure, hearing loss, behavioral problems, cognitive impairment, seizures, encephalopathy, renal disease, microcytic anemia, dental caries, and spontaneous abortions. Blood lead levels typically peak between 18 and 30 months of age.

For children with BLLs of 5 µg/dL (0.2 µmol/L) or greater, the first step is confirmatory testing with a venous sample. Local or state health departments should subsequently be notified to inspect the child's home to detect and remedy any source of lead exposure. Screening children for iron deficiency and initiating ferrous sulfate is also recommended. For BLLs of 5 to 15 µg/dL (0.2-0.7 µmol/L), retesting should occur within 1 to 3 months to ensure the level is not rising. If the BLL is stable or decreasing, the patient should be retested every 3 months with a venous BLL.

PREP Pearls

- For children with a fingerstick lead level of 5 µg/dL (0.2 µmol/L) or greater, a repeat venous sample should be obtained.
- Lead toxicity may occur at any blood lead level and may manifest with gastrointestinal, neurobehavioral, renal, and hematologic symptoms; the vast majority of children with lead toxicity are asymptomatic.
- Universal lead screening is recommended at health supervision visits for children at risk for lead toxicity.

American Board of Pediatrics Content Specification(s)/ Content Area

- Understand the outcomes associated with lead poisoning
- Understand the importance of a screening examination for lead during early periodic screening evaluations
- Recognize the multiple sources of exposure to lead

Suggested Readings

Centers for Disease Control and Prevention, Advisory Committee on Childhood Lead Poisoning Prevention. *Low Level Lead Exposure Harms Children: A Renewed Call for Primary Prevention.* Atlanta, GA: Centers for Disease Control and Prevention; 2012. www.cdc.gov/nceh/lead/ACCLPP/Final_Document_030712.pdf.

Chandran L, Cataldo R. Lead poisoning: basics and new developments. *Pediatr Rev.* 2010;31(10):399-406.

Council on Environmental Health. Prevention of childhood lead toxicity. *Pediatrics.* 2016;138(1):e20151493.

Item 67　Preferred Response: B

While there are a multitude of classes of surface antigens on the red blood cell, the 2 primary classes are ABO and Rh. The ABO group represents surface carbohydrates, while the Rh antigen is a protein. Both groups are genetically determined and inherited in a classic Mendelian manner. Blood type does not seem to impact general health, but it is critically important in the context of receiving a blood transfusion. Red blood cell antigens are highly immunogenic. If a patient is exposed to a foreign red blood cell antigen by receiving mismatched blood, there is a rapid and strong immune response resulting in brisk hemolysis of the transfused blood.

Additionally, it is possible for a mother to become exposed to a foreign red blood cell antigen if it is expressed in a fetus. Because red blood cell antigens are inherited in a Mendelian manner, it is possible for a fetus to express an antigen that the mother does not express (ie, it was inherited from the father). For example, an AA mother and an AB father can produce AB offspring. If there is a fetal-maternal bleed, the mother will be exposed to the B antigen and develop a titer of antibodies to the B antigen that will cross the placenta. This scenario in which a newborn can experience hemolysis as a consequence of a fetal-maternal AB mismatch is known as hemolytic disease of the newborn.

For hemolytic disease of the newborn caused by an Rh mismatch, the immune system of the mother has to be primed through a prior exposure to the Rh antigen. Thus, the first child born with an Rh mismatch may not experience any hemolysis, while subsequent children can experience brisk hemolysis. In this vignette, the mother's history of a fetal loss may represent a prior exposure to an Rh mismatch. In contrast to hemolytic disease of the newborn caused by an Rh mismatch, hemolysis caused by an ABO mismatch does not require a prior maternal exposure to the antigen.

The O blood type is a null antigen and is not immunogenic. The same is true of the Rh-negative group. Given that the newborn in this vignette is experiencing hemolysis, the most likely scenario for hemolysis is an ABO or Rh mismatch in which the newborn expresses a red cell antigen that the mother does not express. The only 2 options provided with such a mismatch are response choices B and D, both of which have Rh mismatches with the newborn expressing the Rh antigen, while the mother does not. Response choice B also shows a positive direct antibody test (a test to assess whether antibodies are present on red blood cells) while response choice D does not. Therefore, response choice B represents the most likely combination of surface antigens to lead to hemolysis.

PREP Pearls

- A direct antibody test (Coombs test) assesses for the presence of antibodies on the surface of red blood cells and will most often be positive in cases of hemolytic disease of the newborn.

- Hemolytic disease of the newborn occurs when the mother develops an antibody titer to a red blood cell antigen expressed on the red blood cells of the fetus but not on her own red blood cells.

- The 2 major groups of red blood cell surface antigens are the ABO group and the Rh group. Both are inherited in a classic Mendelian manner. The O group and the Rh-negative group are null antigens, which are not immunogenic.

American Board of Pediatrics Content Specification(s)/ Content Area

- Recognize the association of ABO or Rh incompatibility with progressive or severe anemia in infants of various ages

Suggested Readings

Dean L. The ABO blood group. In: *Blood Groups and Red Cell Antigens.* Bethesda, MD: National Center for Biotechnology Information; 2005. https://www.ncbi.nlm.nih.gov/books/NBK2267/.

Hendrickson JE, Delaney M. Hemolytic disease of the fetus and newborn: modern practice and future investigations. *Transfus Med Rev.* 2016;30(4): 159-164.

Lauer BJ, Spector ND. Hyperbilirubinemia in the newborn. *Pediatr Rev.* 2011;32(8):341-349.

The girl in the vignette presents with intermittent epistaxis and purulent discharge from her right naris over the past 2 weeks, and her breath is foul-smelling. The most likely explanation for her epistaxis is a nasal foreign body.

Epistaxis occurs commonly in children, especially during the adolescent years. This symptom may be quite distressing to children and their parents, as they are often alarmed by the onset of bleeding and may overestimate the amount of blood loss. A systematic approach to the history and physical examination is key to identifying the small percentage of patients requiring immediate intervention, laboratory evaluation, or subspecialty consultation for further management.

One approach to the differential diagnosis of epistaxis is to classify potential causes as local (which occur much more commonly) versus systemic. Local causes include inflammation, irritation, infection, or trauma. The most common causes include trauma (including nose picking, which is extremely common among children), nasal foreign body, allergic rhinitis, and viral upper respiratory infections. In children presenting with recurrent episodes of unilateral epistaxis associated with mucopurulent nasal drainage and/ or foul-smelling breath, careful physical examination to be performed to identify a nasal foreign body. Local infectious causes—including upper respiratory infection, bacterial rhinitis/sinusitis, and staphylococcal furuncles—may precipitate epistaxis. Structural lesions such as nasal polyps, tumors (both benign and malignant), telangiectasias, and hemangiomas are potential, though less common, local causes of epistaxis.

Although various systemic diseases may lead to nosebleeds in children, these disorders typically present with other associated signs and symptoms. Hematologic disorders that may precipitate epistaxis include leukemias, idiopathic thrombocytopenic purpura, aplastic anemia, von Willebrand disease, platelet dysfunction, and hemophilia or other disorders of coagulation. Toxicity from certain drugs such as warfarin, aspirin, and nonsteroidal anti-inflammatory drugs, may present with epistaxis. Systemic hypertension can, rarely, result in epistaxis in children. Children with systemic infections including congenital syphilis, Dengue fever, and sepsis with disseminated intravascular coagulation may have epistaxis, but will typically display other symptoms. Adolescent girls may be affected by monthly episodes of nasal congestion and epistaxis due to vicarious menstruation, which is thought to be hormonally mediated. Epistaxis is a rare symptom in infants and preambulatory children, and should raise clinical suspicion for a systemic disorder or child abuse.

Juvenile nasopharyngeal angiofibromas are benign tumors that characteristically present in adolescent boys and cause symptoms including nasal obstruction, mucopurulent nasal discharge, and severe epistaxis. It would be unlikely for this lesion to present in a 3-year-old girl, and the symptoms manifested by the girl in the vignette are much more likely to arise from a nasal foreign body.

The term *rhinitis sicca* refers to desiccation of the nasal mucosa, which can arise in dry, cold winter climates or in children who depend on respiratory support systems that expose the nares to dry air (such as nasal cannula or nasal bilevel positive airway pressure). Although rhinitis sicca is a common cause of epistaxis, it is not associated with mucopurulent nasal discharge or foul-smelling breath.

von Willebrand disease is an inherited disorder caused by deficiency or dysfunction of von Willebrand factor, a clotting protein that binds factor VIII. This bleeding disorder may affect up to 1% of the population and can result in epistaxis, but the girl in the vignette has no history of other bleeding or bruising. Furthermore, her nasal discharge and foul-smelling breath would not be explained by von Willebrand disease. Nasal foreign body is a much more common underlying cause of nosebleeds in her age group. In all patients with epistaxis, it is important to inquire about any family history of bleeding disorders.

PREP Pearls

- Children with nasal foreign bodies often present with recurrent episodes of unilateral epistaxis associated with mucopurulent nasal drainage and/or foul-smelling breath.
- Epistaxis is a rare symptom in infants and preambulatory children, and should raise clinical suspicion for a systemic disorder or child abuse.
- Epistaxis is most frequently caused by local inflammation, irritation, infection, or trauma.

American Board of Pediatrics Content Specification(s)/Content Area

- Formulate a differential diagnosis of epistaxis and manage appropriately
- Plan the appropriate evaluation of the various manifestations of epistaxis

Suggested Readings

Delgado EM, Nadel FM. Epistaxis. In: Shaw K, Bachur R, eds. *Fleisher and Ludwig's Textbook of Pediatric Emergency Medicine.* 7th ed. Philadelphia, PA: Wolters Kluwer; 2016;chap 21.

Stoner MJ, Dulaurier M. Pediatric ENT emergencies. *Emerg Med Clin North America*. 2013;31(3):795-801.

| Item 69 | Preferred Response: C |

Systemic lupus erythematosus (SLE) is a chronic inflammatory disease with multisystem involvement that may include skin, joints, kidneys, lungs, nervous system, serosal membranes or other organs. In children, as in adults, SLE is diagnosed based on the Systemic Lupus International Collaborating Clinics (SLICC) criteria, which have been revised and validated from the previously established American College of Rheumatology criteria (Item C69A). The SLICC criteria for SLE diagnosis are more inclusive of patients with heterogeneous manifestations of SLE without major organ involvement. Similar to the girl in the vignette, children with SLE usually present with rash, fever, and arthritis. Children tend to have a more severe clinical course compared with adults with SLE.

Item C69A. Criteria for the Diagnosis of Systemic Lupus Erythematosus.

ACR Criteria	SLICC Clinical Criteria
1. Malar rash	1. Acute cutaneous lupus
2. Photosensitivity	
3. Discoid rash	2. Chronic cutaneous lupus
4. Oral ulcers	3. Oral and nasal ulcers
5. Serositis: pleuritis, pericarditis	4. Serositis
6. Arthritis: nonerosive and nondeforming, involving ≥ 2 joints	5. Joint disease
7. Nephritis	6. Renal
8. Hematologic*: hemolytic anemia with reticulocytosis, leukopenia or lymphopenia on 2 or more occasions, thrombocytopenia	7. Hemolytic anemia
	8. Leukopenia or lymphopenia on 1 or more occasions*
	9. Thrombocytopenia*
9. Neurologic*: seizures, psychosis	10. Neurologic*
	11. Nonscarring alopecia
	SLICC Immunologic Criteria
10. Antinuclear antibody*	Positive titres for:
11. Immunologic: positive LE cell preparation OR antibody to native DNA (anti-dsDNA) OR anti-Smith antibody (anti-Sm) OR False-positive serologic test for syphilis (at least 6 months)	12. ANA
	13. Anti-dsDNA
	14. Anti-Sm
	15. Antiphospholipid
	16. Direct Coombs test
	17. Low complement levels: C3, C4, or CH50
Presence of any ≥4 of the 11 criteria, serially or simultaneously, during any interval of observation	*Presence of ≥4 of the 11 criteria, with at least 1 clinical and 1 immunologic criterion*
	OR biopsy-proven lupus nephritis

* In the absence of offending drugs and associated known metabolic derangements.

Abbreviations: ACR, American College of Rheumatology; ANA, antinuclear antibody; Anti-dsDNA, anti–double-stranded DNA; SLICC, Systemic Lupus International Collaborating Clinics.

Adapted and reprinted with permission from Klein-Gitelman M. Systemic lupus erythematosus (SLE) in children: Clinical manifestations and diagnosis. Sundel R, TePas E. (eds) UpToDate. Wolters-Kluwer. 2018

References:

1. Tan EM, Cohen AS, Fries JF, et al. The 1982 revised criteria for the classification of systemic lupus erythematosus. *Arthritis Rheum* 1982; 25:1271.

2. Hochberg MC. Updating the American College of Rheumatology revised criteria for the classification of systemic lupus erythematosus (letter). *Arthritis Rheum* 1997; 40:1725.

3. Petri M, Orbai AM, Alarcón GS, et al. Derivation and validation of the Systemic Lupus International Collaborating Clinics classification criteria for systemic lupus erythematosus. *Arthritis Rheum* 2012; 64:2677.

A malar butterfly rash, the hallmark of cutaneous SLE (Item C69B) is the most frequent skin manifestation of SLE. The maculopapular, nonpruritic rash typically involves the malar eminences, crossing the nasal bridge and sparing the nasolabial folds. Arthritis in SLE is typically symmetric in both the large and small joints, and frequently involves the knees, wrists, ankles, and fingers. Unlike juvenile idiopathic arthritis (JIA), the arthritis associated with SLE is nonerosive and nondeforming.

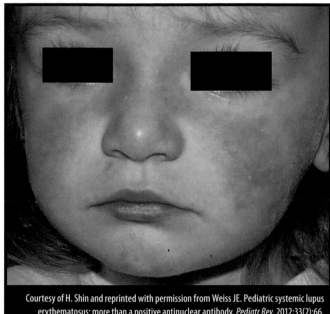

Courtesy of H. Shin and reprinted with permission from Weiss JE. Pediatric systemic lupus erythematosus: more than a positive antinuclear antibody. *Pediatr Rev.* 2012;33(2):66.

Item C69B: Malar rash as seen in cutaneous systemic lupus erythematosus.

Renal involvement, occurring in nearly 75% cases of pediatric SLE, usually develops within the first year of symptom onset, and may present with hematuria, hematuria and proteinuria, nephrotic syndrome, or rapidly progressive glomerulonephritis. Severe disease, with renal biopsy showing focal or diffuse proliferative nephritis, along with immune complex deposition in the mesangium and subendothelial space, is more frequently seen in children than in adults. Aggressive immunosuppressive therapy with high-dose oral corticosteroids (2 mg/kg) or intravenous pulse methylprednisolone (30 mg/kg, max of 1 g) plus more potent immunosuppressive agents (cyclophosphamide or mycophenolate mofetil) is indicated for severe lupus nephritis.

Antineutrophil cytoplasmic (ANCA) vasculitis is a primary small vessel vasculitis, and is rare in the pediatric population. Children most commonly present with microscopic polyangiitis or granulomatosis with polyangiitis (Wegener granulomatosis). Eosinophilic granulomatosis with polyangiitis (Churg-Strauss syndrome) is very rarely seen. Elevated serum titers of antimyeloperoxidase ANCA antibodies (perinuclear pattern) are seen in microscopic polyangiitis, and PR3 ANCA antibodies (cytoplasmic distribution) are present in patients with Wegener granulomatosis. Renal involvement presents with hematuria, hematuria and proteinuria, rapidly progressive glomerulonephritis, or focal segmental glomerulonephritis. Renal biopsy is characterised by paucity of immune complex deposition (pauci-immune), in contrast with SLE where extensive immune complex deposits are seen. Pulmonary capillary inflammation leading to pulmonary hemorrhage is frequent in all forms of ANCA vasculitis. Granulomatous polyangiitis of the upper airways (recurrent epistaxis or sinusitis) and laryngotracheobronchial stenosis are more frequently seen with Wegener granulomatosis. Secondary vasculitis is seen in association with underlying disease such as Henoch-Schönlein purpura (immunoglobulin A vasculitis) and Kawasaki disease (the 2 most common vasculitides seen in children), and SLE.

Chronic idiopathic inflammation of the joints characterizes JIA. The systemic form of JIA (previously called Still disease or systemic juvenile rheumatoid arthritis) presents with daily quotidian (daily, intermittent, high spiking) fever, rash, and polyarticular arthritis. The rash in JIA is macular, with discrete salmon-colored patches that become prominent with fever spikes and fade away as the temperature decreases. Though typically generalized, the rash is often found in the axillae or around the waist. Other manifestations of systemic JIA include serositis, hepatomegaly, splenomegaly, and lymphadenopathy. These are not seen with oligoarticular (most commonly diagnosed) or polyarticular JIA.

Patients with Sjögren syndrome (SS) present with dryness of the mouth and eyes, enlargement of the parotid glands, and an increase in dental caries. Autoimmune-mediated chronic inflammation of the lacrimal and salivary glands leads to the characteristic clinical features. Varied extraglandular manifestation reported in patients with SS may indicate primary SS or a secondary form of SS frequently seen in association with other autoimmune diseases such as JIA and SLE. Elevated titers of anti-Ro/SSA and/or anti-La/SSB antibodies are reported in nearly 80% of patients with primary SS.

PREP Pearls

- A malar butterfly rash is the hallmark and most frequent skin manifestation of cutaneous systemic lupus erythematosus.
- Children tend to have a more severe clinical course than adults with systemic lupus erythematosus.
- Renal involvement occurs in nearly 75% of the pediatric population with systemic lupus erythematosus, usually presenting within the first year of symptoms. This may present with hematuria, hematuria and proteinuria, nephrotic syndrome, or rapidly progressive glomerulonephritis.

American Board of Pediatrics Content Specification(s)/Content Area

- Plan the appropriate management of systemic lupus erythematosus, including recognition of drug-related complications
- Plan the appropriate diagnostic evaluation of systemic lupus erythematosus, and interpret the results appropriately

Suggested Readings

Klein-Gitelman M. Systemic lupus erythematosus (SLE) in children: clinical manifestations and diagnosis. UpToDate.

Petri M, Orbai AM, Alarcón GS, et al. Derivation and validation of the Systemic Lupus International Collaborating Clinics classification criteria for systemic lupus erythematosus. *Arthritis Rheum.* 2012;64:2677-2686.

Sadun RE, Ardoin SP, Schanberg LE. Systemic lupus erythematosus. In: Kliegman RM, Stanton BF, St Geme J, Schor NF, Behrman RE, eds. *Nelson Textbook of Pediatrics.* 20th ed. Philadelphia, PA: Elsevier Saunders; 2016;chap 158:1176-1181.

Tan EM, Cohen AS, Fries JF, et al. The 1982 revised criteria for the classification of systemic lupus erythematosus. *Arthritis Rheum.* 1982; 25:1271-1277.

Weiss JE. Pediatric systemic lupus erythematosus: more than a positive antinuclear antibody. *Pediatr Rev.* 2012;33(2):62-74.

The girl in this vignette is being managed for heart failure and is experiencing persistent symptoms of fatigue and poor growth despite medical management. A patient like this will typically be on diuretics as well as afterload reducers, such as ace inhibitors. If significant symptomatology persists on optimum oral medications, heart transplantation will often be considered. Thirst is a common problem for patients in heart failure. The thirst is caused by diuretic use and the body's desire to hold onto salt and fluid to augment cardiac output. Patients in heart failure are commonly hyponatremic, which complicates their fluid management. Heart failure is a state of sodium and fluid overload, making fluid and sodium restriction logical potential therapies. Although data to support or refute this logic are lacking, the restriction of fluid, sodium, or both are common therapies. Fluid and sodium restriction is far more successful in the inpatient setting than in the outpatient setting because compliance can be difficult.

Given the poor weight gain of this patient, the best choice to control her thirst, of the choices listed, would be with nutritional protein-containing supplements. Juice and water, as hypotonic fluids, will exacerbate hyponatremia. A sports drink with additional sodium would complicate fluid removal given the mechanism of action of diuretics.

PREP Pearls

- Heart failure is a fluid and sodium overload state, and the management of fluid and sodium can be challenging. Treatments can include fluid and sodium restriction and diuretics.
- Weight loss in patients with heart failure can occur in more advanced disease, and supplemental nutrition may be necessary.

American Board of Pediatrics Content Specification(s)/ Content Area

- Plan the dietary management of cardiac disease in a patient who is receiving a fluid-restricted diet

Suggested Readings

Houston BA, Kalathiya RJ, Kim DA, Zakaria S. Volume overload in heart failure: an evidence-based review of strategies for treatment and prevention. *Mayo Clin Proc*. 2015;90(9):1247-1261.

Lindenfeld J, Albert NM, Boehmer JP, et al. HFSA 2010 comprehensive heart failure practice guidelines: section 6. *J Card Fail*. 2010;16(6).

 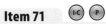

Adolescence is a time of significant physical, cognitive, social, and emotional changes. It can also be a time of great stress in terms of dealing with friends, family, new feelings, and more rigorous schoolwork. Stress is a reaction to anything that is perceived as a challenge or threat. For example, the "fight or flight" response prepares our bodies to deal with a perceived danger. Our bodies prepare to run from danger (ie, fight) by activating our sympathetic nervous system, which causes the adrenal gland to release cortisol and adrenaline. This release causes an increase in heart rate and blood pressure, makes us more alert, tenses our muscles, and slows down digestive functioning. Normally after an immediate stress, our bodies relax and return to a normal state. Individuals who remain stressed for long periods of time may experience medical problems.

Adolescents tend to have different types of stress as compared to adults. Adults tend to be stressed about their jobs, finances, and relationships. Adolescents have a host of stressors that include: dealing with pubertal changes/ensuring their bodies look a certain way; fitting in with their peer group (eg, having the right clothes); experiencing peer pressure (eg, sex, alcohol, drugs); dating; being bullied; and getting into college. These issues might cause prolonged periods of stress that can lead to anxiety, depression, and physical symptoms. Youth with significant anxiety may present with episodes of hyperventilation related to panic attacks. Adolescents will often report muscle tension and spasm in their neck and back and headaches. Headaches may be related to jaw clenching or teeth grinding. Patients may visit their primary care providers with concerns of abdominal pain, diarrhea, constipation, decreased appetite, absent or irregular periods, and fatigue. Other signs of stress include changes in mood, decreased concentration, increased irritability, crying, and anger. Adolescents may try to deal with their stress by sleeping more, or they may have difficulty sleeping. A common response is to isolate oneself from family and friends.

The adolescent in this vignette presents to her primary care provider with headaches; however, she has multiple psychosocial stressors in her life, such as her mother getting a divorce and not doing well in school. She has started isolating herself at home and from her extracurricular activity. The concern for this youth would be to find out how she is addressing her stress and screen her for thoughts of self-harm (suicidal thoughts vs nonsuicidal self-injury). If she is having any suicidal thoughts, a more immediate intervention would be necessary, such as referral to the nearest emergency department for psychiatric evaluation.

Strategies to engage this youth include: finding out if she has someone she is comfortable speaking with about her thoughts and feelings; encouraging her to exercise or get involved in a hobby she enjoys; focus on working on something in which she has some control (ie, improving her grades); and not setting unrealistic expectations for herself.

The other response choices are reasonable steps in management for an adolescent with headache who reports no psychosocial stressors. The adolescent in this vignette has headaches that may be more consistent with tension-type headaches. A trial of a nonsteroidal anti-inflammatory drug may be useful, but does not address the underlying issues related to stress. Magnetic resonance imaging of the brain would rule out an intracranial process (eg, a brain tumor, congenital malformation, or infection) or identify a secondary cause for headaches, if symptoms were increasing in severity or if there were neurologic findings on physical examination. A complete blood cell count and comprehensive metabolic panel would be warranted in patients with fever or vomiting or if there was concern for any other metabolic process.

American Board of Pediatrics Content Specification(s)/ Content Area

- Recognize the clinical findings associated with stress among adolescents

Suggested Readings

Bagnell A. Anxiety and separation disorders. *Pediatr Rev.* 2011;32(10): 440-445.

Chandra A, Batada A. Exploring stress and coping among urban African American adolescents: the Shifting the Lens study. *Prev Chronic Dis.* 2006; 3(2):A40.

Item 72   **Preferred Response: B**

The boy in the vignette has developed acute respiratory distress syndrome (ARDS) due to ingestion of a volatile substance from a plug-in air freshener. Although he is receiving mechanical ventilation and is maintaining adequate ventilation, he remains hypoxic. The best next step in his treatment is to improve alveolar recruitment by increasing positive end-expiratory pressure (PEEP).

Hydrocarbons are organic compounds containing hydrogen and carbon atoms. They appear in a wide variety of household items, including gasoline, kerosene, cleaning products, and propellants from spray bottles. A common source of hydrocarbon toxicity is the oil from plug-in air fresheners, because they are often plugged in at an accessible height and may have a scent intriguing to young children. Certain hydrocarbons are associated with specific toxicities. Carbon tetrachloride, found in some chemical solvents, can cause hepatotoxicity. Several compounds, for example, naphthalene and local anesthetics, can cause methemoglobinemia. Some volatile hydrocarbons are commonly abused by inhalation, that is, "huffing." These cause central nervous system depression via the inhibitory neurotransmitter γ-aminobutyric acid, and lead to euphoria similar to alcohol or narcotic ingestion; they can also lead to dysrhythmia and sudden death due to sensitization of the myocardium to catecholamines.

Although enteral ingestion and systemic absorption of hydrocarbons are harmful, the lung injury resulting from their aspiration is significant. Hydrocarbons are volatile substances with low viscosity and surface tension, which favors aspiration, as opposed to swallowing. When aspirated, low surface tension causes the substance to be distributed over a large surface area in the lungs. As a result, even very small quantities of hydrocarbons can cause severe lung injury. Coughing and vomiting can lead to further aspiration. Therefore, induced emesis, lavage, and activated charcoal are contraindicated. Aspiration of hydrocarbons causes direct injury to airway and alveolar epithelium. It also causes surfactant inactivation and decreased production of surfactant because of injury to type

II alveolar pneumocytes. The decreased quantity and function of surfactant leads to increased alveolar surface tension, alveolar collapse, hypoxia, and increased pulmonary vascular resistance. Lung injury also causes progression of the inflammatory cascade, leading to further surfactant inactivation, edema, increased oxygen diffusion barrier, and direct lung toxicity from inflammatory mediators. Systemic manifestations and other end-organ damage from the inflammatory response syndrome and/or sepsis is also common in severe cases.

Treatment of lung injury from hydrocarbon aspiration is mostly supportive. Hypoxia occurs when alveoli are collapsed or filled with fluid, causing deoxygenated blood originating from the right side of the heart to pass through the lungs without becoming oxygenated. The goal of acute respiratory distress syndrome (ARDS) management is to achieve adequate oxygenation and ventilation while avoiding further trauma from high inflation pressures (barotrauma), high tidal volumes (volutrauma), and the repeated opening and collapsing of lung units (atelectrauma). The evidence-based approach to ARDS in children is the "open lung strategy" in which alveolar recruitment is achieved with airway pressure and positive end-expiratory pressure (PEEP). Strategies include maintaining arterial PO_2 levels of 60 mm Hg or higher, and allowing higher $PaCO_2$ levels to limit inflation pressures as long as the pH is greater than 7.25. The boy in the vignette has a relatively low PEEP, set at 5 cm H_2O, so the best next step is to increase it. Extracorporeal membrane oxygenation is sometimes required for children with severe ARDS, but is reserved for especially refractory cases because of the high risk of the procedure. Helium-oxygen mixture can improve ventilation in diseases of airway obstruction, but is not helpful in improving oxygenation in ARDS.

American Board of Pediatrics Content Specification(s)/ Content Area

- Plan the management of a patient who has ingested or aspirated a substance containing hydrocarbons

Suggested Readings

Heidemann SM, Nair A, Bulut Y, Sapru A. Pathophysiology and management of acute respiratory distress syndrome in children. *Pediatr Clin North Am.* 2017;64(5):1017-1037.

Makrygianni EA, Palamidou F, Kaditis AG. Respiratory complications following hydrocarbon aspiration in children. *Pediatr Pulmonol.* 2016; 51(6):560-569.

Weibrecht KW, Rhyee SH. Acute respiratory distress associated with inhaled hydrocarbon. *Am J Ind Med.* 2011;54(12):911-914.

Vegetarian and vegan diets have become more common; a survey of American adults in 2016 found 8 million people following a vegetarian diet and 3.7 million people following a vegan diet. Personal definitions for vegetarian and vegan diets differ, but typically, vegetarian diets avoid fish, meat, and poultry products, and vegan diets avoid all animal products (including eggs and dairy). Reasons for adhering to vegetarian or vegan diets are individual and may be related to personal health beliefs, political, environmental, or animal-rights beliefs, or religious doctrines.

No data exist in children to support the health benefits of a vegetarian or vegan diet as opposed to an omnivorous diet (containing both animal and plant products). Studies comparing vegetarian or vegan diets to omnivorous diets in adults are difficult to interpret because of lifestyle confounders such as exercise and avoidance of tobacco and alcohol. In adults, vegetarian diets are associated with decreased obesity, hypertension, type 2 diabetes mellitus, and coronary artery disease, but there is no evidence that vegetarian diets independently reduce mortality.

The nutritional adequacy of vegetarian and vegan diets vary markedly from person to person and must be judged individually, based on the variety and amount of nutrients consumed. When plentiful food is available and meals are varied, children consuming vegetarian or vegan diets show normal growth parameters. However, when diets are extremely restricted or poorly planned, children can have nutritional and caloric deficits, leading to suboptimal growth. The greatest risk for suboptimal nutrition occurs during periods of rapid growth. During these times in particular, families should be advised to pay careful attention to ensure sufficient intake of calories, protein, iron, zinc, calcium, vitamin D, cobalamin (vitamin B$_{12}$), long-chain omega-3 fatty acids, and dietary fiber.

Children who consume only vegetarian or vegan diets are at risk for cobalamin (vitamin B$_{12}$) deficiency because it is found only in animal-based food products. Children without sufficient dietary cobalamin should receive vitamin supplementation or regular intake of fortified foods such as certain nutritional yeasts, cereals, and soy products. Niacin (vitamin B$_3$), riboflavin (vitamin B$_2$), and thiamin (vitamin B$_1$) are found in both animal and plant-based foods and are therefore less likely to be deficient in this infant's vegetarian diet.

PREP Pearls

- Children who consume only vegetarian or vegan diets are at risk for cobalamin (vitamin B$_{12}$) deficiency because it is found only in animal-based food products.
- Families of children consuming vegetarian or vegan diets should be advised to pay careful attention to ensure sufficient intake of calories, protein, iron, zinc, calcium, vitamin D, cobalamin (vitamin B$_{12}$), long-chain omega-3 fatty acids, and dietary fiber.
- When plentiful food is available and meals are varied, children consuming vegetarian or vegan diets can achieve normal growth and nutrition.

American Board of Pediatrics Content Specification(s)/ Content Area

- Understand the family and cultural determinants that influence dietary practices and nutrition
- Identify the nutritional complications that can result from vegetarian or vegan diets

Suggested Readings

Lauer B, Spector N. Vitamins. *Pediatr Rev.* 2012;33(8):339-352.

Schurmann S, Kersting M, Alexy U. Vegetarian diets in children: a systematic review. *Eur J Nutr.* 2017;56(5):1797-1817.

Stabler SP. Vitamin B12 deficiency. *N Engl J Med.* 2013;368(2):149-160.

The ill-appearing, unvaccinated boy in this vignette has a clinical picture suggestive of invasive group A streptococcal (GAS) infection after a varicella infection, and is concerning for necrotizing fasciitis (NF). Although NF can be caused by *Staphylococcus aureus*, including methicillin-resistant *S aureus* and other pathogens such as *Clostridium perfringens* and *Clostridium septicum*, the association with varicella is a known risk factor for invasive GAS infection. Primary varicella skin lesions can serve as portal of entry for GAS invasion, and accounted for approximately 15% to 30% of such infections before the routine administration of varicella vaccine in children. Given the significant mortality and morbidity associated with streptococcal NF, emergent surgical exploration for debridement is the best next step in management.

In the United States, the burden of invasive GAS infections is significant. The Centers for Disease Control and Prevention identified 9,557 cases (3.8 cases per 100,000 persons annually) with 1,116 deaths (case-fatality rate of 11.7%) from 2005 through 2012. The highest case-fatality rate was seen in septic shock (45%) followed by streptococcal toxic shock syndrome (STSS; 38%) and NF (29%). The incidence of invasive disease is highest among individuals of age 65 years or older or less than 1 year of age and blacks. Since the addition of the varicella vaccine to the routine childhood immunization series, a steep decline has been observed in the rate of varicella-associated invasive group A streptococcal disease in resource-rich countries. Other risk factors for invasive GAS infection include exposure to other children and household crowding. In some cases, host susceptibility factors may affect the occurrence and severity of invasive GAS infection.

Invasive GAS disease is typically associated with isolation of GAS from the blood or other sterile body site, and may present as STSS with evidence of local soft tissue infection such as NF. The pathogenesis of the severe systemic inflammatory response associated with STSS is related to expression of exotoxins, especially streptococcal pyrogenic exotoxin A. Streptococcal pyrogenic exotoxins represent a family of superantigens that trigger production of proinflammatory cytokines (such as tumor necrosis factor) and result in shock and multiorgan failure.

The onset and clinical course of STSS with NF can be rapidly progressive with shock and multisystem involvement. The clinical presentation of streptococcal NF is characterized by diffuse swelling of an extremity followed by the appearance of bullous lesions, which may initially contain clear fluid but rapidly develop a maroon or violaceous discoloration. Pain, out of proportion to the apparent lesion/area of infection, is a vital early clue for NF. Distinction between cellulitis and NF may be difficult early in the disease presentation.

Necrotizing fasciitis is an emergency that requires urgent surgical exploration or incisional frozen-section biopsy for definitive diagnosis and management. Evaluation by a surgeon should not be delayed for imaging studies. Tissue specimens must be sent for bacterial culture and histopathology. Surgical intervention may vary from resection of all necrotic tissue to radical débridement, or even amputation, depending on the extent and location of the disease. Repeated resection of necrotic tissue may be required to control progressive or persistent infection. In addition to surgical management, aggressive critical care support and antimicrobial therapy with high-dose intravenous penicillin plus a protein-synthesis inhibitor (eg, clindamycin) are required. Clindamycin inhibits enzyme, bacterial toxin, or cytokine production, exhibits a long postantibiotic effect, and has an antimicrobial effect that is unaffected by inoculum size (unlike penicillin). The outcome of STSS with NF may be improved with the use of adjunctive therapy with intravenous immunoglobulin.

PREP Pearls

- Invasive group A streptococcal disease may present as streptococcal toxic shock syndrome with evidence of local soft tissue infection such as necrotizing fasciitis.
- Necrotizing fasciitis is an emergency and requires urgent surgical exploration or incisional frozen-section biopsy for definitive diagnosis and management.
- Varicella skin lesions can serve as a portal of entry for group A streptococcal infection.

American Board of Pediatrics Content Specification(s)/ Content Area

- Recognize the clinical findings associated with necrotizing fasciitis

Suggested Readings

American Academy of Pediatrics. Group A streptococcal infections. In: Kimberlin DW, Brady MT, Jackson MA, Long SS, eds. *Red Book: 2018 Report of the Committee on Infectious Diseases*. 31st ed. Itasca, IL: American Academy of Pediatrics; 2018:748-762.

Frère J, Bidet P, Tapiéro B, et al. Clinical and microbiological characteristics of invasive group A streptococcal infections before and after implementation of a universal varicella vaccine program. *Clin Infect Dis*. 2016;62(1):75-77.

Nelson GE, Pondo T, Toews KA, et al. Epidemiology of invasive group A streptococcal infections in the United States, 2005-2012. *Clin Infect Dis*. 2016;63(4):478-486.

The Apgar scores for the neonate in the vignette are most reflective of her physiologic state at birth. Apgar scores were developed in 1952 by Dr Virginia Apgar as a means to quantitatively describe a neonate's transition to extrauterine life. An Apgar score reflects the neonate's cardiovascular, respiratory, and neurologic state at a specific moment, such as 1 minute after birth. The score is defined by assessment of 5 physical examination findings: heart rate, respiratory rate, reflex irritability, color, and tone. For each component, neonates are scored at regular intervals beginning at 1 minute, 5 minutes, and then continuing every 5 minutes for a period based on their current state. If the Apgar score is less than 7, scores should be assigned for 20 minutes or until the score is greater than 7. Apgar scores may be affected by prematurity, exposure to maternal medication, congenital neurologic conditions, and congenital anomalies.

Apgar scores should not be used to determine the need for resuscitation. All neonates should receive the initial steps of warming, drying, and stimulating immediately after delivery, followed by assessment of heart rate, tone, and respiratory effort to determine whether there is a need for ongoing resuscitation. The Apgar scores of a neonate who requires resuscitation should not be compared with those of a neonate with spontaneous respiration. An increase in Apgar scores between evaluations reflects the neonate's response to resuscitation. For example, in this vignette, the neonate's Apgar scores increased to 7 by 15 minutes after birth reflecting an appropriate response to intubation, chest compressions, and fluid resuscitation. A modified Apgar score that incorporates any resuscitation required has been proposed as an alternative to the traditional Apgar score (Item C75).

Apgar Score				Gestational age_____weeks				
Sign	0	1	2	1 minute	5 minute	10 minute	15 minute	20 minute
Color	Blue or Pale	Acrocyanotic	Completely Pink					
Heart rate	Absent	<100 minute	>100 minute					
Reflex irritability	No Response	Grimace	Cry or Active Withdrawal					
Muscle tone	Limp	Some Flexion	Active Motion					
Respiration	Absent	Weak Cry; Hypoventilation	Good, Crying					
			Total					

Comments:	Resuscitation					
	Minutes	1	5	10	15	20
	Oxygen					
	PPV/NCPAP					
	ETT					
	Chest Compressions					
	Epinephrine					

Reprinted with permission from Watterberg KL, Aucott S, Benitz WE, et al. The Apgar score. *Pediatrics*. 2015;136:820

Item C75: Modified Apgar score.

The correlation between low Apgar scores and long-term adverse neurodevelopmental outcomes is poor. Adverse neurodevelopmental outcomes commonly occur due to asphyxia and impaired gas exchange of varying severity and duration. However, the Apgar score does not assess asphyxia. Although many children with cerebral palsy will have had low Apgar scores, most neonates with low Apgar scores will not have poor long-term outcomes. In addition, Apgar scores do not predict mortality at 1 year of age.

American Board of Pediatrics Content Specification(s)/ Content Area

- Identify the effects of neurologic immaturity on the Apgar score in a very-low-birth-weight infant
- Know the components and significance of the Apgar score

Suggested Readings

Warren JB, Phillipi CA. Care of the well newborn. *Pediatr Rev.* 2012;33:4.

Watterberg KL, Aucott S, Benitz WE, et al. The Apgar score. *Pediatrics.* 2015;136:819.

Item 76   Preferred Response: B

The boy in this vignette has persistent rather than intermittent asthma and needs daily controller therapy in addition to bronchodilators given for acute symptoms. Inhaled corticosteroids are the most effective controller therapy for persistent asthma of any severity. This patient likely has moderate persistent asthma, based on his symptoms of frequent exercise-induced dyspnea and night cough. Low- to medium-dose inhaled steroids would be the first intervention, with escalation of steroid dose or addition of a second controller therapy as the next intervention. The most appropriate second controller therapy would be a leukotriene modifier. Pharmacotherapy should be accompanied by education of the patient and his caregivers about asthma pathophysiology, identification of triggers and recommendations for avoidance, and a written asthma action plan for escalation of therapy with mild and more severe exacerbations.

An oral leukotriene antagonist as primary therapy might be appropriate for mild persistent asthma, but inhaled corticosteroids are the most effective controller therapy and are a better choice in the context of moderate persistent asthma.

An inhaled anticholinergic agent (eg, ipratropium bromide) is appropriate for second-line rescue therapy as a supplement to albuterol for patients in the emergency department with a severe asthma exacerbation or for home therapy in a limited number of patients demonstrated to respond better to ipratropium combined with albuterol than to albuterol alone. Anticholinergic agents are not appropriate for primary controller therapy of asthma.

Oral antihistamines would be beneficial for allergies that may be hidden triggers for this patient, but they are not an effective primary treatment for persistent asthma.

The boy in this vignette has recognized asthma symptoms with viral infections, but likely has other triggers given his subtle symptoms between acute wheezing episodes. Environmental tobacco smoke exposure, allergies, and sources of air pollution (indoors and outdoors) should be addressed as possible unrecognized triggers.

American Board of Pediatrics Content Specification(s)/ Content Area

- Plan appropriate management for wheezing of various etiologies
- Plan the appropriate clinical and diagnostic evaluation of wheezing of various etiologies

Suggested Readings

National Asthma Education and Prevention Program. *Expert Panel Report 3: Guidelines for the Diagnosis and Management of Asthma, Summary Report 2007.* Bethesda, MD: National Institutes of Health; 2007. NIH publication 08-5846. https://www.nhlbi.nih.gov/files/docs/guidelines/asthsumm.pdf.

Rachelefsky G. Inhaled corticosteroids and asthma control in children: assessing impairment and risk. *Pediatrics.* 2009;123(1):353-366.

Wood PR, Hill VL. Practical management of asthma. *Pediatr Rev.* 2009; 30(10):375-385.

Item 77   Preferred Response: B

The girl in this vignette has well-defined areas of hypopigmentation and skin atrophy involving the medial labia majora and the perianal region. The affected skin has a shiny appearance and an area of ecchymosis is present. These physical findings and their distribution are characteristic of lichen sclerosus et atrophicus, also known as lichen sclerosus. Although child sexual abuse may produce bruising, hypopigmentation and atrophy would not be present. Both irritant contact dermatitis and vulvovaginitis may cause postinflammatory hypopigmentation, but the abnormal pigmentation would not be so well demarcated and bruising would be absent.

Lichen sclerosus is an uncommon chronic inflammatory disease of unknown cause that usually affects the anogenital region. It occurs most often in women, but 5% to 15% of cases occur in children, almost exclusively girls younger than 7 years. Lichen sclerosus begins as small pink or white papules that coalesce to form plaques. Ultimately, the lesions become atrophic and appear as shiny ivory-colored areas of hypopigmentation in a figure-of-8 or hourglass distribution surrounding the vulva, perineum, and anus (Item C77). The skin may be wrinkled, and blisters (sometimes hemorrhagic) may occur. Patients may experience dysuria, painful defecation, constipation, or bleeding. In boys, involvement usually is limited to the foreskin, causing it to become sclerotic and difficult to retract.

There is no cure for lichen sclerosus but many cases involute at or before puberty. First-line treatment usually is with a medium- to high-potency topical steroid. Many clinicians initiate therapy with an ultrapotent (group 1) agent like clobetasol propionate or betamethasone dipropionate, tapering the frequency of application or potency as the condition improves. Once control is achieved, the topical steroid is withdrawn and maintenance therapy with a topical calcineurin inhibitor is often begun.

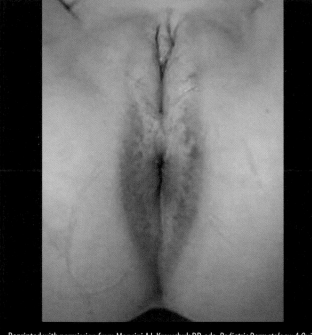

Reprinted with permission from Mancini AJ, Krowchuk DP, eds. *Pediatric Dermatology: A Quick Reference Guide*. 3rd ed. Elk Grove Village, IL: American Academy of Pediatrics; 2016:720.

Item C77: Circumferential hypopigmented atrophic patches in a figure-of-eight configuration characteristic of lichen sclerosis.

PREP Pearls

- Although primarily a disease of women, lichen sclerosus may occur in children, especially girls.
- Occasionally, the lesions of lichen sclerosus may be confused with lesions of child sexual abuse.
- Typical lichen sclerosus lesions are shiny, wrinkled, ivory-colored atrophic patches located in a figure-of-8 or hourglass distribution surrounding the vulva, perineum, and anus. Blisters may occur.

American Board of Pediatrics Content Specification(s)/ Content Area

- Recognize the clinical findings associated with lichen sclerosis, and manage appropriately

Suggested Readings

American Academy of Pediatrics Section on Dermatology. Lichen sclerosus et atrophicus (LSA). In: Mancini AJ, Krowchuk DP, eds. *Pediatric Dermatology: A Quick Reference Guide*. 3rd ed. Elk Grove Village, IL: American Academy of Pediatrics; 2016:719-723.

Tong LX, Sun GS, Teng JMC. Pediatric lichen sclerosus: a review of the epidemiology and treatment options. *Pediatr Dermatol*. 2015;32(5): 593-599.

The girl in this vignette has Turner syndrome. The test most likely to reveal the diagnosis is a karyotype. Turner syndrome results from a missing or structurally abnormal X chromosome. About half of girls with Turner syndrome have a 45,X karyotype. The other half have a karyotype with a portion of an X chromosome missing or rearranged, or a karyotype that contains mosaicism, for example 45,X/46,XX. Features of Turner syndrome displayed by the girl in this vignette include small size at birth, history of recurrent otitis media, difficulty with math, short stature with declining growth velocity, epicanthal folds, high-arched palate, and multiple nevi.

Turner syndrome occurs in 1 of 2,500 live female births. Prenatally, cystic hygroma may be present. Clinical features in infancy may include small birth size, lymphedema, and evidence of congenital heart disease. Short stature is apparent in childhood and may be the only presenting feature. Turner syndrome should be considered in all girls with short stature. Common physical features include ptosis, epicanthal folds, low-set prominent ears, neck webbing, low posterior hairline, shortened fourth metacarpals, broad chest with widely spaced nipples, and multiple nevi. Bicuspid aortic valve, coarctation of the aorta, partial anomalous pulmonary venous return, and aortic root dilatation are associated cardiac anomalies. Primary ovarian failure is common and manifests as delayed puberty or abnormal pubertal progression. Gonadotropins (luteinizing hormone and follicle-stimulating hormone) are elevated around the age of typical pubertal onset. Renal anomalies (eg, horseshoe kidney) and skeletal anomalies (scoliosis, pes planus, high upper-to-lower segment ratio) are common. Intelligence is usually normal but difficulties in math and visual-spatial skills are common. Girls with Turner syndrome are at increased risk for developing autoimmune thyroid disease and celiac disease. Current guidelines outline screening recommendations at diagnosis and throughout life for individuals with Turner syndrome.

In the evaluation of declining growth velocity, an insulin-like growth factor-1 level would be indicated to evaluate for growth hormone deficiency, and a thyroid-stimulating hormone level would be indicated to evaluate for hypothyroidism. These tests would not reveal the diagnosis of Turner syndrome. The insulin-like growth factor-1 level would be normal. Girls with Turner syndrome do, however, have an increased incidence of autoimmune hypothyroidism. Brain magnetic resonance imaging would be indicated for any biochemical evidence of pituitary hormone deficiencies or indications of a central nervous system problem.

PREP Pearls

- Primary ovarian failure is common in Turner syndrome and manifests as delayed puberty or abnormal pubertal progression.
- Turner syndrome should be considered in all girls with short stature.

Suggested Readings

Gravholt CH, Andersen NH, Conway GS, et al; International Turner Syndrome Consensus Group. Clinical practice guidelines for the care of girls and women with Turner syndrome: proceedings from the 2016 Cincinnati International Turner Syndrome Meeting. *Eur J Endocrinol.* 2017;177(3):G1-G70.

Loscalzo ML. Turner syndrome. *Pediatr Rev.* 2008;29(7):219-227.

Item 79   Preferred Response: C

The girl in the vignette has the infantile form of Tay-Sachs disease, an autosomal recessive metabolic disorder caused by hexosaminidase A deficiency. Tay-Sachs disease presents as a neurodegenerative disorder with loss of motor skills, increased weakness, decreased alertness, and increased startle response between 3 and 6 months of age, after an initial period of normal development. The clinical syndrome evolves to include seizures, blindness, spasticity, and ultimately death, typically by the age of 4 years. Physical examination findings include a cherry-red spot of the fovea centralis of the macula of the retina (Item C79), normal-sized liver and spleen, hyperreflexia, ankle clonus, and diffuse muscular hypotonia. There is also a juvenile form with adult onset, slower progression, and neurologic findings including progressive dystonia, motor neuron disease, and spinocerebellar degeneration.

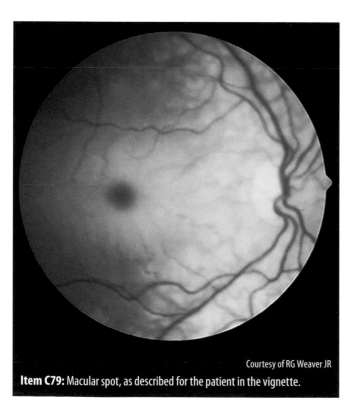

Courtesy of RG Weaver JR

Item C79: Macular spot, as described for the patient in the vignette.

Tay-Sachs disease is a lysosomal storage disorder with increasing systemic storage of a glycosphingolipid, GM2 ganglioside. Diagnosis relies on the demonstration of low to absent levels of β-hexosaminidase A enzymatic activity with normal to high levels of the β-hexosaminidase B isoenzyme in leukocyte enzyme testing. Molecular testing is performed via gene mutation analysis for the *HEXA* gene. Individuals of Ashkenazi Jewish ethnicity could have a carrier rate of up to 1 in 30 for Tay-Sachs disease, warranting carrier screening during preconceptual counseling.

There is no cure for Tay-Sachs disease at this time. Management is mainly supportive involving adequate nutrition and hydration, treating infections, and controlling seizures.

A cherry-red spot can also be seen in infantile Gaucher disease (GD), GM1 gangliosidosis, galactosialidosis, Niemann-Pick disease type A, and Sandhoff disease. A child with GD, Wolman disease, and mucopolysaccharidosis type 1 would present with hepatosplenomegaly unlike the girl in the vignette, who has a normal-sized liver and spleen. Children with mucopolysaccharidosis type 1, also known as Hurler syndrome, present with coarsening of the facies, progressive skeletal dysplasia, macroglossia, and corneal clouding, in addition to neurodegenerative progression. Gaucher disease presents with enlarged liver and spleen, osteopenia, focal lytic or sclerotic lesions of the bone, lung disease, and anemia with thrombocytopenia. Type 1 GD lacks central nervous system findings, while types 2 and 3 have progressive neurologic decline.

Wolman disease, also known as lysosomal acid lipase deficiency, presents with infantile-onset malabsorption because of the storage of cholesterol esters and triglycerides in hepatic macrophages that leads to hepatomegaly, liver disease, and adrenal gland calcification/adrenal cortical insufficiency. Infants typically do not live past age 1 year. Enzyme replacement therapy is available for GD, Wolman disease, and mucopolysaccharidosis type 1.

PREP Pearls

- Diagnosis of Tay-Sachs disease relies on the demonstration of low to absent levels of β-hexosaminidase A enzymatic activity in the white blood cells, with normal to high levels of the β-hexosaminidase B isoenzyme.

- Physical examination findings of Tay-Sachs disease include a cherry-red spot of the fovea centralis of the macula of the retina, normal-sized liver and spleen, hyperreflexia, ankle clonus, and diffuse muscular hypotonia.

- Tay-Sachs disease is an autosomal recessive metabolic disorder caused by hexosaminidase A deficiency, which presents as a neurodegenerative disorder. After an initial period of normal development in early infancy, there is loss of motor skills, increased weakness, decreased alertness, and increased startle response between 3 and 6 months of age.

American Board of Pediatrics Content Specification(s)/
Content Area

- Recognize the clinical features associated with Tay-Sachs disease
- Plan the appropriate immediate and long-term management of Tay-Sachs disease, while considering the long-term prognosis

Suggested Readings

ACOG Committee on Genetics. ACOG Committee Opinion No. 442: preconception and prenatal carrier screening for genetic diseases in individuals of Eastern European Jewish descent. *Obstet Gynecol.* 2009; 114:950-953.

Bley AE, Giannikopoulos OA, Hayden D, Kubilus K, Tifft CJ, Eichler FS. Natural history of infantile G(M2) gangliosidosis. *Pediatrics.* 2011;128(5): e1233-1241.

Kaback MM, Desnick RJ. Tay-Sachs disease. *GeneReviews.* https://www. ncbi.nlm.nih.gov/books/NBK1218/.

Wang RY, Bodamer OA, Watson MS, Wilcox WR; on behalf of the ACMG Work Group on Diagnostic Confirmation of Lysosomal Storage Diseases. ACMG Standards and Guidelines— Lysosomal storage diseases: diagnostic confirmation and management of presymptomatic individuals. http://www.acmg.net/StaticContent/PPG/Lysosomal_storage_diseases__ Diagnostic.15.pdf.

Item 80 — Preferred Response: D

Pediatric clinicians' ability to correctly identify developmental delays by questioning caregivers and observing the child (termed "surveillance") has high specificity; that is, experienced pediatric clinicians, like the colleague in the vignette, rarely suspect a development delay where there is none. However, surveillance is not sensitive for more subtle developmental problems. Therefore, failing to use validated developmental screening tools in infants and young children at specific ages increases the risk of missed diagnoses and treatment delays. The American Academy of Pediatrics recommends developmental screening at 9, 18, and 24 or 30 months, and screening specifically for autism at 18 and 24 months.

In 2009, less than one-half of pediatricians reported routine use of developmental screening tools. This proportion has likely risen since then because of concerted quality improvement efforts and increased reimbursement among insurers. In 2016, a total of 45 state Medicaid programs were providing reimbursement for developmental screening in primary care settings. Quality improvement efforts, like the work described in this vignette, achieve screening rates of over 80%.

Developmental screening tools can be broad, covering several developmental domains, or narrow, covering select conditions (eg, autism) or areas (eg, social-emotional development). The Ages and Stages Questionnaire-3 (ASQ-3) and the Parents' Evaluation of Developmental Status (PEDS) are commonly used parent-report tools in primary care. The ASQ-3 involves caregivers reporting age-specific milestones whereas the PEDS elicits caregivers' concerns in different areas. The Parents' Evaluation of Developmental Status: Developmental Milestones (PEDS:DM) is an age-specific milestone checklist designed to accompany the PEDS. These screening tools are compared in Item C80. Both the ASQ-3 and the PEDS plus PEDS:DM have acceptable psychometric properties for identifying infants and children most likely to have delays that qualify them for developmental services.

Item C80. Comparison of Common Developmental Screening Tools*.

Local Conditions	ASQ-3	PEDS plus PEDS:
Type of measure	Parent report with observable skills	Parent report with concerns plus observable skills
Scores produced	Age-specific cutoffs in 5 developmental domains	Refer/no refer using 5 pathways based on predictive developmental and behavioral concerns plus age-specific cutoffs
Number of items scored	30	16-18
Time to administer	10-20 min	5-10 min
Ages	1 mo-5.5 years; there are different tools for each age	0-7 years; all ages receive the same tool (PEDS) with age-specific developmental milestone items

Abbreviations: ASQ-3, Ages and Stages Questionnaire-3; PEDS, Parents' Evaluation of Developmental Status; PEDS-DM, Parents' Evaluation of Developmental Status: Developmental Milestones.

* Both tools are available in English and Spanish; have clear interpretation guidelines; use language at the 4th-5th grade reading level; and can be scored by a paraprofessional with proper training (eg, medical assistant).

Courtesy of J. VanCleave

The Modified Checklist for Autism in Toddlers-Revised With Follow Up (M-CHAT-R/F) is a 2-stage screening tool for autism. It is a 20-item measure written at the 4th to 6th grade level. It is validated in children aged 16 to 30 months. There are follow-up questions to elicit more detail for each item; these questions should be asked of caregivers when an item's response signals a concern for autism.

Developmental screening tools can identify infants and children at risk for developmental delays. Children with borderline scores and children referred based on screening results but found not to qualify for services should be re-screened more frequently than children comfortably in the "pass" range. There are several reasons a child may have developmental delays; therefore, a concerning screen should prompt the clinician to investigate whether social factors or organic factors (eg, an underlying genetic, neurological, or nutritional disorder) are involved. Referral to community support services (eg, nurse home-visiting program or Head Start program) may be helpful. A closer look at growth, birth history, or family history may provide direction for a diagnostic evaluation.

PREP Pearls

- Broad developmental screening tools do not adequately screen for autism; an autism-specific screening tool should be administered separately.
- Children with borderline scores and children referred for evaluation for services but found not to qualify are high risk and should be closely monitored and screened more frequently.
- Routine use of developmental tools in children aged 0 to 5 years identifies 2- to 6-times more children with suspected delays, compared to surveillance alone.

- Understand the factors that can cause variations in the normal developmental sequence and recognize their associated features

- Understand the uses and limitations of various developmental screening tools

Suggested Readings

Marks KP, LaRosa AC. Understanding developmental-behavioral screening measures. *Pediatr Rev.* 2012;33(10):448-458.

Robins DL, Casagrande K, Barton M, Chen CM, Dumont-Mathieu T, Fein D. Validation of the Modified Checklist for Autism in Toddlers, Revised With Follow-up (M-CHAT-R/F). *Pediatrics.* 2014;133(1):37-45.

Item 81   Preferred Response: D

The best isolation precaution to use when caring for the infant in this vignette with cytomegalovirus infection is universal precautions. The *Guideline for Isolation Precautions: Preventing Transmission of Infectious Agents in Healthcare Settings* from the Centers for Disease Control and Prevention recommends standard (universal) precautions for patients infected with cytomegalovirus, including standard precautions for pregnant health care workers.

Universal or standard precautions are routine practices that should be followed by all health care workers in all clinical settings. A fundamental component of universal precautions is hand hygiene. Hand hygiene is the most important element in preventing transmission of pathogens in health care settings. Additional measures in universal precautions include the use of personal protective equipment (PPE) in high-risk situations. Gloves should be used if there is the potential for contact with blood or body fluids, mucous membranes, nonintact skin, or infected material. Gowns may be needed for anticipated contact with blood or body fluids. Face protection, such as masks and goggles or face shields are recommended for procedures that can generate splashes of body fluids or aerosols, and masks are recommended for procedures that require sterile technique.

Transmission-based precautions are additional measures to prevent pathogen transmission when universal precautions may not be sufficient. When transmission-based precautions are needed, they should always be used in addition to universal precautions. The principal routes of transmission addressed by transmission-based precautions are contact, droplet, and airborne.

Contact precautions are used as a preventative measure for organisms transmitted through direct or indirect contact for which universal precautions alone would not interrupt transmission. Organisms for which contact precautions are used include *Staphylococcus aureus* and herpes simplex virus. Additionally, contact precautions are used for multidrug-resistant organisms and for specific clinical scenarios, such as excessive wound drainage or diarrhea. To prevent transmission of such pathogens to skin or clothing, an additional barrier in the form of gloves and gowns is used whenever there will be contact with the patient or the patient's environment. Hand hygiene should be performed prior to donning PPE; gloving is not a substitute for hand hygiene. Personal protective equipment should be put on upon room entry and removed prior to exit. Hand hygiene should follow removal of PPE. Additionally, equipment used to care for a patient on contact isolation should be dedicated to that patient or disposable.

Droplet precautions are used as a preventative measure for infections transmitted by the respiratory route, including infections caused by influenza virus, adenovirus, rhinovirus, and *Bordetella pertussis*. Droplet transmission occurs when respiratory particles from an infected individual travel short distances and make contact with the mucous membranes of a susceptible host. To prevent droplet transmission, facial protection, in the form of a mask is required.

Airborne precautions are used as a preventative measure for infections transmitted by the airborne route, including tuberculosis, measles, and varicella infections. Fine particles of these pathogens can remain infective over time and can travel long distances, in contrast to the droplets generated in patients with pathogens that require droplet precautions. Therefore, specialized masks (N95 or higher level respirator) and air handling and ventilation systems are used in the setting of airborne precautions.

PREP Pearls

- Hand hygiene is the most important element in preventing transmission of pathogens in health care settings.

- Transmission-based precautions, including contact, droplet, and airborne precautions, are additional measures to prevent transmission of pathogens for which universal precautions may not be sufficient.

- Universal precautions are routine practices, including hand hygiene and use of personal protective equipment in prescribed scenarios, that should be followed by all health care workers in all clinical settings.

American Board of Pediatrics Content Specification(s)/ Content Area

- Understand the appropriate use of universal, airborne, droplet, and contact precautions

Suggested Readings

American Academy of Pediatrics. Isolation precautions. In: Kimberlin DW, Brady MT, Jackson MA, Long SS, eds. *Red Book: 2018 Report of the Committee on Infectious Diseases.* 31st ed. Itasca, IL: American Academy of Pediatrics; 2018:148-157.

Siegel JD, Rhinehart E, Jackson M, Chiarello L; Healthcare Infection Control Practices Advisory Committee. 2007 Guideline for isolation precautions: preventing transmission of infectious agents in healthcare settings. *Am J Infect Control.* 2007;35(10 suppl 2):S65-S164.

The child in the vignette has Klippel-Feil syndrome, with congenital fusions of the cervical vertebrae. Many children with Klippel-Feil syndrome have associated abnormalities including congenital heart disease, vertebral fusions at other levels, and hearing loss. Children with vertebral anomalies often have associated renal anomalies. Sprengel deformity, a congenital elevation of the scapula, is present in about 15% to 20% of individuals with Klippel-Feil syndrome. Item C82 shows a short neck in a child with Klippel-Feil syndrome. Most children with cervical vertebral fusions do not experience symptoms. However, primary care providers should ask about the presence of neck and arm pain and neurologic symptoms such as paresthesias, numbness, and weakness during health supervision visits for children with this syndrome. The physical examination should include a complete neurologic examination to assess strength, muscle tone, and reflexes.

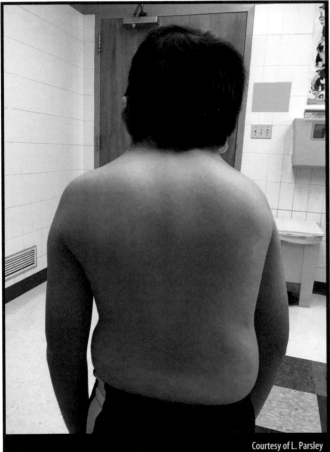

Courtesy of L. Parsley

Item C82: Short, webbed neck in a child with Klippel-Feil syndrome and Sprengel deformity.

Evaluation for this 4-year-old girl should include a thorough history and physical examination, including careful cardiac auscultation. The family should be asked about any history of speech and language delay and concerns about the girl's hearing. Because renal abnormalities can be clinically silent, renal ultrasonography should be performed for all children with Klippel-Feil syndrome. Thoracolumbar radiography should be performed to look for additional vertebral fusions and associated scoliosis. Consultation with neurosurgery should be considered prior to clearance for contact sports participation.

Magnetic resonance imaging (MRI) of the spine is indicated when the history or physical examination findings suggest spinal cord or nerve root compression, or when radiographs show signs of spinal canal narrowing or instability. Before undergoing anesthesia or participating in contact sports, children with Klippel-Feil syndrome should undergo flexion and extension lateral cervical radiography to look for evidence of instability.

Echocardiography would be indicated if there were concern for congenital heart disease based on history or physical examination. Vertebral artery ultrasonography is used to look for decreased blood flow, which is not associated with Klippel-Feil syndrome.

PREP Pearls

- Children with vertebral anomalies should undergo renal ultrasonography to look for underlying renal anomalies.
- Klippel-Feil is a syndrome of congenital cervical vertebral fusions. Most individuals with this syndrome have decreased cervical motion.
- Sprengel deformity, a congenital elevation of the scapula, is present in about 15% to 20% of individuals with Klippel-Feil syndrome.

American Board of Pediatrics Content Specification(s)/ Content Area

- Recognize the clinical and radiologic findings associated with Klippel-Feil syndrome

Suggested Readings

Loder R. The cervical spine. In: Weinstein SL, Flynn HM, eds. *Lovell & Winter's Pediatric Orthopaedics.* 7th ed. Philadelphia: Lippincott Williams and Wilkins; 2013;chap 21:821-893.

Samartzis D, Herman J, Lubicky JP, Shen FH. Sprengel's deformity in Klippel-Feil syndrome. *Spine.* 2007;32(18):e512-e516.

Tracy MR, Dormans JP, Kusumi K. Klippel-Feil syndrome: clinical features and current understanding of etiology. *Clin Orthop Relat Res.* 2004;(424):183-190.

The newborn in the vignette has a caput succedaneum, which is most likely associated with cranial molding. Caput succedaneum is localized superficial edema of the scalp most likely due to venous congestion from cervical pressure on the presenting part during delivery or the use of vacuum extraction. It is bruising/swelling resulting from an accumulation of blood and serum above the periosteum and below the skin from prolonged pressure. Because it is exterior to the periosteum, the swelling may extend across suture lines and across the midline. It may be associated with erythema, petechiae, and ecchymoses of overlying skin, but is not usually associated with a falling hematocrit, underlying linear skull fracture, or low platelet count. Caput succedaneum is usually a benign condition that presents at birth and resolves within a few days without treatment. If ecchymosis is extensive, hyperbilirubinemia or anemia may develop. Rarely reported complications include necrotic lesions, scarring, alopecia, or infection.

Pediatric health care providers must be able to distinguish among caput succedaneum, cephalohematoma, and subgaleal hemorrhage in the newborn. Item C83 depicts the anatomic difference between these extradural fluid collections.

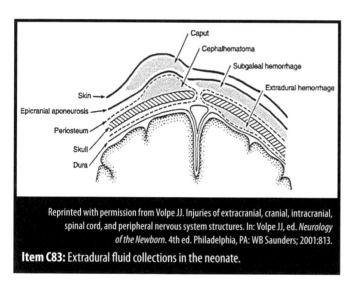

Reprinted with permission from Volpe JJ. Injuries of extracranial, cranial, intracranial, spinal cord, and peripheral nervous system structures. In: Volpe JJ, ed. *Neurology of the Newborn*. 4th ed. Philadelphia, PA: WB Saunders; 2001:813.

Item C83: Extradural fluid collections in the neonate.

Cephalohematoma is a subperiosteal hemorrhage localized to the surface of 1 cranial bone. A cephalohematoma is more likely to occur with prolonged labor or instrument-assisted delivery. It is clinically distinguishable from caput succedaneum because it presents as a unilateral swelling with sharply demarcated boundaries that do not cross the suture lines, the swelling is slower in onset (usually first noticed several hours to days after birth), and there is little if any overlying discoloration of skin. Also, the resolution of a cephalohematoma is slower than that of a caput. They generally resorb spontaneously within a few weeks, but may calcify and remain as a bony prominence for 3 to 4 months. It is important to note that an underlying skull fracture, usually linear and not depressed, may be found in 10% to 25% of cases of cephalohematoma.

Subgaleal hemorrhage is a collection of blood beneath the epicranial aponeurosis and above the periosteum of the skull, which can extend the length of the occipitofrontalis muscle. This condition occurs more commonly with vacuum-assisted delivery. The mechanism of injury may be secondary to a linear skull fracture and/or shearing of the emissary veins between the scalp and dural sinuses as a result of traction on the scalp during delivery. A subgaleal hemorrhage presents as a fluctuant mass that increases in size soon after birth. Bleeding can be extensive and lead to hemorrhagic shock and hyperbilirubinemia. A primary hereditary coagulopathy or secondary consumptive coagulopathy may be present.

PREP Pearls

- Bleeding from a subgaleal hemorrhage can be extensive and lead to hemorrhagic shock and hyperbilirubinemia.
- Caput succedaneum is an accumulation of blood and serum above the periosteum and below the skin from prolonged pressure during parturition that leads to bruising and swelling of the scalp.
- The localized superficial edema of caput succedaneum may cross the midline and suture lines, whereas the subperiosteal hemorrhage of a cephalohematoma is localized to the surface of 1 cranial bone.

American Board of Pediatrics Content Specification(s)/ Content Area

- Distinguish between caput succedaneum, cephalohematoma, and subgaleal hemorrhage

Suggested Readings

Akangire G, Carter B. Birth injuries in neonates. *Pediatr Rev.* 2016;37(11): 451-462.

Lauren H, Campbell DE. Physical examination of the newborn. In: McInerny TK, Adam HM, Campbell DE, DeWitt TG, Foy JM, Kamat DM, eds. *American Academy of Pediatrics Textbook of Pediatric Care.* 2nd ed. Elk Grove Village, IL: American Academy of Pediatrics; 2017:802-819.

Paller AS, Mancini AJ. Cutaneous disorders of the newborn: cephalohematoma, caput succedaneum. In: *Hurwitz Clinical Pediatric Dermatology.* 5th ed. Philadelphia, PA: Elsevier; 2016;chap 2:13.

Infectious diarrhea is common in pediatric patients. In the majority of cases, supportive care is indicated, and antimotility agents are not recommended. The infant in this vignette has an acute, but resolving, diarrheal illness and positive test results for norovirus and *Clostridium difficile*. The clinical presentation is consistent with an infectious gastroenteritis, with several sick contacts at day care. He received intravenous fluids on the first day of his illness. His diarrhea has started to improve, and he is tolerating liquids without difficulty. Thus, supportive care is indicated.

The positive *C difficile* test result may be difficult to interpret in this age group. Roughly 40% of neonates younger than 1 month are colonized with *C difficile*. At 6 months of age, 30% of infants are colonized. By age 3 years, colonization rates approach adult colonization rates, which range between 0% and 3%. Given this infant's improvement in symptoms, the lack of antibiotic exposure, and the absence of frequent hospitalizations, the positive *C difficile* test result is likely to reflect colonization and not infection. Typically, testing in this age group would not be indicated unless there were risk factors for *C difficile* colitis, including antibiotic use and frequent hospitalizations.

There are many potential causes of infectious enteritis or colitis in this infant. Norovirus and rotavirus are commonly encountered viral causes of gastroenteritis in the United States. Rotavirus infection can cause significant morbidity and mortality, particularly in underdeveloped countries. It generally manifests during the winter season and can lead to severe dehydration. Norovirus is a common foodborne illness and generally presents with less severe vomiting and diarrhea compared with rotavirus. In addition to *C difficile*, bacterial causes of acute diarrhea include *Salmonella, Shigella, Campylobacter jejuni*, and *Escherichia coli* O157:H7. These bacterial causes generally present with severe watery diarrhea, and hematochezia is often reported. Treatment for *Salmonella, Shigella*, and *Campylobacter* is generally reserved for patients with underlying medical conditions or severe disease. Treatment for *C difficile* colitis includes removal of concurrent antibiotic therapy (if applicable). The use of metronidazole (first-line), vancomycin, or fecal microbiota transplant (for refractory disease) may be considered.

Loperamide (an antimotility agent) is not indicated in the treatment of infectious diarrhea, given the potential risk of ileus or toxic megacolon. Metronidazole and vancomycin would be reasonable treatment options for *C difficile* infection, however it is unlikely that this infant has true *C difficile* colitis. In addition, his symptoms are beginning to improve with supportive care only.

PREP Pearls

- *Clostridium difficile* colonization is common in infants and children younger than 3 years.
- Antimotility agents are not recommended for management of infectious diarrhea.
- In most cases of infectious diarrhea, the diarrhea is self-resolving and supportive care is recommended.

American Board of Pediatrics Content Specification(s)/ Content Area

- Identify the pathogens commonly associated with infectious diarrhea in patients of various ages
- Apply age-appropriate guidelines in the use of anti-diarrhea medicines
- Plan the appropriate diagnostic evaluation for *Clostridium difficile* infection

Suggested Readings

American Academy of Pediatrics Policy Statement, Committee on Infectious Diseases. *Clostridium difficile* infection in infants and children. *Pediatrics*. 2013;131(1):196-200.

CaJacob NJ, Cohen MB. Update on diarrhea. *Pediatr Rev*. 2016;37(8):313-322.

Item 85 (I-C) **Preferred Response: B**

Dizziness, loss of balance, and lower body temperature are all associated with acute alcohol intoxication, whereas increased heart rate is a sign of alcohol withdrawal. Alcohol is a central nervous system depressant and its use/abuse results in both physiologic and behavioral effects.

The physiologic effects of acute alcohol intoxication include decreased heart rate, lower blood pressure, and lower body temperature. Nausea, vomiting, dizziness, drowsiness, impaired short-term memory, slurred speech, loss of balance, and ataxia may occur. Severe intoxication can cause respiratory depression and coma. Symptoms of alcohol withdrawal occur 5 to 24 hours after reduction of alcohol intake and may last 2 to 7 days. Signs of alcohol withdrawal include tachycardia, sweating, fever, tremors, seizures, elevated blood pressure, vomiting, and diarrhea.

Behavioral effects of acute alcohol intoxication include talkativeness, euphoria, irritability, and anxiety. Alcohol may cause adolescents to feel relaxed and at ease in social situations and thus prompt additional drinking. Alcohol withdrawal can cause insomnia, irritability, craving, disorientation, and hallucinations.

Alcohol is the drug most commonly used by youth, with most 12th grade students reporting that they have used alcohol. A tool such as the 6-item CRAFFT can be used to identify the adolescent in this vignette as at risk for alcohol abuse. The CRAFFT tool is a mnemonic acronym of the first letters of key words in the screening questions: car, relax, alone, friends (or family), forgetting, and trouble. This adolescent boy has multiple key behaviors (ie, having ridden in a car driven by someone who had been using alcohol, uses alcohol to relax, uses alcohol while alone, and told by a friend that he should cut down on his drinking). Additional items are forgetting things done while using alcohol and getting in trouble while using alcohol. Endorsement of 2 or more CRAFFT behaviors should prompt further assessment.

PREP Pearls

- Signs of alcohol withdrawal include tachycardia, sweating, fever, tremors, seizures, elevated blood pressure, vomiting, and diarrhea.
- Symptoms of alcohol withdrawal occur 5 to 24 hours after reduction of alcohol intake and may last 2 to 7 days.
- The physiologic effects of acute alcohol intoxication include decreased heart rate, lower blood pressure, and lower body temperature.

American Board of Pediatrics Content Specification(s)/ Content Area

- Identify the major physiologic consequences associated with alcohol use/abuse
- Recognize the major behavioral consequences of alcohol use/abuse

Suggested Readings

Adger H Jr, Saha S. Alcohol use disorders in adolescents. *Pediatr Rev.* 2013; 34(3):103-113.

Committee on Substance Abuse; Kokotailo PK. Alcohol use by youth and adolescents: a pediatric concern. *Pediatrics.* 2010;125(5):1078-1087.

Legano L. Alcohol. *Pediatr Rev.* 2007;28(4):153-155.

Ocampo AMS, Knight JR. Substance use in adolescence. In: Augustyn M, Zuckerman B, Caronna EB, eds. *The Zuckerman Parker Handbook of Developmental and Behavioral Pediatrics for Primary Care.* 3rd ed. Philadelphia, PA: Wolters Kluwer; 2011:366-372.

Item 86 — Preferred Response: D

The boy in the vignette, with myelomeningocele, has new symptoms of back and leg pain and decreased ambulation. Myelomeningocele is a static problem, so new symptoms suggest a new process. The 2 most likely causes for his symptoms are tethered cord and increased intracranial pressure due to shunt failure. Because computed tomography of his head showed no change from previous imaging, the most likely cause is tethered cord. The best diagnostic test for suspected tethered cord is magnetic resonance imaging of the spine. Chronic urinary tract infection may cause back pain but would not cause limitations in ambulation.

Myelomeningocele is a neural tube defect in which the spinal cord and the meninges protrude out from the spinal canal to the surface of the skin. It is typically repaired at birth, and the defect does not worsen or change over time. Myelomeningocele is commonly associated with Chiari II malformation and hydrocephalus, strabismus, learning disabilities, seizures, bowel and bladder dysfunction, latex allergy, and tethered cord. Myelomeningocele and Chiari II malformation are generally diagnosed antenatally, but tethered cord may not present until years later, especially during periods of growth. Symptoms of tethered cord include back or leg pain and worsening of gait, as in the boy in the vignette. There may also be a change in bowel or bladder function, progressive scoliosis, new contractures, or worsening limb atrophy.

PREP Pearls

- In children with myelomeningocele, tethered cord may not present until the child is older, particularly during periods of growth.
- Myelomeningocele is a static problem, so new symptoms suggest a new process.
- Symptoms of tethered cord may include back or leg pain, worsening of gait, change in bowel or bladder function, progressive scoliosis, new contractures, or worsening limb atrophy.

American Board of Pediatrics Content Specification(s)/ Content Area

- Recognize other abnormalities commonly associated with myelomeningocele
- Recognize the clinical manifestations of and complications associated with spinal dysraphism, and manage appropriately

Suggested Readings

Bui CJ, Tubbs RS, Oakes WJ. Tethered cord syndrome in children: a review. *Neurosurg Focus.* 2007;23(2):E2.

Liptak GS, Dosa NP. Myelomeningocele. *Pediatr Rev.* 2010;31(11):443-450.

Item 87 — Preferred Response: C

The otoscopic image (Item C87A) for the girl in this vignette shows a cholesteatoma, a benign skin tumor typically located in the middle ear and mastoid space. Clinical suspicion of a cholesteatoma should arise when otoscopic examination of the tympanic membrane reveals a vague, irregular white mass that may resemble tympanosclerosis and may protrude from the tympanic membrane with or without recurrent otorrhea. Although cholesteatomas are benign skin growths, they can be destructive to the surrounding tissues of the middle ear, causing necrosis of ossicles, hearing loss, and infection of the middle ear, mastoid, and meninges. These infections can be serious and occasionally fatal. Congenital cholesteatomas may occur but are less common than acquired cholesteatomas, which result from a history of prolonged eustachian tube dysfunction, retraction pockets, and chronic middle ear effusion and inflammation (otitis media). Patients with cholesteatomas should be referred to an otolaryngologist. Most cholesteatomas require surgical treatment. Oral or topical antibiotics and ear lavage will not definitively resolve cholesteatomas.

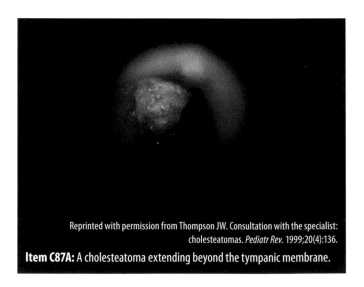

Reprinted with permission from Thompson JW. Consultation with the specialist: cholesteatomas. *Pediatr Rev.* 1999;20(4):136.

Item C87A: A cholesteatoma extending beyond the tympanic membrane.

Diseases of the middle ear include eustachian tube dysfunction, middle ear effusion, and chronic serous otitis media. Otitis media with effusion typically occurs after an episode of acute otitis media and may persist for weeks to months. However, unlike acute otitis media, signs of infection, such as fever and otalgia, are absent. When symptoms are present, they manifest most commonly as hearing loss, ear fullness, and balance problems. Otoscopic findings of middle ear disease include a retracted tympanic membrane (Item C87B), effusion with or without air fluid levels behind the tympanic membrane (Item C87C), opacification of the tympanic membrane, and impaired tympanic membrane mobility when positive pressure is applied via pneumatic otoscopy.

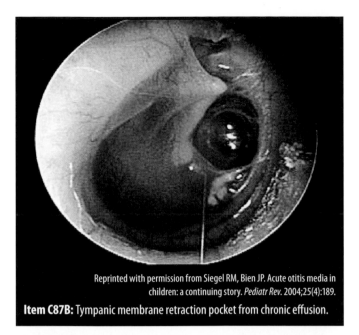

Reprinted with permission from Siegel RM, Bien JP. Acute otitis media in children: a continuing story. *Pediatr Rev.* 2004;25(4):189.

Item C87B: Tympanic membrane retraction pocket from chronic effusion.

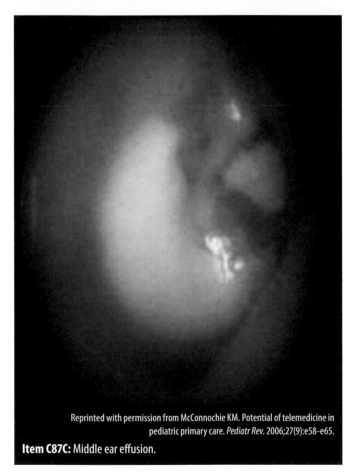

Reprinted with permission from McConnochie KM. Potential of telemedicine in pediatric primary care. *Pediatr Rev.* 2006;27(9):e58-e65.

Item C87C: Middle ear effusion.

Risk factors for the development of recurrent or chronic middle ear disease include a family history of otitis media, formula feeding (instead of breastfeeding), prolonged bottle use, adenoidal hypertrophy, secondhand smoke exposure, day care attendance, and low socioeconomic status. Allergic

rhinitis may be associated with middle ear disease (as demonstrated in observational studies), but treatment with antihistamines and intranasal glucocorticoids is not beneficial. Gastroesophageal reflux disease has not been proven to cause middle ear disease. Complications of prolonged middle ear disease include development of retraction pockets, hearing loss, tympanosclerosis, and cholesteatoma.

PREP Pearls

- Complications of prolonged middle ear disease include development of retraction pockets, hearing loss, tympanosclerosis, and cholesteatoma.
- Most cholesteatomas require surgical treatment.
- Patients with persistent otorrhea and/or a white mass behind the tympanic membrane should be referred to an otolaryngologist for further evaluation and management.

American Board of Pediatrics Content Specification(s)/Content Area

- Recognize the various etiologies of diminished tympanic membrane mobility
- Recognize the clinical findings and complications associated with middle ear disease other than otitis media
- Understand risk factors associated with the development of recurrent or chronic middle ear disease

Suggested Readings

American Academy of Family Physicians; American Academy of Otolaryngology-Head and Neck Surgery; American Academy of Pediatrics Subcommittee on Otitis Media with Effusion. Clinical practice guideline: otitis media with effusion. *Pediatrics.* 2004;113(5):1412-1429.

Gould JM, Matz PS. Otitis media. *Pediatr Rev.* 2010;41(3):102-116.

Rosenfeld RM, Shin JJ, Schwartz SR, et al. Clinical practice guideline: otitis media with effusion (update). *Otolaryngol Head Neck Surg.* 2016; 154(1):s1-s41.

Thompson JW. Consultation with the specialist: cholesteatomas. *Pediatr Rev.* 1999;20(4):134-136.

Item 88   Preferred Response: D

The adolescent in this vignette has heavy menstrual bleeding and iron deficiency anemia as manifested by a microcytic anemia. The iron deficiency suggests that the menorrhagia is a chronic problem. The differential diagnosis for menorrhagia can be broadly classified as dysfunctional uterine bleeding or as a function of a bleeding diathesis. Bleeding diatheses, in turn, can be classified as platelet-related or coagulation factor–related. Platelet-related bleeding can be caused by an inadequate number of platelets or inadequate platelet function. The patient in this vignette has a normal platelet count. For coagulation factor–related bleeding, the intrinsic, extrinsic, and common coagulation pathways can be assessed by measuring the prothrombin time and partial thromboplastin time (Item C88), which are normal for the patient in this vignette. Therefore, she does not have a deficiency of coagulation factors in the intrinsic, extrinsic, or common pathways (ie, factors II-XII).

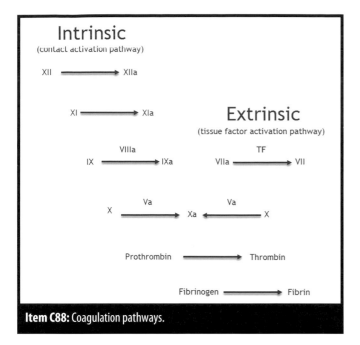

Intrinsic
(contact activation pathway)

XII ⟶ XIIa

XI ⟶ XIa

Extrinsic
(tissue factor activation pathway)

VIIIa
IX ⟶ IXa

TF
VIIa ⟶ VII

Va   Va
X ⟶ Xa ⟵ X

Prothrombin ⟶ Thrombin

Fibrinogen ⟶ Fibrin

Item C88: Coagulation pathways.

Von Willebrand disease (vWD) is the most common bleeding disorder and results from decreased function or absence of von Willebrand factor (vWF), a linking factor that allows functional platelets to bind to connective tissue proteins to form a clot. Following injury to the endothelium of a blood vessel, vWF binds specifically to collagen types I and III. Additionally, vWF carries factor VIII in the blood, so a deficiency of vWF can result in lower levels of factor VIII in the plasma. Von Willebrand disease has multiple phenotypes ranging from mild to severe bleeding disorders that mirror the degree of dysfunction or absence of vWF. There are several different types of vWD, including types 1, 2A, 2B, 2M, 2N, and 3. The evaluation for vWD includes tests for vWF antigen and activity, which are commercially available as a test panel. The patient in this vignette has both low vWF antigen level and activity. Her abnormal bleeding combined with her mother's bleeding history suggests a heritable vWD. The relatively mild bleeding phenotype suggests that she has type I disease, which manifests as a deficiency of functional vWF. Thus, her bleeding is most likely caused by a deficiency of a protein involved in platelet adhesion to collagen.

PREP Pearls

- The prothrombin time will be prolonged if there is a deficiency of coagulation factors in the extrinsic (factor VII) or common pathways (factors V, X, II), while the partial thromboplastin time will be prolonged if there is a deficiency of coagulation factors in the intrinsic (factors VIII, IX, XI, XII) or common pathways.
- Von Willebrand disease is diagnosed through testing von Willebrand factor antigen and activity.
- Von Willebrand disease is the most common bleeding disorder and results from decreased function or absence of von Willebrand factor.

American Board of Pediatrics Content Specification(s)/ Content Area

- Recognize the clinical findings associated with von Willebrand disease
- Plan the appropriate management of von Willebrand disease

Suggested Readings

Cooper S, Takemoto C. Von Willebrand disease. *Pediatr Rev.* 2014;35(3): 136-137.

Gray SH, Emans SJ. Abnormal vaginal bleeding in adolescents. *Pediatr Rev.* 2007;28(5):175-182.

Rodriguez V, Warad D. Pediatric coagulation disorders. *Pediatr Rev.* 2016; 37(7):279-291.

Item 89	Preferred Response: A

The injury sustained by the boy in the vignette is best described as a greenstick fracture of his left radius. A greenstick-type injury is the most common fracture pattern seen in children, accounting for up to half of all fractures in children younger than 12 years. The typical mechanism of a greenstick fracture is a fall onto an outstretched hand. The pliable nature of pediatric bones makes them less likely to break into comminuted fragments when an injury force is sustained. With greenstick injuries, the affected long bone bends before it breaks, with the thick and active periosteum remaining intact on 1 side. The bony cortex is typically disrupted on the convex side of the fracture, while it remains intact on the concave side. On plain radiographs, bones with greenstick injuries often resemble an immature, or "green" tree branch, which breaks in a similar manner when bent.

Angulation and rotation of greenstick fractures are common, but these fractures are never displaced, because the intact cortex maintains apposition at the fracture site and bone ends are not separated. To restore anatomic alignment, the fracture often must be completed. Inadequate reduction of the deformity or persistent bowing of the bone can result in abnormal bone growth and loss of function. Greenstick fractures with angulation of more than 15 degrees require closed reduction, immobilization in a splint, and orthopedic follow-up. The long-term prognosis for these fractures is generally good; complications are rare in children because of the remarkable capacity of their bones to rapidly heal and remodel.

The pattern of injury seen on this boy's radiographs is not consistent with that of a metaphyseal corner fracture. Metaphyseal corner fractures, also known as "bucket-handle" fractures, occur when a child's extremity is pulled or twisted forcibly, or when a child is shaken. They result from periosteal avulsion of bone and cartilage secondary to violent twisting forces or downward pull on an extremity. These fractures are frequently bilateral. Children with metaphyseal corner fractures are often asymptomatic. These fractures should always raise suspicion for child abuse.

The fracture sustained by the boy in the vignette does not involve the physeal region of the bone, and therefore cannot be classified as a Salter-Harris type I or a Salter-Harris type IV injury. Fractures that are described using the Salter-Harris classification system must involve the physis, or "growth plate" region of a bone. Growth plate injuries constitute nearly 20% of all pediatric skeletal injuries. The Salter-Harris system for classifying physeal injuries is based on the extent of involvement of the physis, epiphysis, and joint. Physeal damage due to trauma may disrupt bone growth and carries the potential for limb length discrepancies at the injured site in 1% to 10% of cases. A Salter-Harris type I fracture indicates bony injury across the physis only, with no fracture through the adjacent metaphyseal or epiphyseal regions. These types of fractures generally heal well with few complications. When suspected, Salter-Harris type I fractures should be immobilized, and children should be referred for orthopedic follow-up.

Salter-Harris type IV fractures cross through 3 regions of bone: the epiphysis, physis, and metaphysis. It is imperative for anatomic alignment of these fractures to be properly restored to avoid disturbances in growth and normal joint function. Orthopedic consultation should generally be obtained for children with Salter-Harris type IV injuries.

PREP Pearls

- Greenstick fractures with angulation of more than 15 degrees require closed reduction, immobilization in a splint, and orthopedic follow-up. To restore anatomic alignment, the fracture often must be completed.

- Greenstick-type injury is the most common fracture pattern seen in children, accounting for up to half of fractures in children younger than 12 years. The typical mechanism is a fall onto an outstretched hand.

- With greenstick injuries, the affected long bone bends before it breaks, with the thick and active periosteum remaining intact on 1 side.

American Board of Pediatrics Content Specification(s)/ Content Area

- Recognize the clinical and radiographic findings associated with a greenstick fracture

Suggested Readings

Chasm RM, Swencki SA. Pediatric orthopedic emergencies. *Emerg Med Clin North Am.* 2010;28:907-926.

Jones C, Wolf M, Herman M. Acute and chronic growth plate injuries. *Pediatr Rev.* 2017;38(3):129-138.

Thompson R, Kim-YJ, Lee L. Musculoskeletal trauma. In: Shaw K, Bachur R, eds. *Fleisher and Ludwig's Textbook of Pediatric Emergency Medicine.* 7th ed. Philadelphia, PA: Lippincott Williams & Wilkins; 2015;chap 119: 1195-1237.

Item 90   **Preferred Response: B**

For the boy in this vignette, the best next step is to evaluate a first-morning urine specimen for protein. A urine protein-creatinine ratio greater than 0.2 in a first-morning sample is abnormal. The boy's normal growth parameters, physical examination, and blood pressure place him at low risk for underlying chronic kidney disease. Fever is the most likely cause of his proteinuria noticed 6 months ago. However, a repeat urinalysis is important, because persistent asymptomatic proteinuria may be the only finding in the early stages of chronic kidney disease.

The American Academy of Pediatrics (AAP) does not recommend urinalysis as part of routine health visits. Screening urinalysis should be considered for children at high risk for chronic kidney disease. Prematurity, hydronephrosis, hypertension, diabetes mellitus, history of acute renal failure/glomerulonephritis or Henoch-Schöenlein purpura, children with sickle cell disease or trait, elevated body mass index (>97th percentile), and family history of renal disease or nephrolithiasis are risk factors for chronic kidney disease in children.

Urine dipstick testing for protein appears positive when urine albumin secretion is more than 300 mg/day. Normal urine albumin secretion is less than 30 mg/day. Persistent dipstick-positive proteinuria or a urine protein-creatinine ratio higher than 0.2 is considered abnormal, and indicates renal pathology requiring further evaluation by a pediatric nephrologist. Proteinuria can result from a range of causes, from benign to significant renal pathology. Differentiation between benign and pathologic causes is important because proteinuria may be the only indication of renal disease in some patients. However, detailed evaluation should be limited to patients suspected of having renal pathology of clinical significance.

Benign causes of proteinuria include orthostatic proteinuria and conditions associated with transient proteinuria such as fever, stress, exercise, cold, and abdominal surgery. A urine dipstick analysis should be repeated after the resolution of conditions associated with transient proteinuria. In adolescents, isolated asymptomatic proteinuria is most frequently associated with orthostatic proteinuria (OP), a benign condition with no adverse effect on renal function. Orthostatic proteinuria occurs when children are active and disappears when they are supine/asleep for at least 2 hours. To confirm OP, a first-morning urine sample is needed. It is important that the child collect the urine sample immediately upon waking, because even a small amount of activity can lead to proteinuria.

Twenty-four hour urine collection for proteinuria, though still performed in adults, is not routinely performed in children. Studies have shown that the urine protein-creatinine ratio in a first-morning urine sample is as sensitive as 24-hour urine collection for detecting pathologic proteinuria. According to the Kidney Disease Outcomes Quality Initiative guidelines from the National Kidney Foundation, it is not usually necessary to obtain timed/24-hour urine collections for evaluating proteinuria in adults or children.

Renal ultrasonography could be considered after proteinuria has been confirmed on a first-morning urinalysis. This imaging may show increased echogenicity of the parenchyma consistent with renal disease (nonspecific changes in acute or chronic renal failure) or congenital anomalies associated with chronic kidney disease. Congenital abnormalities noted on renal ultrasonography such as hydronephrosis (unilateral versus bilateral), increased echogenicity of renal parenchyma, abnormal renal size (small or enlarged), cysts, or bladder abnormalities determine the diagnosis and management in children with chronic kidney disease.

PREP Pearls

- A first-morning urine sample should be obtained to confirm proteinuria identified in a patient with no signs or symptoms of renal disease. Studies have shown that the urine protein-creatinine ratio in a first-morning urine sample is as sensitive as 24-hour urine collection for detecting pathologic proteinuria.
- Orthostatic proteinuria occurs when the patient is active (random urine sample) and disappears when the patient is supine/asleep for at least 2 hours (first-morning sample).
- Persistent dipstick-positive proteinuria or a urine protein-creatinine ratio higher than 0.2 is abnormal.

American Board of Pediatrics Content Specification(s)/ Content Area

- Plan the appropriate clinical and laboratory evaluation of proteinuria
- Identify the possible causes of proteinuria

Suggested Readings

Hains D, Spencer JD. Use of urinalysis and urine culture in screening; In: McInerny TK, Adam HM, Campbell DE, DeWitt TG, Foy JM, Kamat DM, eds. *American Academy of Pediatrics Textbook of Pediatric Care.* 2nd ed. Elk Grove Village, IL: American Academy of Pediatrics; 2017:225-228.

Hogg RJ, Portman RJ, Milliner D, Lemley KV, Eddy A, Ingelfinger J. Evaluation and management of proteinuria and nephrotic syndrome in children: recommendations from a pediatric nephrology panel established at the National Kidney Foundation conference on proteinuria, albuminuria, risk, assessment, detection, and elimination (PARADE). *Pediatrics.* 2000;105(6):1242-1249.

Sebestyen JF, Alon US. The teenager with asymptomatic proteinuria: think orthostatic first. *Clin Pediatr.* 2011;50:179-182.

Item 91   Preferred Response: A

An appropriately sized blood pressure cuff is imperative to obtaining an accurate blood pressure measurement (Item C91A). The cuff bladder width should be 40% of the arm circumference as measured at a point that is midway between the olecranon and the acromion. From a practical standpoint, this will result in a cuff that covers 80% to 100% of the circumference of the arm and two-thirds of the length (See Daniels SR. Consultation with the specialist. The diagnosis of hypertension in children: an update. *Pediatr Rev.* 1997;18(4):131-135).

When inflating the cuff, continue to inflate 20 mm Hg past the point where the radial pulse is no longer palpated. Deflate at a rate of 2 to 3 mm Hg per second while auscultating the brachial artery.

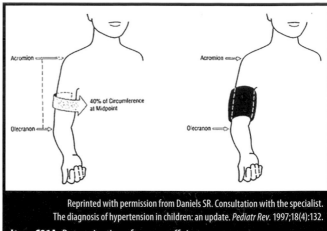

Reprinted with permission from Daniels SR. Consultation with the specialist. The diagnosis of hypertension in children: an update. *Pediatr Rev.* 1997;18(4):132.

Item C91A: Determination of proper cuff size.

All children aged 3 years and older should have a blood pressure measured during every visit to their provider. Children under 3 years of age should have their blood pressure measured if they have a predisposing condition (Item C91B). Pediatric blood pressure interpretation comes from percentiles based on the child's age, sex, and height. A systolic and diastolic blood pressure below the the 90th percentile for age, sex, and height is normal. Prehypertension (systolic or diastolic) is at or above the 90th percentile but below the 95th percentile. Stage I hypertension is at or above the 95th percentile but lower than the 99th percentile. Stage II hypertension is greater than the 99th percentile. These measurements should occur on at least 3 separate visits at least several weeks apart.

Item C91B. Comorbid Conditions Requiring a Blood Pressure Measurement in Children Younger Than Age 3 Years.

Past Medical History	Bone marrow transplant
	Low birthweight
	Malignancy
	Neonatal Intensive Care Unit stay
	Prematurity
	Recurrent urinary tract infection
	Solid organ transplant
Current Medical Conditions	Congenital heart disease
	Genitourinary abnormalities
	Hematuria
	Increased intracranial pressure
	Proteinuria
	Renal disease
	Systemic illness associated with hypertension
Medications	Taking medications known to increase blood pressure
Family History	Congenital kidney disease

Courtesy of S. Guralnick

PREP Pearls

- Blood pressure measurements should be interpreted based on percentiles for sex, age, and height.
- To obtain a meaningful blood pressure reading, the guidelines for proper measurement must be followed: use a cuff bladder width that is 40% of arm circumference; place cuff midway between olecranon and acromion; inflate the cuff to 20 mm Hg above the point at which the pulse is no longer palpated; and deflate the cuff no faster than 2 to 3 mm Hg per second.

American Board of Pediatrics Content Specification(s)/ Content Area

- Understand the appropriate technique, including appropriate cuff size, for measuring blood pressure
- Understand when to screen for an increased blood pressure and how to interpret the results

Suggested Readings

Brady TM. Hypertension. *Pediatr Rev.* 2012;33(12):541-542.

Daniels SR. Consultation with the specialist. The diagnosis of hypertension in children: an update. *Pediatr Rev.* 1997;18(4):131-135.

Item 92 **Preferred Response: D**

Cultural competence is the ability to effectively interact with people of different cultures and meet their social, cultural, and linguistic needs. The United States is rich with diversity and immigrant populations. For providers to deliver the best health care possible, it is important to build rapport and be aware of cultural norms and differences. If a provider cannot effectively communicate with the patient or their parent/guardian, important information may be miscommunicated.

This vignette describes a common scenario. The adolescent may have been born in the United States or learned English in school, whereas his mother may not have had the opportunity or desire to learn English. The use of a medical interpreter assists in providing respect to the parent, building rapport, assessing the mother's knowledge regarding eating disorders, and ensuring that information is not miscommunicated. In this situation, the adolescent may not want his mother to know what is being discussed and translate something different from what the provider described, which could have devastating results. It is best to use a neutral qualified interpreter and not the patient, other family members, or friends.

Being a culturally competent provider requires the consideration of immigration status, education level, socioeconomic status, beliefs, and family structure. Patient care can be affected if these factors are not considered. Medicine is its own culture, and the medical culture might not coincide with the cultural beliefs of a patient and their family. For example, perhaps a family matriarch makes medical decisions for a child and not the child's parents; or it may be culturally inappropriate to discuss a diagnosis with a child or adolescent; or a family might not believe in "Western medicine" and trust complementary or alternative medicine instead. If beliefs regarding medical diagnosis and treatment are not explored, it may hinder a provider's ability to negotiate with a family.

Providers may use the following steps to provide culturally competent care:

- Describe the medical condition and treatment in terms the patient and family can understand and in their native language. Use a medical interpreter (in person, by phone, or by video). When using an in-person medical interpreter, always maintain eye contact with the patient or family member.
- Prioritize treatment options.
- Determine the patient and parent priorities.
- Describe the plan of care.
- Determine if the patient and parents accept the plan of care.
- If the patient and parent are in conflict about the devised treatment plan, provide more information and renegotiate.

The adolescent in this vignette has bradycardia and orthostatic changes that are a manifestation of malnutrition caused by weight loss related to an eating disorder. He would benefit from laboratory studies to assess for electrolyte abnormalities and rule out other organic causes of weight loss such as inflammatory bowel disease and thyroid dysfunction. Increasing his daily caloric intake is crucial to improving his heart rate and weight. Eating disorders are mental health conditions with medical complications, so it would be helpful to involve a psychiatrist to address his thoughts regarding food and his body image. However, the best next step for this patient is the use of an interpreter to discuss the medical complications of an eating disorder.

If his mother does not understand the severity of his medical condition because of a language barrier and miscommunication, it may potentially delay the appropriate treatment and have devastating results.

PREP Pearls

- Identify cultural beliefs of the patient and their family that may influence acceptance of treatment plans.
- Never use the patient as the medical interpreter.
- Use qualified trained medical interpreters to obtain history and discuss medical diagnoses and treatment plans.

American Board of Pediatrics Content Specification(s)/ Content Area

- Understand the various cultural issues that could affect medical care

Suggested Readings

Kodjo C. Cultural competence in clinician communication. *Pediatr Rev.* 2009;30(2):57-63.

Lewis C. Immigrant adolescents and young adults. In: Neinstein LS, Katzman DK, Callahan ST, Gordon CM, Joffe A, Rickert VI, eds. *Neinsteins's Adolescent and Young Adult Health Care: a Practical Guide.* 6th ed. Philadelphia, PA: Wolters Kluwer; 2016:652-656.

The infant in the vignette had an episode in which he started choking, changed color, and appeared to stop breathing. The episode resolved, and the infant otherwise does not have any risk factors for sudden death. The most likely explanation for the event is a brief resolved unexplained event (BRUE), which was previously referred to as "apparent life-threatening event" (ALTE).

The term BRUE refers to an episode in which an infant younger than 1 year of age exhibits 1 or more of the following: (1) cyanosis or pallor; (2) apnea, hypopnea, or irregular breathing; (3) hypertonia or hypotonia; and (4) altered mental status. In 2016, the American Academy of Pediatrics published BRUE clinical practice guidelines, which provided diagnosis and management recommendations based on the likelihood of an underlying disorder or subsequent events. The guidelines also recommended replacing the term ALTE with BRUE, to decrease the subjectivity in taking the history, remove the implication of a life-threatening event, and emphasize that the event has resolved.

The diagnosis of BRUE requires that there be no known cause of the event. There are many causes for such events that would not qualify as BRUE, such as acquired or congenital disorders of the airway, cardiovascular disease, gastroesophageal reflux disease, central nervous system pathology, nonaccidental trauma, intercurrent illness, and metabolic conditions (Item C93A). Intercurrent illness may be heralded by viral symptoms such as fever, congestion, or persistent respiratory signs or symptoms. Abnormal physical findings at the time of assessment may indicate an underlying disorder. A thorough history should be taken to delineate the details of the event, and to screen for factors that would indicate an underlying disorder.

Several characteristics differentiate infants' risks of having a recurrent BRUE event. Infants younger than 2 months, those born at less than 32 weeks' gestational age with corrected gestational age less than 45 weeks, and those who had a previous event are considered to be at higher risk. Patient factors associated with a lower risk of recurrent BRUE include age greater than 60 days, duration of the event less than 1 minute, no history of cardiopulmonary resuscitation (CPR) by a trained medical provider during the event, and no concerning historical or physical examination features. Infants classified as being at higher risk and those for whom the diagnosis of BRUE is excluded are considered outside the scope of the guidelines.

Management recommendations for patients at lower risk for BRUE are presented in 4 categories:
- "should" provide education for caregivers and resources for CPR training to caregivers.
- "may" include pertussis testing, 12-lead electrocardiography, and brief monitoring with continuous pulse oximetry and serial observations.
- "should not" obtain laboratory testing; perform radiography, electroencephalography, or echocardiography; initiate home cardiorespiratory monitoring; prescribe medications.
- "need not" obtain viral respiratory testing, urinalysis, blood glucose, serum bicarbonate, or serum lactate testing, or neuroimaging; or admit to hospital strictly for cardiorespiratory monitoring (Item C93B).

Anomalous left coronary artery can manifest at any age, particularly in infancy, and can cause congestive heart failure, arrhythmia, and sudden death. This diagnosis is not likely in this vignette, because the historical symptoms and physical examination findings of coronary insufficiency or congestive heart failure are not present.

The 6-second periods of apnea that the boy exhibits are consistent with periodic breathing, a normal newborn respiratory pattern that is not associated with choking, gagging, or color change.

Although seizure is a possible explanation for the event, it is less likely than BRUE, given the absence of predisposing conditions, the rapid return to normal state, and the boy's otherwise low-risk stratification.

PREP Pearls

- Patients experiencing a brief resolved unexplained event–like event with a concerning history or physical examination findings may fall outside of the definition and scope of the clinical guideline recommendations for brief resolved unexplained event.

- Patients presenting after a brief resolved unexplained event who meet lower-risk criteria do not require electroencephalography, neuroimaging, or laboratory testing.

- The term "brief resolved unexplained event" has replaced "apparent life threatening event." This change was implemented to decrease the subjectivity in event history taking, remove the implication that the event was life-threatening, and emphasize that the events are fully resolved.

American Board of Pediatrics Content Specification(s)/Content Area

- Recognize the clinical findings of an brief resolved unexplained event (BRUE), and manage appropriately
- Identify risk factors associated with sudden infant death syndrome
- Counsel parents regarding prevention of sudden infant death syndrome

Suggested Readings

Bommel N, Kannarkatt S. Case 5: BRUE in an infant found to have feeding difficulties. *Pediatr Rev.* 2017;38:535.

Tieder JS, Bonkowsky JL, Etzel RA, et al; Subcommittee on Apparent Life Threatening Events. Brief resolved unexplained events (formerly apparent life-threatening events) and evaluation of lower-risk infants. *Pediatrics* 2016;137(5). pii: e20160591.

Zwemer E, Claudius I, Tieder J. Update on the evaluation and management of brief resolved unexplained events (previously apparent life-threatening events). *Rev Recent Clin Trials.* 2017;12(4):233-239.

Item C93A. BRUE Definition and Factors for Inclusion and Exclusion.

	Includes	Excludes
Brief	Duration <1 min; typically 20–30 s	Duration ≥1 min
Resolved	Patient returned to his or her baseline state of health after the event	At the time of medical evaluation:
	Normal vital signs	Fever or recent fever
	Normal appearance	Tachypnea, bradypnea, apnea
		Tachycardia or bradycardia
		Hypotension, hypertension, or hemodynamic instability
		Mental status changes, somnolence, lethargy
		Hypotonia or hypertonia
		Vomiting
		Bruising, petechiae, or other signs of injury/trauma
		Abnormal weight, growth, or head circumference
		Noisy breathing (stridor, sturgor, wheezing)
		Repeat event(s)
Unexplained	Not explained by an identifiable medical condition	Event consistent with GER, swallow dysfunction, nasal congestion, etc
		History or physical examination concerning for child abuse, congenital airway abnormality, etc
Event Characterization		
Cyanosis or pallor	Central cyanosis: blue or purple coloration of face, gums, trunk	Acrocyanosis or perioral cyanosis
	Central pallor: pale coloration of face or trunk	Rubor
Absent, decreased, or irregular breathing	Central apnea	Periodic breathing of the newborn
	Obstructive apnea	Breath-holding spell
	Mixed obstructive apnea	
Marked change in tone (hyper- or hypotonia)	Hypertonia	Hypertonia associated with crying, choking, or gagging due to GER or feeding problems
	Hypotonia	Tone changes associated with breath-holding spell
		Tonic eye deviation or nystagmus
		Tonic-clonic seizure activity
		Infantile spasms
Altered responsiveness	Loss of consciousness	Loss of consciousness associated with breath-holding spell
	Mental status change	
	Lethargy	
	Somnolence	
	Postictal phase	

Abbreviations: BRUE, brief resolved unexplained event; GER, gastroesophageal reflux.

Reprinted with permission from Tieder, JS, Bonkowsky, JL, Etzel, RA, et al. Brief Resolved Unexplained Events (Formerly Apparent Life-Threatening Events) and Evaluation of Lower-Risk Infants. *Pediatrics* 2016;137, page e3.

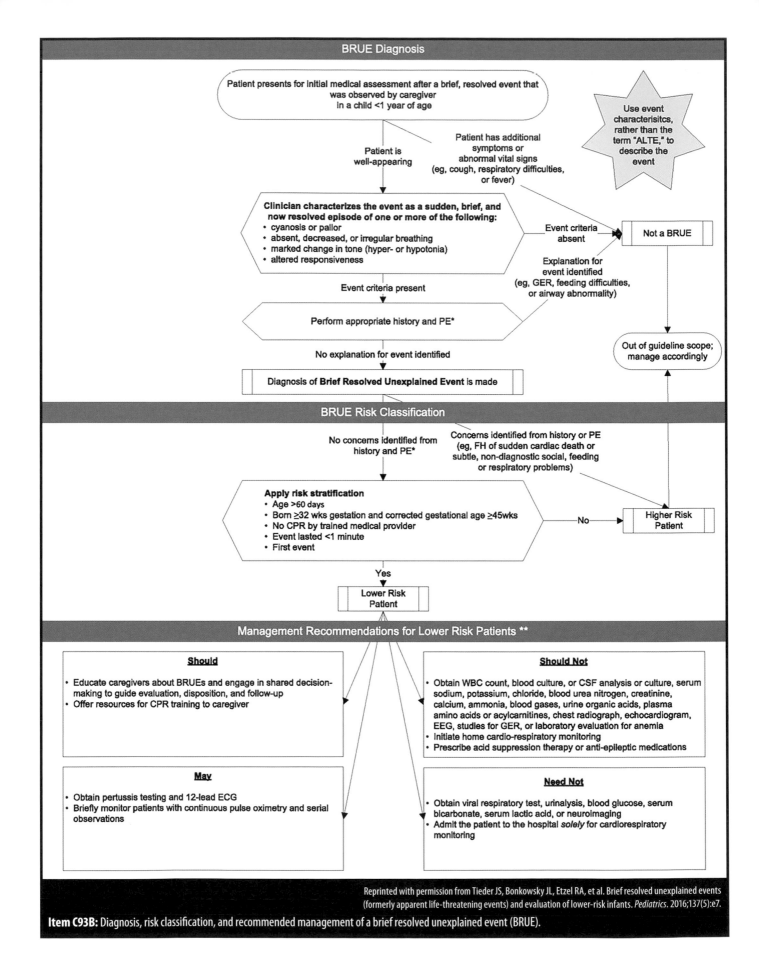

BRUE Diagnosis

Patient presents for initial medical assessment after a brief, resolved event that was observed by caregiver in a child <1 year of age

Use event characterisitcs, rather than the term "ALTE," to describe the event

Patient is well-appearing

Patient has additional symptoms or abnormal vital signs (eg, cough, respiratory difficulties, or fever)

Clinician characterizes the event as a sudden, brief, and now resolved episode of one or more of the following:
- cyanosis or pallor
- absent, decreased, or irregular breathing
- marked change in tone (hyper- or hypotonia)
- altered responsiveness

Event criteria absent → Not a BRUE

Explanation for event identified (eg, GER, feeding difficulties, or airway abnormality)

Event criteria present

Perform appropriate history and PE*

No explanation for event identified

Diagnosis of **Brief Resolved Unexplained Event** is made

Out of guideline scope; manage accordingly

BRUE Risk Classification

No concerns identified from history and PE*

Concerns identified from history or PE (eg, FH of sudden cardiac death or subtle, non-diagnostic social, feeding or respiratory problems)

Apply risk stratification
- Age >60 days
- Born ≥32 wks gestation and corrected gestational age ≥45wks
- No CPR by trained medical provider
- Event lasted <1 minute
- First event

No → Higher Risk Patient

Yes

Lower Risk Patient

Management Recommendations for Lower Risk Patients **

Should
- Educate caregivers about BRUEs and engage in shared decision-making to guide evaluation, disposition, and follow-up
- Offer resources for CPR training to caregiver

Should Not
- Obtain WBC count, blood culture, or CSF analysis or culture, serum sodium, potassium, chloride, blood urea nitrogen, creatinine, calcium, ammonia, blood gases, urine organic acids, plasma amino acids or acylcarnitines, chest radiograph, echocardiogram, EEG, studies for GER, or laboratory evaluation for anemia
- Initiate home cardio-respiratory monitoring
- Prescribe acid suppression therapy or anti-epileptic medications

May
- Obtain pertussis testing and 12-lead ECG
- Briefly monitor patients with continuous pulse oximetry and serial observations

Need Not
- Obtain viral respiratory test, urinalysis, blood glucose, serum bicarbonate, serum lactic acid, or neuroimaging
- Admit the patient to the hospital *solely* for cardiorespiratory monitoring

Reprinted with permission from Tieder JS, Bonkowsky JL, Etzel RA, et al. Brief resolved unexplained events (formerly apparent life-threatening events) and evaluation of lower-risk infants. *Pediatrics.* 2016;137(5):e7.

Item C93B: Diagnosis, risk classification, and recommended management of a brief resolved unexplained event (BRUE).

Item 94 — Preferred Response: B

The boy in this vignette has a corneal abrasion, for which the most appropriate treatment is antibiotic ophthalmic drops. Anesthetic or corticosteroid ophthalmic drops and eye patching are contraindicated.

Corneal abrasions typically result from eye trauma, sometimes relatively minor trauma such as the sand that was thrown into this boy's eye. Corneal abrasions can also be caused by inappropriately prolonged contact lens use. Because the cornea is highly innervated, corneal abrasions can be quite painful. Patients may experience tearing, photophobia, or a foreign body sensation. It may feel difficult for them to open the affected eye. Corneal abrasion in young infants may present with inconsolable crying or fussiness.

Conjunctival injection and tearing may be present. If a corneal abrasion is suspected, fluorescein staining should be performed to visualize corneal epithelial defects. If a retained foreign body is identified, it should be removed with saline irrigation or a cotton swab. Patients with corneal abrasions should not have significant vision loss, hyphema, corneal opacity, or an irregular, dilated, or fixed pupil; these findings warrant urgent ophthalmologic evaluation.

Treatment for corneal abrasions includes pain control and infection prevention. Pain control is usually achieved with oral analgesics, although a several-day course of topical nonsteroidal anti-inflammatory ophthalmic drops can be used in patients without other ocular pathology. Ophthalmic antibiotic drops or ointments are indicated for infection prevention. Antipseudomonal coverage is indicated for corneal abrasions associated with prolonged contact lens use.

Ophthalmic anesthetic drops should not be prescribed because they can delay healing, mask worsening symptoms, and can be toxic to the corneal epithelium with repeated administration. Ophthalmic corticosteroid drops should not be used because they may delay healing and increase susceptibility to infection. Although patching had, in the past, been recommended in the treatment of corneal abrasions, a Cochrane meta-analysis showed that patching does not improve pain control and may prolong healing time.

Follow-up may not be necessary for patients with uncomplicated small abrasions if their symptoms resolve as expected, within 24 to 48 hours. Patients with larger abrasions, abrasions associated with contact lens use, or severe or nonresolving pain should be seen for follow-up within 2 to 4 days.

PREP Pearls

- Anesthetic or corticosteroid ophthalmic drops or eye patching are contraindicated in the management of corneal abrasions.
- Corneal abrasions should be treated with topical antibiotics and either oral analgesics or a short course of topical nonsteroidal anti-inflammatory drugs.
- If a corneal abrasion is suspected, fluorescein staining should be performed to visualize corneal epithelial defects.
- Symptoms of corneal abrasion include eye pain, foreign body sensation, tearing, photophobia, and eye redness.

American Board of Pediatrics Content Specification(s)/Content Area

- Plan the appropriate initial and follow-up management of a corneal abrasion
- Plan the appropriate clinical evaluation of a suspected foreign body in the eye
- Recognize the clinical findings associated with corneal abrasion in patients of various ages

Suggested Readings

Aguilera ZP, Chen PL. Eye pain in children. *Pediatr Rev.* 2016;37(10):418-425.

Browner EA. Corneal abrasions. *Pediatr Rev.* 2012;33(6):285-286.

Lim CH, Turner A, Lim BX. Patching for corneal abrasion. *Cochrane Database Syst Rev.* 2016;7:CD004764.

Wipperman JL, Dorsch JN. Evaluation and management of corneal abrasions. *Am Fam Physician.* 2013;87(2):114-120.

Item 95 — Preferred Response: C

Mumps virus is the most likely cause of orchitis in the adolescent boy described in the vignette. He developed acute testicular pain and swelling during the course of an upper respiratory tract illness, with bilateral submaxillary swelling. His college roommates have developed a similar illness. This raises concern for an outbreak of mumps infection. Of the various viral pathogens that can cause parotid gland inflammation, such as parainfluenza virus, Epstein-Barr virus, cytomegalovirus, and human immunodeficiency virus, only the mumps virus has the potential for epidemic spread. The boy's clinical presentation is not consistent with a sexually transmitted disease (such as *Neisseria gonorrheae or Chlamydia trachomatis* infection) or an invasive bacterial infection (such as *Haemophilus influenzae* type b). Serious infections due to *H influenzae* type b almost exclusively occur in unvaccinated children younger than 4 years of age.

Mumps is an acute, communicable, vaccine-preventable systemic illness that commonly affects children. It is caused by the mumps virus, an enveloped, negative-sense RNA virus that belongs to the Paramyxoviridae family. Mumps only affects humans. Transmission occurs via direct contact with respiratory tract secretions, droplets, or contaminated fomites. The incubation period is usually 15 to 24 days, with a median of 19 days. Patients are contagious from 1 to 2 days before the onset of parotid swelling to several days thereafter.

During the prodromal period of mumps infection, a mild, nonspecific illness may occur with symptoms of low-grade fever, headache, and malaise. Development of unilateral or bilateral salivary gland swelling, typically parotitis, occurs in 95% of patients with symptomatic disease. The parotid gland swelling is painful, progressive over a few days, and can last up to 1 week. Mumps infection may be asymptomatic in approximately one-third of cases. Complications of mumps include orchitis and meningitis. Orchitis is reported in 15% to 30% of postpubertal men with mumps infection; it typically develops 4 to 8 days after the onset of parotitis. Most cases of orchitis have associated epididymitis. Cerebrospinal fluid pleocytosis may be noted in approximately 50% of cases, but 90% of patients remain asymptomatic. Before the introduction of the measles-mumps-rubella (MMR) vaccine, aseptic meningitis due to the mumps virus was a frequent cause of viral meningitis in high-income countries. Unusual complications include hearing loss, myocarditis, and nephritis.

Mumps is typically a self-limited illness. Most patients recover completely by 2 weeks after symptom onset. Long-term sequelae are rare. If the diagnosis of mumps is suspected, consultation with an infectious disease specialist or state or local health department is recommended for further diagnostic evaluation. The diagnosis is confirmed by virus isolation and detection of MuV nucleic acid by reverse-transcriptase polymerase chain reaction in buccal swab, saliva, or cerebrospinal fluid specimens or serology (presence of mumps-specific immunoglobulin M antibody).

In the United States, a 2-dose age-appropriate MMR vaccine series is currently recommended as part of a routine childhood immunization series. Effectiveness is approximately 88% (range, 66%–95%). By 2005, routine implementation of the 2-dose MMR vaccine series had resulted in a 99% reduction in reported cases of mumps in the United States. However, recent outbreaks of mumps among adolescents and young adults in highly immunized populations in resource-rich countries, including the United States, have led to public health concern and renewed strategies for control. Several mumps outbreaks have occurred on college campuses involving students with high rates of 2-dose MMR vaccine coverage (>90%). In 1 outbreak, students who reported receipt of a 2nd dose of MMR vaccine at 13 years of age or older were at increased risk for mumps infection compared to those who received a third immunization. Factors contributing to the resurgence of mumps may include waning vaccine-induced immunity among adolescents and young adults and an increased pool of susceptible individuals in overcrowded settings, such as college campuses.

In the setting of large mumps outbreaks, the Centers for Disease Control and Prevention has recommended consideration of a third dose of MMR vaccine. During a recent outbreak among vaccinated students at a major American university, public health investigators implemented a 3rd dose of MMR vaccine for outbreak control; students who received the 3rd dose showed a 60% to 78% reduction in mumps risk compared with students who had received only 2 doses.

PREP Pearls

- Complications of mumps include orchitis and meningitis
- Development of unilateral or bilateral salivary gland swelling, typically parotitis, is a characteristic feature of mumps.
- In the setting of large mumps outbreaks, the Centers for Disease Control and Prevention has recommended consideration of a third dose of MMR vaccine.

American Board of Pediatrics Content Specification(s)/ Content Area

- Recognize the clinical features and complications associated with mumps

Suggested Readings

American Academy of Pediatrics. Mumps. In: Kimberlin DW, Brady MT, Jackson MA, Long SS, eds. *Red Book: 2018 Report of the Committee on Infectious Diseases*. 31st ed. Itasca, IL: American Academy of Pediatrics; 2018:567-573.

Cardemil CV, Dahl RM, James L, et al. Effectiveness of a third dose of MMR vaccine for mumps outbreak control. *N Engl J Med*. 2017;377(10):947-956.

Hviid A, Rubin S, Mühlemann K. Mumps. *Lancet*. 2008;371(9616):932-944.

Immediately after any adverse event resulting in harm to a patient, counseling services should be made available to the providers involved. It is increasingly recognized that providers, including trainees, involved in such an event become "second victims." They are haunted by mistakes, real or perceived. Debriefing sessions and counseling should be offered to those involved to prevent unhealthy coping mechanisms.

In 2008, the National Academy of Medicine (formerly Institute of Medicine) published a landmark report on medical errors in health care in the United States. The report estimated that 44,000 patients die annually because of preventable errors. In response, health care systems throughout the country began to examine their practices with a focus on systems changes that could decrease the risk of medical errors. Providers have changed how and when they disclose adverse events. Historically, these events were not uniformly revealed to patients and their families. Currently, full disclosure of medical errors has become the standard of practice in the United States. Disclosure should be timely and include all involved parties. Providers should consider offering an apology without placing blame. In addition, there should be a systematic evaluation of the medical error to understand the contributing factors and identify means of prevention for the future.

In this vignette, changing the TPN ordering guidelines may be of benefit to the system as a whole, but will not help the medical team. In the absence of negligence, disciplinary action is not warranted. In this case, the TPN was ordered correctly. Therefore, education on the components of TPN would not be helpful.

PREP Pearls

- Counseling services should be offered to health-care providers after an adverse event to ensure healthy coping.
- Debriefing sessions may offer a safe space in which members of the medical team can begin to process their feelings after an adverse event.
- Providers involved in an adverse event resulting in harm to a patient may become second victims.

American Board of Pediatrics Content Specification(s)/ Content Area

- Use appropriate methods of support for physicians and other health-care providers after an error producing medical harm occurs
- Use appropriate means to disclose medical errors to patients
- Apply appropriate methods of support for patients and their families after an error producing medical harm occurs

Suggested Readings

Leonard MS. Patient safety and quality improvement: medical errors and adverse events. *Pediatr Rev*. 2010;31:151.

McDonnell WM, Neuspiel DR; for the Committee on Medical Liability and Risk Management and Council on Quality Improvement and Patient Safety. Disclosure of adverse events in pediatrics. *Pediatrics*. 2016;138(6):1-6.

Pereira-Argenziano L, Levy FH. Patient safety and quality improvement: terminology. *Pediatr Rev*. 2015;36:403.

The infant in this vignette is well and has a peripheral cyanosis best defined as acrocyanosis. The mother should be provided with an explanation of the pathophysiology and reassurance that he is well. Acrocyanosis can be exacerbated by elevated blood hemoglobin level and cold exposure.

In a well infant or child with only peripheral cyanosis, there is no indication for admission to the hospital or monitoring. Normal oxygen saturation and normal cardiovascular and pulmonary examination findings are reassuring for a lack of underlying cardiorespiratory pathology in a previously well child. The most common causes of cyanosis in the well child are acrocyanosis, cold exposure, and Raynaud phenomenon.

Cyanosis alone, without findings to suggest organ system damage or nonaccidental trauma, is not consistent with child abuse. If an infant with cyanosis is irritable or has unusual bruises, then there would potentially be concern for abuse.

There is nothing in the history or examination findings that suggests underlying cardiac or pulmonary disease that would necessitate a radiograph or electrocardiogram. The lack of central cyanosis suggests good central perfusion and adequate cardiac function. Extrapulmonary causes of cyanosis include congenital heart disease. If the infant in this vignette had a low peripheral oxygen saturation, heart murmur, or single S_2, an electrocardiogram would be appropriate as the first line of evaluation.

Even if the child is not entirely well appearing, the presence of normal oxygen saturation is reassuring for minimal or no pathology. Other causes of cyanosis in this group include diffuse pigmentary lesions, extensive tattoos, or clothing dye that has transferred to the skin. If the child has a normal oxygen saturation but appears ill, consideration must be given for septic shock, cardiogenic shock, or critical polycythemia. In children with decreased peripheral oxygen saturation, the primary cause of cyanosis is critical cardiorespiratory illness. A decision algorithm for cyanosis in children is shown in Item C97.

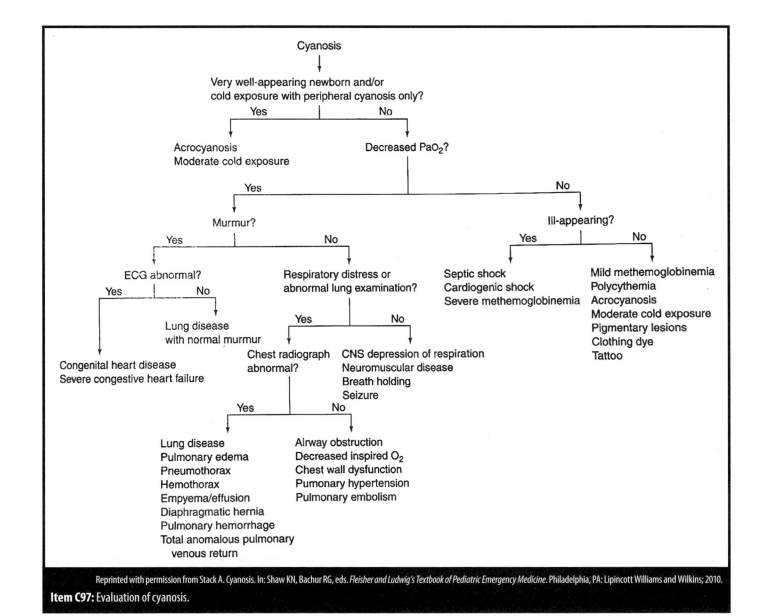

Reprinted with permission from Stack A. Cyanosis. In: Shaw KN, Bachur RG, eds. *Fleisher and Ludwig's Textbook of Pediatric Emergency Medicine.* Philadelphia, PA: Lipincott Williams and Wilkins; 2010.

Item C97: Evaluation of cyanosis.

American Board of Pediatrics Content Specification(s)/ Content Area

- Identify the common extrapulmonary causes of cyanosis
- Plan the appropriate clinical and laboratory evaluation of cyanosis

Suggested Readings

Baptist EC, Kwak J. Visual diagnosis: a 7-month-old girl with cyanotic spells. *Pediatr Rev.* 2015;36(10):e35-e38.

Fleck DE, Hoeltzel MF. Hand and food color change: diagnosis and management. *Pediatr Rev.* 2017;38(11):511-519.

Tingelstad J. Consultation with the specialist: nonrespiratory cyanosis. *Pediatr Rev.* 1999;20(10):350-352.

Item 98	Preferred Response: C

The patient in this vignette has erythema, scaling, and hypopigmentation of the alar creases, findings typical of seborrheic dermatitis in adolescents and young adults. Atopic dermatitis may involve the face but lesions usually are concentrated around the eyes and mouth with sparing of the perinasal region. The absence of a history of atopic dermatitis also argues against this diagnosis. Periorificial dermatitis may involve the perinasal area but rarely is limited to this region. In addition, lesions are erythematous papules or pustules, often with background erythema (Item C98). Although the patient's lesions are scaling, there is no border elevation or central clearing as would be expected in tinea corporis (also called tinea faciei when located on the face).

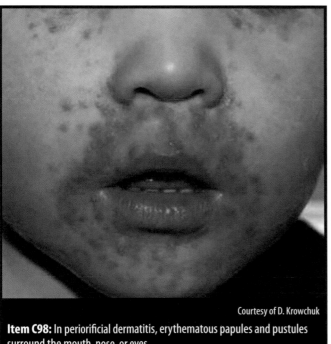

Courtesy of D. Krowchuk

Item C98: In periorificial dermatitis, erythematous papules and pustules surround the mouth, nose, or eyes.

Seborrheic dermatitis is a chronic and relapsing inflammatory disorder that affects areas in which sebaceous glands are concentrated. It is especially common in adolescents and young adults in whom sebaceous gland activity is greatest. Although the cause is not fully understood, it may be the result of an inflammatory response to the yeasts of the genus *Malassezia*. Typical findings are scaling of the scalp (ie, dandruff) or scaling and erythema of the eyebrows, eyelids, glabella, alar or retroauricular creases, beard or sideburn areas, or ear canals.

For affected areas of the skin, treatment is with a low-potency topical corticosteroid (eg, hydrocortisone 1% or 2.5%) or an agent active against yeast (eg, clotrimazole, miconazole nitrate, or ketoconazole) applied twice daily as needed. Scalp involvement is treated with an antiseborrheic shampoo containing pyrithione zinc, selenium sulfide, or ketoconazole. If facial skin is also involved, patients may be advised to allow some of the shampoo to contact affected areas and then rinse. If signs of scalp inflammation are present (eg, erythema or erosions), a topical corticosteroid solution (eg, fluocinolone acetonide 0.1%) may be applied at bedtime if needed.

American Board of Pediatrics Content Specification(s)/ Content Area

- Recognize the clinical findings associated with seborrheic dermatitis, and manage appropriately

Suggested Readings

American Academy of Pediatrics Section on Dermatology. Seborrheic dermatitis. In: Mancini AJ, Krowchuk DP, eds. *Pediatric Dermatology: A Quick Reference Guide.* 3rd ed. Elk Grove Village, IL: American Academy of Pediatrics; 2016:341-346.

Okokon EO, Verbeek JH, Ruotsalainen JH, Ojo OA, Bakhoya VN. Topical antifungals for seborrheic dermatitis. *Cochrane Database Syst Rev.* 2015;5:CD008138.

Item 99	Preferred Response: B

The boy in this vignette has trisomy 21, an enlarged thyroid, and a relatively low heart rate of 62 beats/min. The most likely cause of his examination findings is Hashimoto thyroiditis with hypothyroidism. Hashimoto thyroiditis, autoimmune thyroid disease, is the most common cause of thyroid enlargement in children and occurs with increased frequency in children with trisomy 21. His relatively low heart rate is suggestive of associated hypothyroidism.

Graves disease is another cause of thyroid enlargement and occurs with increased frequency in trisomy 21. However, hyperthyroidism is seen in Graves disease. The boy in this vignette shows no evidence of hyperthyroidism. Multinodular goiter and simple colloid goiter are also potential etiologies of thyroid enlargement but are much more rare causes in this age group and in individuals with trisomy 21.

Hashimoto thyroiditis, including thyroid enlargement, can occur with normal thyroid function, especially early in the disease process, or with hypothyroidism. Rarely, a transient hyperthyroid phase is detected; this phase is caused by the release of stored thyroid hormone with the initial autoimmune insult to the gland. This hyperthyroid phase is called hashitoxicosis. Thyroid peroxidase and thyroglobulin antibodies are markers of Hashimoto thyroiditis and can aid in the diagnosis.

Thyroid ultrasonography is not indicated in the evaluation of thyroid enlargement or Hashimoto thyroiditis unless there is asymmetry of the thyroid gland, a palpable nodule, or cervical lymphadenopathy. The American Academy of Pediatrics Section on Endocrinology added the following recommendation to the Choosing Wisely guidelines in 2017: "Avoid routinely ordering thyroid ultrasounds in children who have simple goiters or autoimmune thyroiditis." Thyroid ultrasonography often reveals incidental nodules that require further evaluation for thyroid cancer. Although there is an increased risk of thyroid cancer in the setting of Hashimoto thyroiditis, the overall incidence remains very low. An incidental finding of a thyroid nodule can cause unnecessary anxiety and medical costs. There is no evidence that early detection of thyroid cancer in a nodule before it becomes palpable improves outcomes.

As with the boy in this vignette, Hashimoto thyroiditis, especially when the associated hypothyroidism is mild, is often asymptomatic. Symptoms of acquired hypothyroidism may include fatigue, constipation, dry skin, brittle hair, and in female individuals, menstrual irregularities.

Children with trisomy 21 are at increased risk for both congenital hypothyroidism and acquired autoimmune hypothyroidism (Hashimoto thyroiditis). Therefore, thyroid screening tests are recommended at birth, 6 months, 12 months, and annually thereafter.

PREP Pearls

- Children with trisomy 21 are at increased risk for congenital hypothyroidism and acquired autoimmune thyroid disease. Thyroid screening tests are recommended at birth, 6 months, 12 months, and annually thereafter.
- Hashimoto thyroiditis, autoimmune thyroid disease, is the most common cause of thyroid enlargement in children.
- Thyroid ultrasonography is not routinely recommended in the evaluation of Hashimoto thyroiditis or simple goiter.

American Board of Pediatrics Content Specification(s)/ Content Area

- Understand the natural history of Hashimoto thyroiditis

Suggested Readings

American Academy of Pediatrics. Section on Endocrinology. Five things physicians and patients should question. http://www.choosingwisely.org.

Bull MJ; Committee on Genetics. Health supervision for children with Down syndrome. *Pediatrics*. 2011;128(2):393-406.

Diaz A, Lipman Diaz EG. Hypothyroidism. *Pediatr Rev*. 2014;35(8):336-347.

Item 100 **Preferred Response: B**

Hepatic dysfunction beginning within the first week after birth, after the introduction of breast milk or cow milk–based formula is highly suggestive of galactosemia. Immediate implementation of a lactose-restricted diet is imperative within the first 10 days after birth to abate the symptoms and reduce the risk of long-term complications. Classic galactosemia presents with feeding problems, failure to thrive, progressive hepatic dysfunction, bleeding, cataracts, and *Escherichia coli* sepsis in neonates after a lactose-containing diet is introduced. If a lactose-restricted diet is not provided rapidly, liver failure/cirrhosis, sepsis, and death can occur. Even with adequate treatment, children are at risk for speech apraxia, developmental delays, motor function abnormalities, and premature ovarian insufficiency. Affected children should also receive supplemental calcium, vitamin D, and vitamin K to prevent reduced bone mineralization and bleeding. Routine monitoring performed by a geneticist should include measurement of erythrocyte galactose-1-phosphate and urinary galactitol levels, and evaluation for cataracts, speech and developmental delays, osteopenia, and premature ovarian insufficiency.

Galactosemia is an autosomal recessive inborn error of metabolism diagnosed via detection of elevated erythrocyte galactose-1-phosphate concentration, reduced erythrocyte galactose-1-phosphate uridylyltransferase (GALT) enzyme activity, and biallelic gene mutations in the *GALT* gene. Nearly 100% of infants with classic galactosemia are detected in newborn screening programs.

A gluten-free diet is indicated for treatment of celiac disease. Celiac disease is an autoimmune disorder that occurs in children and adults who are genetically predisposed to small intestinal villus damage when gluten-containing foods are ingested. This leads to bloating, abdominal pain, nausea/vomiting, and malabsorption of nutrients. Gluten is found in wheat, rye, and barley.

A phenylalanine-free diet is indicated for children and adults with phenylketonuria, also known as phenylalanine hydroxylase (PAH) deficiency. A deficiency in PAH leads to severe intellectual disability, musty odor, reduced skin and hair pigmentation, epilepsy, and Parkinson-like features in untreated individuals. If a low-protein diet and a Phe-free medical formula are introduced in early infancy, the child will grow up with normal intellectual function or only mild cognitive deficits. No physical examination findings or laboratory abnormalities (including hepatic dysfunction) are present in early infancy. Newborn screening routinely includes screening for PAH deficiency, because it is related to a form of intellectual disability that is highly preventable with effective treatment when introduced early in life.

A protein-restricted diet is recommended for a number of inborn errors of metabolism, including phenylketonuria, organic acidurias, and urea cycle disorders. Galactosemia does not warrant a protein-restricted diet.

PREP Pearls

- Classic galactosemia presents with feeding problems, failure to thrive, progressive hepatic dysfunction, bleeding, cataracts, and *Escherichia coli* sepsis in infants once a lactose-containing diet is introduced. If a lactose-restricted diet is not provided rapidly, liver failure/cirrhosis, sepsis, and death can occur.
- Hepatic dysfunction beginning within the first week after birth, after the introduction of breast milk or cow milk–based formula, is highly suggestive of galactosemia. Immediate implementation of a lactose-restricted diet is imperative within the first 10 days after birth to abate the symptoms and reduce the risk of long-term complications.
- Newborn screening includes evaluation for galactosemia, so that rapid treatment may be initiated.

American Board of Pediatrics Content Specification(s)/Content Area

- Plan the appropriate immediate and long-term management of galactosemia, while considering the long-term prognosis
- Recognize the clinical features associated with galactosemia
- Recognize the laboratory features associated with galactosemia

Suggested Readings

Berry GT. Classic galactosemia and clinical variant galactosemia. *GeneReviews.* https://www.ncbi.nlm.nih.gov/books/NBK1518/.

Grady NEG, Millard D. Congenital galactosemia. *Neoreviews.* 2017;18(4):e228-e233.

Palermo L, Geberhiwot T, MacDonald A, Limback E, Hall SK, Romani C. Cognitive outcomes in early-treated adults with phenylketonuria (PKU): a comprehensive picture across domains. *Neuropsychology.* 2017;31(3):255-267.

Welling L, Bernstein LE, Berry GT; Galactosemia Network (GalNet). International clinical guideline for the management of classical galactosemia: diagnosis, treatment, and follow-up. *J Inherit Metab Dis.* 2017;40(2):171-176.

Item 101   Preferred Response: B

The 12-month-old girl in this vignette is meeting developmental milestones for gross and fine motor skills. Playing peek-a-boo and stranger anxiety are appropriate cognitive milestones at this age as well. However, pointing at objects and identifying familiar caregivers by a name (eg, "dada" or "mama") are skills that should be present by 12 months. Such deficits may represent a delay in language development.

Development builds on skills previously attained. For example, in gross motor skill acquisition, an infant who cannot yet sit well will be unlikely to start standing. By age 12 months, infants typically are able to pull to stand and to cruise on furniture; some, but not all, will start to take a few independent steps.

By 12 months of age, cognitive development is demonstrated by the recognition of objects as tools and a sense of object permanence, as evidenced by the infant playing peek-a-boo and becoming upset when familiar caregivers leave the room. Cognitive development is facilitated by gains in fine motor skills. Infants at 12 months of age no longer explore objects orally as much; instead, they manipulate objects in their hands to examine them in more detail and with a longer attention span. During their second year, they start to use objects in their hands as tools (eg, a crayon to draw), further combining fine motor and cognitive skills.

Between 10 and 18 months, infants begin to realize that people and things have names. The use of "dada" and "mama" early in life is reinforced by parents' positive expressions such that the infant eventually begins to use these labels specifically for them. The infant also begins to understand "no," and by age 12 months many infants can understand several dozen words and follow a simple command if a gesture is used to reinforce it.

Around this time, infants begin to point to desired objects as a way to get adults to retrieve the object. Eventually the infant uses vocalization when pointing, and begins to point to objects simply to get an adult's attention (eg, an airplane flying overhead) or to get the adult to name the object. Because of this, pointing is an important component of language development.

Infants with delays in language development should be assessed for hearing loss. Babbling will develop in the absence of hearing, but without hearing the use of specific sounds for caregivers and objects will not develop.

A clinician's concern about development is highly specific for a developmental delay. A 12-month-old infant who does not crawl, drags one side while crawling, cannot stand with support, does not search for objects that are hidden, has no single words, or does not use gestures or pointing should prompt concern for a developmental delay.

PREP Pearls

- A 12-month-old should be able to crawl and stand with support. Failing to meet these milestones should prompt concern for a gross motor delay.
- A 12-month-old should search for objects that are hidden, have at least one single word, and use gestures or pointing. Failing to meet these milestones should prompt concern for a cognitive or language developmental delay.

American Board of Pediatrics Content Specification(s)/Content Area

- Evaluate the cognitive and behavioral developmental progress/status of an infant at 12 months of age
- Evaluate the motor developmental progress/status of an infant at 12 months of age

Suggested Readings

Johnson CP, Blasco PA. Infant growth and development. *Pediatr Rev.* 1997;18(7):224-242.

McQuiston S, Kloczko N. Speech and language development: monitoring process and problems. *Pediatr Rev.* 2011;32(6):230-239.

Item 102 — Preferred Response: D

The girl in this vignette is most at risk for hepatocellular carcinoma (HCC). Chronic infection with hepatitis B virus puts an infected individual at risk of serious liver disease including cirrhosis, hepatic failure, and HCC.

Chronic infection with hepatitis B virus increases the lifetime risk of developing hepatocellular carcinoma by 100 fold. The likelihood of developing chronic hepatitis B infection is inversely related to the age at which infection was acquired. Ninety percent of infants that acquired infection perinatally or in their first year develop chronic infection, compared to 5% to 10% of older children and adults. To screen for sequelae of infection, individuals with chronic hepatitis B infection should have regular screening with abdominal ultrasonography and determination of serum aminotransferase and α-fetoprotein levels. All patients with suspected or known chronic hepatitis B infection should be followed by a pediatric gastroenterologist.

Risk factors for HCC in the setting of hepatitis B virus infection include viral load, hepatitis B e antigen positivity, co-infection with hepatitis C virus or HIV, degree of liver injury, presence of cirrhosis, male sex, use of alcohol, and consumption of aflatoxins in diet. The peak incidence of HCC in the setting of chronic hepatitis B infection is in the fifth decade. However, HCC can develop in childhood.

Biliary carcinomas are rare in the United States, occurring in 1 to 2 per 100,000 persons. The peak incidence is in the 50- to 70-year-old age range. Biliary carcinomas have been more strongly associated with hepatitis C virus infection compared to hepatitis B virus infection, although they are less common than HCC in this setting. Other risk factors for biliary carcinomas include primary sclerosing cholangitis, choledochal cysts, chronic intrahepatic stone disease, Lynch syndrome (hereditary nonpolyposis colorectal cancer), and biliary papillomatosis.

Hepatic sarcomas arise from supportive tissues in the liver and typically occur in middle-aged or older patients. They are rare and not associated with hepatitis B virus infection.

Hepatoblastoma is the most common liver malignancy of early childhood. The majority of hepatoblastomas present within the first 2 years of age. Development of hepatoblastoma is associated with several syndromes, including Beckwith-Wiedemann syndrome, rather than with hepatitis B virus infection.

PREP Pearls

- Chronic infection with hepatitis B virus increases the lifetime risk of developing hepatocellular carcinoma by 100 fold.
- Chronic infection with hepatitis B virus puts an infected individual at risk of serious liver disease including cirrhosis, hepatic failure, and hepatocellular carcinoma.
- To screen for sequelae of infection, individuals with chronic hepatitis B infection should have regular screening with abdominal ultrasonography and determination of serum aminotransferase and α-fetoprotein levels.

American Board of Pediatrics Content Specification(s)/ Content Area

- Understand the risks associated with perinatally acquired hepatitis B virus infections

Suggested Readings

American Academy of Pediatrics. Hepatitis B. In: Kimberlin DW, Brady MT, Jackson MA, Long SS, eds. *Red Book: 2018 Report of the Committee on Infectious Diseases*. 31st ed. Itasca, IL: American Academy of Pediatrics; 2018:401-427

Christenson J, Manaloor J. Hepatitis A, B, and C. *Pediatr Rev*. 2016;37(10):426-438.

Jonas MM. Hepatitis B virus infection in children. *Clin Liver Dis*. 2013;2(1):41-44.

Pan C, Zhang J. Natural history and clinical consequences of hepatitis B virus infection. *Int J Med Sci*. 2005;2(1):36-40

Item 103 — Preferred Response: D

Intoeing is common in young children and can arise as a result of 1 or more variations in lower extremity alignment. The child in the vignette has intoeing as a result of internal tibial torsion, which is thought to be due to variations in intrauterine position. The tibia rotates inward relative to the femur and patella. With the patella facing anteriorly, the foot and ankle will be rotated medially. Item C103A shows a child with tibial torsion; his right foot is rotated internally relative to the thigh. Internal tibial torsion is often unilateral or, when bilateral, more severe on 1 side. Internal tibial torsion typically resolves spontaneously. Bracing with a bar-and-shoe device, reverse last shoes (designed to pull the forefoot into an abducted position), or shoe inserts have not been shown to accelerate the resolution of tibial torsion. Therefore, the best next step in management for this girl would be to reassure her parents.

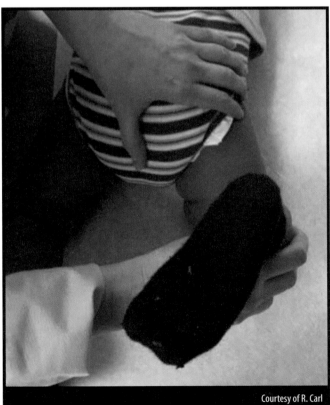

Courtesy of R. Carl

Item C103A: Tibial torsion; note this patient's right foot is rotated internally relative to the thigh.

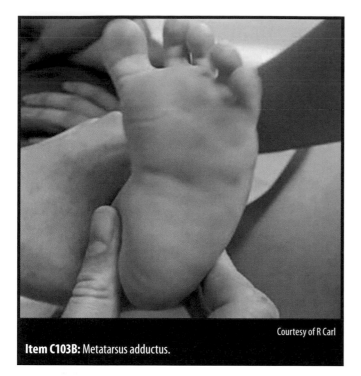

Item C103B: Metatarsus adductus.

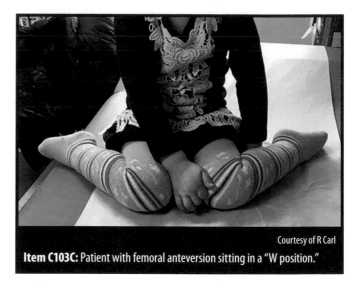

Item C103C: Patient with femoral anteversion sitting in a "W position."

Metatarsus adductus is a common cause of intoed position in infants (Item C103B). The forefoot rests in an adducted position, leading to a rounded appearance of the lateral border of the foot. Metatarsus adductus results from pressure on the foot due to intrauterine positioning. In most cases, metatarsus adductus improves without treatment. Bracing and stretching do not appear to hasten correction. Orthopaedic surgery referral is warranted for children with metatarsus adductus when the foot position is rigid (ie, the foot cannot be stretched into a neutral position) or for severe deformity that persists beyond 6 to 9 months of age.

Children with external tibial torsion usually present with out-toeing during the preschool and early school age years. External tibial torsion may worsen with growth.

With femoral anteversion, the femoral heads and neck have 'excessive' anterior rotation. This allows for increased internal rotation and decreased external rotation of the hips. Children with femoral anteversion tend to walk with the hips rotated inward, leading to intoeing. Parents may report that affected children sit in a 'W-position' (Item C103C). Unlike metatarsus adductus and tibial torsion, femoral anteversion is almost always bilateral and symmetric. Braces, special shoes, and shoe inserts do not alter the natural history of this variant, which tends to correct gradually by the preadolescent years.

For internal and external tibial torsion and femoral anteversion, surgical correction is considered in rare cases, when children at or near skeletal maturity experience pain and/or significant gait disturbance. Physical therapy may be indicated for gait training in school-aged children with functional limitations. Therapy may improve gait mechanics but does not alter the natural history of these normal variations in lower extremity alignment.

PREP Pearls

- Braces, casting, shoe inserts, and physical therapy do not accelerate correction of internal tibial torsion or femoral anteversion.
- Metatarsus adductus, internal tibial torsion, and femoral anteversion are normal developmental variants that lead to the appearance of intoeing, and typically do not require treatment.

American Board of Pediatrics Content Specification(s)/Content Area

- Recognize the clinical findings associated with tibial torsion

Suggested Readings

Rerucha CM, Dickison C, Baird DC. Lower extremity abnormalities in children. *Am Family Physician.* 2017;96(4):226-233

Sarwark JF, LaBella CR, eds. *Pediatric Orthopaedics and Sports Injuries: A Quick Reference Guide.* 2nd ed. Elk Grove Village, IL: American Academy of Pediatrics; 2014

Sielatycki JA, Hennrikus WL, Swenson RD, Fanelli MG, Reighard CJ, Hamp JA. In-toeing Is often a primary care orthopedic condition. *J Pediatr.* 2016;177:297-301.

Item 104   Preferred Response: D

The radiographs (Item C104) demonstrate multiple magnets that have been ingested by the boy in the vignette. The spaces between the magnets are suggestive of bowel wall entrapment, so an urgent surgical consult is warranted. A history of magnet ingestion is often unclear or unknown, because the event is usually not witnessed. In this case, the subtle changes in appetite and stooling history, along with mild but notable tenderness to palpation on examination should raise concern. Obtaining plain radiography is the appropriate first step; more than 1 view is necessary to avoid misclassifying multiple stacked magnets as a single magnet. Given the radiographic findings demonstrating multiple magnets and suggestion of bowel entrapment along with clinical symptoms, immediate evaluation by a pediatric surgeon is the recommended next step.

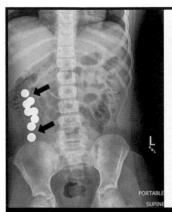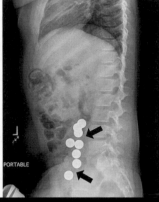

Reprinted with permission from Green SS. Ingested and aspirated foreign bodies. *Pediatr Rev.* 2015;(10):430-437.

Item C104: Spaces (arrows) between the magnets suggest bowel wall entrapment.

Timing is critically important in the management of magnet ingestions. If one can be assured that only a single magnet was ingested, conservative management with close monitoring may be appropriate. Most will progress through the gastrointestinal tract without complication. However, in a case such as this with multiple magnets ingested, subtle symptoms, mild abnormalities on the physical examination, and radiographic features concerning for mural entrapment, it is not appropriate to delay treatment while awaiting serial abdominal radiography results or attempts to encourage natural passage through the gastrointestinal tract via enemas or oral laxatives. The potential complications are too severe. The attraction of 2 or more magnets or a magnet to other metal objects across the walls of adjacent loops of bowel can lead to ischemia, necrosis, perforation, fistula development, bowel obstruction, intussusception, or volvulus.

The management of magnet ingestion depends on the number, location, and type of magnet(s) ingested, with consideration of the time since ingestion. The task force of the North American Society of Pediatric Gastroenterology, Hepatology, and Nutrition developed an algorithm to guide management decisions as published in Kramer et al.

PREP Pearls

- The attraction of 2 or more ingested magnets or a magnet to other metal objects across the walls of adjacent loops of bowel can lead to severe complications, including ischemia, necrosis, perforation, fistula development, bowel obstruction, intussusception, or volvulus.
- Urgent surgical consultation is recommended if there are clinical or radiographic findings suggestive of bowel entrapment or perforation.

American Board of Pediatrics Content Specification(s)/ Content Area

- Plan the management of a patient who has ingested a magnet

Suggested Readings

Green SS. Ingested and aspirated foreign bodies. *Pediatr Rev.* 2015;36(10):430-437.

Kramer RE, Lerner DG, Lin T, et al. Management of ingested foreign bodies in children: a clinical report of the NASPGHAN Endoscopy Committee. *J Pediatr Gastroenterol Nutr.* 2015;60(4):562-574. doi: 10.1097/ MPG.xxxxxxxxxxxxxxxx

Larsen CD, King MA. Abdominal pain and vomiting in a 4-year-old boy. *Pediatr Rev.* 2015;36(3):132-134.

Item 105	Preferred Response: B

The neonate in this vignette has trisomy 21 with associated duodenal atresia. Most neonates with duodenal atresia have a history of polyhydramnios identified by prenatal ultrasonography. The persistent bilious emesis in the context of a sunken or scaphoid abdomen is suggestive of a proximal small bowel obstruction. The abdominal radiograph in this vignette demonstrates the presence of a "double bubble," resulting from the dilated stomach and duodenal bulb.

Duodenal atresia occurs in approximately 1 in 10,000 births and is more common in children with trisomy 21 (25%-40% of patients with duodenal atresia will also have trisomy 21). It is also more common in children with other congenital anomalies including VACTERL association (vertebral defects, anal atresia, cardiac defects, tracheoesophageal fistula, renal anomalies, and limb abnormalities), malrotation, and biliary tract disorders. Prenatal ultrasonography can suggest the diagnosis with the presence of polyhydramnios and/or a double bubble. Duodenal atresia generally presents within the first 24 to 48 hours after birth, with persistent emesis and/or bilious emesis with radiographic evidence of a double bubble. Management includes bowel decompression and surgical repair (duodeno-duodenostomy or duodenojejunostomy). Long-term complications, outside of other possible congenital anomalies, are rare.

Malrotation is another congenital small bowel anomaly, occurring prenatally due to abnormal intestinal rotation and fixation. Asymptomatic malrotation is relatively common (up to 1 in 200 live births), with symptomatic malrotation occurring in 1 of 6,000 live births. Like duodenal atresia, malrotation can also be associated with other congenital anomalies. Presentation of malrotation can vary significantly and may not be diagnosed until adulthood, or it can be found as an incidental finding during autopsy. Infants with symptomatic malrotation may present with small bowel obstruction due to midgut volvulus; early recognition and diagnosis is essential because delay in surgical intervention can result in bowel necrosis and significant morbidity and mortality. Diagnosis is often made with an upper gastrointestinal series, demonstrating abnormal positioning of the duodenojejunal junction (normally located at the level of the ligament of Treitz). Item C105 demonstrates an upper gastrointestinal series with malrotation (duodenum does not cross vertebral bodies) and volvulus ("corkscrew" of the small intestine). Management may vary depending on symptoms and type of malrotation. The presence of a midgut volvulus requires emergent surgical intervention. When malrotation is found incidentally, surgical consultation is warranted to determine if the Ladd procedure may be appropriate to prevent midgut volvulus.

Although many gastrointestinal (and nongastrointestinal) diseases and conditions can cause vomiting, the presence of bilious emesis, severe abdominal pain and vomiting (particularly without diarrhea), fever, lethargy, and/or abdominal distention should prompt consideration of a bowel obstruction. Initial evaluation may include laboratory evaluation, radiographs (acute abdominal series), ultrasonography, and surgical consultation. Infants and young children with bowel obstruction can present with more subtle signs and symptoms (for example, intussusception may present in infants and young children with mental status changes and irritability).

While both cow milk protein allergy and gastroesophageal reflux disease can present with vomiting, bilious emesis would not be a common feature; in addition, the early and severe nature of these symptoms for the neonate in this vignette make these diagnoses less likely. Hirschsprung disease would present with large bowel obstruction, delayed passage of meconium, and a very distended abdomen.

PREP Pearls

- Duodenal atresia presents within the first 1 to 2 days after birth with vomiting and minimal abdominal distention and is often associated with other congenital anomalies.
- Early recognition of small bowel obstruction is essential; signs of bowel obstruction can include vomiting, abdominal pain, abdominal distention, fever, and lethargy.

American Board of Pediatrics Content Specification(s)/ Content Area

- Recognize the clinical features associated with malrotation, and manage appropriately
- Plan the evaluation of the acute onset of vomiting as a result of obstruction in children of various ages
- Recognize the clinical features associated with duodenal atresia, and manage appropriately

Suggested Readings

Morris G, Kennedy A Jr, Cochran W. Small bowel congenital anomalies: a review and update. *Curr Gastroenterol Rep*. 2016;18(4):16.

Parashette KR, Croffie J. Vomiting. *Pediatr Rev*. 2013;34(7):307-321.

Item 106   Preferred Response: A

The girl in this vignette has attention-deficit/hyperactivity disorder (ADHD) and is being treated with a long-acting methylphenidate that is effective in providing sufficient coverage of her symptoms. The primary issue to address is emotionality when the effect of the medication wears off in the late afternoon. After ensuring that there are no other factors that better explain the symptoms (eg, hunger, fatigue), the most appropriate next step is to add an afternoon dose of a short-acting methylphenidate. A switch to a morning dose of short-acting methylphenidate does not provide the necessary length of coverage during the day. Although switching to a mixed salts of amphetamine preparation or to an α-agonist are reasonable approaches, the girl's parents would like to continue with the same medication if possible. In this case, the addition of a short-acting methylphenidate to address the emotionality in the later afternoon should be tried before switching medications.

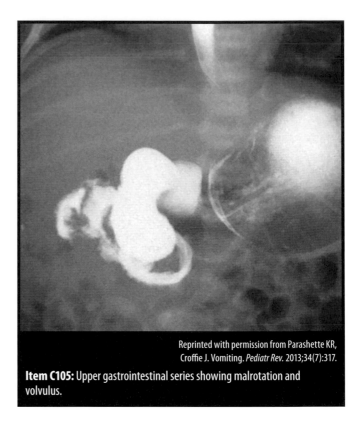

Reprinted with permission from Parashette KR, Croffie J. Vomiting. *Pediatr Rev*. 2013;34(7):317.

Item C105: Upper gastrointestinal series showing malrotation and volvulus.

Attention-deficit/hyperactivity disorder has a prevalence of 5% to 10% and is a chronic neurodevelopmental disorder defined by developmentally inappropriate levels of inattention, hyperactivity, and impulsivity, with functional impairment from these symptoms in at least 2 environments (eg, home, school, work, extracurricular activities). The diagnosis of ADHD is based on meeting the criteria outlined in the *Diagnostic and Statistical Manual of Mental Health Disorders* (Fifth Edition). Sufficient symptoms (6 of 9 for children up to 17 years of age; 5 of 9 for individuals 17 years of age and older) in the categories of inattention and/or hyperactivity/ impulsivity are required. These symptoms need to have been present for more than 6 months, been present before 12 years of age, and resulted in impairment in multiple environments. The behaviors need to be beyond what is expected for the child's developmental age.

During the evaluation process, it is essential to gather information from the child's primary caregivers about symptoms and functioning at home and from other adults in the child's life (eg, teachers, coaches, employers) about symptoms and functioning in other environments (eg, school, sports, work). Areas to ask about include academics, relationships, family life, and daily activities. It is also important to ask about the impact of symptoms on the child's self-esteem. Specific rating scales for ADHD (eg, Vanderbilt rating scales) can be helpful for obtaining this information. A physical examination should be paired with the comprehensive history to identify other medical, developmental, or mental health problems that may underlie or coexist with ADHD. The differential diagnosis of ADHD includes seizure disorder, sleep-disordered breathing, vision or hearing impairment, developmental delay, mental health problems, and autism spectrum disorder. A coexisting condition, such as oppositional defiant disorder, learning disability, anxiety, and tic disorder, is present in most children with ADHD. Laboratory studies and neuroimaging are typically not needed unless the evaluation of other suspected conditions requires them.

In most patients, ADHD is a chronic condition that persists into adolescence and adulthood. Parents and their children should be educated about the diagnosis, treatment options, natural history, and prognosis for ADHD. Evidence-based treatments for ADHD include behavioral management and pharmacological treatment. Effective behavioral management interventions emphasize structure, routine, and consistency and include behavioral parent training and behavioral classroom management. Classroom accommodations and behavior report cards can be useful in supporting children in school and may be formally implemented under Section 504 of the Rehabilitation Act of 1973.

Dopamine and norepinephrine are involved in communication in the prefrontal cortex and striatum, areas of the brain affected by ADHD. Medications that are effective in treating ADHD include stimulant medications (ie, methylphenidate, amphetamine preparations), α-agonists (ie, guanfacine, clonidine), and a norepinephrine-reuptake inhibitor (ie, atomoxetine). These medications improve relevant dopamine and/or norepinephrine signaling. Stimulants are considered first-line treatment because of the strength of their evidence base. They are available in multiple formulations (eg, liquid, capsule, tablet, transdermal patch) and with different durations of action (eg, short acting, intermediate acting, long acting). Nonstimulant medications (eg, atomoxetine, guanfacine, clonidine) are typically used when there is poor response or significant adverse effects with stimulant medication, concerns about substance/medication abuse, significant tics, or parental preference.

PREP Pearls

- A coexisting condition, such as oppositional defiant disorder, learning disability, anxiety, and tic disorder, is present in most children with attention-deficit/hyperactivity disorder.
- Attention-deficit/hyperactivity disorder has a prevalence of 5% to 10% and is a chronic neurodevelopmental disorder defined by developmentally inappropriate levels of inattention, hyperactivity, and impulsivity with functional impairment from these symptoms in at least 2 environments.
- Attention-deficit/hyperactivity disorder is a chronic condition that persists into adolescence and adulthood in most patients. Parents and their children should be educated about the diagnosis, treatment options, natural history, and prognosis.
- Nonstimulant medications (atomoxetine, guanfacine, clonidine) are typically used when there is poor response or significant adverse effects with stimulant medication, concerns about substance/medication abuse, significant tics, or parental preference.

American Board of Pediatrics Content Specification(s)/Content Area

- Understand the neurochemical basis of ADHD
- Plan the appropriate management of ADHD
- Plan the appropriate diagnostic evaluation of ADHD

Suggested Readings

Feldman HM, Reiff MI. Attention deficit-hyperactivity disorder in children and adolescents. *N Engl J Med*. 2014;370(9):838-846.

Floet AM, Scheinet C, Grossman L. Attention-deficit/hyperactivity disorder. *Pediatr Rev*. 201;31(2):56-69.

Subcommittee on Attention-Deficit/Hyperactivity Disorder, Steering Committee on Quality Improvement and Management. ADHD: clinical practice guideline for the diagnosis, evaluation, and treatment of attention-deficit/hyperactivity disorder in children and adolescents. *Pediatrics*. 2011;128(5):1007-1022.

Item 107	Preferred Response: D

The girl in the vignette has a family history suggestive of hereditary hemorrhagic telangiectasia (HHT). This is an autosomal dominant disorder characterized by the presence of arteriovenous malformations (AVMs) in the brain, lungs, liver, gastrointestinal tract, pancreas, and spinal cord, and telangiectasias in the skin and mucosa. People with HHT often have headaches and epistaxis starting in childhood; telangiectasias may not appear until adolescence or early adulthood. Although headaches and epistaxis are common in children, because of her family history, this girl's epistaxis raises concern for HHT and she should be referred for a genetics evaluation. If she is diagnosed with HHT, screening for AVMs and other complications of HHT will need to be discussed. Screening recommendations are being updated based on new literature, so discussion with a geneticist or other specialist in HHT is the best next step.

For the girl in the vignette, who is only having nosebleeds, pulmonary function tests and echocardiography are not indicated at this time. If HHT is ultimately diagnosed, echocardiography with bubble study may eventually be performed to look for evidence of a pulmonary AVM. Without any cutaneous findings, referral to dermatology would not be the best next step for the girl in this vignette.

Cerebral AVMs are often clinically silent until there is an intracranial hemorrhage. Arteriovenous malformations are the most common cause of pediatric hemorrhagic stroke. Before rupturing, AVMs can cause hemiparesis, vision loss, seizures, or other neurologic deficits. Symptoms may be seen because of the mass effect of the AVM on brain tissue, or there may be a vascular steal effect, depriving the local brain tissue of blood supply and causing progressive neurologic deficits. A vein of Galen aneurysmal malformation can present in the neonatal period or in infancy with congestive heart failure because of the large blood volume that is shunted directly back into the right heart. Prominent facial veins, hydrocephalus, and cranial or orbital bruits may also be present.

PREP Pearls

- A vein of Galen aneurysmal malformation can present in the neonatal period or in infancy with congestive heart failure because of the large blood volume that is shunted directly back into the right heart.
- Cerebral arteriovenous malformations are often clinically silent until there is an intracranial hemorrhage.
- Hereditary hemorrhagic telangiectasia is an autosomal dominant disorder characterized by the presence of arteriovenous malformations in the brain, lungs, liver, gastrointestinal tract, pancreas, and spinal cord, and telangiectasias in the skin and mucosa.

Suggested Readings

McDonald J, PyeritzRE. Hereditary hemorrhagic telangiectasia. *GeneReviews* https://www.ncbi.nlm.nih.gov/books/NBK1351/.

Sims ME. Arteriovenous malformation presenting as intracranial hemorrhage in a preterm infant. *NeoReviews*. 2016;17(11):e665-e666.

Item 108 — Preferred Response: B

Evaluation of a testicular mass should always begin with ultrasonography, which is both sensitive and specific, and can delineate between a testicular neoplasm and a nonmalignant process. Because bilateral disease occurs in about 2% to 4% of patients with testicular masses, bilateral ultrasonography should be performed even if an obvious mass is not palpated in the contralateral testis. If a tumor is suspected after ultrasonography has been performed, referral to a pediatric oncologist and/or urologist is indicated. Additional evaluation may include measurement of tumor markers, such as lactate dehydrogenase, β-human chorionic gonadotropin (elevated in choriocarcinoma and seminoma), and α-fetoprotein (elevated in yolk sac cells). Obtaining a testosterone level would not differentiate the cause of the testicular mass because testosterone is not a tumor marker of testicular cancer. While all sexually active teenagers should undergo screening for gonorrhea and chlamydia infections, these tests would not determine the cause of the testicular mass.

Testicular cancer is most common among males aged 15 to 34 years. Risk factors associated with testicular cancer are a family history of testicular cancer and a personal history of cryptorchidism, gonadal dysgenesis, testicular atrophy, Klinefelter syndrome, or human immunodeficiency virus. White men are 4.5 times more likely to develop testicular cancer than African American men.

PREP Pearls

- If further evaluation of a testicular mass is necessary after a thorough history and physical examination, ultrasonography is the method of choice.
- Risk factors associated with testicular cancer are a family history of testicular cancer and a personal history of cryptorchidism, gonadal dysgenesis, testicular atrophy, Klinefelter syndrome, or human immunodeficiency virus.

Suggested Readings

Adelman WP, Joffe A. Consultation with the specialist. *Pediatr Rev.* 2005;26(9):341-344.

Agarwal PK, Palmer JS. Testicular and paratesticular neoplasms in prepubertal males. *J Urol.* 2006;176(3):875-881.

Blair RJ. Testicular and scrotal masses. *Pediatr Rev.* 2014;35(10):450-451.

Item 109 — Preferred Response: D

Lymph is a straw-colored fluid that leaks from the vasculature. This extravascular fluid is captured in valved lymph vessels that carry it proximally into lymph ducts, which ultimately drain back into the subclavian veins. The largest lymph duct is the thoracic duct. As the lymph flows proximally, it filters through lymph nodes. Lymph nodes are highly structured aggregates of lymphocytes. Lymph contains any foreign antigens that may be present in the blood stream. As the lymph filters through lymph nodes, foreign antigens are detected, and lymphocytes that are specific for that foreign antigen are activated and replicate.

An enlarged lymph node (often defined as > 1 cm) is referred to as lymphadenopathy. Lymphadenopathy can be physiologic or pathologic. Physiologic lymphadenopathy is referred to as reactive adenopathy and represents expansion of the lymphocyte population within a lymph node as a consequence of activation by a foreign antigen. As the foreign infection is controlled and the antigens are removed from the lymph, the lymph node will usually return to its normal size. Pathologic lymphadenopathy can be infectious or malignant. Infectious lymphadenopathy occurs when the lymph node itself becomes infected by an organism, which can be viral, bacterial, or fungal. Lymphadenopathy caused by an infection of the lymph node is called infectious lymphadenitis. Malignant lymphadenopathy occurs when a lymphocyte within the lymph node undergoes malignant transformation and replicates (lymphoma) or when malignant cells from elsewhere in the body become trapped in a lymph node and ultimately replicate and replace the normal lymph node architecture.

Reactive lymphadenopathy is typically painless, and the lymph nodes are firm but not hard, and often freely movable. Infectious lymphadenitis most often presents with an enlarged, tender lymph node with overlying erythema. Malignant lymphadenopathy often presents with painless lymph node enlargement, and the enlarged nodes are hard and often matted down. Both infectious lymphadenitis and malignant lymphadenopathy often present with other systemic symptoms.

The patient in this vignette has an infectious source (acne vulgaris with an inflamed pimple) and a painless, freely movable, enlarged lymph node. The enlarged lymph node is on the same side as the pimple and shares its anatomic drainage pattern. It is therefore most likely that the patient has a reactive lymphadenopathy secondary to an infection with a skin organism, such as *Staphylococcus aureus*. The absence of systemic symptoms and the physical examination findings make the other options unlikely.

American Board of Pediatrics Content Specification(s)/ Content Area

- Plan the appropriate clinical evaluation of acute cervical lymphadenopathy
- Plan the appropriate management of chronic cervical lymphadenopathy
- Plan the appropriate management of acute cervical lymphadenopathy
- Identify the age-related etiology of chronic cervical lymphadenopathy
- Formulate a differential diagnosis of cervical lymphadenopathy

Suggested Readings

Gaddey HL, Riegel AM. Unexplained lymphadenopathy: evaluation and differential diagnosis. *Am Fam Physician*. 2016;94(11):896-903

Ilia N. Buhtoiarov. Pediatric lymphoma. *Pediatr Rev*. 2017;38(9):410-423.

Sahai S. Lymphadenopathy. *Pediatr Rev*. 2013;34(5):216-227.

Item 110   **Preferred Response: C**

The adolescent boy in the vignette presents with pain at the site of a left ankle lesion, which is most likely caused by a black widow spider bite. His vital signs are normal and he has no pain proximal to his ankle. He has already cleansed the lesion. The next best step in management is prescription of an oral analgesic.

Though there are thousands of spider species, only 2 species in the United States, black widow and brown recluse spiders, are dangerous. Recommended management for most other spider bites involves only local wound care.

The bite of the black widow spider (*Latrodectus mactans)* is the leading cause of death from spider bites in the United States. As shown in Item Q110, black widow spiders are shiny black in appearance with a bright red hourglass-shaped marking on their abdomens. Their venom contains a neurotoxin that stimulates myoneural junctions, nerves, and nerve endings. Clinical manifestations resulting from black widow spider bites typically include generalized muscle pain and rigidity, developing 1 to 8 hours after the bite. The pain is crampy and may be felt in the abdomen, flanks, chest, and thighs. Affected children may also experience nausea, vomiting, chills, respiratory distress, urinary retention, and priapism. Death from cardiovascular collapse may result, with small children being particularly at risk.

Any child with severe pain and muscle rigidity after a spider bite should be suspected to have toxicity from a *Latrodectus* bite. Some experts recommend treatment with *Latrodectus* antivenin in all small children (<40 kg) with a confirmed black widow spider bite. However, this treatment is not required in older children with normal vital signs and only local muscle pain at the bite site. Treatment with an analgesic for pain would be the best management for children such as the boy in the vignette who have normal vital signs, no signs of systemic toxicity, and pain localized only to the bite site.

Spiders from the *Loxosceles reclusa* (brown recluse) species produce a cytotoxic venom containing a substance similar to hyaluronidase. Children with brown recluse bites can display a spectrum of manifestations at the bite site, from minor local reactions (pain, erythema, and a blister at the bite site) to development of extensive tissue necrosis and ulceration. Affected children may also develop influenza-like symptoms (fever, chills, malaise, arthralgias, nausea, vomiting), intravascular hemolysis, disseminated rash, hematuria, and renal failure.

Management of brown recluse spider bites varies with the clinical severity of the bite. Bites with no associated necrosis or necrosis less than 2 cm require local wound care and observation only, while those associated with extensive necrosis may require surgical debridement, antibiotic treatment, and eventual skin grafting. Studies have demonstrated no significant benefit from treatment with steroids, heparin, dapsone, or hyperbaric oxygen therapy. Antivenin is not commercially available for the treatment of brown recluse spider bites.

There is no proven role for either antibiotic therapy or corticosteroid therapy for patients with black widow spider bites. Therefore, treatment of the boy in the vignette with these agents would not be indicated. Because the boy in the vignette weighs more than 40 kg, has only mild pain, and is systemically well with normal vital signs, he does not need to be referred to an emergency department for *Latrodectus* antivenin therapy at this time.

American Board of Pediatrics Content Specification(s)/ Content Area

- Plan the appropriate management of a spider bite

Suggested Readings

Seeyave DM, Brown KM. Environmental emergencies, radiation emergencies, bites and stings. In: Shaw K, Bachur R, eds. *Fleisher and Ludwig's Textbook of Pediatric Emergency Medicine*. 7th ed. 2015;chap 98:718-759

Item 111   **Preferred Response: D**

The neonate in the vignette has Potter syndrome associated with autosomal recessive polycystic kidney disease (ARPKD). Potter syndrome/Potter sequence, or oligohydramnios sequence presents with characteristic features in the neonate caused by oligohydramnios. These features include pulmonary hypoplasia (presenting with respiratory distress in the newborn), facial appearance (pseudoepicanthus, flattened ears and nose, recessed chin), skeletal abnormalities (hemivertebrae, sacral agenesis), ophthalmologic malformations (eg, cataracts, lens prolapse), and limb abnormalities (club feet and hip dislocation).

Oligohydramnios is diagnosed when the amniotic fluid volume is less than expected for gestational age. This may occur secondary to abnormal renal development with resulting decreased urine output, or premature, prolonged rupture of membranes. Before 16 weeks of gestation, amniotic fluid volume is dependent on transmembrane flow. After 16 weeks of gestation, decreased fetal urinary excretion due to disorders of renal development will lead to oligohydramnios. This results in pulmonary hypoplasia; normal amniotic fluid levels are required for lung development between 16 and 28 weeks of gestation. Management of Potter syndrome is dependent on the associated anomalies; the severity of pulmonary hypoplasia usually determines the prognosis.

Potter syndrome is not inherited; however, the causative renal abnormalities may be inherited. Investigation may reveal a family history of renal disease (eg, autosomal recessive polycystic kidney disease [ARPKD], mutations in *RET*, *UPK3A* gene leading to hereditary renal dysplasia/agenesis). Potter syndrome has not been associated with maternal substance abuse or maternal hypertension.

In children with ARPKD, ultrasonography demonstrates large and echogenic kidneys with decreased corticomedullary differentiation. Macrocysts are not typically seen. Hepatomegaly and increased hepatic echogenicity are usually seen in severe cases of ARPKD, indicating associated congenital hepatic fibrosis. Liver involvement is almost always seen in children with ARPKD, presenting as malformation of the developing biliary ducts. Initially liver function is normal, with portal hypertension, liver enlargement, and injury developing over time.

PREP Pearls

- Potter syndrome/Potter sequence or oligohydramnios sequence is a set of characteristic features in the neonate caused by oligohydramnios.
- The characteristic features of Potter syndrome include pulmonary hypoplasia (respiratory distress in the newborn), facial appearance (pseudoepicanthus, flattened ears and nose, recessed chin), and limb abnormalities (club feet and hip dislocation).
- The severity of pulmonary hypoplasia usually determines the prognosis in children with Potter syndrome.

American Board of Pediatrics Content Specification(s)/ Content Area

- Recognize the renal findings associated with Potter syndrome (pulmonary hypoplasia)

Suggested Readings

Gupta S. Potter syndrome. https://emedicine.medscape.com/article/983477-overview#a5

National Center for Advancing Translational Sciences, National Institutes of Health. Potter sequence.

Item 112 **Preferred Response: A**

The National Cholesterol Education Program's Expert Report (1992) made recommendations for screening and treating hypercholesterolemia in children. These guidelines were updated in 2011 by the Expert Panel on Integrated Guidelines for Cardiovascular Health and Risk Reduction in Children and Adolescents of the National Heart, Lung, and Blood Institute. Important changes have been made in concert with the increasing incidence of obesity and other cardiovascular risks in children.

The screening process for lipid disorders is based on age, other cardiovascular health risks, and family history. A positive family history is defined as early coronary heart disease in a first-degree relative. In this context "early" is considered to be age 55 years or younger for a man and age 65 years or younger for a woman. Diseases included are heart attack, angina, coronary intervention (either surgical or percutaneous catheterization laboratory intervention), stroke, or sudden cardiac death. Such a family history is an independent risk factor for the development of cardiovascular disease.

Recent studies have demonstrated a statistically significant association between high lipid levels in later childhood and early adult cardiovascular disease. Additionally, it is normal for lipid levels to decrease during puberty. Therefore, children later in childhood but before puberty should have universal screening of their lipid levels. The guidelines now state that universal screening should take place between the ages of 9 and 11 years and then again at age 17 to 21 years. No routine screening should take place at any other age group in pediatrics. Children with a positive family history or a moderate- or high-risk medical condition (Item C112) should be screened at ages 2 to 8 years and 12 to 16 years with 2 fasting lipid profiles. (See Expert Panel on Integrated Guidelines for Cardiovascular Health and Risk Reduction in Children and Adolescents for more information.) The average of these 2 results should be used to dictate next steps.

Item C112. Special Risk Conditions.

High risk
T1DM and T2DM
Chronic kidney disease/end-stage renal disease/post–renal transplant
Post-orthotopic heart transplant
Kawasaki disease with current aneurysms
Moderate Risk
Kawasaki disease with regressed coronary aneurysms
Chronic inflammatory disease (systemic lupus erythematosus, juvenile rheumatoid arthritis)
HIV infection
Nephrotic syndrome

Reprinted with permission from the Expert Panel on Integrated Guidelines for Cardiovascular Health and Risk Reduction in Children and Adolescents; National Heart, Lung, and Blood Institute. Expert Panel on Integrated Guidelines for Cardiovascular Health and Risk Reduction in Children and Adolescents: summary report. *Pediatrics.* 2011:128(suppl 5):S240.

Most people with atherosclerotic disease are asymptomatic. In more extreme cases, there can be physical examination findings suggestive of lipid deposition, such as corneal arcus and planar, tuberous, or tendinous xanthomas. Xanthomas, which are lipid deposition over tendons, are yellow-orange, nonpainful, and common on the elbows and knees.

The lipoprotein analysis for the boy in this vignette should be performed now because of his significant family history. It is not appropriate to wait to make this assessment.

PREP Pearls

- Children and adolescents with a family history of premature cardiovascular disease secondary to hypercholesterolemia need a lipoprotein analysis.
- Most patients with hypercholesterolemia are asymptomatic.
- Universal screening for lipid disorders should occur between 9 and 11 years of age.

American Board of Pediatrics Content Specification(s)/Content Area

- Know the risk factors associated with hypercholesterolemia/hyperlipidemia
- Know the risk factors associated with coronary artery disease
- Recognize the clinical features associated with hypercholesterolemia/hyperlipidemia, and evaluate appropriately

Suggested Readings

Expert Panel on Integrated Guidelines for Cardiovascular Health and Risk Reduction in Children and Adolescents; National Heart, Lung, and Blood Institute. Expert Panel on Integrated Guidelines for Cardiovascular Health and Risk Reduction in Children and Adolescents: summary report. *Pediatrics.* 2011;128(suppl 5):S213-S255.

NCEP Expert Panel on Blood Cholesterol Levels in Children and Adolescents. National Cholesterol Education Program (NCEP): highlights of the report of the Expert Panel on Blood Cholesterol Levels in Children and Adolescents. *Pediatrics.* 1992;89(3):495-501

Starc TJ, Deckelbaum RJ. Evaluation of hypercholesterolemia in childhood. *Pediatr Rev.* 1996;17(3):94-97.

Item 113   Preferred Response: D

The adolescent in this vignette has a history of migraines with aura, which is an absolute contraindication for any combined hormonal contraceptive (CHC) method, including oral contraceptive pills (OCP) and the contraceptive patch. She has been taking an appropriate dose of ibuprofen, which has had minimal effect on reducing her symptoms. A trial of a different nonsteroidal anti-inflammatory drug, such a naproxen, is unlikely to have a significant effect on her menstrual cramps. The next step in treatment would be a trial of a hormonal method, and a progestin only method would be an ideal choice with this patient's medical history. A progestin only pill will cause amenorrhea due to thinning of the uterine lining and ultimately decrease the number of menstrual periods she has, thus eliminating her menstrual cramps.

There are a variety of contraceptive options available for both contraceptive and noncontraceptive purposes.

According to the Centers for Disease Control and Prevention (CDC), the pregnancy rate and birth rate for teenagers between 15 and 19 years of age has steadily declined between 1990 and 2009. Some of the decline in teenage pregnancy rates is caused by the availability of more effective forms of contraception, such as intrauterine devices (IUDs) and the progestin only implant, which are effective for several years and decrease issues with compliance. Many teenagers under-utilize these methods, do not have access to them, or still choose to use condoms or the withdrawal method as their primary form of contraception.

Intrauterine devices are the most widely used contraceptive method worldwide. It was previously thought that nulliparous women were not eligible for an IUD because of increased risk of pelvic inflammatory disease. However, numerous studies have demonstrated that IUDs are the most efficacious and safe method for women regardless of parity. There are several US Food and Drug Administration (FDA)–approved IUDs available for use in the United States: the copper IUD and hormonal (progestin only) IUDs. Copper-containing IUDs have been available in the United States since 1988 and are ideal for a woman who does not want to take hormones. A sterile foreign body reaction in the uterus inhibits sperm motility and creates a hostile environment for sperm and ova. It has no effect on ovulation and is approved to stay in place for 10 years, but has been found to remain effective up to 12 years. Adverse effects of the non-hormonal IUD include heavier menstrual flow and increased menstrual cramping. The progestin-only IUDs have varying levels of progestin and work by thickening cervical mucus and thinning the endometrial lining. The progestin (levonorgestrel) has varying effects on inhibiting ovulation. The progestin-only IUDs have varying doses of levonorgestrel, which correspond to length of effectiveness (range, 3 to 7 years). All of the progestin IUDs decrease menstrual flow, and it is a common side effect to become amenorrheic after 1 year of use. A hormonal IUD can also be used for the treatment of dysmenorrhea and heavy menstrual flow. Intrauterine devices can easily be removed at any time, and fertility returns after removal. The failure rates for all IUDs are less than 1% (0.2%-0.8%). Some women with levonorgestrel IUDs may have intermittent spotting.

Another type of long-acting reversible contraceptive is the subdermal progestin implant. It is a 4-cm radio-opaque rod that is inserted under the skin on the medial aspect of the upper arm. It contains 68 mg of etonogestrel, releases 60 μg of hormone daily, and is effective for 3 years. The mechanism of action is similar to hormone-containing IUDs. Insertion requires that a provider complete the company-sponsored training on insertion and removal. The failure rate is 0.05%.

Medroxyprogesterone is the progestin-only injectable contraceptive. It has 2 forms (intramuscular, 150-mg dose; subcutaneous, 104-mg dose) and requires an injection once every 3 months. Its mechanism of action is similar to the other progestin-only methods mentioned above. Many adolescents favor this method because it is not detectable once injected.

Progestin only pills are ideal for adolescents who may have a contraindication to an estrogen-containing compound but desire to take a daily pill. These pills have the same mechanism of action as the progestin-only IUDs. Adolescents taking these pills must be diligent in taking the pill at the same time every day because the effect of the progestin will decrease after 24 hours and will lead to breakthrough bleeding and, if used for contraception, method failure.

All of the progestin-only methods can be associated with some irregular bleeding and eventually cause amenorrhea, which is important to discuss with the adolescent who may want to have a monthly period. Medroxyprogesterone in particular is associated with 2 potential adverse effects, weight gain (up to 5 lbs after one year of consecutive use and up to 8 lbs after 2 years of consecutive use) and loss of bone mineral density. There is a black box warning for medroxyprogesterone related to bone mineral density associated with decreased hip and spine bone density. The reduction in bone density can be reversed once use is discontinued and is more severe in patients with less weight-bearing activities (ie, an adolescent who uses a wheelchair). It is important to counsel young women on medroxyprogesterone about calcium and vitamin D supplementation. All of the progestin-only methods are great options for young women with chronic conditions in which estrogen-containing compounds would be contraindicated when taken in combination with certain antiepileptics, antiretrovirals, and antibiotics. Progestin-only methods are also used to treat catamenial (menstrual-associated) epilepsy and suppress menstruation in patients with physical and mental disabilities.

The CHC options include OCPs, the contraceptive patch, and vaginal ring, all of which have varying amounts of estrogen and progestin. The OCP is the most commonly used contraceptive method in the United States. These methods have more frequent dosing than the progestin only methods discussed above. The OCP requires daily dosing, the patch must be changed weekly, and the vaginal ring must be changed once every 3 weeks. Because these methods are more dependent on the adolescent being responsible for dosing, they have a higher failure rate and greater chance for poor adherence. The CHC options work by inhibiting ovulation and thickening cervical mucus. Aside from contraception, these methods are often used to regulate menstrual cycles/decrease menstrual flow, treat endometriosis and dysmenorrhea, and correct abnormal testosterone levels associated with polycystic ovarian syndrome and acne. The CHC options are also protective against both ovarian and uterine cancers.

The main risk of CHC methods is the risk of a venous thromboembolism. A full list of the absolute contraindications for all contraceptive methods can be reviewed in the CDC summary chart of US medical eligibility criteria for contraceptive use. A few of the absolute contraindications for CHC method use include a prior history of venous thromboembolism, migraine headache with aura, uncontrolled hypertension (systolic blood pressure > 160 mm Hg; diastolic blood pressure > 100 mm Hg), hepatocellular disease, thrombogenic mutations, current or past history of cerebrovascular event, and current breast cancer. A table showing different contraception methods is shown in Item C113.

PREP Pearls

- Contraceptives are used for a variety of medical issues aside from contraception.
- Long-acting reversible contraception methods, which include intrauterine devices and implants, are the most effective methods of contraception.
- The US Medical Eligibility Criteria for Contraceptive Use is useful in determining which methods are best for patients with and without chronic medical conditions.

American Board of Pediatrics Content Specification(s)/Content Area

- Understand the non-contraceptive benefits of oral contraceptives
- Identify relative and absolute contraindications to the use of oral contraceptives
- Understand the forms of contraception available to adolescents and their associated effectiveness and complications
- Understand factors associated with contraceptive use or lack of use in adolescents

Suggested Readings

Centers for Disease Control and Prevention. Summary chart of U.S. medical eligibility criteria for contraceptive use, 2010. https://www.cdc.gov/reproductivehealth/unintendedpregnancy/pdf/legal_summary-chart_english_final_tag508.pdf.

Curtis KM, Tepper NK, Jatlaoui TC, et al. U.S. Medical eligibility criteria for contraceptive use, 2016. *MMWR Recomm Rep.* 2016;65(3):1-103.

Nickles MC, Alderman E. Noncontraceptive use of contraceptive agents. *Pediatr Rev.* 2014;35(6):229-242.

Upadhya K. Contraception for adolescents. *Pediatr Rev.* 2013;34(9):384-393.

BIRTH CONTROL GUIDE

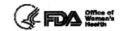

Most Effective

Methods	Number of pregnancies expected per 100 women*	Use	Some Risks	
Sterilization Surgery for Women	less than 1	Onetime procedure Permanent	• Pain • Bleeding • Infection or other complications after surgery • Ectopic (tubal) pregnancy	
Surgical Sterilization Implant for Women	less than 1	Onetime procedure Waiting period before it works Permanent	• Mild to moderate pain after insertion • Ectopic (tubal) pregnancy	
Sterilization Surgery for Men	less than 1	Onetime procedure Waiting period before it works Permanent	• Pain • Bleeding • Infection	
Implantable Rod	less than 1	Inserted by a healthcare provider Lasts up to 3 years	• Changes in bleeding patterns • Weight gain • Breast and abdominal pain	
IUD Copper	less than 1	Inserted by a healthcare provider Lasts up to 10 years	• Cramps • Bleeding • Pelvic inflammatory disease • Infertility • Tear or hole in the uterus	
IUD w/ Progestin	less than 1	Inserted by a healthcare provider Lasts up to 5 years	• Irregular bleeding • No periods • Abdominal/pelvic pain • Ovarian cysts	
Shot/Injection	6	Need a shot every 3 months	• Bone loss • Bleeding between periods • Weight gain	• Nervousness • Abdominal discomfort • Headaches
Oral Contraceptives (Combined Pill) "The Pill"	9	Must swallow a pill every day	• Nausea • Breast Tenderness • Headache	• Rare: high blood pressure, blood clots, heart attack, stroke
Oral Contraceptives (Progestin only) "The MiniPill"	9	Must swallow a pill every day	• Irregular bleeding • Headache • Breast tenderness	• Nausea • Dizziness
Oral Contraceptives Extended/Continuous Use "The Pill"	9	Must swallow a pill every day.	• Risks are similar to other oral contraceptives (combined) • Light bleeding or spotting between periods	
Patch	9	Put on a new patch each week for 3 weeks (21 total days). Don't put on a patch during the fourth week.	• Exposure to higher average levels of estrogen than most oral contraceptives	
Vaginal Contraceptive Ring	9	Put the ring into the vagina yourself. Keep the ring in your vagina for 3 weeks and then take it out for one week.	• Vaginal discharge • Discomfort in the vagina • Mild irritation • Risks are similar to oral contraceptives (combined)	
Diaphragm with Spermicide	12	Must use every time you have sex.	• Irritation • Allergic reactions	• Urinary tract infection • Toxic shock
Sponge with Spermicide	12-24	Must use every time you have sex.	• Irritation • Allergic reactions	• Hard time removing • Toxic shock
Cervical Cap with Spermicide	17-23	Must use every time you have sex.	• Irritation • Allergic reactions	• Abnormal Pap test • Toxic shock
Male Condom	18	Must use every time you have sex. Except for abstinence, latex condoms are the best protection against HIV/AIDS and other STIs.	• Allergic reactions	
Female Condom	21	Must use every time you have sex. May give some protection against STIs.	• Irritation • Allergic reactions	
Spermicide Alone	28	Must use every time you have sex.	• Irritation • Allergic reactions • Urinary tract infection	

Least Effective

U.S. Food and Drug Administration.

Item C113: Birth Control Guide.

The boy in the vignette has many of the complications of prematurity, including chronic lung disease, intraventricular hemorrhage with hydrocephalus, and necrotizing enterocolitis. Because an obstruction was encountered below the vocal cords with a 3.0-mm endotracheal tube, but a 2.5-mm tube passed easily, the most likely cause of respiratory failure in this child is subglottic stenosis. The most appropriate service to consult is otolaryngology.

Upper airway obstruction can occur either above, below, or at the glottis (Item C114). Supraglottic obstruction can be caused by oropharyngeal pathology such as retrognathia and adenotonsillar hypertrophy, laryngomalacia, and epiglottitis. Subglottic obstruction can be caused by laryngotracheitis (croup), bacterial tracheitis, complete tracheal ring, laryngeal web, and subglottic stenosis. Glottic airway obstruction is caused by vocal cord dysfunction or paralysis. Extrathoracic airway obstruction tends to cause inspiratory stridor, because the highly negative intrathoracic pressure required to draw air into the lungs causes the obstructed area to collapse during inspiration. In contrast, intrathoracic airway obstruction tends to cause expiratory wheezing, because the positive intrathoracic pressure required to push air out of the lungs causes the obstructed airway to collapse during expiration. However, biphasic obstructive sounds can occur in any pathology if moderately severe, and minimal air entry and less sound may occur if the obstruction is extreme.

The procedure of direct laryngoscopy and endotracheal intubation itself carries several risks. Laryngoscopy can be traumatic to the upper airway structures, because manipulation of the tongue and epiglottis with a laryngoscope blade can cause bleeding and swelling. Multiple attempts, an uncontrolled setting, untrained providers, and forcefulness can make complications more likely. Vagal stimulation can occur during laryngoscopy, and in unstable patients, can cause bradycardia (and in some cases, cardiac arrest), intracranial hypertension, and pulmonary hypertensive crisis.

Cardiopulmonary interactions that occur during positive pressure ventilation, before and after intubation, can cause decreased right ventricular preload, increased right ventricular afterload, and decreased left ventricular afterload. Premedication with adequate sedation and neuromuscular blockade can lessen the chances of patient movement and laryngospasm, and increase the chances of successful intubation. However, with sedatives there is a risk of hypotension. Because no ventilation occurs during the laryngoscopy itself, hypoxia and hypercarbia may ensue if the endotracheal tube is not inserted in a timely manner. Thus, depending on the needs and stability of the patient, care must be taken before the procedure to ensure adequate preload, preoxygenation, proper personnel, and optimal choice of sedatives and neuromuscular blocking agents.

Aspiration is a possibility if the child has a full stomach. In that circumstance, rapid sequence intubation can be considered, in which bag-valve-mask ventilation is not performed while sedation and neuromuscular blockade is being induced. However, the risk is very high in unstable patients and in those with intracranial hypertension because of the possibility of hypoxic cardiac arrest and herniation, respectively.

The narrowest part of a child's airway is the subglottic area. Contact of an endotracheal tube with airway structures can cause inflammation and subsequent scarring and stenosis. Circumstances that exacerbate airway injury include prolonged intubation, multiple or traumatic intubation attempts, inappropriately large-diameter endotracheal tubes, and inadequate sedation during intubation. Infants, especially those who are premature, are particularly vulnerable, because airway obstruction exponentially increases as inner diameter decreases. Undetected subglottic stenosis can occur, as in the child in the vignette, only to be unmasked by an intercurrent illness, and can manifest as severe respiratory failure.

While general surgeons can perform a tracheostomy, the procedure is not always necessary. Referral to an otolaryngologist is important for the diagnosis and treatment of severe subglottic stenosis. Although the child in the vignette has chronic lung disease of prematurity and the physical findings of patent ductus arteriosus, his respiratory failure is not likely from pulmonary or cardiac causes.

Item C114. Common Causes of Upper Airway Obstruction.

Variable	Laryngomalacia	Supraglottitis (Epiglottitis)	Laryngotracheitis (Croup)	Bacterial Tracheitis
Affected site	Supraglottis	Supraglottis	Subglottis	Trachea
Common ages	2-4 weeks, resolves around 18 months	2-6 years	6-36 months	3 months to 6 years
Onset	Slow	Rapid	Slow	Rapid
Stridor	Inspiratory	Inspiratory, biphasic	Biphasic	Biphasic
Toxic appearance	Uncommon	Yes	Uncommon	Yes
Drooling	No	Yes	No	No
Hoarseness	No	Uncommon	Yes	Possible
Cough	No	Systolic	Yes	Yes
Microbiology	None	Bacterial: *Haemophilus influenzae*, *Streptococcus pneumoniae*, β-hemolytic streptococci, *Staphylococcus aureus*	Viral; parainfluenza	Bacterial: *S aureus*, *S pneumoniae*, *H influenzae*, *Moraxella catarrhalis*

Reprinted with permission from Virbalas J, Smith L. Upper airway obstruction. *Pediatr Rev*. 2015;36(2):63.

American Board of Pediatrics Content Specification(s)/ Content Area

- Understand the potential complications associated with endotracheal intubation
- Plan the appropriate ventilatory support for patients with various conditions
- Recognize the clinical features of acute respiratory distress syndrome, including associated sequelae

Suggested Readings

Sarnaik AP, Clark JA, Sarnaik AA. Respiratory distress and failure. In: Klicgman RM, Stanton BF, St Geme J, Schor NF, eds. *Nelson Textbook of Pediatrics*. 20th ed. Philadelphia, PA: Elsevier; 2015:528-545

Thomas RE, Rao SC, Minutillo C, Vijayasekaran S, Nathan EA. Severe acquired subglottic stenosis in neonatal intensive care graduates: a case-control study [published online ahead of print September 2]. *Arch Dis Child Fetal Neonatal Ed.* 2017.

Virbalas J, Smith L. Upper airway obstruction. *Pediatr Rev.* 2015;36;62.

Item 115   **Preferred Response: C**

The boy in this vignette ingested an unclear number of iron-containing prenatal vitamins. He is at significant risk for toxicity, and therefore requires evaluation and monitoring, including a measurement of his serum iron concentration. Neither activated charcoal nor gastric lavage with bicarbonate is indicated. Although the boy may eventually require deferoxamine, it would not be appropriate to administer it at this point given the lack of severe symptoms and an unclear ingestion history.

Pediatric iron ingestions are common, with approximately 11,000 cases reported annually in the United States. Most are accidental exposures, typically occurring in toddlers and young children. The main source of the ingested iron is prenatal vitamins. Most prenatal multivitamins contain 60 to 65 mg of elemental iron, which is much higher than the 15 to 18 mg in a typical multivitamin. Serious iron ingestions are becoming less common in the United States because of regulations regarding packaging. Intentional ingestions are more commonly seen in teenagers and young adults.

Peak serum iron levels occur within 2 to 3 hours after therapeutic dosing. With ingestions of supratherapeutic doses, peak serum levels are not seen until 4 to 6 hours after ingestion. Patients who have ingested less than 20 mg/kg

of elemental iron are typically asymptomatic. Ingestions of greater than 60 mg/kg of elemental iron are associated with severe toxicity. Ingestions between 20 and 60 mg/kg of elemental iron cause variable symptoms, with some patients remaining asymptomatic and others showing signs of serious toxicity. Deaths have been reported after ingestions of 60 to 300 mg/kg of elemental iron.

Iron toxicity has 5 predictable phases, as shown in Item C115.

Item C115. Phases of Iron Toxicity.

Phase	Timing	Symptoms
Gastrointestinal phase	30 min - 6 h	Abdominal pain, nausea, vomiting, diarrhea, hematemesis, melena, lethargy, shock, metabolic acidosis
Latent phase	6-24 h	Apparent recovery
Shock and metabolic acidosis	6-72 h	Cardiovascular toxicity (shock, pallor, tachycardia, hypotension), coagulopathy, acute respiratory distress syndrome, renal dysfunction, metabolic acidosis, gastrointestinal hemorrhage
Hepatotoxicity and hepatic necrosis	12-96 h	Hepatic injury
Bowel obstruction	2-8 wk	Bowel obstruction, typically at the gastric outlet

Courtesy of I Larson.

All children with suspected iron ingestion must be evaluated for symptoms of toxicity, including subtle signs of hypovolemia and metabolic acidosis. Serum iron concentration and electrolyte levels should be measured in all patients with signs of toxicity, unknown ingestion amounts, or ingestions of more than 40 mg/kg of elemental iron. Serum iron concentration is most useful if measured within the first 4 to 6 hours after ingestion, but may not correlate with the severity of illness because the test measures free plasma iron rather than intracellular iron. Children who have ingested more than 40 mg/kg of elemental iron or who have severe symptoms should also undergo abdominal radiography to evaluate for radiopaque pills in the gastrointestinal tract.

The treatment of iron toxicity includes symptomatic management and supportive care, with attention to volume resuscitation. Children with a significant number of radiopaque pills identified on radiography may benefit from gastrointestinal decontamination, including gastric lavage or whole bowel irrigation. Intravenous deferoxamine should be considered in children with severe symptoms, a significant number of radiopaque pills on radiography, or a peak serum iron concentration greater than 500 µg/dL (90 µmol/L). Deferoxamine is a chelating agent that binds ferric iron in the blood to create water-soluble ferrioxamine, which is then excreted in urine. Activated charcoal does not bind iron well and is therefore not recommended to treat iron ingestion, and gastric lavage with bicarbonate is not recommended because of the large volumes required.

American Board of Pediatrics Content Specification(s)/Content Area

- Plan the management of a patient who has ingested iron pills

Suggested Readings

Chang TP, Rangan C. Iron poisoning: a literature-based review of epidemiology, diagnosis, and management. *Pediatr Emerg Care.* 2011;27(10):978-985.

Perrone J. Iron. In: Hoffman RS, Howland MA, Lewin NA, Nelson LS, Goldfrank LR, eds. *Goldfrank's Toxicologic Emergencies.* 10th ed. New York, NY: McGraw Hill Education; 2015:chap 46

Item 116   Preferred Response: C

The adolescent girl described in the vignette exhibits signs and symptoms consistent with a diagnosis of infectious mononucleosis (IM), which is most frequently associated with primary Epstein-Barr virus (EBV) infection. Epstein-Barr virus is a ubiquitous human γ-herpesvirus that infects more than 95% of the global population by adulthood. The B lymphocytes are the primary cellular target of EBV resulting in a lifelong, latent infection. Individuals between the ages of 15 and 24 years are at highest risk of developing IM, with an overall incidence of approximately 500 cases per 100,000 persons annually in the United States. In adolescents, transmission typically occurs via exposure to infected saliva and rarely via a sexual route. In preadolescents, the mode of transmission is unknown.

In young children, primary EBV infection is often asymptomatic. In adolescents and young adults, primary EBV infections frequently manifest as IM, which is characterized by fever, malaise or fatigue, pharyngitis, and cervical lymphadenopathy. An enlarged spleen may be palpable in 15% to 65% of cases during the first 3 weeks of illness. Uncommon manifestations include palatal petechiae, bilateral upper eyelid edema, and rash (in 3%-15% of cases). The classic morbilliform rash associated with acute IM is noted during the first days of illness. It primarily involves the trunk and spares the extremities, and resolves within 1 to 6 days of illness. The rash can also be macular, petechial, scarlatiniform, urticarial, or erythema multiforme.

The laboratory diagnosis of acute EBV infection is based on serology. Heterophile antibody tests (eg, Paul-Bunnell test or slide agglutination reaction test) primarily detect immunoglobulin M (IgM), and are approximately 85% sensitive in the diagnosis of IM in older children and adolescents during the first 2 weeks of illness. Heterophile antibodies are often absent in children younger than 4 years of age. A complete blood cell count may show marked lymphocytosis with an elevated number of atypical lymphocytes during the second week of illness. In a patient with symptoms and signs consistent with a diagnosis of acute IM, the detection of more than 10% atypical lymphocytes on a peripheral blood smear in conjunction with a positive heterophile antibody test result is diagnostic of acute EBV infection. Measurement of EBV-specific antibody titers is recommended for definitive diagnosis of EBV IM, especially in young children or patients with heterophile antibody–negative IM. The detection of IgM antibody against viral capsid antigen in the absence of antibodies against Epstein-Barr nuclear antigen confirms the diagnosis of recent acute EBV infection. The differential diagnosis of IM includes primary human immunodeficiency virus, human herpesvirus 6, cytomegalovirus, and *Toxoplasma gondii* infection.

The natural history of EBV IM in most patients is characterized by recovery over a period of weeks without sequelae. However, severe complications can occur. Hematologic complications include hemolytic anemia, thrombocytopenia, aplastic anemia, disseminated intravascular coagulation, and hemophagocytic lymphohistiocytosis (HLH). Neurologic complications include aseptic meningitis, encephalitis, optic neuritis, facial nerve palsy, transverse myelitis, and Guillain-Barré syndrome. Other unusual but potentially life-threatening complications include splenic rupture, upper airway obstruction due to severe tonsillar enlargement, and myocarditis. Epstein-Barr virus has been associated with solid tumors (eg, Burkitt lymphoma, nasopharyngeal carcinoma) and lymphoproliferative disorders in immunocompromised patients (eg, transplant recipients, patients with human immunodeficiency virus). Severe or fatal IM can occur in men with X-linked lymphoproliferative syndrome.

Supportive care is the mainstay of treatment for acute, uncomplicated EBV IM. Corticosteroids are not indicated for uncomplicated IM, given the risk of adverse effects. However, a short-course of steroids (1 mg/kg per day of oral prednisone; maximum, 20 mg/day for 1 week) should be considered for complicated disease, such as significant tonsillar enlargement with impending airway obstruction, massive splenomegaly, myocarditis, hemolytic anemia, or HLH. In addition to steroids, treatment of life-threatening HLH may warrant additional immunosuppressive regimens (eg, cyclosporine).

Patients with IM who are treated with antibiotics, especially amoxicillin or ampicillin, can develop a distinctive morbilliform rash. Compared with the spontaneous EBV exanthem, ampicillin-induced rash in individuals with EBV IM typically occurs within 1 week of treatment initiation and is more severe and generalized, involving the face, neck, trunk, extremities, and sometimes the palms and soles.

Although antiviral agents, such as acyclovir or ganciclovir, show in vitro activity against EBV, there is no proven clinical benefit in EBV IM affecting previously healthy individuals as described in the vignette. Given the risk of splenic rupture during the first 3 weeks of illness, patients must be counseled about avoidance of contact and collision sports until at least 4 weeks after symptom onset, when there has been complete recovery and the spleen is not palpable.

PREP Pearls

- Adolescents and young adults with primary Epstein-Barr virus infections frequently present with infectious mononucleosis (IM) characterized by fever, malaise or fatigue, pharyngitis, and cervical lymphadenopathy.
- In a patient with symptoms of IM, the detection of more than 10% atypical lymphocytes on a peripheral blood smear in conjunction with a positive heterophile antibody test is diagnostic of acute Epstein-Barr virus infection.
- Supportive care is the mainstay of treatment for acute, uncomplicated EBV IM.

American Board of Pediatrics Content Specification(s)/ Content Area

- Plan the management of a patient with acute or uncomplicated infectious mononucleosis
- Understand the epidemiology of Epstein-Barr virus
- Understand the importance of host factors in the outcome of Epstein-Barr virus infection

Suggested Readings

American Academy of Pediatrics. Epstein-Barr virus infections (infectious mononucleosis). In: Kimberlin DW, Brady MT, Jackson MA, Long SS, eds. *Red Book: 2018 Report of the Committee on Infectious Diseases.* 31st ed. Itasca, IL: American Academy of Pediatrics; 2018:334-338

Jenson HB. Epstein-Barr virus. *Pediatr Rev.* 2011;32(9):375-384.

Pinninti S, Hough-Telford C, Pati S, Boppana S. Cytomegalovirus and Epstein-Barr virus infections. *Pediatr Rev.* 2016;37(6):223-234.

Item 117   Preferred Response: D

Based on her clinical presentation of bilious emesis and radiographic findings of dilated loops of bowel, the neonate in the vignette has jejunal atresia. Among the response choices, the most likely cause is maternal cigarette smoking during pregnancy. Maternal cigarette smoking may also cause poor growth in utero leading to low birthweight. The differential diagnosis for bilious emesis in a neonate includes malrotation with volvulus, duodenal or jejunal atresia, duodenal or jejunal web, Hirschsprung disease, and meconium ileus. Although necrotizing enterocolitis must be considered, it is less common among neonates born at term.

The pathogenesis of small bowel atresia varies based on location. Jejunal and ileal atresia result from impaired vascular supply, which leads to localized ischemia. In theory, nicotine from cigarette smoking causes vasoconstriction, leading to relative hypoxia and infarction. Jejunal and ileal atresia have also been associated with maternal cocaine use. These defects typically are not associated with other congenital anomalies.

Duodenal atresia, with an incidence ranging from 0.5 to 1 per 10,000 live births, occurs because of failed or incomplete recanalization of the duodenum after the seventh week of gestation. Twenty-five percent to 30% of cases of duodenal atresia are associated with trisomy 21. Duodenal atresia frequently occurs with other congenital anomalies, such as congenital heart disease, annular pancreas, malrotation, and renal anomalies. The diagnosis may be suggested by a double bubble sign on plain abdominal radiography.

Advanced maternal age, congenital rubella syndrome, and exposure to levetiracetam are not associated with congenital intestinal anomalies. Congenital rubella syndrome typically presents with deafness, cataracts, congenital heart disease, and low birthweight.

PREP Pearls

- Duodenal atresia is caused by failed or incomplete recanalization of the intestine during development.
- Jejunal and ileal atresia result from impaired vascular supply leading to ischemia.
- Maternal cigarette use during pregnancy is associated with low birthweight and intestinal anomalies, specifically jejunal and ileal atresia.

American Board of Pediatrics Content Specification(s)/ Content Area

- Recognize the effects of maternal smoking on a fetus

Suggested Readings

Bales C, Liacouras CA. Intestinal atresia, stenosis and malrotation. In: Kliegman RM, Stanton BF, St Geme JW, Schor NF, eds. *Nelson Textbook of Pediatrics.* 20th ed. Philadelphia, PA: Saunders Elsevier; 2016:1800-1804.

Chandran L, ChitkaraM. Vomiting in children: reassurance, red flag, or referral? *Pediatr Rev.* 2008;29;183.

Item 118   Preferred Response: B

The girl in this vignette has normal examination findings, other than tachypnea and irritability, and there is no supportive data to suggest a cardiac or respiratory source of her tachypnea. Therefore, the most likely etiology is metabolic. Of the response choices, metabolic acidosis from salicylate ingestion is the most likely cause for her tachypnea.

The girl does not have fever or primary upper respiratory signs or symptoms that might suggest respiratory syncytial virus infection. A family history of diabetes is only helpful if the child has symptoms of diabetic ketoacidosis, but the normal urinalysis results make this unlikely. Although apple juice is acidic, it is difficult to ingest enough to produce systemic acidosis.

In the presence of tachypnea when there is no fever, signs of respiratory distress or acute respiratory compromise, or cardiac abnormalities, a search for a metabolic cause of the tachypnea will be the most helpful.

Multiple factors affect respiratory rate, and the range of normal respiratory rate is fairly broad, particularly in younger children. Tachypnea may be one of the first signs of respiratory distress and should be evaluated. Fever is probably the most common cause of tachypnea, and the elevated respiratory rate may resolve with a decrease in body temperature. Other causes of tachypnea include airway reactivity, cardiac and intrapulmonary processes, upper airway obstruction, and metabolic derangement. For a 4-year-old, the average respiratory rate is about 25 breaths/min, and the range may be from 15 to 35 breaths/min. For newborns, a normal respiratory rate may be as high as 55 breaths/min or as low as 20 breaths/min. By one year of age, the average respiratory rate is around 30 breaths/min but the normal range is still very broad.

PREP Pearls

- In the presence of tachypnea when there is no fever, respiratory distress, acute respiratory compromise, or cardiac abnormalities, a metabolic cause of the tachypnea should be sought.
- There is a broad range in normal for respiratory rate, especially in infants and young children.

American Board of Pediatrics Content Specification(s)/Content Area

- Plan the appropriate clinical and diagnostic evaluation of tachypnea of various etiologies
- Recognize the various factors that influence respiratory rate
- Recognize normal breathing patterns in patients of various ages

Suggested Readings

Bloomfield D. Tachypnea. *Pediatr Rev.* 2002;23(8):294-295.

Harris C, Homnick DN. The pulmonary physical exam. In: Light MJ, Blaisdell CJ, Homnick DN, Schechter MS, Weinberger MM, eds. *Pediatric Pulmonology.* Elk Grove Village, IL: American Academy of Pediatrics; 2011:77-88

Item 119   Preferred Response: C

The boy in this vignette has X-linked hypophosphatemic rickets (XLH), the most common form of familial hypophosphatemic rickets. His knee radiograph shows metaphyseal widening and fraying, consistent with rickets. His biochemical profile is consistent with XLH.

X-linked hypophosphatemic rickets is characterized by renal phosphate wasting and impaired stimulation of 1α-hydroxylase that normally occurs in response to low phosphorus levels. In unaffected individuals, low phosphorus levels stimulate 1α-hydroxylase, resulting in increased conversion of 25-hydroxyvitamin D to 1,25-dihydroxyvitamin D, the activated form of vitamin D. Thus in XLH, the 1,25-dihydroxyvitamin D level is inappropriately normal (it should be high).

Treatment of XLH is with phosphorus and calcitriol (1,25-dihydroxyvitamin D). The phosphorus is given in 4 or 5 daily doses for more consistent serum phosphorus levels. Calcitriol is given twice daily. Optimizing the phosphorus and calcitriol doses while avoiding complications of therapy can be challenging.

Mutations in *PHEX* cause XLH, which is inherited in an X-linked dominant manner. De novo mutations can occur. Renal phosphate wasting results from elevated levels of the phosphaturic compound fibroblast growth factor–23, which also prevents the normal stimulation of 1α-hydroxylase by low phosphorus levels, so that 1,25-dihydroxyvitamin D levels are inappropriately normal. The low phosphorus level, inappropriately normal 1,25-dihydroxyvitamin D level, and normal parathyroid hormone (PTH) level of the boy in this vignette are consistent with XLH. Tubular reabsorption of phosphate, if calculated, would also be low. The PTH level is normal because calcium is not affected in this disorder prior to therapy. The high alkaline phosphatase level is a nonspecific marker of rickets.

Calcium and cholecalciferol (vitamin D3) is the treatment for nutritional rickets caused by vitamin D deficiency, which is characterized by a low 25-hydroxyvitamin D level, high PTH level (caused by total body calcium depletion), normal or low calcium level, low phosphorus level (caused by PTH-induced renal phosphate wasting), and high alkaline phosphatase level.

Calcium and calcitriol (1,25-dihydroxyvitamin D) is the treatment for rickets caused by 1α-hydroxylase deficiency. In this deficiency, the level of 1,25-dihydroxyvitamin D is low, resulting in a low calcium level, high PTH level, and low phosphorus level.

Phosphorus and calcium is the treatment for metabolic bone disease of prematurity, which is caused by inadequate calcium and phosphorus intake for normal bone mineralization. Vitamin D does not play a significant role in metabolic bone disease of prematurity. Item C119 summarizes the biochemical abnormalities in these conditions.

Item C119. Biochemical Abnormalities in Various Etiologies of Rickets.

Condition	Calcium	Phosphorus	Parathyroid Hormone	Alkaline Phosphatase	25-Hydroxy-vitamin D	1,25-Dihydroxy- vitamin D
Vitamin D deficiency	Normal or Low	Low	High	High	Low	Variable
X-linked hypophosphatemic rickets	Normal	Low	Normal	High	Normal	Normal
1α-hydroxylase deficiency	Low	Low	High	High	Normal	Low
Metabolic bone disease of prematurity	Normal	Low	High	High	NA	High

Abbreviation: NA, not applicable.

Courtesy of K. Vogt.

Clinical symptoms of hypophosphatemia often do not occur until the serum phosphorus level is less than 1 mg/dL (0.32 mmol/L). Phosphorus is important as a component of cell membranes, ATP, and 2,3-diphosphoglycerate in red blood cells, which plays a role in oxygen delivery. Symptoms of hypophosphatemia include muscle weakness, encephalopathy, cardiomyopathy, and hemolysis. Chronic hypophosphatemia results in decreased bone mineralization.

PREP Pearls

- Biochemically, X-linked hypophosphatemic rickets is characterized by a low phosphorus level, an inappropriately normal 1,25-dihydroxy vitamin D level, normal parathyroid hormone and calcium levels, and a high alkaline phosphatase level.
- Treatment of X-linked hypophosphatemic rickets is with phosphorus and calcitriol (activated vitamin D or 1,25-dihydroxyvitamin D).
- X-linked hypophosphatemic rickets is characterized by renal phosphate wasting and impaired stimulation of 1α-hydroxylase that normally occurs in response to low phosphorus levels.

American Board of Pediatrics Content Specification(s)/Content Area

- Plan the appropriate management of familial hypophosphatemic rickets
- Recognize the clinical and laboratory features associated with hypophosphatemia

Suggested Readings

Greenbaum LA. Rickets and hypervitaminosis D. In: Kliegman RM, Stanton BF, St. Geme JW, Schor NF, eds. *Nelson Textbook of Pediatrics.* 20th ed. Philadelphia, PA: Elsevier; 2016:331-341

Pavone V, Testa G, Gioitta Iachino S, Evola FR, Avondo S, Sessa G. Hypophosphatemic rickets: etiology, clinical features and treatment. *Eur J Orthop Surg Traumatol.* 2015;25(2):221-226.

Ramakrishnan R, Fuchs J, Singhal G. Case 1: growth failure and abnormal radiographs in a 3-year-old girl. *Pediatr Rev.* 2016;37(8):348-350.

US National Library of Medicine. Hereditary hypophosphatemic rickets. Genetics Home Reference website. https://ghr.nlm.nih.gov/condition/hereditary-hypophosphatemic-rickets.

Item 120 — Preferred Response: C

The infant in the vignette has spinal muscular atrophy (SMA), which results from progressive degeneration and loss of anterior horn cells in the spinal cord and the brain stem nuclei. Children present with symmetric muscle weakness beginning proximally then moving distally, hypotonia, areflexia/hyporeflexia, and tongue fasciculations. The facial muscles are relatively spared; however, suck and swallow capabilities are typically affected. Fasciculations of the tongue are seen in most children, which is a defining physical examination finding not commonly seen in pediatric neuromuscular disorders. As the disease advances, the child develops a bell-shaped chest and paradoxical respirations because of intercostal muscle weakness with relative preservation of the diaphragm musculature. This is known as "abdominal breathing." Diaphragmatic involvement will occur later in the disease course, resulting in full-time ventilator dependency or death.

Spinal muscular atrophy is a predominantly autosomal recessive neuromuscular disorder with 5 subtypes:
- SMA 0: Prenatal onset with infantile death
- SMA I: Onset <6 months of age with lifespan of ≥2 years
- SMA II: Onset at 6-18 months, 70% alive at 25 years of age
- SMA III: Onset >18 months, normal lifespan
- SMA IV: Adulthood onset, normal lifespan

There is one X-linked form of SMA.

The infant in the vignette likely has SMA type I, given the age at symptom onset and clinical findings. Diagnosis of SMA is established by history, physical examination, and the presence of biallelic pathogenic gene variants in *SMN1* on molecular analysis, most commonly an exon 7 deletion. The number of copies, ranging from 0 to 5, of the *SMN2* gene, can modify the phenotype. The more copies of *SMN2*, the milder the phenotype.

Treatment is supportive at this time; there is no cure. Close monitoring of the child's nutritional state, respiratory function, and orthopedic status, with reassessment at least every 6 months is recommended, with appropriate interventions such as gastrostomy tube or noninvasive ventilator support, as the child's condition worsens. New approaches and treatments are being investigated, including upregulating the *SMN2* gene protein product to alter the natural history of the motor neuron degeneration via antisense oligonucleotides which are single-stranded RNA molecules that target complementary sequences in the SMN2 transcript that lead to inclusion of exon 7 increasing the full-length of the SMN protein. This has demonstrated substantial promise for the treatment of this disorder.

Duchenne muscular dystrophy is an X-linked recessive disorder presenting with progressive proximal muscular weakness and calf hypertrophy in boys. Creatine kinase levels are 10 times that of normal. Symptoms present in early childhood, typically between 3 and 5 years of age, with wheelchair dependency occurring before age 13 years. Dilated cardiomyopathy occurs during the second decade of life, and is the leading cause of morbidity and mortality. Heterozygous female carriers are also at risk for dilated cardiomyopathy.

Prader Willi syndrome presents in the neonate with global hypotonia, poor suck, hypogonadism, and characteristic facial features that include bitemporal narrowing of the head, almond-shaped eyes, elongated face, and thin upper lip. It is characterized by feeding difficulties and poor weight gain in early infancy, with the transition to excessive eating and morbid obesity in early to late childhood. Diagnosis is made via DNA methylation testing of the parent-specific imprinting critical region for Prader Willi (PWCR) on chromosome 15.

Zellweger syndrome is an autosomal recessive peroxisomal biogenesis disorder that presents in the newborn period with global hypotonia, poor feeding, seizures, liver cysts with dysfunction, and distinctive facies. Typical facial dysmorphology includes flattened facies, large anterior fontanelle, broad nasal bridge, and widely spaced sutures. Affected infants typically die in the first year after birth.

An infant with Duchenne muscular dystrophy, Prader Willi syndrome, or Zellweger syndrome will not have tongue fasciculations.

PREP Pearls

- Children with spinal muscular atrophy present with symmetric muscle weakness beginning proximally then moving distally, hypotonia, areflexia/hyporeflexia, and tongue fasciculations with sparing of the facial musculature.
- Duchenne muscular dystrophy is an X-linked recessive disorder presenting in boys typically between 3 and 5 years of age with progressive proximal muscular weakness, calf hypertrophy, and creatine kinase levels 10 times normal. Wheelchair dependency typically occurs before age 13 years.
- Spinal muscular atrophy is an autosomal recessive neuromuscular disorder with 5 subtypes, which results from progressive degeneration and loss of anterior horn cells in the spinal cord and the brain stem nuclei.

American Board of Pediatrics Content Specification(s)/ Content Area

- Understand the inheritance pattern in a patient who has a neuromuscular disorder (eg, muscular dystrophy, spinal muscular atrophy

Suggested Readings

Bowerman M, Becker CG, Yáñez-Muñoz RJ, et al; UK SMA Research Consortium. Therapeutic strategies for spinal muscular atrophy: SMN and beyond. *Dis Model Mech*. 2017;10(8):943-954.

Parente V, Corti S. Advances in spinal muscular atrophy therapeutics. *Ther Adv Neurol Disord*. 2018 Feb 5;11:1756285618754501.

Prior TW, Finanger E. Spinal muscular atrophy. *GeneReviews*. https://www.ncbi.nlm.nih.gov/books/NBK1352.

Wang CH, Finkel RS, Bertini ES, et al; Participants of the International Conference on SMA Standard of Care. Consensus statement for standard of care in spinal muscular atrophy. *J Child Neurol*. 2007;22(8)1027-1049.

Item 121   Preferred Response: D

The child in this vignette will likely benefit most from watchful waiting, rather than referral for tonsillectomy. He does not meet the criteria for tonsillectomy based on infection frequency (Item C121A). For the child in the vignette, there is insufficient evidence to support the use of prophylactic cephalosporin. Children thought to have frequent recurrent episodes of group A *Streptococcus* (GAS) pharyngitis are often chronic carriers of GAS who are experiencing repeated viral infections.

Item C121A. Paradise criteria for tonsillectomy.*

Criterion	Definition
Minimum frequency of sore throat episodes	7 or more in the preceding year, or
	5 or more in each of the preceding 2 years, or
	3 or more in each of the preceding 3 years
Clinical features (in addition to sore throat)	Temperature > 38°C, or
	Cervical lymphadenopathy (tender nodes or >2 cm), or
	Tonsillar exudate, or
	Positive culture for Group A *Streptococcus*

*Assumes episodes were treated with appropriate antibiotics and documented in the medical record.

Adapted and reprinted with permission from Baugh RF, Archer SM, Mitchell RB, et al; American Academy of Otolaryngology-Head and Neck Surgery Foundation. Clinical practice guideline: tonsillectomy in children. *Otolaryngol Head Neck Surg*. 2011;144(1 suppl):S8.

Tonsillectomy and adenotonsillectomy are among the most common surgical procedures in children and adolescents. The most common indication for these procedures has shifted from recurrent GAS pharyngitis to obstructive sleep apnea syndrome (OSAS). The prevalence of OSAS ranges from 1.2% to 5.7%. The American Academy of Pediatrics recommends that primary care clinicians universally screen for OSAS at health supervision visits by asking caregivers if their child snores, because snoring is a nearly universally present symptom in OSAS. If affirmative, the primary care clinician should further explore the likelihood of OSAS based on signs and symptoms that are more specific to the disorder (Item C121B). Not all snoring indicates OSAS, and occasional snoring with upper respiratory infections, as in the child in this vignette, is less concerning for the syndrome.

Item C121B. Symptoms and Signs of Obstructive Sleep Apnea Syndrome.

History
Frequent snoring (more than 3 nights per week)
Labored breathing during sleep
Gasps/snorting noises/observed episodes of apnea
Sleep enuresis
Sleeping in a seated position or with the neck hyperextended
Cyanosis
Headaches on awakening
Daytime sleepiness
Attention-deficit/hyperactivity disorder
Learning problems
Physical examination
Underweight or overweight
Tonsillar hypertrophy
Adenoidal facies
Micrognathia/retrognathia
High-arched palate
Failure to thrive
Hypertension

Reprinted with permission from Marcus CL, Brooks LJ, Draper KA, et al; American Academy of Pediatrics. Diagnosis and management of childhood obstructive sleep apnea syndrome. *Pediatrics*. 2012;130(3):579.

While eliciting associated signs and symptoms is helpful in separating snoring children at low risk of having OSAS, polysomnography remains the only reliable diagnostic tool for this condition. It is recommended that children suspected of having OSAS undergo this test prior to adenotonsillectomy. Polysomnography requires overnight testing in a specialized laboratory and is expensive. It is often inconvenient for families, and long wait times are common. If polysomnography is not available, referral to an otolaryngologist or sleep specialist for further evaluation is recommended. Alternative but less accurate strategies, such as overnight oximetry, sleep videos, daytime nap polysomnography, and clinical questionnaires, are sometimes used in lieu of polysomnography.

Adenotonsillectomy is the first-line treatment for nearly all children with OSAS. Children who are obese demonstrate less improvement in symptoms, but adenotonsillectomy is still generally preferred over alternatives, including continuous positive airway pressure. Adenotonsillectomy has a complication rate of approximately 20%, with respiratory compromise and postoperative hemorrhage being the most common complications. Velopharyngeal insufficiency occurs in about 1 in 1,200 cases, and death occurs in about 1 or 2 in 30,000 cases. Children with risk factors for complications, such as craniofacial abnormalities, severe obesity, and age younger than 3 years, should be observed overnight on an inpatient unit after surgery.

Adenotonsillectomy alone is usually effective for OSAS, but children should be evaluated 6 to 8 weeks after surgery to ensure resolution of symptoms. For children at high risk for persistent OSAS, including children with markedly abnormal preoperative polysomnography, obesity, or continued symptoms after surgery, a repeat polysomnogram and/or referral to a sleep specialist is recommended.

Tonsillectomy for recurrent severe throat infections is controversial. The 2011 American Academy of Otolaryngology-Head and Neck Surgery guideline for tonsillectomy in children recommends tonsillectomy for patients meeting the Paradise criteria (Item C121A); the child in this vignette does not meet these criteria. While tonsillectomy is very effective in reducing the frequency of episodes of severe pharyngitis, most children meeting the Paradise criteria but who did not undergo tonsillectomy in controlled trials experienced a natural reduction in the frequency and severity of throat infections. The 2012 Infectious Disease Society of America guideline for GAS infections does not recommend tonsillectomy solely to reduce the frequency of such infections, given the natural decrease in infection frequency and the difficulty identifying GAS carriers (in whom antibiotics are generally not warranted).

Less common indications for tonsillectomy include recurrent peritonsillar abscess, recurrent throat infections in the setting of multiple antibiotic allergies, concern for tonsillar malignancy, and halitosis. Less common indications for adenoidectomy alone include recurrent sinusitis and otitis media with effusion where repeat tympanostomy tube insertion is required.

PREP Pearls

- Adenotonsillectomy has a complication rate of about 20%; however, most complications are short term and the procedure is overall well tolerated.
- Adenotonsillectomy is the first-line therapy for obstructive sleep apnea syndrome.
- Tonsillectomy for recurrent, severe throat infections should be limited to patients meeting strict criteria; watchful waiting is appropriate in most cases.

American Board of Pediatrics Content Specification(s)/ Content Area

- Understand the indications for an adenoidectomy and the resulting effects on nasal function, sleep physiology, and eustachian tube function
- Recognize complications associated with tonsillectomy and/or adenoidectomy, including those associated with velopharyngeal insufficiency
- Understand the indications for a tonsillectomy

Suggested Readings

Baugh RF, Archer SM, Mitchell RB, et al; American Academy of Otolaryngology-Head and Neck Surgery Foundation. Clinical practice guideline: tonsillectomy in children. *Otolaryngol Head Neck Surg.* 2011;144(1 suppl):S1-S30.

Marcus CL, Brooks LJ, Draper KA, et al; American Academy of Pediatrics. Diagnosis and management of childhood obstructive sleep apnea syndrome. *Pediatrics.* 2012;130(3):576-584.

Shulman ST, Bisno AL, Clegg HW, et al. Clinical practice guideline for the diagnosis and management of group A streptococcal pharyngitis: 2012 update by the Infectious Diseases Society of America. *Clin Infect Dis.* 2012;55(10):1279-1282.

Item 122 (I-C) (P) (SBP) (S)   **Preferred Response: B**

The medical error presented in this vignette is best described as a nonintercepted error. The omission of drug monitoring was not previously recognized (or intercepted), and it reached the patient yet it did not result in harm.

A medical error is an act that has the potential to cause patient harm, regardless of whether harm reaches the patient (Item C122). A medical error that results in harm to the patient is considered a preventable adverse event. Medical errors that do not cause harm to the patient are known as potential adverse events or near misses. There are 2 types of potential adverse events: intercepted and nonintercepted. An intercepted error is recognized and corrected before it reaches the patient. A nonintercepted error actually reaches the patient but does not result in harm.

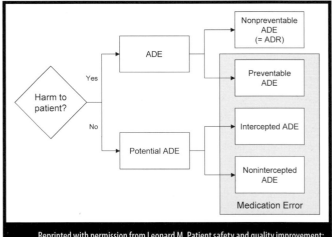

Reprinted with permission from Leonard M. Patient safety and quality improvement: medical errors and adverse events. *Pediatr Rev.* 2010;31(4):152.

Item C122: The relationship between medication errors, adverse drug events, and harm. Abbreviations: ADE, adverse drug event; ADR, adverse drug reaction.

An error of commission occurs when an incorrect action is taken. In contrast, an error of omission occurs when a correct action is not taken. In this vignette, failing to perform drug monitoring would be considered an error of omission.

A sentinel event is an unexpected event that threatens or results in serious injury or death. Both adverse events and potential adverse events may qualify as sentinel events. Sentinel events are not necessarily the result of medical errors, because they may occur as a result of nonpreventable events.

American Board of Pediatrics Content Specification(s)/ Content Area

- Understand and apply the definition of a near-miss event
- Understand and apply the definition of a medical error
- Understand and apply the definition of a sentinel event

Suggested Readings

Committee on Medical Liability and Risk Management and Council on Quality Improvement and Patient Safety. Disclosure of adverse events in pediatrics. *Pediatrics*. 2016;138(6):1-6.

Leonard M. Patient safety and quality improvement: medical errors and adverse events. *Pediatr Rev*. 2010;31(4):151-158.

Item 123   **Preferred Response: C**

The athlete in the vignette is experiencing fatigue and abdominal cramping. Her core temperature, respiratory rate, and heart rate are elevated. She is able to articulate her symptoms and does not appear to have mental status changes. Her clinical presentation is consistent with heat exhaustion.

Over the past 2 decades, data from research on thermoregulation have demonstrated that children do not have increased susceptibility to heat illness. Several environmental and external factors can contribute to the development of heat illness including heat, humidity, extra layers of clothing and padding, and the intensity and length of the exercise performed. While rates of heat illness increase with extreme temperatures and humidity, it is important to remember that heat illness can occur with moderate temperatures as well. Intrinsic risk factors include poor conditioning, obesity, and recent acute illness (especially illness that leads to dehydration, eg, viral gastroenteritis).

To mitigate the risk of heat illness, athletes should have access to appropriate fluids and should be encouraged to take frequent breaks in hot, humid conditions. Activity organizers should consider shortening or cancelling outdoor recreational events in extreme heat conditions. Coaches should be aware of the importance of having athletes gradually increase activity and amount of equipment to acclimatize to hot, humid conditions. Several factors contribute to the high rates of heat illness in football players: there is typically a higher proportion of overweight/obese athletes, practices begin in the summer, players wear thick padding, and many teams hold 2 practices per day in the preseason. Physicians who provide medical coverage for events should be able to identify and treat heat illness, and should promote awareness of these conditions for coaches, players, families, and school officials. For events that take place in hot, humid conditions, organizers should have means of rapid cooling available and an emergency action plan in place.

When evaluating an athlete with possible heat illness, physicians should ideally obtain a rectal temperature to determine core temperature. Individuals affected by heat stroke exhibit mental status changes and a core temperature higher than 40°C. These athletes may have impaired ability to sweat and often have hot, dry skin. When heat stroke is suspected, health care providers should initiate rapid cooling by immersing the athlete in cold water until he or she becomes more responsive and core temperature is below 39°C. Ice packs and cold towels can be used, but will not cool as effectively as immersion. Heat stroke affects multiple organ systems, and can lead to organ failure and death if not treated promptly.

Exercise-associated muscle cramps are very common in runners and may be associated with heat illness. Although there are several theories about possible causes of muscle cramps (eg, electrolyte imbalance, dehydration), the cause is unknown. Poor conditioning is a risk factor for heat illness. Neither heat illness nor exercise-associated muscle cramps would explain the elevated temperature noted in the athlete in the vignette.

American Board of Pediatrics Content Specification(s)/ Content Area

- Plan the appropriate evaluation of heat illness, and manage appropriately
- Understand the mechanisms of heat-related illness, including age-related factors
- Recognize the clinical findings associated with heat illness, including complications

Suggested Readings

Bergeron MF, Devore C, Rice SG. Policy statement: climatic heat stress and exercising children and adolescents. *Pediatrics*. 2011;128(3):e741-747.

Yeargin SW, Kerr ZY, Casa DJ, et al. Epidemiology of exertional heat illnesses in youth, high school, and college football. *Med Sci Sports Exerc*. 2016;48(8):1523-1529.

Item 124   **Preferred Response: A**

The decision to keep the girl's confidence and respect her privacy, after informing her of her legal rights and offering resources, is an example of the application of the principle of autonomy. Health care professionals are often faced with ethical dilemmas in caring for abused or neglected children and adolescents. It is important for medical providers to be familiar with the mandatory reporting laws of the state and country in which they practice. The age of the patient and the type of abuse or neglect will determine the next step in management, including reporting to authorities.

When faced with ethical dilemmas, the 4 principles often referred to in medical decision making are:

- Autonomy: Allowing or enabling patients to make their own informed decisions about which health care interventions they will or will not receive
- Beneficence: The obligation to act for the benefit of others; to do good
- Nonmaleficence: The obligation to minimize or eliminate harm
- Justice: The obligation to treat others equally and to distribute benefits and burdens fairly

In this case, the 18-year-old girl is legally an adult; therefore, she has control over the decision about whether to share information with her parents or the authorities. She should be informed that grabbing or pushing by her boyfriend that leaves bruising may be considered physical abuse and his yelling may qualify as verbal abuse. These behaviors may precede more severe emotional, verbal, physical, or sexual abuse. It is the provider's responsibility to ensure that the girl is making an informed decision when choosing not to report, as well as to offer information regarding community resources that aid victims of intimate partner violence. Building a trusting relationship with this young adult and scheduling a follow-up visit are critical. Routine screening of all adolescents and young adults for intimate partner violence is recommended as a part of the health supervision visit.

PREP Pearls

- When faced with ethical dilemmas, the 4 principles often referred to in medical decision making are:
  - Autonomy: Allowing or enabling patients to make their own informed decisions about which health care interventions they will or will not receive
  - Beneficence: The obligation to act for the benefit of others; to do good
  - Nonmaleficence: The obligation to minimize or eliminate harm
  - Justice: The obligation to treat others equally and to distribute benefits and burdens fairly
- Routine screening of all adolescents and young adults for intimate partner violence is recommended as a part of the health supervision visit.

American Board of Pediatrics Content Specification(s)/Content Area

- Recognize and apply ethical principles regarding the issue of intimate-partner violence
- Recognize and apply ethical principles regarding the issues of physical and mental abuse

Suggested Readings

Fisher MA. Ethics for the pediatrician: caring for abused children. *Pediatr Rev.* 2011;32(7):373-e78.

Opel DJ, Olson ME. Ethics for the pediatrician: bioethics education and resources. *Pediatr Rev.* 2012;33(8):370-373.

Thackeray JD, Hibbard R, Dowd MD and the Committee on Child Abuse and Neglect, and the Committee on Injury, Violence, and Poison Prevention. Intimate partner violence: the role of the pediatrician. *Pediatrics* 2010;125(5);1094-1100.

The adolescent girl in this vignette has signs and symptoms consistent with acute cholecystitis (inflammation of the gallbladder) including fever, right upper quadrant abdominal pain, and a positive Murphy sign (pain halting inspiration during deep palpation of the right upper quadrant). Ultrasonography is the most helpful initial diagnostic test for acute cholecystitis, because it will identify gallstones, gallbladder wall thickening, and edema. Cholecystitis most often occurs due to the presence of gallstones (cholelithiasis), and cholecystectomy is indicated for treatment.

Cholelithiasis is most commonly found in asymptomatic children, generally as an incidental finding. However, some children may be symptomatic and show signs of colicky, sharp pain in the right upper quadrant, most commonly experienced after eating a fatty meal. Although laboratory findings can suggest cholelithiasis (elevated levels of transaminases, γ-glutamyltransferase, and alkaline phosphatase), the diagnosis is made by ultrasonographic examination of the gallbladder. Cholecystectomy may be indicated with symptomatic cholelithiasis and in asymptomatic individuals with sickle cell disease or other chronic hemolytic anemias. In addition to hemolytic anemia, obesity and long-term parenteral nutrition are risk factors for formation of gallstones.

Choledocholithiasis (common bile duct gallstones) can present with right upper quadrant abdominal pain, fever, jaundice, acholic stools, and dark urine. Choledocholithiasis can result in cholangitis, thus emergent gastroenterology and surgical consultation is warranted for biliary decompression. Cholecystectomy is indicated in cases of choledocholithiasis.

Cholescintigraphy (commonly known as a HIDA scan) can demonstrate poor gallbladder function but cannot specifically diagnose cholecystitis. Computed tomography of the abdomen is unnecessary in this case, as gallstones are most often radiolucent. An upper gastrointestinal series is not indicated as there is clinical evidence (history and examination) of cholecystitis.

PREP Pearls

- The presence of jaundice and acholic stools with cholelithiasis should prompt consideration of choledocholithiasis.
- The risk for cholelithiasis is highest in children with chronic hemolytic anemia, obesity, or long-term exposure to parenteral nutrition.
- Ultrasonography is the preferred diagnostic modality for suspected cholelithiasis, cholecystitis, or choledocholithiasis.

American Board of Pediatrics Content Specification(s)/Content Area

- Recognize the clinical features associated with choledocholithiasis
- Identify the risk factors associated with the development of cholelithiasis
- Recognize the clinical features associated with cholecystitis

Suggested Readings

Guralnick S. Cholelithiasis and cholecystitis. *Pediatr Rev.* 2009;30(9):368-369.

Rothstein DH, Harmon CM. Gallbladder disease in children. *Semin Pediatr Surg.* 2016;25(4):225-231.

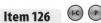
Gifted children demonstrate superior abilities, skills, or talent in areas such as intelligence, music, athletics, or art. With an IQ greater than 2 standard deviations above the mean (ie, >130), the boy in this vignette is a cognitively gifted child who will most likely need educational enrichment activities. Through activities that increase the breadth and depth of covered content, the boy's parents and teachers can address his intellectual needs and nurture him in developing his areas of interest or skill.

Children who are cognitively gifted tend to develop language and vocabulary early, demonstrate excellent memory and problem-solving skills, and have an advanced sense of humor. They tend to be curious, sensitive, perfectionistic, and emotionally intense. Gifted children commonly have asynchronous development; social-emotional development may be less advanced than cognitive development. This asynchronous development must be considered when determining academic placement. Options for gifted children include early kindergarten entry, pull-out programs, curriculum modifications, accelerated classes, and grade advancement. In general, early kindergarten entry and grade advancement are not recommended unless the gifted child's social and behavioral development also align with that of the potential classmates. Opportunities for socialization and supports for social-emotional development should be provided if needed.

Although behavioral problems may occur when a gifted child is not being challenged, it is important to recognize that giftedness may be accompanied by conditions such as attention-deficit/hyperactivity disorder, autism spectrum disorder, and learning disabilities. Further evaluation to assess for other diagnoses is warranted prior to considering evidence-based treatments such as behavioral management and/or medication management for attention-deficit/hyperactivity disorder.

Parents may focus their efforts in seeking opportunities and services for their gifted child. This places pressure on the gifted child and decreases the child's time for interacting with peers and for being independent. This also leaves less time, attention, and resources for other family members. Pediatricians should caution parents about these possible outcomes and counsel them to ensure that each child in the family receives one-on-one attention and is treated according to his or her distinct needs. In addition, just like their siblings, gifted children should be expected to comply with household chores and rules.

Pediatricians can support the family of a gifted child by:
- Helping the family access standardized testing to identify their child as gifted
- Educating the family on the likelihood and impact of uneven development
- Identifying possible coexisting conditions
- Guiding families in decisions about education and activities
- Guiding families on parenting their gifted child while fostering healthy family relationships

Helpful resources for parents and professionals include the National Association for Gifted Children (www.nagc.org) and the Council for Exceptional Children (http://www.cec.sped.org).

PREP Pearls

- Although behavioral problems may occur when a gifted child is not being challenged, it is important to recognize that giftedness may be accompanied by conditions such as attention-deficit/hyperactivity disorder, autism spectrum disorder, and learning disabilities.
- Gifted children commonly have asynchronous development; social-emotional development may be less advanced than cognitive development.
- Intellectually gifted children can be nurtured by providing educational enrichment in areas of interest or skill via activities with increased breadth and depth of covered content.

American Board of Pediatrics Content Specification(s)/Content Area

- Understand the effects of gifted children on family dynamics
- Provide anticipatory guidance with respect to management of a gifted child

Suggested Readings

Jaffe AC. The gifted child. *Pediatr Rev*. 2000;21(7):240-242.

Liu YH, Lien J, Kafka T, Stein MT. Discovering gifted children in practice. *J Dev Behav Pediatr*. 2005;26(5):366-269.

Rosenberg MD, Robokos D, Kennedy RF. The gifted child. *Pediatr Rev*. 2010;31(1):41-43.

Item 127 **Preferred Response: C**

The girl in the vignette has acute right cranial nerve VII palsy. When no underlying cause is found, this is called Bell palsy. The recommended treatment of pediatric Bell palsy is a course of oral steroids, based on adult studies showing that oral steroid treatment is associated with quicker recovery and a higher likelihood of complete recovery.

Amoxicillin would only be beneficial in this setting if there were signs of acute otitis media. Ophthalmology referral is recommended for patients with Bell palsy, to make sure the cornea is protected until recovery of full eye closure, but does not directly influence recovery of cranial nerve function. Similarly, speech therapy may be helpful but does not have a direct effect on recovery.

Bell palsy presents with acute onset of unilateral facial weakness involving all the branches of cranial nerve VII, including the temporal branches that innervate the frontalis muscles of the forehead. There may be a prodrome of ear pain or disturbances in hearing. Other symptoms can include hyperacusis, impaired lacrimation, and diminished taste, all ipsilateral to the side of facial weakness. Facial sensation remains normal.

The physical examination finding in Bell palsy is weakness in the upper and lower face. It is important to differential Bell palsy from a central nervous system disorder, such as an acute stroke, that only affects the lower face. To assess upper facial strength, the child should be asked to raise her eyebrows, or to visually track an object upward when holding her head still. When she tries to look upward, the forehead wrinkles will be diminished on the side of facial weakness, indicating that the temporal branches of the facial nerve are involved, confirming a peripheral nerve (cranial nerve VII) palsy. If the forehead wrinkles symmetrically, then a central nervous system cause is most likely.

Management of acute cranial nerve VII palsy starts with clinical assessment for underlying causes, based on the history and physical examination. Causes of acute cranial nerve VII palsy include infections (acute otitis media, meningitis, Lyme disease, human immunodeficiency virus seroconversion, varicella zoster, herpes simplex virus), trauma, structural lesions (cholesteatoma, brainstem tumor), granulomatous disease (tuberculosis, sarcoidosis), hypertension, leukemia, and lymphoma. If an underlying cause is suspected, laboratory or imaging studies may be needed. In areas in which Lyme disease is endemic, serologic studies may be conducted without any other symptoms of Lyme disease being present. For a child with a first instance of Bell palsy with no signs, symptoms, or risk factors for specific causes of acute cranial nerve VII palsy, further diagnostic testing is not necessary. The recommended treatment of Bell palsy is oral steroids; treatment is most effective if started within 3 days of symptom onset. Consideration of antivirals and empiric treatment for Lyme disease can be made on a case-by-case basis.

PREP Pearls

- In Bell palsy, forehead wrinkles are diminished ipsilateral to the facial weakness.
- The recommended treatment for Bell palsy is oral steroids; treatment is most effective if started within 3 days of symptom onset. Antivirals and empiric treatment for Lyme disease can be considered on a case-by-case basis.

American Board of Pediatrics Content Specification(s)/ Content Area

- Recognize the clinical findings associated with Bell palsy, and manage appropriately

Suggested Readings

Engström M, Berg T, Stjernquist-Desatnik A, et al. Prednisolone and valaciclovir in Bell's palsy: a randomised, double-blind, placebo-controlled, multicentre trial. *Lancet Neurol.* 2008;7(11):993.

Madhok VB, Gagyor I, Daly F, et al. Corticosteroids for Bell's palsy (idiopathic facial paralysis). *Cochrane Database Syst Rev.* 2016;7:CD001942.

Nigrovic NE, Thompson AD, Fine AM, Kimia A. Clinical predictors of Lyme disease among children with a peripheral facial palsy at an emergency department in a Lyme disease–endemic area. *Pediatrics.* 2008;122(5):e1080-e1085.

Item 128 — Preferred Response: C

The American Academy of Pediatrics recommends exclusive breastfeeding for 6 months and continuation of breastfeeding (along with solid foods) until the first year of age or longer as desired by the mother and infant. The provision of human milk to term and preterm infants reduces the incidence of childhood infections, allergic disease, and some autoimmune diseases, as well as improves neurodevelopmental outcomes and reduces the risk of sudden infant death syndrome. While each species has a unique composition of milk, human milk provides the optimal nutritional composition for infants through 12 months of age. As compared to cow milk, human milk contains more available iron and carbohydrate, less protein and calcium, and similar amounts of fat.

With the exception of infant formula, cow milk should not be introduced until 12 months of age due to the risk of gastrointestinal bleeding, iron-deficiency anemia, and excessive renal solute load. Because cow milk is intended for calves, protein and minerals (such as sodium, potassium, calcium, chloride, and phosphorus) essential for the higher growth velocity, are significantly higher than human milk. As a result, the renal solute load in cow milk is high and may lead to dehydration and hypernatremia in infants, especially during illnesses. Furthermore, the iron content of cow milk is low and poorly absorbed. Cow milk can also cause gastrointestinal bleeding in infants, which may lead to iron deficiency.

PREP Pearls

- As compared to cow milk, human milk contains more available iron and carbohydrate, less protein and calcium, and similar amounts of fat.
- With the exception of infant formula, cow milk should not be introduced until 12 months of age because of the risk of gastrointestinal bleeding, iron deficiency anemia, and excessive renal solute load.

American Board of Pediatrics Content Specification(s)/ Content Area

- Understand the appropriate age at which cow milk should be introduced into the diet
- Understand the qualitative and quantitative differences between human milk and cow milk

Suggested Readings

DiMaggio DM, Cox A, Porto AF. Updates in infant nutrition. *Pediatr Rev.* 2017;38(10):449-462.

Martin CR, Ling PR, Blackburn GL. Review of infant feeding: key features of breast milk and infant formula. *Nutrients.* 2016;8(5):279.

Michaelsen KM. Cows' milk in complementary feeding. *Pediatrics.* 2000;106(5):1302-1303.

Item 129 — Preferred Response: D

The boy in this vignette has asymptomatic laboratory abnormalities of the coagulation profile, with a mildly prolonged prothrombin time (PT) and partial thromboplastin time (PTT). His history is remarkable for having received prolonged treatment with third-generation cephalosporin antibiotic prophylaxis for ureteral reflux. This history must raise concern for a coagulation disorder caused by vitamin K deficiency.

Vitamin K is critical for the synthesis of factors II, VII, IX, and X. Factor VII is in the extrinsic pathway, factor IX in the intrinsic pathway, and factors II and X are in the common pathway (Item C129). As such, vitamin K deficiency results in both a prolonged PT and PTT. Some vitamin K (phylloquinone [vitamin K_1]) is derived through the ingestion of green leafy vegetables, but an important isoform of vitamin

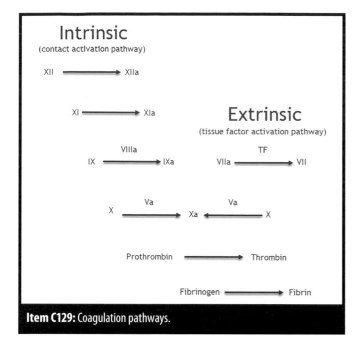

Intrinsic
(contact activation pathway)

Extrinsic
(tissue factor activation pathway)

Item C129: Coagulation pathways.

K (menaquinones [vitamin K_2]) is dependent on synthesis or modification by gut bacteria. Thus, any disruption of the microbiome of the gut can result in vitamin K deficiency. The boy in this vignette has received a prolonged course of antibiotics with a third-generation cephalosporin. This treatment has likely altered his gut microbiome, and this disruption has manifested as vitamin K deficiency with a resultant prolongation of the PT and PTT. This deficiency can be corrected through the administration of 2.5 mg of vitamin K orally, with subsequent doses repeated daily as needed. If prophylactic antibiotics are required for an extended period of time, prophylactic vitamin K replacement can be considered.

Although an acquired factor V deficiency can occur through the development of anti-factor V antibodies or liver dysfunction, anti-factor V antibodies are very rare, and there is no history to suggest liver dysfunction. Factor VII deficiency would result in a prolonged PT but not a prolonged PTT. Hypofibrinogenemia would result in a bleeding phenotype, but would not prolong the PT or the PTT.

PREP Pearls

- For children on long-term antibiotic therapy or prophylaxis, vitamin K deficiency can be prevented through the administration of vitamin K orally once weekly.
- Gut bacteria synthesize vitamin K_2, an important isoform of vitamin K. Disruption of the gut microbiome (eg, by broad-spectrum antibiotics) can result in vitamin K deficiency.

American Board of Pediatrics Content Specification(s)/ Content Area

- Recognize the presenting signs and symptoms of hemorrhagic disease of the newborn in an infant who did not receive vitamin K, and manage appropriately
- Recognize the signs, symptoms, and causes of vitamin K deficiency, and manage appropriately
- Plan appropriate vitamin K administration for a newborn infant

Suggested Readings

Lauer B, Spector N. Vitamins. *Pediatr Rev.* 2012;33(8):339-351.

Rodriguez V, Warad D. Pediatric coagulation disorders. *Pediatr Rev.* 2016;37(7):279-291.

Zimmerman B, Valentino LA. Hemophilia: in review. *Pediatr Rev.* 2013;34(7):289-294.

Item 130 Ⓢ **Preferred Response: B**

The boy in the vignette has a small chin laceration that will require the placement of 2 simple sutures. The anticipated laceration repair procedure should be brief and minimally painful, given that a topical anesthetic gel is being used. Minimal sedation (anxiolysis) is the most appropriate level of sedation for this procedure, and intranasal midazolam is the most appropriate medication option.

For healthy infants and children requiring only minimal sedation (anxiolysis) for an anticipated procedure, midazolam is a frequently used, effective pharmacologic option. This agent can be administered orally, intranasally, intravenously, and rectally. For children undergoing brief, minimally painful procedures, administration of midazolam intranasally or orally obviates the need for establishment of intravenous access (which can also be a painful, anxiety-provoking procedure). Nitrous oxide is another effective option for minimal sedation in children.

Some children may experience significant anxiety and distress when faced with even a relatively simple and minimally painful procedure, despite the use of topical anesthetics and nonpharmacologic calming and distraction techniques. Procedural sedation and analgesia (PSA) includes the use of pharmacologic agents to alleviate anxiety, control procedure-related pain, and facilitate sedation for children during procedures and diagnostic tests. Pediatric providers involved with arranging and administering PSA must determine the most appropriate level of sedation for a given procedure in each patient. An ideal plan for sedation should adequately allay a child's fear and anxiety, achieve the child's cooperation, and provide immobilization to the degree required for the procedure, reduce pain and discomfort, induce amnesia, and maintain the child's safety. Minimal sedation, the sedation level indicated for the patient in the vignette, allows children to converse and respond normally to verbal commands and does not impair the integrity of the airway or cardiorespiratory function. Other levels of PSA, which are often discussed as a continuum, include moderate sedation, deep sedation, and general anesthesia. A thorough assessment should be completed before any procedural sedation in any patient.

Many nonpharmacologic techniques, such as the use of distraction, guided imagery, hypnosis, relaxation, parental presence, coaching, and education regarding the procedure, have been shown to help children cope with medical procedures. These strategies should be used in combination with appropriate analgesic and anxiolytic agents. Adequate preparation of the child and caregiver(s) involved is an essential step in performing any medical procedure. Use of an analgesic and/or sedative agent does not eliminate the need to properly prepare the patient and his/her caregiver(s). Clear, calming communication and nonpharmacologic modalities should be incorporated throughout any procedure to minimize a child's discomfort and anxiety.

Intramuscular morphine would not be the best medication option for the boy in the vignette. Morphine is a narcotic analgesic that relieves pain and may cause sedation in some children (especially when used in higher doses). However, the primary effect of morphine is alleviation of pain and not sedation. For the boy in the vignette, the pain associated with his laceration and suture placement should be controlled by the topical anesthetic agent that was applied to the wound. Administration of an anxiolytic medication, rather than a systemic analgesic, is most appropriate in this case.

Both intravenous etomidate and intravenous propofol would provide a deeper level of sedation than necessary for the boy in the vignette. They are rapidly acting, potent sedatives that are indicated for patients requiring deeper levels of sedation for more prolonged and/or painful procedures. These medications can have a significant impact on airway integrity and cardiorespiratory function in children. Therefore, they should only be administered by providers who are trained and skilled in their administration as well as necessary rescue procedures.

PREP Pearls

- Individualized procedural sedation goals include allaying fear and anxiety, achieving cooperation and immobilization, reducing pain and discomfort, inducing amnesia, and maintaining safety.
- Minimal sedation allows children to converse and respond normally to verbal commands, and does not impair airway integrity or cardiorespiratory function.
- Using an analgesic and/or sedative agent does not eliminate the need to properly prepare children and their caregivers for a procedure. Clear, calming communication and nonpharmacologic modalities should be used to minimize the patient's discomfort and anxiety.

American Board of Pediatrics Content Specification(s)/ Content Area

- Understand the appropriate use of sedative analgesia
- Understand the appropriate use of minimal sedation (anxiolytic)

Suggested Readings

Caglar D, Kwun R, Haines CJ. Pediatric procedural sedation and analgesic in the emergency department. *Pediatr Emerg Med Rep.* 2011;16(8):93.

Gozal D, Gozal Y. Pediatric sedation/anesthesia outside the operating room. *Curr Opin Anaesthesiol.* 2008;21:494-498.

Item 131   Preferred Response: B

For patients such as the adolescent boy in the vignette, there will usually be a recognizable and apparent cause for the gross hematuria, unlike those presenting with asymptomatic microscopic hematuria. A detailed history, physical examination, and urinalysis generally provide information to guide the investigation for the underlying cause of gross hematuria (Item C131A). Bright red hematuria is usually indicative of lower urinary tract bleeding, whereas glomerular hematuria (as in nephritis) is commonly described as cola, tea, or brown

colored. An estimate of blood loss cannot be made based on urinary color change because even 1 mL of blood per liter of urine can induce a visible color change in urine.

Item C131A. Diagnosis of gross hematuria.

Clues/History	Possible Diagnosis
Lower tract symptoms (dysuria, urgency, frequency, suprapubic pain)	UTI
Recent illness (pharyngitis, impetigo, viral illness)	Postinfectious glomerulonephritis
Abdominal pain	UTI, HSP, crystalluria/stone
Concurrent illness	IgAN
Extreme exertion, influenza	Rhabdomyolysis
Arthralgias	HSP, SLE
Diarrhea (± bloody)	HUS
Cough, hemoptysis	Vasculitis
Hearing loss	Alport disease
Nail or patellar abnormalities	Nail patella syndrome
Sickle cell disease	Glomerulonephritis, papillary necrosis
Drugs (diuretics, cyclophosphamide)	Stones, hemorrhagic cystitis
Birth asphyxia	Renal vein thrombosis
Physical Findings	
Suprapubic pain	UTI
Flank pain	IgAN, stones, renal vein thrombosis, pyelonephritis
Rash (purpura, petechiae)	HSP, SLE, HUS, bleeding dyscrasia, abuse
Edema	Glomerulonephritis, nephrotic syndrome
Abdominal mass	Wilms tumor, hydronephrosis, cystic kidney disease
Conjunctivitis, pharyngitis	Adenovirus (hemorrhagic cystitis)
Meatal stenosis	Infection, trauma
Nail or patellar abnormalities	Nail patella syndrome
Family History	
Hematuria	Benign familial hematuria, thin basement membrane disease
Hearing loss or prominent history of renal failure in males	Alport syndrome
Cystic kidney disease	Autosomal dominant polycystic kidney disease
Nail/patellar abnormalities	Nail patella syndrome
Sickle cell disease or trait	

Abbreviations: HSP, Henoch-Schönlein purpura; HUS, hemolytic-uremic syndrome; IgAN, immunoglobulin A nephropathy; SLE, systemic lupus erythematosus; UTI, urinary tract infection.

Reprinted with permission from Massengil SF. Hematuria. *Pediatr Rev.* 2008;29(10):345

Urinary tract infection, meatal/perineal irritation, trauma, crystalluria, and nephrolithiasis are common causes of gross hematuria in children. The presence of blood clots with dysuria indicates cystitis. Cystitis, or inflammation of the urinary bladder, may occur alone (uncomplicated) or in association with pyelonephritis (complicated). One of the most important risk factors for the development of acute cystitis, especially in female patients, is sexual intercourse. Risk factors for cystitis with pyelonephritis include anatomic or physiologic abnormalities associated with incomplete bladder emptying, indwelling urinary catheters, and associated diagnoses such as malignancy or diabetes mellitus. Bacteria from the intestinal tract colonize the periurethral area and urinary tract (eg, bacteria, fungi, viruses, parasites), and are the usual etiologic agents for cystitis. Gram-negative bacteria, such as *Escherichia coli*, account for nearly 90% of cases of uncomplicated cystitis.

Children presenting with asymptomatic gross hematuria usually require evaluation for the underlying etiology (Item C131B). This includes a urinalysis with microscopy (to differentiate between RBC and heme pigments), urine calcium-creatinine ratio (for hypercalciuria), serum creatinine and C3 levels (for nephritis), renal ultrasonography (for congenital anomalies or bladder mass), and hemoglobin electrophoresis (for sickle cell disease). The adolescent boy in the vignette has asymptomatic bright red hematuria of 1 day's duration, suggestive of lower urinary tract bleeding. The differential diagnosis for this child includes infection (cystitis), hypercalciuria, congenital renal anomalies, or bladder mass.

Cystoscopy is rarely indicated for children presenting with hematuria (gross or microscopic); it is helpful in evaluating patients with a bladder mass identified on ultrasonography or a history of urethral trauma. In cases of gross hematuria associated with a history of trauma, computed tomography (CT) of the abdomen and pelvis is indicated. Children with nephrolithiasis may present with varying degrees of flank pain; discomfort with the severe colicky pain radiating to the flank is most commonly seen with large and/or obstructing calculi. These children may have dysuria with associated infection or hypercalciuria. Renal ultrasonography is the preferred initial imaging modality for suspected nephrolithiasis. Although spiral CT is the most sensitive test for renal stones, the risk of radiation exposure must be balanced with the benefit of detecting small stones that might be missed on renal ultrasonography.

Children with a history of perineal and meatal irritation may present with gross hematuria; management includes supportive care and reassurance. Children with glomerulonephritis may present with edema or a history suggestive of an underlying autoimmune disorder (joint pains and swelling, fatigue, malaise, oral ulcers, or skin rash).

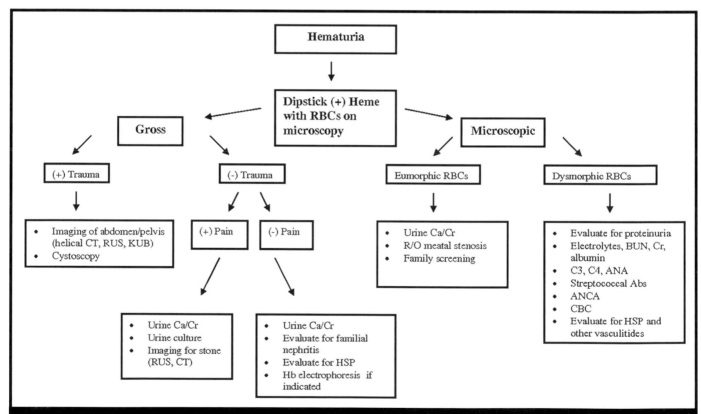

Reprinted with permission from Massengil SF. Hematuria. *Pediatr Rev.* 2008;29(10):344.

Item C131B: Algorithm for evaluation of hematuria. Abbreviations: ANA, antinuclear antibody; ANCA, antineutrophil cytoplasmic antibody; Abs, antibodies; BUN, blood urea nitrogen; C, complement; Ca, calcium; CBC, complete blood count; Cr, creatinine; CT, computed tomography scan; HSP, Henoch-Schönlein purpura; Hb, hemoglobin; KUB, kidney ureter-bladder radiograph; RBC, red blood cell; R/O, rule out; RUS, renal ultrasonography.

American Board of Pediatrics Content Specification(s)/ Content Area

- Plan the appropriate clinical evaluation of red urine of non-hematogenous origin
- Formulate a differential diagnosis of gross hematuria
- Recognize the disorders associated with hematuria
- Plan the appropriate clinical evaluation of gross hematuria

Suggested Readings

Massengil SF. Hematuria. *Pediatr Rev.* 2008;29(10):342-348.

Item 132   **Preferred Response: D**

The patient in this vignette has pericarditis, for which nonsteroidal anti-inflammatory drugs (NSAIDs) are the treatment of choice.

The etiology of acute pericarditis can be viral, bacterial, rheumatologic, idiopathic, drug induced, or oncologic. Acute pericarditis can also be caused by uremia or occur after cardiac surgery. Viral causes include coxsackievirus, echovirus, adenovirus, Epstein-Barr virus, influenza virus, and HIV. Patients with viral pericarditis can have myocardial involvement. Bacterial pericarditis can be caused by *Staphylococcus aureus*, *Haemophilus influenzae*, and tuberculosis. Patients with bacterial pericarditis can be quite toxic.

Regardless of the underlying etiology, acute pericarditis presents with chest pain that is typically substernal and sharp. The pain is exacerbated by inspiration and often improved by sitting upright and leaning forward. Some patients experience scapular pain given the involvement of the phrenic nerve. A pericardial friction rub is pathognomonic but not found in every patient. It is a scratchy, high-pitched, to-and-fro sound caused by the pericardial surfaces rubbing together. Markers of inflammation, such as white blood cell count, erythrocyte sedimentation rate, and C-reactive protein level, are typically elevated. Patients with myocardial involvement can have elevated troponin levels.

Electrocardiography can reveal classic findings including diffuse ST segment elevation and PR segment depression initially, followed by normalization of these findings, then widespread T-wave inversions and finally normalization of the T waves. If there is a large pericardial effusion, electrocardiography may demonstrate low-voltage QRS complexes. Chest radiography can have normal findings or show lung or mediastinal disease (from an underlying cause) or cardiomegaly in the case of a large pericardial effusion. Echocardiography can have normal findings or demonstrate a pericardial effusion.

Management of pericarditis includes diagnosing and managing any underlying cause. The typical frontline pharmacologic therapy is NSAIDs to treat the associated chest pain

and inflammation. For persistent pain or effusion, colchicine is an accepted next step in therapy. Some providers will use glucocorticoids for chronic pain, inflammation, or effusion that persists after use of NSAIDs and/or colchicine.

There is no role for cardiac catheterization in the management of pericarditis. Glucocorticoids are not a first-line therapeutic option in pericarditis but may have a role when NSAIDs and colchicine have failed. Intravenous immunoglobulin may have a role in the treatment of myocarditis but not pericarditis.

American Board of Pediatrics Content Specification(s)/ Content Area

- Recognize pathogens commonly associated with pericarditis
- Recognize the clinical findings associated with pericarditis and plan appropriate initial management
- Understand the natural history of pericarditis

Suggested Readings

Blanco CC, Parekh JB. Pericarditis. *Pediatr Rev.* 2010;31(2):83-84.

Reddy SR, Singh HR. Chest pain in children and adolescents. *Pediatr Rev.* 2010;31(1):e1-e9.

Item 133   **Preferred Response: A**

This vignette provides an example of a scenario where confidentiality cannot be maintained. The patient has been drinking alcohol regularly, driving intoxicated, and has no insight into his behavior and how it may affect himself and others. In the provider's opinion, this is potential harm to self (alcohol poisoning or a motor vehicle collision while intoxicated) and potential harm to others (driving intoxicated). In this situation, it would be appropriate to break confidentiality and discuss the alcohol abuse with the patient's mother so that resources can be provided to assist the patient. It is unlikely for any adolescent to follow through with treatments or services without parental involvement if they do not believe they have a health-related issue.

The other response choices are reasonable, but will not protect this adolescent's health and safety. Making a safety contract with an adolescent who feels he has control over his behavior and no insight into his situation will not ensure he stops drinking and driving. The contract may be signed in effort to convince the provider to not disclose information to a parent. A blood alcohol level and urine toxicology screen could provide useful information in regard to how much the patient is drinking as well as if other substances are being used. This could provide further evidence in support of an intervention and the need for parental involvement. Lastly, providing brochures on drug and alcohol rehabilitation programs to an adolescent with no concern for his behavior is unlikely to make a significant impact.

Confidentiality is the protection of personal information and an important concept in caring for adolescents. Providers who take care of adolescent patients must be aware of federal and state laws regarding the protection of confidential health information and informed consent. Confidentiality should be explained at the beginning of an initial health care visit so that both the patient and parent are aware that it is recommended the provider speak to an adolescent alone, and that the conversation is considered confidential. Parents should be informed that the purpose of the confidential interview is not to alienate them, but to build trust between the provider and the adolescent. This trust is crucial because if the adolescent does not feel secure that health-related information they share with the physician will be kept in confidence, they may not answer questions honestly, seek medical care, or develop trust in the health care system. Adolescents and parents should be encouraged to foster open lines of communication with one another to discuss topics that may be uncomfortable.

There are circumstances in which confidentiality must be broken, and it is important that the adolescent and parent are aware of situations in which this may occur. Situations that may require a breach of confidentiality include harm to self (ie, suicide), harm to others (ie, homicide), or harm inflicted by others (ie, physical or sexual abuse).

Health care providers are mandated reporters, for minors, of the following:

- Child abuse or endangerment (physical, sexual, or emotional abuse)
- Consensual sex (dependent on state laws), based on age at first sexual activity; age difference between partners; and, in certain states (eg, Texas), if partners are the same sex
- Suicidal thoughts or attempts
- Homicidal thoughts or attempts
- Sexually transmitted infections (state health departments)
- Injuries from criminal acts such as gunshot and stab wounds
- Parental notification for specific medical services such as abortion in certain states (eg, Texas)

It helps to be transparent with the adolescent that there are other circumstances when confidentiality cannot be maintained based on the provider's judgement or circumstances outside of the provider's control. It is the provider's responsibility to disclose to the adolescent that confidentiality needs to be broken if there is a perceived threat to their health and safety and that it is not a punishment. A breach in confidentiality should only occur in effort to benefit the adolescent. Circumstances outside of the provider's control in which confidential information may be shared include parents gaining access to medical records, billing statements that document tests that have been ordered, and communication from insurance companies. The adolescent should be involved in how information is shared with a parent, who shares the information, and how much detail is disclosed if confidentiality cannot be maintained. Some adolescents will become angered with the provider that confidential information will be shared with a parent, while others will be relieved that a dialogue will be started so that they can get help pertaining to their particular need.

PREP Pearls

- A breach in confidentiality should only be done to benefit the health or safety of an adolescent or if there is concern about harm to others.
- Adolescents are more likely to disclose information to providers who discuss confidentiality.
- Be transparent regarding situations that warrant a breach in confidentiality. Laws regarding confidentiality may vary by state.

American Board of Pediatrics Content Specification(s)/Content Area

- Understand when a parent must be notified about an adolescent's medical condition

Suggested Readings

Ford C, English A, Sigman G. Confidential health care for adolescents: position paper of the Society for Adolescent Medicine. *J Adolesc Health.* 2004;35(2):160-167.

Levy SJ, Williams JF; AAP Committee on Substance Use and Prevention. Substance use screening, brief intervention, and referral to treatment. *Pediatrics.* 2016;138(1):e20161211.

Item 134 **Preferred Response: A**

The child in the vignette has suffered a severe traumatic brain injury. Despite maximal medical and surgical therapy, he shows no brain activity. The formal clinical examination for brain death, including physical examination and apnea test, was consistent with brain death. This was repeated 12 hours later with the same results. With this information, death by neurologic criteria (ie, brain death) should be declared.

Throughout most of human existence, death occurred after the cessation of breathing and circulation. Several decades ago, with the advent of mechanical ventilation and contemporary critical care, it became possible to sustain organ function for long periods without any brain function and thus without any capacity to participate in the human experience. In 1968, a committee from Harvard University published a report on the "irreversible coma." The report's recommendations were gradually adopted by many institutions and evolved into what is now known as brain death criteria. In 1981, the United States President's Commission released the Uniform Determination of Death Act (UDDA) establishing 2 paths to the determination of death, 1) by neurologic criteria or 2) by circulatory criteria. Death was defined as either the irreversible cessation of circulatory or respiratory functions or irreversible cessation of all functions of the entire brain, including the brainstem.

The American Academy of Pediatrics published formal guidelines for determining brain death in children and neonates in 1987, with an update in 2011. Prerequisites for brain death testing include an absence of neurologic function with a known, irreversible cause of coma. A potentially treatable cause of coma, such as hypotension, hypothermia, toxic substances, metabolic disturbances, sedatives, or neuromuscular blocking agents, must not be present. Electrolytes out of the normal range and antiepileptic medications within the therapeutic range may be present, as long as they are not likely to affect the results of the examination. Two independent examinations, each including a physical examination and apnea test, are required to make the declaration of brain death. The examinations must occur 12 hours apart for infants and children between 31 days and 18 years of age and 24 hours apart for term neonates of 37 weeks of gestation up to 30 days of age. Details on how to conduct the clinical examination and apnea test are shown in Item C134.

Item C134. Brain death examination for infants and children.

Brain Death Examination for Infants and Children
Two physicians must perform independent examinations separated by specified intervals.

Age of Patient	Timing of first exam	Inter-exam. interval
Term newborn 37 weeks gestational age and up to 30 days old	☐ First exam may be performed 24 hours after birth OR following cardiopulmonary resuscitation or other severe brain injury	☐ At least 24 hours ☐ Interval shortened because ancillary study (section 4) is consistent with brain death
31 days to 18 years old	☐ First exam may be performed 24 hours following cardiopulmonary resuscitation or other severe brain injury	☐ At least 12 hours OR ☐ Interval shortened because ancillary study (section 4) is consistent with brain death

Section 1. PREREQUISITES for brain death examination and apnea test

A. IRREVERSIBLE AND IDENTIFIABLE Cause of Coma (Please check)

☐ Traumatic brain injury   ☐ Anoxic brain injury   ☐ Known metabolic disorder   ☐ Other (Specify)

B. Correction of contributing factors that can interfere with the neurologic examination	Examination One		Examination Two	
a. Core Body Temp is over 95° F (35° C)	☐ Yes	☐ No	☐ Yes	☐ No
b. Systolic blood pressure or MAP in acceptable range (Systolic BP not less than 2 standard deviations below age appropriate norm) based on age	☐ Yes	☐ No	☐ Yes	☐ No
c. Sedative/analgesic drug effect excluded as a contributing factor	☐ Yes	☐ No	☐ Yes	☐ No
d. Metabolic intoxication excluded as a contributing factor	☐ Yes	☐ No	☐ Yes	☐ No
e. Neuromuscular blockade excluded as a contributing factor	☐ Yes	☐ No	☐ Yes	☐ No

☐ If ALL prerequisites are marked YES, then proceed to section 2, OR
☐ _____ confounding variable was present. Ancillary study was therefore performed to document brain death. (Section 4).

Section 2. Physical Examination (Please check) NOTE: SPINAL CORD REFLEXES ARE ACCEPTABLE	Examination One Date/ time:		Examination Two Date/ Time:	
a. Flaccid tone, patient unresponsive to deep painful stimuli	☐ Yes	☐ No	☐ Yes	☐ No
b. Pupils are midposition or fully dilated and light reflexes are absent	☐ Yes	☐ No	☐ Yes	☐ No
c. Corneal, cough, gag reflexes are absent	☐ Yes	☐ No	☐ Yes	☐ No
Sucking and rooting reflexes are absent (in neonates and infants)	☐ Yes	☐ No	☐ Yes	☐ No
d. Oculovestibular reflexes are absent	☐ Yes	☐ No	☐ Yes	☐ No
e. Spontaneous respiratory effort while on mechanical ventilation is absent	☐ Yes	☐ No	☐ Yes	☐ No

☐ The _____ (specify) element of the exam could not be performed because _____.
Ancillary study (EEG or radionuclide CBF) was therefore performed to document brain death. (Section 4).

Section 3. APNEA Test	Examination One Date/ Time	Examination Two Date/ Time
No spontaneous respiratory efforts were observed despite final PaCO$_2$ ≥ 60 mm Hg and a ≥ 20 mm Hg increase above baseline. (Examination One) No spontaneous respiratory efforts were observed despite final PaCO$_2$ ≥ 60 mm Hg and a ≥ 20 mm Hg increase above baseline. (Examination Two)	Pretest PaCO$_2$: _____ Apnea duration: _____ min Posttest PaCO$_2$: _____	Pretest PaCO$_2$: _____ Apnea duration: _____ min Posttest PaCO$_2$: _____

Apnea test is contraindicated or could not be performed to completion because _____.
Ancillary study (EEG or radionuclide CBF) was therefore performed to document brain death. (Section 4).

Section 4. ANCILLARY testing is required when (1) any components of the examination or apnea testing cannot be completed; (2) if there is uncertainty about the results of the neurologic examination; or (3) if a medication effect may be present. Ancillary testing can be performed to reduce the inter-examination period however a second neurologic examination is required. Components of the neurologic examination that can be performed safely should be completed in close proximity to the ancillary test	Date/Time: _____	
☐ Electroencephalogram (EEG) report documents electrocerebral silence OR	☐ Yes	☐ No
☐ Cerebral Blood Flow(CBF) study report documents no cerebral perfusion	☐ Yes	☐ No

Section 5. Signatures

Examiner One

I certify that my examination is consistent with cessation of function of the brain and brainstem. Confirmatory exam to follow.

_____   _____
(Printed Name)   (Signature)

_____   _____   _____   _____
(Specialty)   (Pager #/License #)   (Date mm/dd/yyyy)   (Time)

Examiner Two

☐ I certify that my examination☐ and/or ancillary test report ☐confirms unchanged and irreversible cessation of function of the brain and brainstem. The patient is declared brain dead at this time.
Date/Time of death: _____

_____   _____
(Printed Name)   (Signature)

_____   _____   _____   _____
(Specialty)   (Pager #/License #)   (Date mm/dd/yyyy)   (Time)

Reprinted with permission from Nakagawa TA, Ashwal S, Mathur M, Mysore M; Society of Critical Care Medicine, Section on Critical Care and Section on Neurology of American Academy of Pediatrics; Child Neurology Society. Guidelines for the determination of brain death in infants and children: an update of the 1987 task force recommendations. *Pediatrics.* 2011;128(3):e735

Both physical examinations and apnea tests for the boy in the vignette are consistent with brain death, therefore, death should be declared. Ancillary testing, that is, cerebral blood flow scanning or electroencephalography, may be performed if any component of the physical examination or apnea testing cannot be performed. However, they should not be performed if the clinical testing can be completed, because results can conflict.

Recommending withdrawal of life-sustaining therapies is not the correct response, because death should be declared before that is done. Recovering organs for transplantation after brain death is appropriate, but only after declaring death and then obtaining consent from the family for organ recovery. Once death is declared, if organ retrieval is not planned, the machines sustaining breathing and circulation should be discontinued; no recommendation or consent is required.

PREP Pearls

- Brain death should be declared after 2 independent examinations, including a physical examination and apnea testing, are consistent with brain death.
- When determining brain death, ancillary testing, (ie, cerebral blood flow scanning and electroencephalography), should be performed only if any component of the physical examination or apnea testing cannot be performed.

American Board of Pediatrics Content Specification(s)/ Content Area

- Recognize and apply ethical decision-making when caring for critically ill patients
- Recognize and apply ethical principles surrounding the issue of brain death

Suggested Readings

Greer DM, Varelas P, Haque S, Wijdicks E. Variability of brain death determination guidelines in leading US neurologic institutions. *Neurology.* 2008;0:284-289.

Lewis A, Varelas P, Greer D. Prolonging support after brain death: when families ask for more. *Neurocrit Care.* 2016;24:481-487.

Nakagawa TA, Ashwal S, Mathur M, Mysore M; Society of Critical Care Medicine, Section on Critical Care and Section on Neurology of American Academy of Pediatrics; Child Neurology Society. Guidelines for the determination of brain death in infants and children: an update of the 1987 task force recommendations. *Pediatrics.* 2011;128:e720-e740.

Item 135   Preferred Response: C

The neonate in this vignette has Stickler syndrome, a connective tissue disorder otherwise known as hereditary arthro-ophthalmopathy. Patients typically have characteristic orofacial anomalies, including a flattened midface, depressed nasal bridge, short nose, anteverted nares, and micrognathia. Palatal abnormalities, including cleft lip, cleft palate, and/or bifid uvula, may be seen. Other associated symptoms include severe myopia, cataracts, retinal detachment, hearing loss, and joint hypermobility. Stickler syndrome is not associated with atrial septal defects, agenesis of the corpus callosum, or hydronephrosis.

The embryonic palate develops between the 4th and 13th weeks of gestation, as neural crest cells migrate and cause fusion of the facial prominences. Palatal clefts can involve the soft palate, hard palate, and/or alveolar ridge. Clefts can be syndromic (ie, associated with additional structural abnormalities arising away from the palate or with a known syndrome) or nonsyndromic (ie, isolated). Patients with a cleft palate may also have a cleft lip. Although fewer than 15% of cleft lips are syndromic, roughly 50% of cleft palates that are not associated with a cleft lip are syndromic.

A bifid uvula may be a marker of an underlying submucosal cleft palate, in which the oral mucosa is intact but the underlying musculature is misaligned and not attached properly at the midline. Although most older infants, children, and adults with a submucosal cleft palate are asymptomatic, some will present with velopharyngeal insufficiency and associated speech abnormalities. Neonates with submucosal cleft palates may have feeding difficulties and poor weight gain because of an inability to generate sufficient negative pressure when breastfeeding. Bifid uvula can also be associated with Loeys-Dietz syndrome and 22q11 deletion syndrome.

PREP Pearls

- A bifid uvula may be a marker of an underlying submucosal cleft palate. Submucosal cleft palates can cause breastfeeding difficulties and poor weight gain in neonates and velopharyngeal insufficiency and associated speech abnormalities in older children and adults.
- Stickler syndrome is a connective tissue disorder characterized by ocular abnormalities (myopia, cataracts, and/or retinal detachment), midface abnormalities (flattened midface, depressed nasal bridge, short nose, anteverted nares, micrognathia, and cleft palate), hearing loss, and joint hypermobility.

American Board of Pediatrics Content Specification(s)/ Content Area

- Identify conditions associated with a bifid uvula

Suggested Readings

Burg ML, Chai Y, Yao CA, Magee W, Figueiredo JC. Epidemiology, etiology, and treatment of isolated cleft palate. *Front Physiol.* 2016;7:67.

Khan M, Ullah H, Naz S, et al. A revised classification of the cleft lip and palate. *Can J Plastic Surg.* 2013;21(1):48-50.

Robin NH, Moran RT, Ala-Kokko L. Stickler syndrome. *GeneReviews.*

Item 136   Preferred Response: B

Ocular toxocariasis is the most likely diagnosis in the girl described in the vignette, based on her unilateral vision loss, retinal lesion, eosinophilia, history of geophagia, and contact with puppies. Ocular toxocariasis (also called "ocular larva migrans") is caused by the zoonotic parasite *Toxocara canis* (dog roundworm), and less commonly, *Toxocara cati* (cat roundworm). The disease is endemic throughout the United States, affecting up to 14% of the population; the prevalence of symptomatic disease among seropositive individuals is unknown.

Dogs and cats are the primary hosts for *Toxocara*, with humans acting as incidental hosts. The infection is acquired when children unintentionally ingest eggs that were excreted in the soil (eg, sandboxes, playgrounds) by infected puppies. *Toxocara* eggs become infective within 2 to 4 weeks and can remain viable in soil for months to years, especially in hot, humid environments. Other risk factors for infection include contact with puppies or a history of pica. An uncommon infection, toxocariasis typically affects children because of their poor hygiene and play habits. After ingestion, *Toxocara* eggs hatch and release larvae that penetrate the intestinal mucosa and migrate to the liver, lungs, heart, muscle (visceral larva migrans), and eyes (ocular larva migrans). The larval migration into tissues is associated with a severe inflammatory response, producing clinical symptoms and eosinophilia.

The clinical spectrum of toxocariasis can range from asymptomatic infection in most cases to 2 well-defined syndromes, visceral larva migrans (VLM) and ocular larva migrans (OLM).Children with VLM are usually younger (2-7 years of age) than children with OLM. Ocular larva migrans commonly presents with unilateral vision loss or strabismus without systemic symptoms. Common ophthalmologic signs of OLM include chorioretinitis, subretinal granulomatous mass/scar, vitritis, scotoma endophthalmitis, motile chorioretinal nematode, optic papillitis, and keratitis. Ocular disease can be severe, resulting in permanent vision loss. Children with VLM often present with fever, abdominal pain, cough, or wheezing. Clinical and laboratory manifestations include hepatomegaly, leukocytosis, persistent eosinophilia, and hypergammaglobulinemia. Eosinophilia is less common in OLM than VLM. Rare manifestations include pneumonia, myocarditis, and meningoencephalitis.

In suspected cases of OLM or VLM, the diagnosis may be confirmed by serology using an enzyme immunoassay to detect *Toxocara* antibodies in serum, though a positive test result does not necessarily indicate current, active infection. Toxocara enzyme immunoassay has been reported to have a sensitivity of 78% and a specificity of 92% at a titer of 1:32 or higher. It is less sensitive for the diagnosis of OLM. In rare instances, the definitive diagnosis of toxocariasis is made by detection of the larvae in tissue biopsy specimens (eg, liver).

Treatment options for OLM include topical or systemic corticosteroids to reduce inflammation, and surgery. Antiparasitic therapy may be used, but may not result in eradication of the parasite from the eyes. In contrast, for patients with VLM, albendazole is the recommended treatment; systemic corticosteroids may be considered in severe disease (eg, myocarditis).

Measures to reduce the risk of toxocariasis include good hand hygiene after soil contact, timely disposal of pet feces, routine deworming of dogs and cats, and increased awareness of the disease among pet owners. There is no role for prophylactic antiparasitic therapy for exposed people. Toxocariasis is regarded as one of the neglected parasitic infections and is currently targeted by the Centers for Disease Control and Prevention for public health action.

Other parasitic infections including cysticercosis, trichuriasis, and trichinosis can cause moderate to severe secondary eosinophilia, but the clinical presentation of the child described in the vignette is most consistent with a diagnosis of ocular toxocariasis.

PREP Pearls

- Manifestations of ocular toxocariasis include chorioretinitis, subretinal granulomatous mass/scar, vitritis, scotoma, and endophthalmitis.
- Ocular larva migrans should be suspected in a child who presents with unilateral vision loss and retinal lesions with a history of contact with dogs (especially puppies).
- Ocular toxocariasis (also called ocular larva migrans) is caused most commonly by the zoonotic parasites *Toxocara canis* (dog roundworm).

American Board of Pediatrics Content Specification(s)/ Content Area

- Understand the epidemiology of *Toxocara*
- Recognize the clinical features associated with *Toxocara* infestation

Suggested Readings

American Academy of Pediatrics. Toxocariasis, ocular toxocariasis. In: Kimberlin DW, Brady MT, Jackson MA, Long SS, eds. *Red Book: 2018 Report of the Committee on Infectious Diseases*. 31st ed. Itasca, IL: American Academy of Pediatrics; 2018:808-809.

Centers for Disease Control and Prevention (CDC). Ocular toxocariasis—United States, 2009-2010. *MMWR Morb Mortal Wkly Rep*. 2011;60:734-736.

Woodhall DM, Fiore AE. Toxocariasis: a review for pediatricians. *J Pediatric Infect Dis Soc*. 2014;3:154-159.

Item 137   Preferred Response: D

The neonate in the vignette has evidence of a butterfly vertebra, patent foramen ovale, esophageal atresia, and an abnormal digit. The most likely diagnosis is VACTERL, an association of *v*ertebral anomalies, *a*nal atresia, *c*ardiac anomalies, *t*racheo*e*sophageal fistula, *r*enal anomalies, and *l*imb anomalies. VACTERL is diagnosed based on the presence of 3 of these major anomalies. To date, no genetic mutation has been identified for the VACTERL association.

During normal development, at 4 weeks, the foregut separates into the dorsal and ventral foregut. Esophageal atresia (EA) occurs when there is improper separation of the esophagus from the trachea. Esophageal atresia most commonly occurs with a tracheoesophageal fistula. Neonates with EA typically present with poor feeding, nonbilious emesis, and increased oral secretions. To diagnose EA, a nasogastric tube should be inserted and a lateral radiograph obtained to document the tube's position in the esophageal pouch.

CHARGE syndrome is characterized by *c*oloboma, *h*eart defect, *a*tresia choanae, *r*etarded growth, *g*enitourinary abnormality, and *e*ar anomalies. The clinical diagnosis is based on the presence of 4 of the aforementioned major criteria or 3 major and 3 minor criteria. It is caused by a mutation in the *CHD7* gene and is inherited in an autosomal dominant manner.

22q11.2 deletion syndrome (with varying presentations previously labeled as DiGeorge syndrome, Shprintzen syndrome, velocardiofacial syndrome, and conotruncal anomaly face syndrome) is characterized by cardiac anomalies, hypoparathyroidism, abnormal palate, and immune dysfunction. Affected children may have developmental delays and are at risk for psychiatric disorders such as schizophrenia in adulthood.

Fanconi anemia is characterized by pancytopenia and short stature. Affected children may also have café au lait spots (55%) and upper limb anomalies (43%). Fanconi anemia is inherited in an autosomal recessive manner and results from chromosomal fragility.

American Board of Pediatrics Content Specification(s)/ Content Area

- Recognize the clinical and laboratory features associated with tracheoesopheal fistula in a newborn infant

Suggested Readings

Hudson A, Trider CL, Blake K. CHARGE syndrome. *Pediatr Rev.* 2017;38;56.

Pereira E, Marion R. Chromosome 22q11.2 deletion syndrome. *Pediatr Rev.* 2015;36;270.

Ross AJ. Intestinal obstruction in the newborn. *Pediatr Rev.* 1994;15;338.

PREP Pearls

- Esophageal atresia typically presents with poor feeding, nonbilious emesis, and increased oral secretions.
- Most neonates with esophageal atresia also have a tracheoesophageal fistula.
- VACTERL association consists of *v*ertebral anomalies, *a*nal atresia, *c*ardiac defects, *t*racheo*e*sophageal atresia, *r*enal anomalies and *l*imb anomalies.

Item 138   **Preferred Response: A**

The boy in this vignette most likely has moderate persistent asthma based on his constellation of symptoms in conjunction with an obstructive pattern on spirometry. A forced expiratory volume in 1 second of less than 80% predicted for age in the presence of a normal forced vital capacity defines moderate persistent asthma per the most recent guidelines. Use of inhaled corticosteroids is the most effective first-line management for persistent asthma of any severity. Second-line or additive management might include a leukotriene modifier.

Asthma Action Plan

For: _____ Doctor: _____ Date: _____

Doctor's Phone Number_____ Hospital/Emergency Department Phone Number _____

GREEN ZONE

Doing Well

- No cough, wheeze, chest tightness, or shortness of breath during the day or night
- Can do usual activities

And, if a peak flow meter is used,

Peak flow: more than _____
(80 percent or more of my best peak flow)

My best peak flow is: _____

Before exercise

Take these long-term control medicines each day (include an anti-inflammatory).

Medicine	How much to take	When to take it
□ _____	□ 2 or □ 4 puffs_____	5 minutes before exercise

YELLOW ZONE

Asthma Is Getting Worse

- Cough, wheeze, chest tightness, or shortness of breath, or
- Waking at night due to asthma, or
- Can do some, but not all, usual activities

-Or-

Peak flow: _____ to _____
(50 to 79 percent of my best peak flow)

First Add: quick-relief medicine—and keep taking your GREEN ZONE medicine.
_____ (short-acting beta₂-agonist) □ 2 or □ 4 puffs, every 20 minutes for up to 1 hour □ Nebulizer, once

Second If your symptoms (and peak flow, if used) return to GREEN ZONE after 1 hour of above treatment:
□ Continue monitoring to be sure you stay in the green zone.

-Or-

If your symptoms (and peak flow, if used) do not return to GREEN ZONE after 1 hour of above treatment:
□ Take:_____ (short-acting beta₂-agonist) □ 2 or □ 4 puffs or □ Nebulizer

□ Add:_____ (oral steroid) mg per day For _____(3–10) days

□ Call the doctor □ before/ □ within_____ hours after taking the oral steroid.

RED ZONE

Medical Alert!

- Very short of breath, or
- Quick-relief medicines have not helped, or
- Cannot do usual activities, or
- Symptoms are same or get worse after 24 hours in Yellow Zone

-Or-

Peak flow: less than _____
(50 percent of my best peak flow)

Take this medicine:

□ _____ (short-acting beta₂-agonist) □ 4 or □ 6 puffs or □ Nebulizer

□ _____ (oral steroid) mg

Then call your doctor NOW. Go to the hospital or call an ambulance if:
- You are still in the red zone after 15 minutes AND
- You have not reached your doctor.

DANGER SIGNS
- Trouble walking and talking due to shortness of breath
- Lips or fingernails are blue

- Take □ 4 or □ 6 puffs of your quick-relief medicine AND
- Go to the hospital or call for an ambulance _____ NOW!
  (phone)

See the reverse side for things you can do to avoid your asthma triggers.

Reprinted from the National Institutes of Health

Item C138-1: Asthma Action Plan template.

Leukotriene modifiers may be used as primary treatment for mild persistent asthma in situations where parents refuse inhaled steroids or where the child will not use a metered-dose inhaler or nebulizer for steroids. It is also appropriate as secondary or add-on therapy for more severe asthma, especially in the context of allergy as comorbidity.

Oral albuterol is not indicated as a controller therapy for persistent asthma and is rarely used as rescue therapy. Albuterol can be delivered by inhalation with equal or greater efficacy and fewer adverse effects as a rescue medication.

Although this boy has symptoms of upper respiratory allergies, and allergen exposure may be playing a role in the severity of his asthma, use of topical nasal steroids or oral antihistamines is not the primary intervention for his asthma.

In addition to providing pharmacotherapy and an explanation of medication actions and appropriate uses, this child and his family should also understand what his triggers are and how to avoid them, as well as have a written asthma action plan and education regarding asthma physiology.

Additionally, families may appreciate visual aids that serve as reminders. Examples of these tools are shown in Item C138-1 and Item C138-2.

PREP Pearls

- Inhaled corticosteroids are the most effective primary controller therapy for asthma of any severity.
- Leukotriene modifiers may be used as primary treatment for mild persistent asthma or as secondary or add-on therapy for more severe asthma, especially in the context of allergy as comorbidity.

American Board of Pediatrics Content Specification(s)/ Content Area

- Understand the role of leukotriene antagonists in the management of asthma
- Plan appropriate outpatient management of a patient with asthma (eg, self-assessment, education, pulmonary function testing, drug therapy, asthma action plans)

How To Control Things That Make Your Asthma Worse

This guide suggests things you can do to avoid your asthma triggers. Put a check next to the triggers that you know make your asthma worse and ask your doctor to help you find out if you have other triggers as well. Then decide with your doctor what steps you will take.

Allergens

☐ **Animal Dander**
Some people are allergic to the flakes of skin or dried saliva from animals with fur or feathers.
The best thing to do:
- Keep furred or feathered pets out of your home.
If you can't keep the pet outdoors, then:
- Keep the pet out of your bedroom and other sleeping areas at all times, and keep the door closed.
- Remove carpets and furniture covered with cloth from your home. If that is not possible, keep the pet away from fabric-covered furniture and carpets.

☐ **Dust Mites**
Many people with asthma are allergic to dust mites. Dust mites are tiny bugs that are found in every home—in mattresses, pillows, carpets, upholstered furniture, bedcovers, clothes, stuffed toys, and fabric or other fabric-covered items.
Things that can help:
- Encase your mattress in a special dust-proof cover.
- Encase your pillow in a special dust-proof cover or wash the pillow each week in hot water. Water must be hotter than 130° F to kill the mites. Cold or warm water used with detergent and bleach can also be effective.
- Wash the sheets and blankets on your bed each week in hot water.
- Reduce indoor humidity to below 60 percent (ideally between 30—50 percent). Dehumidifiers or central air conditioners can do this.
- Try not to sleep or lie on cloth-covered cushions.
- Remove carpets from your bedroom and those laid on concrete, if you can.
- Keep stuffed toys out of the bed or wash the toys weekly in hot water or cooler water with detergent and bleach.

☐ **Cockroaches**
Many people with asthma are allergic to the dried droppings and remains of cockroaches.
The best thing to do:
- Keep food and garbage in closed containers. Never leave food out.
- Use poison baits, powders, gels, or paste (for example, boric acid). You can also use traps.
- If a spray is used to kill roaches, stay out of the room until the odor goes away.

☐ **Indoor Mold**
- Fix leaky faucets, pipes, or other sources of water that have mold around them.
- Clean moldy surfaces with a cleaner that has bleach in it.

☐ **Pollen and Outdoor Mold**
What to do during your allergy season (when pollen or mold spore counts are high):
- Try to keep your windows closed.
- Stay indoors with windows closed from late morning to afternoon, if you can. Pollen and some mold spore counts are highest at that time.
- Ask your doctor whether you need to take or increase anti-inflammatory medicine before your allergy season starts.

Irritants

☐ **Tobacco Smoke**
- If you smoke, ask your doctor for ways to help you quit. Ask family members to quit smoking, too.
- Do not allow smoking in your home or car.

☐ **Smoke, Strong Odors, and Sprays**
- If possible, do not use a wood-burning stove, kerosene heater, or fireplace.
- Try to stay away from strong odors and sprays, such as perfume, talcum powder, hair spray, and paints.

Other things that bring on asthma symptoms in some people include:

☐ **Vacuum Cleaning**
- Try to get someone else to vacuum for you once or twice a week, if you can. Stay out of rooms while they are being vacuumed and for a short while afterward.
- If you vacuum, use a dust mask (from a hardware store), a double-layered or microfilter vacuum cleaner bag, or a vacuum cleaner with a HEPA filter.

☐ **Other Things That Can Make Asthma Worse**
- Sulfites in foods and beverages: Do not drink beer or wine or eat dried fruit, processed potatoes, or shrimp if they cause asthma symptoms.
- Cold air: Cover your nose and mouth with a scarf on cold or windy days.
- Other medicines: Tell your doctor about all the medicines you take. Include cold medicines, aspirin, vitamins and other supplements, and nonselective beta-blockers (including those in eye drops).

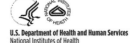
U.S. Department of Health and Human Services
National Institutes of Health

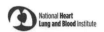
National Heart Lung and Blood Institute

For More Information, go to: www.nhlbi.nih.gov

NIH Publication No. 07-5251
April 2007

Item C138-2: Asthma Action Plan template.

Suggested Readings

Centers for Disease Control and Prevention. Asthma. http://www.cdc.gov/asthma.

National Asthma Education and Prevention Program. *Expert Panel Report 3: Guidelines for the Diagnosis and Management of Asthma, Summary Report 2007.* Bethesda, MD: National Institutes of Health; 2007. NIH publication 08-5846.

Wood PR, Hill VL. Practical management of asthma. *Pediatr Rev.* 2009; 30(10):375-385.

Item 139	Preferred Response: C

The adolescent boy in this vignette has Klinefelter syndrome, which occurs in about 1 of 600 male newborns and is diagnosed by a karyotype showing 47,XXY. The patient's history of language delay, tall stature for his family, low upper-to-lower segment ratio (relatively long legs), and abnormal puberty are consistent with Klinefelter syndrome. In early adolescence, a normal upper-to-lower segment ratio is around 1. (The lower segment is measured from the pubic symphysis to the floor. The upper segment is calculated by subtracting the lower segment from total height). Individuals with Klinefelter syndrome have disproportionately long legs and are at higher risk for language delay and learning problems. Primary testicular failure (primary hypogonadism) with small firm testes and abnormal puberty are prominent features of Klinefelter syndrome. Accordingly, pubic hair development for the patient in this vignette is discordant with his testicular development. His pubic hair development is primarily a manifestation of adrenarche and adrenal androgen secretion, rather than testosterone secretion from the testes. Gynecomastia occurs secondary to the hypogonadism.

Echocardiography would aid in the diagnosis of Marfan syndrome, a connective tissue disorder caused by mutations in *FBN1*, which encodes the fibrillin-1 protein. Marfan syndrome can affect the aortic root, causing enlargement and even aortic dissection. Features of Marfan syndrome include a tall, thin body habitus and long arms (arm span is greater than height), legs, and fingers (arachnodactyly), as well as other skeletal abnormalities (eg, scoliosis, pectus abnormality, crowded teeth), hyperflexibility, striae, and eye abnormalities (eg, myopia, dislocated lens). Marfan syndrome occurs in about 1 of 5,000 people.

An insulin-like growth factor-1 (IGF-1) level would aid in the diagnosis of growth hormone excess. Growth hormone–secreting pituitary adenomas are rare in pediatrics. The high levels of growth hormone result in increased IGF-1 production in the liver. Measurement of IGF-1 is preferable given its greater stability compared to random growth hormone levels.

A serum homocysteine level would aid in the diagnosis of homocystinuria. Classic homocystinuria is a rare metabolic disorder affecting about 1 in 200,000 people. It is caused by accumulation of homocysteine from a lack of cystathionine β-synthase activity. The excess homocysteine and its metabolites result in clinical manifestations including myopia, lens dislocation, osteopenia, intellectual disability, developmental delays, seizures, failure to thrive in early childhood, and megaloblastic anemia. A tall, thin body habitus with long, arms, legs, and fingers is characteristic of individuals with homocystinuria.

Other etiologies of tall stature include precocious puberty, familial tall stature, and other genetic syndromes (eg, Sotos syndrome). Precocious puberty causes early growth acceleration and tall stature during childhood, but final adult height may be compromised because of early cessation of growth. Familial tall stature is tall stature that is consistent with the genetic potential of having tall parents. It is the most common etiology of tall stature. These children are otherwise healthy and grow with normal height velocity along a height percentile as expected for their parents' heights.

The evaluation of tall stature should include a history of birth size, any developmental abnormalities, and parents' heights and pubertal timing. Physical examination should include examination of the growth chart, evaluation of body proportions (upper-to-lower segment ratio, arm span), pubertal staging, presence of gynecomastia, and search for evidence of an underlying genetic condition (skeletal abnormalities, striae, dysmorphic features). A bone age radiograph can help to narrow the differential diagnosis. Laboratory evaluation and further testing should be directed by patient history and physical examination findings.

PREP Pearls

- Familial tall stature is the most common etiology of tall stature.
- Features of Klinefelter syndrome include tall stature with disproportionately long legs, primary hypogonadism with small firm testes, gynecomastia, and language delay.

American Board of Pediatrics Content Specification(s)/Content Area

- Differentiate among the causes of tall stature
- Plan the appropriate diagnostic evaluation of tall stature

Suggested Readings

Albuquerque EV, Scalco RC, Jorge AA. Management of endocrine disease: diagnostic and therapeutic approach of tall stature. *Eur J Endocrinol.* 2017;176(6):R339-R353.

Braun LR, Marino R. Disorders of growth and stature. *Pediatr Rev.* 2017;38(7):293-304.

Zargham S, Crotty JE. Tall stature. *Pediatr Rev.* 2014;35(12):538-539.

Item 140	Preferred Response: B

The girl in the vignette has 22q11.2 deletion syndrome, also known as velocardiofacial syndrome or DiGeorge syndrome. Hypocalcemia occurs in 17% to 60% of affected patients. Calcium homeostasis tends to normalize with age, but may recur in late childhood or adulthood especially during periods of illness, stress, or pregnancy. Calcium supplementation is sometimes warranted. Consumption of carbonated drinks or alcohol may worsen hypocalcemia.

Common associated findings in children with this disorder include congenital heart disease, palatal abnormalities, characteristic facial dysmorphology, learning difficulties, renal anomalies, and immune deficiency (Item C140A). Facial dysmorphology consists of hooded upper eyelids, ocular hypertelorism, squared off or overfolded helices, bulbous nasal tip with nasal dimple, and hypoplastic alae nasae.

Item C140A. Clinical Findings by Organ System in 22q11.2 Deletion.

Organ System			
Cardiac (74%)	*Mainly conotruncal defects*		
	• Atrial septal defect	• Tetralogy of Fallot	• Vascular ring
	• Interrupted aortic arch	• Truncus arteriosus	• Ventricular septal defect
Palatal abnormalities (69%)	• Bifid uvula	• Submucosal cleft palate	
	• Cleft palate	• Velopharyngeal incompetence	
Gastrointestinal	• Gastrointestinal anomalies	• Constipation	• Feeding and swallowing difficulties
	• Atresias		
	• Hirschsprung disease		
	• Imperforate anus		
	• Intestinal malrotation		
Endocrinologic	• Celiac disease	• Growth hormone deficiency	• Hypothyroidism
	• Graves disease	• Hypocalcemia (50%)	• Vitiligo
Neurologic	• Central nervous system anomalies, including tethered cord		
	• Seizures		
Renal	• Absent uterus	• Hydronephrosis	• Inguinal hernia
	• Cryptorchidism	• Hypospadias	• Multicystic/dysplastic kidneys
	• Duplicated kidney	• Horseshoe kidney	• Renal agenesis
Ophthalmologic	• Anophthalmia	• Ptosis	• Strabismus
	• Posterior embryotoxon	• Sclerocornea	• Tortuous retinal vessels
Neurobehavioral	• Anxiety	• Learning difficulties (70-90%)	• Social interaction difficulties
	• Attention deficit disorder	• Perseveration	
	• Autism (20%)	• Psychiatric disorders, especially schizophrenia (25%)	
Skeletal	• Clubfeet	• Polydactyly	• Vertebral anomalies
	• Craniosynostosis	• Scoliosis	
Facial dysmorphology	• Bulbous nasal tip with nasal dimple	• Hypoplastic alae nasae	• Squared off or overfolded helices
	• Hooded upper eyelids	• Ocular hypertelorism	
Autoimmune	• Autoimmune cytopenias	• Graves disease	• Juvenile rheumatoid arthritis
Other	• Asymmetric crying facies	• Hearing loss (conductive and sensorineural)	• Laryngotracheoesophageal anomalies
	• Enamel hypoplasia	• Immune deficiency (77%)	

Adapted and reprinted with permission from McDonald-McGinn DM, Emanuel BS, Zackai EH. 22q11.2 deletion syndrome. *GeneReviews*.

Congenital heart disease in these children often manifests as conotruncal defects, including tetralogy of Fallot, perimembranous ventricular septal defect, truncus arteriosus, or interrupted aortic arch. Palatal deformities can range from velopharyngeal incompetence to cleft palate. Additional clinical findings can include feeding and swallowing problems, gastrointestinal and laryngotracheoesophageal anomalies, hearing loss, growth hormone deficiency, seizures, central nervous system anomalies, skeletal abnormalities (club feet, scoliosis, vertebral anomalies), renal abnormalities, ophthalmologic problems, thyroid problems, hypocalcemia, psychiatric disorders, autism, and enamel hypoplasia. Autoimmune disease commonly occurs with 22q11.2 deletion, especially juvenile rheumatoid arthritis, hypothyroidism, Graves disease, and autoimmune cytopenias. The cytopenias are less common than is hypocalcemia.

Diagnosis of 22q11.2 deletion syndrome can be made with fluorescence in situ hybridization analysis for the submicroscopic deletion of chromosome 22, high-resolution karyotype, or a chromosomal microarray. Baseline evaluations recommended at the time of diagnosis are noted in Item C140B.

Treatment for 22q11.2 deletion syndrome entails a multidisciplinary approach tailored to the individual's specific presentation. The health-care team will consist of a combination of medical disciplines as well as speech pathology and early intervention specialists. Growth hormone may be required if poor growth, in association with growth hormone deficiency, is present. Sixty percent of affected adults have a psychiatric disorder (schizophrenia, anxiety, and depression) that will warrant a psychiatrist. The thyroid profile should be monitored annually because of the risk of thyroid dysfunction.

Item C140B. Baseline Evaluations at Time of Diagnosis of 22q11.2 Deletion Syndrome.

Evaluations at Diagnosis

- Assess for feeding problems, including gastroesophageal reflux and swallowing dysfunction
- Audiology evaluation
- Baseline cardiac evaluation, including chest radiograph, echocardiogram, and electrocardiogram
- Cervical spine films for children over age 4 years of age (6-view)
- Chest radiograph for vertebral anomalies
- Clinical evaluation of the palate
- Close follow-up of growth to look for possible growth hormone deficiency
- Complete blood cell count with differential; possibly T- and B-cell subsets if low absolute lymphocyte count
- Early intervention referral by 1 year of age
- Evaluate need for a psychologist or psychiatrist if any evidence of anxiety, psychosis, or mood problems
- Hematology evaluation if a bleeding disorder is suspected
- Immunology evaluation including flow cytometry, immunoglobulins, and T-cell function
- Measurement of serum ionized calcium and intact parathyroid hormone level; if abnormal, consult endocrinology
- Ophthalmology evaluation
- Renal ultrasonography
- Speech and language assessment by one year of age
- Thyroid-stimulating hormone level

Adapted and reprinted with permission from McDonald-McGinn DM, Emanuel BS, Zackai EH. 22q11.2 deletion syndrome. *GeneReviews*.

Hypercalcemia, hypercalciuria, and hypothyroidism are commonly associated with Williams syndrome. Pancytopenia is associated with Fanconi anemia and X-linked dyskeratosis congenita. Thrombocytopenia can be seen with thrombocytopenia absent radius syndrome and Wiskott-Aldrich syndrome.

PREP Pearls

- 22q11.2 deletion syndrome, also known as velocardiofacial syndrome or DiGeorge syndrome, is associated with hypocalcemia in 17% to 60% of patients and thyroid dysfunction.
- Common clinical findings with 22q11.2 deletion syndrome include congenital heart disease, palatal abnormalities, characteristic facial dysmorphology, learning difficulties, renal anomalies, and immune deficiency.
- Diagnosis of 22q11.2 deletion syndrome can be made with fluorescence in situ hybridization analysis for the submicroscopic deletion of chromosome 22, high-resolution karyotype, or a chromosomal microarray.

American Board of Pediatrics Content Specification(s)/ Content Area

- Recognize the features of velocardiofacial syndrome and plan appropriate diagnostic evaluation

Suggested Readings

Bassett AS, McDonald-McGinn DM, Devriendt K, et al; International 22q11.2 Deletion Syndrome Consortium. Practical guidelines for managing patients with 22q11.2 deletion syndrome. *J Pediatr.* 2011;159(2):332-339.e1.

McDonald-McGinn DM, Emanuel BS, Zackai EH. 22q11.2 deletion syndrome. *GeneReviews.* https://www.ncbi.nlm.nih.gov/books/NBK1523/.

Pereira E, Marion R. Chromosome 22q11.2 deletion syndrome. *Pediatr Rev.* 2015;36(6):270-272.

Item 141   Preferred Response: B

The girl in this vignette demonstrates clinical signs and symptoms consistent with Kawasaki disease (KD). A complete blood cell count with differential, comprehensive metabolic panel, C-reactive protein level, erythrocyte sedimentation rate, and urinalysis will add to the diagnosis and guide treatment. Kawasaki disease is associated with vasculitis of coronary and other medium-sized, extraparenchymal arteries. Early initiation of treatment with intravenous immunoglobulin and high-dose aspirin can mitigate long-term effects on coronary vessels.

The etiology of KD remains unknown. There is no gold-standard diagnostic test; thus, the diagnosis is based on clinical and laboratory criteria. Kawasaki disease should be suspected in a child with a fever, typically greater than 39°C, for at least 5 days' duration. The diagnosis is made from the fever along with other signs and symptoms as described by Newberger et al (http://circ.ahajournals.org/content/110/17/2747). More than 90% of children with KD have bilateral, nonexudative, limbic-sparing conjunctivitis (Item C141). A diffusely erythematous oropharynx with cracked lips and a strawberry tongue are often seen, but oral ulcers and tonsillar exudate are not typical for KD. The hands and feet are often swollen early in the course, and a desquamating rash on distal fingers and toes is common. Bullae and vesicles are not typically seen.

Clinical features including arthritis and arthralgia, vomiting and diarrhea, abdominal pain, extreme irritability, testicular swelling, and a desquamating rash in the groin, are

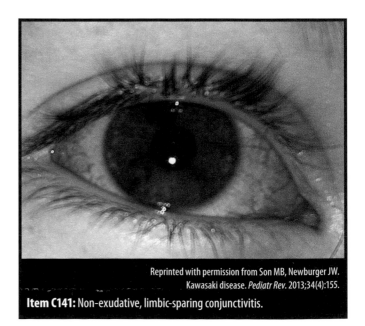

Reprinted with permission from Son MB, Newburger JW. Kawasaki disease. *Pediatr Rev.* 2013;34(4):155.

Item C141: Non-exudative, limbic-sparing conjunctivitis.

associated with KD and can mimic other conditions. Children with suspected KD based on clinical and/or laboratory findings should undergo echocardiography to assess for coronary artery abnormalities and overall heart function. If coronary abnormalities are seen, the child should be treated for KD, regardless of whether all criteria are met.

Infants and children with some criteria for KD, but not quite meeting the clinical case definition, should be assessed for "incomplete KD." Nearly all children with KD have elevated inflammatory markers. Therefore, children with a C-reactive protein level less than 3.0 mg/dL (286 nmol/L) and erythrocyte sedimentation rate less than 40 mm/h should be evaluated daily for continued fever and change in laboratory values. If peeling of the distal hands or feet is seen, echocardiography should be performed. If the C-reactive protein level is 3.0 mg/dL (286 nmol/L) or greater or the erythrocyte sedimentation rate is 40 mm/h or greater, the clinician should assess for whether the child meets other laboratory criteria (http://circ.ahajournals.org/content/110/17/2747). For those with fewer than 3 other criteria, echocardiography is recommended. If vascular changes are seen on echocardiography, treatment is recommended. If no changes are seen, echocardiography should be repeated if fever persists. If 3 or more other laboratory criteria are met, the child should undergo echocardiography and be treated for KD. For infants 6 months of age and younger who have had at least 7 days of fever without other clinical criteria, laboratory testing should be done to determine if laboratory criteria for KD are met.

Viral and bacterial infections, particularly adenovirus infection and streptococcal pharyngitis, may also present in a similar fashion to KD and should be excluded before treating for KD. Therefore, a broad viral respiratory panel and rapid antigen testing for streptococcal pharyngitis may be helpful; however, positive results alone do not exclude KD. While Epstein-Barr virus infection can present similarly to KD, a heterophile antibody test has a high false-negative rate in younger children. Because the child in this vignette has no respiratory symptoms and is fully immunized, chest radiography and blood culture are not indicated. A typically developing 3-year-old should be able to report dysuria; in the absence of dysuria, a urinary tract infection is less likely. A serum measles IgM antibody test and, in certain circumstances, viral culture from a nasopharyngeal sample can diagnose measles. However, measles prevalence is much less likely in this vaccinated child and in the absence of an epidemic; decisions around testing for measles in this context should be done in consultation with public health officials.

PREP Pearls

- Infants younger than 6 months with Kawasaki disease can present with fever and few or no accompanying clinical features. Echocardiography is recommended in these infants with fever for 7 or more days and elevated inflammatory marker levels.
- Kawasaki disease should be suspected in a child with fever for several days, even when signs and symptoms less common in Kawasaki disease (eg, headache, vomiting) are present.

American Board of Pediatrics Content Specification(s)/Content Area

- Recognize the clinical findings associated with Kawasaki disease
- Plan the appropriate diagnostic evaluation of Kawasaki disease, and interpret the results

Suggested Readings

Newburger JW, Takahashi M, Gerber MA, et al. Diagnosis, treatment, and long-term management of Kawasaki disease: a statement for health professionals from the Committee on Rheumatic Fever, Endocarditis and Kawasaki Disease, Council on Cardiovascular Disease in the Young. American Heart Association. *Circulation*. 2004;110(17):2751. (http://circ.ahajournals.org/content/110/17/2747)

Son MB, Newburger JW. Kawasaki disease. *Pediatr Rev*. 2013;34(4):151-162.

Item 142   Preferred Response: C

The boy in this vignette has fever, tenderness over the proximal right femur with pain in the right hip, and elevated markers of inflammation. Osteomyelitis is the most likely diagnosis, and the best initial imaging study for this patient is radiography of the pelvis. Although bony changes in osteomyelitis are not evident in radiographs until 2 to 3 weeks after the onset of illness, other pathology associated with bone pain must be ruled out.

The diagnostic evaluation of osteomyelitis starts with a comprehensive history and physical examination. The history should include duration of symptoms, preceding trauma, personal or family history of staphylococcal disease, and animal exposures. A thorough physical examination is critical in identifying the location of disease, given that the site of the disease process may not be readily apparent. Further diagnostic evaluation includes a combination of laboratory tests and radiologic studies. Laboratory tests should include blood cultures, complete blood cell counts, and inflammatory markers (erythrocyte sedimentation rate, C-reactive protein). The first-line imaging study is radiography, which can exclude items on the differential diagnosis including fractures and osseous tumors. The bony changes caused by osteomyelitis are not apparent in radiographs until 2 to 3 weeks after the onset of illness. Therefore, the definitive radiologic study in the acute setting is magnetic resonance imaging. Although computed tomography and bone scan can be useful, they both have the drawback of radiation exposure. Ultrasonography can be helpful in evaluation for joint effusions, which can be present in the setting of osteomyelitis as a reactive effusion in a joint adjacent to the site of osteomyelitis or as concurrent septic arthritis.

Staphylococcus aureus is the most frequently isolated organism in osteomyelitis. Other pathogens include *Streptococcus pyogenes* and *Streptococcus pneumoniae*. In children younger than 4 years, *Kingella kingae* should be on the differential. Additionally, in patients with sickle cell disease or with pertinent exposures, *Salmonella* species should be considered.

The management of osteomyelitis always includes antibiotics but often requires a combination of medical and surgical management. Antibiotics used to treat osteomyelitis should have adequate bone penetration. Empiric antibiotics should be directed against the possible etiologic agents (namely *S aureus*), then narrowed based on organism identification and antimicrobial susceptibility results. Every attempt should be made to determine the organism by blood culture, surgical specimens, or bone biopsy. Antibiotics that are effective against *K kingae* should also be included for young children, and antibiotics against *Salmonella* species should be included in patients with sickle cell disease. Antibiotics are administered initially via the parenteral route, and if feasible they are converted to the oral route. In acute hematogenous osteomyelitis, the typical duration of antibiotic therapy is 4 to 6 weeks.

PREP Pearls

- *Staphylococcus aureus* is the leading cause of osteomyelitis.
- In acute hematogenous osteomyelitis, the typical duration of antibiotic therapy is 4 to 6 weeks, initially via the parenteral route followed by transition to oral therapy, if feasible.
- The diagnostic evaluation of osteomyelitis always starts with a comprehensive history and physical examination, followed by laboratory tests (blood cultures, complete blood cell counts, and inflammatory markers) and radiologic studies (radiography followed by magnetic resonance imaging).

American Board of Pediatrics Content Specification(s)/ Content Area

- Plan the appropriate diagnostic evaluation of osteomyelitis, with attention to the sequence with which positive findings become evident on imaging studies
- Identify the etiology of osteomyelitis in patients of various ages
- Plan the appropriate management of osteomyelitis in patients of various ages

Suggested Readings

Conrad D. Acute hematogenous osteomyelitis. *Pediatr Rev*. 2010; 31:(11)464-471.

Peltola H, Paakkonen M. Acute osteomyelitis in children. *N Engl J Med*. 2014;370:(14)352-360.

Item 143 　　　　　　　　　Preferred Response: C

The boy in the vignette had an episode of unresponsiveness accompanied by muscle jerking, with a very rapid recovery. He did not have a postictal phase with lethargy or confusion. His history suggests a syncopal episode with myoclonic jerks rather than a seizure. The trigger for this episode is unclear. His mother has a history of similar episodes, which could indicate an inherited ion channel disorder predisposing him to arrhythmia such as long QT syndrome or catecholaminergic polymorphic ventricular tachycardia. Although neurocardiogenic (vasovagal) and situational syncope (eg, due to micturition, defecation, or the sight of blood) are more common than cardiogenic syncope due to arrhythmia, the boy should be evaluated by a cardiologist given the unclear etiology of his syncope and his family history. If this evaluation does not reveal an underlying cardiac disorder, the boy could be cleared for basketball participation.

Head injury, such as concussion, should also be included in the differential diagnosis for this child's episode of unresponsiveness. Myoclonic activity can be seen in association with concussion. Individuals with concussion can be returned to physical activity in a stepwise fashion, once asymptomatic for 24 to 48 hours, gradually increasing the intensity and difficulty of activity each day if they do not experience increased symptoms. Because the boy had a rapid recovery and is currently asymptomatic with normal physical examination findings, concussion is unlikely.

In a child with a suspected seizure, neurology evaluation, including electroencephalography, laboratory studies, and neuroimaging may be warranted. However, seizure activity would not preclude participation in basketball. Children with seizure disorders are less likely to participate in sports and physical activity than their siblings. Physicians should look for ways to promote safe sports participation for children with epilepsy. Certain sports, such as swimming, diving, archery, and powerlifting, may pose a high risk to an athlete with a poorly controlled seizure disorder (and potentially to teammates and officials). Therefore, individuals with frequent seizures, despite appropriate treatment with antiepileptic medications, should have an individualized evaluation with discussion of appropriate types of activity and ways to mitigate risk.

PREP Pearls

- Certain sports, such as swimming, diving, archery, and powerlifting, may pose a high risk to an athlete with a poorly controlled seizure disorder.
- Having a seizure disorder, even when poorly controlled, is not an absolute contraindication to sports participation.
- Syncope with myoclonic jerks may be mistaken for seizure activity.

American Board of Pediatrics Content Specification(s)/ Content Area

- Understand the guidelines for sports participation for patients who have a seizure disorder

Suggested Readings

Anderson JB, Willis M, Lancaster H, Leonard K, Thomas C. The evaluation and management of pediatric syncope. *Pediatr Neurol*. 2016;55:6-13.

Bernhardt DT, Roberts WO, eds. *Preparticipation Physical Evaluation*. 4th ed. Elk Grove Village, IL: American Academy of Pediatrics; 2010.

Wong J, Wirrell E. Physical activity in children/teens with epilepsy compared with that in their siblings without epilepsy. *Epilepsia*. 2006;47(3):631-639.

Item 144 　　　　　　　　　Preferred Response: C

Standard deviation (SD) is a measure of dispersion; it measures the variability of data around the mean. A small SD indicates that data points are clustered close to the mean; a higher SD indicates a wider range of values. In samples with a normal distribution (bell-shaped curve), 68% of the values fall within 1 SD and 95% of the values fall within 2 SD above and below the mean (Item C144).

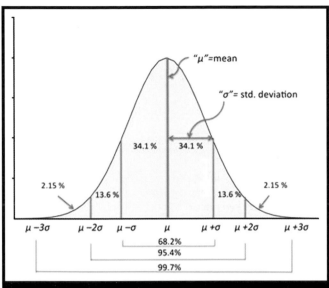

"μ"=mean

"σ"= std. deviation

34.1 %　34.1 %

2.15 %　13.6 %　13.6 %　2.15 %

μ −3σ　μ −2σ　μ −σ　μ　μ +σ　μ +2σ　μ +3σ

68.2%
95.4%
99.7%

Reprinted with permission from Smith TK, Johnson SB. Research and statistics: distribution, variability, and statistical significance. *Pediatr Rev*. 2010;31(10):432.

Item C144: Illustration of normal distribution.

Midparental height is an important calculation to perform when determining normal variability in stature and it provides a good estimate of a child's genetic adult height potential. The calculation for midparental height is:

- For girls, the average of (father's height - 13 cm or 5 inches) + mother's height
- For boys, the average of (mother's height + 13 cm or 5 inches) + father's height

The child's projected height is then compared with the midparental height range. If a child with short stature has a projected height that falls within 2 SDs of this value (by definition, 95% of the time, the value will fall within this range from the mean), then the child's height is within the expected range, given genetic potential. If so, the child probably has familial short stature, which is considered a normal variant. If the child's projected height falls outside this range, then other causes of short stature should be considered.

The midparental height for the girl in the vignette is the average of (5'7" - 5") + 5'2" = 5'2". If she has familial short stature, given an SD of 1.67 inches, 95% of the time, a girl in this situation will have a final height between 4'10.7" and 5'5.3".

PREP Pearls

- A small standard deviation indicates that data points are clustered close to the mean; a higher standard deviation indicates a wider range of values.
- In samples with a normal distribution (bell-shaped curve), 68% of the values fall within 1 standard deviation and 95% of the values fall within 2 standard deviations above and below the mean.
- Standard deviation is a measure of dispersion; it measures the variability of data around the mean.

American Board of Pediatrics Content Specification(s)/ Content Area

- Understand standard error in the interpretation of results
- Understand standard deviation in the interpretation of results
- Understand confidence interval in the interpretation of results

Suggested Readings

Braun LR, Marino R. Disorders of growth and stature. *Pediatr Rev*. 2017;38(7)293-304.

Smith TK, Johnson SB. Research and statistics: distribution, variability and statistical significance. *Pediatr Rev*. 2010;31(10);431-432.

Soyemi K. Choosing the right statistical test. *Pediatr Rev*. 2012;33(5)e38-e44.

Tanner JM, Goldstein H, Whitehouse RH. Standards for children's height at ages 2-9 years allowing for heights of parents. *Arch Dis Child*. 1970;45(244):755762.

Item 145　　　　　　　　　**Preferred Response: A**

The boy in this vignette likely has an atypical pneumonia, possibly due to *Mycoplasma*. Thus, the test most likely to be helpful is one that would rapidly identify *Mycoplasma* antigen, such as a polymerase chain reaction (PCR) from nasal washing. The long time course with progression of cough from dry to wet and the presence of mild wheezing suggest *Mycoplasma* or another atypical organism. Lack of fever and adenopathy makes Epstein-Barr virus unlikely, and the course of the illness lasting several weeks makes other acute respiratory viruses less likely. Lack of fever and systemic toxicity makes bacterial pneumonia unlikely, and thus a sputum Gram stain and culture will not be helpful. Given the history of recent pertussis immunization it is not likely that he has pertussis, even an atypical pertussis commonly found in the underimmunized adolescent population.

In the preschool population, *Mycoplasma* is a possible but uncommon cause of pneumonia. In older children and adolescents it is underappreciated because of its relatively protean manifestations. Viral pathogens are most often implicated in preschool children and are also common in older children. According to the *Red Book*, 10% of *Mycoplasma*-infected school-aged children will develop pneumonia. The presentation is usually that of persistent cough with rales and/or wheezing. The cough is initially dry, but may become productive persisting for up to 4 weeks. In most situations, treatment of *Mycoplasma* will not change the course of the illness. However, in older children with atypical pneumonia who are ill enough to require hospitalization, the use of a macrolide antibiotic to shorten the course of illness is appropriate. In addition, droplet isolation precautions and good hand washing will limit the spread of the organism.

Historically, *Mycoplasma* disease has been diagnosed retrospectively by measuring the rise in IgM antibody titers, which peak at 3 to 6 weeks after initial infection and may last for up to several months. The PCR test is available commercially and has both sensitivity and specificity of 80% to 100% when performed on respiratory secretions. The correlation of suggestive symptoms with a positive PCR result is still not absolutely diagnostic, as *Mycoplasma* organisms can colonize the airway and produce positive PCR results for several weeks after an infection. Therefore, a positive result does not guarantee current symptomatic infection, and the diagnosis is usually made based on clinical findings, or retrospectively by a rise in IgM-specific antibody titer.

PREP Pearls

- Antibiotics will usually not change the course of a *Mycoplasma* infection; but, use of a macrolide antibiotic is appropriate in older children who require hospitalization.
- *Mycoplasma* infection should be considered in school-aged children and adolescents with a prolonged cough.

American Board of Pediatrics Content Specification(s)/ Content Area

- Understand the epidemiology of *Mycoplasma pneumoniae*
- Plan appropriate management for a patient with *Mycoplasma pneumoniae* infection
- Recognize the clinical features associated with *Mycoplasma pneumoniae* infection
- Plan the appropriate diagnostic evaluation of *Mycoplasma pneumoniae* infection

Suggested Readings

American Academy of Pediatrics. *Mycoplasma pneumoniae* and other *Mycoplasma* species infections. In: Kimberlin DW, Brady MI, Jackson MA, Long SS, eds. *Red Book: 2018 Report of the Committee on Infectious Diseases.* 31st ed. Itasca, IL: American Academy of Pediatrics; 2018:573-575.

Wank K, Gill P, Perera R, Thomson A, Mant D, Harnden A. Clinical symptoms and signs for the diagnosis of *Mycoplasma pneumoniae* in children and adolescents with community-acquired pneumonia. *Cochrane Database Syst Rev.* 2012;10:CD009175.

Item 146　　　　　　　**Preferred Response: B**

The girl in this vignette has intellectual disability (ID), defined by significant delays in both cognitive and adaptive functioning. The causes of ID include congenital infections (eg, cytomegalovirus, rubella, toxoplasmosis), central nervous system infections (eg, meningitis, encephalitis), trauma, malignancy, genetic abnormalities (eg, trisomy 21, fragile X syndrome), inborn errors of metabolism, and teratogens (eg, alcohol, illicit and prescription drugs, lead, radiation). Ethanol is the most common teratogen causing ID.

Fetal alcohol spectrum disorder encompasses a range of adverse effects associated with prenatal alcohol exposure (eg, fetal alcohol syndrome, partial fetal alcohol syndrome, alcohol-related birth defects, alcohol-related neurodevelopmental disorder, neurobehavioral disorder associated with prenatal alcohol exposure). Full fetal alcohol syndrome includes differences in growth (ie, weight and/or height ≤ 10th percentile), physical features (eg, smooth philtrum, thin upper lip, small palpebral fissures), and central nervous system abnormalities (eg, microcephaly, seizures, ID, learning disabilities, attention-deficit/hyperactivity disorder). Moderate to heavy alcohol consumption during pregnancy is associated with greater risk of fetal alcohol syndrome; however, there are no known safe limits of alcohol consumption during pregnancy.

Identifying the cause of ID can help with family planning, identifying associated medical risks, accessing support systems, and relieving families of guilt or anxiety about presumed causes of their child's ID. In the case of inborn errors of metabolism, treatment may be available.

PREP Pearls

- Full fetal alcohol syndrome includes differences in growth (ie, weight and/or height ≤10th percentile), physical features (eg, smooth philtrum, thin upper lip, small palpebral fissures), and central nervous system abnormalities (eg, microcephaly, seizures, intellectual disability, learning disabilities, attention-deficit/ hyperactivity disorder).
- Moderate to heavy alcohol consumption during pregnancy is associated with greater risk of fetal alcohol syndrome; however, there are no known safe limits of alcohol consumption during pregnancy.
- The causes of intellectual disability include congenital infections (eg, cytomegalovirus, rubella, toxoplasmosis), central nervous system infections (eg, meningitis, encephalitis), trauma, malignancy, genetic abnormalities (eg, trisomy 21, fragile X syndrome), inborn errors of metabolism, and teratogens (eg, alcohol, illicit and prescription drugs, lead, radiation).

American Board of Pediatrics Content Specification(s)/ Content Area

- Identify common infectious causes of intellectual disabilities
- Identify common teratogenic causes of intellectual disabilities

Suggested Readings

Oji-Mmuo CN, Corr TE, Doheny KK. Addictive disorders in women: the impact of maternal substance use on the fetus and newborn. *Neoreviews.* 2017;18(10):e576-e586.

Shea SE. Intellectual disability (mental retardation). *Pediatr Rev.* 2012;33(3):110-121.

Williams JF, Smith VC; Committee on Substance Abuse. Fetal alcohol spectrum disorders. *Pediatrics.* 2015;136(5):e1395-e1406.

Item 147　　　　　　　**Preferred Response: B**

The boy in the vignette has global developmental delay and infantile spasms. The lesion his mother had on her forehead was most likely a Shagreen patch, and the boy's cousins have autism and seizures. Taken together with the boy's clinical presentation, it is very likely that the boy and his family members have tuberous sclerosis. The dermatologic finding associated with tuberous sclerosis in an infant is Ash-leaf spots, which are flat, white, oval macules.

Flat, brown macules with an irregular border (cafe au lait spots) are seen in neurofibromatosis; they can also occur in isolation (without any underlying neurocutaneous syndromes). A raised, red papule with a well-demarcated border (hemangioma) and raised, flesh-colored papules with an indentation in the center (molluscum contagiosum) are not associated with developmental delay or infantile spasms.

Early treatment of infantile spasms, within the first 2 weeks of onset, is associated with improved long-term developmental outcome, so early recognition and diagnosis are critical. Treatment of infantile spasms in the setting of tuberous sclerosis is usually with the anticonvulsant vigabatrin. For all other causes, initial treatment is usually a course of high-dose steroids. It is critically important to evaluate infants with infantile spasms for tuberous sclerosis so that the best treatment can be initiated as soon as possible.

A minority of children with infantile spasms will have a favorable outcome. Outcome is most closely related to the level and rapidity of seizure control and the underlying diagnosis. The best chance of a favorable outcome is in cases of cryptogenic infantile spasms, when no underlying disorder is found. For the boy in the vignette, who probably has tuberous sclerosis, a favorable outcome is less likely.

PREP Pearls

- Outcome in infantile spasms is most closely related to the underlying diagnosis and to early treatment and control of seizures.
- Patients with infantile spasms should be evaluated for signs of tuberous sclerosis including flat, white, oval macules (Ash-leaf spots).

American Board of Pediatrics Content Specification(s)/ Content Area

- Recognize the clinical findings associated with infantile spasms
- Understand the prognosis of infantile spasms

Suggested Readings

O'Callaghan FJ, Lux AL, Darke K, et al. The effect of lead time to treatment and of age of onset on developmental outcome at 4 years in infantile spasms: evidence from the United Kingdom Infantile Spasms Study. *Epilepsia*. 2011;52(7):1359-1364.

Shields D; Child Neurology Foundation Disorder Directory. Infantile spasms. http://www.childneurologyfoundation.org/disorders/infantile-spasms/.

Item 148   Preferred Response: C

The adolescent girl in this vignette has a microfissure in her ear canal and a perforated tympanic membrane caused by aggressive cleaning with a cotton-tipped applicator, usage of which should be avoided. This trauma predisposed her to develop acute otitis externa complicated by a perforated tympanic membrane. Additional risk factors for developing otitis externa include prolonged exposure to water. Bacterial pathogens commonly associated with otitis externa include *Pseudomonas aeruginosa* and *Staphylococcus aureus*. Initial treatment of otitis externa includes pain management and selection of an appropriate antimicrobial agent. For uncomplicated otitis externa in which the tympanic membrane remains intact, antimicrobial treatment consists of a topical preparation. A 2010 Cochrane review found no difference in topical antibiotic preparations in terms of cure rates, and there was insufficient evidence that the addition of a corticosteroid improved outcomes. For cases of otitis externa in which the tympanic membrane is not intact, aminoglycosides (neomycin and gentamicin) should be avoided because of the associated ototoxicity in the middle ear.

In complicated or severe cases of otitis externa, such as coexisting acute otitis media, lymphadenitis, or facial cellulitis, or in patients who are immunocompromised and at

risk for developing necrotizing otitis externa with extension to osteomyelitis, oral or intravenous antibiotics are recommended. If purulent otorrhea obstructs visualization of the tympanic membrane, it may be necessary to gently remove the obstruction manually or with light suction. However, performing a lavage without visualizing the tympanic membrane is contraindicated and may necessitate a referral to an otolaryngologist. Additionally, if edema has extended beyond 50% narrowing of the ear canal, it may be prudent to use a medication wick (one-fourth inch ribbon gauze) to ensure appropriate delivery of the antibiotic therapy to the auditory canal epithelium. During treatment of otitis externa, instructions should be provided to keep the area dry and refrain from prolonged exposure to water, such as swimming.

PREP Pearls

- A 2010 Cochrane review found that there was insufficient evidence to add corticosteroids to topical antibiotic preparations.
- Aminoglycosides should be avoided in the treatment of otitis externa with nonintact tympanic membrane because of ototoxicity.
- Microfissures from trauma predispose patients to otitis externa. Aggressive cleaning with cotton-tipped applicators may cause perforations of the tympanic membrane.

American Board of Pediatrics Content Specification(s)/ Content Area

- Recognize the clinical findings associated with foreign body in the external ear canal
- Recognize pathogens commonly associated with otitis externa
- Plan the appropriate initial and prophylactic management of otitis externa

Suggested Readings

Kaushik V, Malik T, Saeed SR. Interventions for acute otitis externa. *Cochrane Database Syst Rev.* 2010;20(1):CD004740.

Long M. Otitis externa. *Pediatr Rev.* 2013;(34)3:143-144.

Rosenfeld RM, Schwartz SR, Cannon CR, et al. Clinical practice guideline: acute otitis externa. *Otolaryngol Head Neck Surg.* 2014;150(1 suppl):S1-S4.

Item 149   Preferred Response: C

The 18-month-old patient in this vignette presents with a microcytic anemia and excessive milk consumption. Although the most obvious and well-recognized consequence of iron deficiency is anemia, the best-studied non-hematologic consequence of iron deficiency is an effect on cognition. Therefore, the patient in this vignette is at increased risk for developing neurocognitive changes.

It may be helpful to visualize the red blood cell as a sac filled with hemoglobin. The more hemoglobin there is in the red blood cell, the more full the sac gets. A deficiency of any component of the hemoglobin molecule will therefore result in a smaller volume of the red blood cell. The size of red blood cells is measured by the mean corpuscular volume. The 2 primary components of hemoglobin that can be deficient are heme or the globin protein. To form hemoglobin, the 4 globin subunits must bind to a molecule of heme, which is dependent on iron. Iron deficiency will therefore result in deficiency of heme, which will result in a deficiency of hemoglobin, and ultimately a microcytic anemia. Although the patient in this vignette could theoretically have a variant of thalassemia, his excessive milk consumption strongly suggests iron deficiency. He should receive a complete evaluation for iron deficiency, including measurement of the serum iron level, total iron binding capacity, and serum ferritin level. Iron replacement therapy for iron deficiency can be given orally or intravenously. Oral iron replacement should be taken on an empty stomach with an acidic or neutral fluid. It is therefore most appropriate to take iron with water or orange juice. Oral replacement should include 2 to 4 mg of elemental iron per kilogram of weight daily. Ferrous sulfate is 20% elemental iron. Serum iron levels should be rechecked after 3 months of therapy and should then be continued for an additional 3 months once they have completely normalized. Intravenous iron therapy is both safe and effective and is a reasonable alternative if oral iron is not tolerated.

Iron deficiency does not increase the risk for leukemia or severe aplastic anemia. Although milk protein allergy can lead to iron deficiency, iron deficiency does not increase the risk for milk protein allergy.

PREP Pearls

- Iron-deficiency anemia is associated with health problems including neurocognitive changes.
- Microcytic anemia can be caused by a deficiency of globin (ie, a thalassemia variant) or a deficiency of heme, which is iron dependent.
- Oral iron replacement should be given on an empty stomach with water or orange juice, and the dose should be 2 to 4 mg/kg/day of elemental iron.

American Board of Pediatrics Content Specification(s)/ Content Area

- Recognize the normal variations in hemoglobin concentration and mean corpuscular volume during childhood
- Distinguish between a disorder of erythrocyte production and a disorder of erythrocyte destruction based on laboratory results
- Understand the etiology of iron deficiency
- Recognize the laboratory findings associated with microcytic anemia
- Identify non-hematologic effects of iron deficiency

Suggested Readings

Baker RD, Greer FR; Committee on Nutrition American Academy of Pediatrics. Diagnosis and prevention of iron deficiency and iron deficiency anemia in infants and young children (0–3 years of age). *Pediatrics.* 2010;126(5):1040-1050.

DeLoughery TG. Microcytic anemia. *N Engl J Med.* 2014;371:1324-1331.

Wang M. Iron deficiency and other types of anemia in infants and children. *Am Fam Physician.* 2016;93(4):270-278.

Item 150   Preferred Response: D

The 17-year-old girl in the vignette presents with lethargy, bradycardia, slowed and shallow respirations, and miosis following an unwitnessed toxic ingestion. Although her clinical history, the smell of alcohol on her breath and clothing, and serum ethanol level confirms that she has recently consumed ethanol, a serum ethanol level of 50 mg/dL is unlikely to have the effect on her cardiorespiratory status and pupillary examination that is being currently observed. Her clinical findings suggest opioid toxicity; therefore, administration of intravenous naloxone would be the best next management step for her.

Although it is important for pediatric providers to recognize the signs and symptoms of ethanol intoxication, understanding that ethanol may mask toxicity caused by ingestion of other drugs is equally important. Most toxic ingestions in preschool-aged children are unintentional, occur due to developmentally normal exploratory behavior, and involve small amounts of a single agent. In contrast, toxic exposures in adolescents are much more likely to be intentional and involve multiple drugs (polypharmacy). Drug abuse, experimental risk-taking behaviors, and mood disorders with suicidal ideation place adolescents at risk for poisoning from multiple substances.

Adolescents who are intoxicated may present to medical attention after intentional or unintentional overdoses, suicide attempts, changes in mental status/behavior, or with injuries sustained as a result of the effects of drugs and/or alcohol. Historical information provided by these patients may not be reliable, due either to their unwillingness and/or inability to accurately disclose the types and amounts of toxins involved. Clinicians should ask other household members about all medications, vitamin and mineral supplements, herbal and folk remedies, alcoholic beverages, illicit substances, and household chemicals present in the home. Adolescents may also have access to drugs and other toxins in their school, work, or recreational environments. For adolescents presenting acutely after a toxic ingestion, family members, friends, and/or paramedics can sometimes provide important information about open containers, empty bottles, spilled contents, drug paraphernalia, or suicide notes at the scene.

Providers caring for children presenting after presumed ethanol intoxication should maintain a high index of suspicion for the coingestion of other toxic substances. The nonspecific symptoms of depressed level of consciousness, labile behavior, nausea, vomiting, and ataxia, commonly seen in patients with ethanol intoxication, can also be caused by other dangerous toxins. Although toxicology screening is generally unnecessary for children presenting after unintentional ingestions who have clinical findings that are consistent with the history, it *is* indicated in situations in which the possibility of a potentially harmful coingestion exists. Few early signs may be present after ingestion of harmful doses of some toxic substances, and these signs can be "masked" by the presence of other toxins, such as ethanol. Furthermore, specific antidotes for substances used with ethanol may be available and should be given as early as possible in the patient's clinical course.

Urine toxicology screening provides qualitative data about the recent use of a limited number of substances, typically drugs of abuse. These screens are relatively inexpensive and provide rapid results (usually within 1 hour). Although they provide no information about timing or quantity of ingestion, the information obtained may help clinicians make sense of patients' clinical findings, anticipate their clinical course and potential for withdrawal, and determine disposition. Serum toxicologic testing provides quantitative data. This is important in the diagnosis and management of ingestion of several drugs and medications, including acetaminophen and salicylates. Clinicians should become familiar with the specific drugs tested for at their institutions. It is important to understand that a negative urine and/or serum toxicology screen cannot definitively rule out a toxic ingestion; the screens used at most centers cannot detect every agent that a child may have been exposed to.

Activated charcoal is indicated as the decontamination agent of choice for many poisonings, but it would not be the best next step for the girl in this vignette. Although her gag reflex is currently intact, her lethargy and shallow respirations, as well as the possibility that her neurologic status could become further compromised, place her at risk for aspiration of oral charcoal. Activated charcoal would not have a benefit in alleviating the effects of the girl's ethanol ingestion, because toxic alcohols are known to be very poorly adsorbed by charcoal. Furthermore, the exact time and nature of her ingestion is unknown, so it is uncertain whether activated charcoal would be effective in blocking the absorption of other toxins. Finally, the constellation of clinical findings in this girl suggests possible intoxication with opioids, and naloxone is the antidote of choice for opioid toxicity.

Intravenous dextrose would not be the best next management step for this girl. Her serum glucose level is normal. Intravenous fomepizole is the antidote of choice for ethylene glycol and methanol toxicity. Although ingestion of these substances cannot be excluded in the girl in the vignette, her clinical signs and symptoms are much more suggestive of a mixed opioid/ethanol exposure.

PREP Pearls

- Although toxicology screening is generally unnecessary for children presenting after unintentional ingestions with clinical findings consistent with the history, it can be useful when the possibility of a potentially harmful coingestion exists.

- Providers caring for children with presumed ethanol intoxication should maintain a high index of suspicion for the coingestion of other toxic substances.

- Toxic ingestions in preschool-aged children are typically unintentional, occur due to developmentally normal exploratory behavior, and involve small amounts of a single agent. Toxic exposures in adolescents are much more likely to be intentional and involve multiple drugs.

American Board of Pediatrics Content Specification(s)/ Content Area

- Recognize the signs and symptoms of ethanol intoxication, and manage appropriately
- Understand that ethanol intoxication may mask toxicity caused by ingestion of other drugs

Suggested Readings

Adger H Jr, Shonali S. Alcohol use disorders in adolescents. *Pediatr Rev.* 2013;34:103-114.

Legano L. Alcohol. *Pediatr Rev.* 2007;28;153-155.

Item 151   **Preferred Response: B**

The goal of maintenance intravenous (IV) fluid administration is to provide fluids and electrolytes that meet the daily metabolic needs of patients unable to take fluids and nutrition orally. The absence of any signs of dehydration, normal electrolyte and renal function values, and refusal of oral intake together indicate that maintenance IV fluid, rather than rehydration therapy, is appropriate for this girl.

In children, the most frequently used guidelines for IV fluid therapy are based on the Holliday and Segar method, which estimates fluid and electrolyte needs based on caloric energy expenditures of hospitalized children. Maintenance fluids replace all insensible and sensible fluid losses. Energy expenditure of 100 kcal is associated with 100 mL of water loss. In hospitalized children, daily energy expenditure is estimated at 100 kcal/kg and translates into 100 mL/kg sensible and insensible fluid loss. Electrolyte losses are estimated at 2 to 3 mEq for sodium and chloride and 1 to 2 mEq for potassium per 100 mL of fluid loss. For higher weights, fluid requirements do not show the same proportional increase.

Maintenance fluid requirements for hospitalized children, based on the Holliday and Segar method, are:

≤10 kg = 100 mL/kg OR 4 mL/kg per hour
>10 kg - 20 kg = 1,000 mL/day + 50 mL/kg for weight >10 kg
    OR
    40 mL/h + 2 mL/kg/h for weight >10 kg
>20 kg = 1,500 mL/day + 20 mL/kg for weight >20 kg
    OR
    60 mL/h + 1 mL/kg/h for weight > 20 kg

For the girl in the vignette, with a weight of 10 kg, daily energy expenditure of 100 kcal × 10 kg = 1,000 kcal = 1,000 mL of fluid loss per day. This would be accompanied by sodium and chloride loss = 20 to 30 mEq/day and potassium loss = 10 to 20 mEq/day. These losses translate into maintenance fluid requirements of 1,000 mL/day (40 mL/h). For patients who weigh more than 60 kg, fluid replacements of 100 mL/h or 2,400 mL/day are recommended.

PREP Pearls

- Electrolyte losses are estimated at 2 to 3 mEq for sodium and chloride and 1 to 2 mEq for potassium per 100 mL of fluid loss.

- Energy expenditure to meet daily metabolic needs is estimated at 100 kcal/kg and is associated with 100 mL/kg sensible and insensible fluid loss.

- Maintenance intravenous fluids aim to provide fluids and electrolytes to meet the daily metabolic needs of patients unable to take fluids orally.

American Board of Pediatrics Content Specification(s)/ Content Area

- Identify the physiologic requirements for sodium and potassium in patients of various ages

Suggested Readings

Mahajan P. Fluids and electrolytes in clinical practice. In: McInerny TK, Adam HM, Campbell DE, DeWitt TG, Foy JM, Kamat DM, eds. *American Academy of Pediatrics Textbook of Pediatric Care*. 1st ed. Elk Grove Village, IL: American Academy of Pediatrics; 2009:471-480.

The patient in this vignette had syncope during exercise or physical activity, which should raise suspicions of a cardiac etiology. This concerning history is often difficult to elicit. Of the response choices listed, electrocardiography is the most likely to reveal the diagnosis.

Syncope is an acute and transient loss of consciousness that resolves without intervention. Syncope can have neurally mediated, situational, neurologic, psychogenic, or cardiac causes (Item C152A).

Cardiac syncope can be a result of structural heart disease, arrhythmias, or myocardial dysfunction (Item C152B). These etiologies can result in decreased cardiac output leading to decreased cerebral perfusion and syncope. Prolonged cardiac syncope can cause ischemic injury and sudden death. Cardiac syncope can occur without any preceding symptoms but can also be preceded by chest pain or tachycardia.

Given that the adolescent girl in this vignette had syncope during exercise, cardiogenic syncope should be at the top of the differential diagnosis. Although electroencephalography,

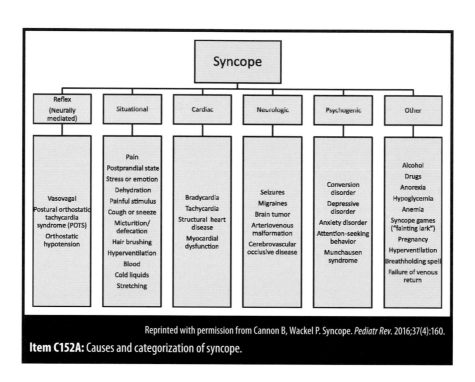

Reprinted with permission from Cannon B, Wackel P. Syncope. *Pediatr Rev.* 2016;37(4):160.

Item C152A: Causes and categorization of syncope.

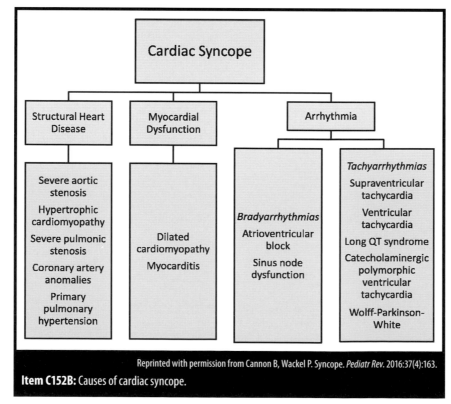

Reprinted with permission from Cannon B, Wackel P. Syncope. *Pediatr Rev.* 2016;37(4):163.

Item C152B: Causes of cardiac syncope.

orthostatic blood pressure measurements, and a serum glucose level may be part of a syncope evaluation, the history implies that a cardiac evaluation is most likely to reveal the diagnosis.

PREP Pearls

- Cardiac causes of syncope include structural heart disease, arrhythmia, or myocardial dysfunction.
- Syncope that occurs during exercise is concerning for a cardiac cause.

American Board of Pediatrics Content Specification(s)/Content Area

- Recognize the cardiac causes of syncope

Suggested Readings

Cannon B, Wackel P. Syncope. *Pediatr Rev.* 2016;37(4):159-168.

Willis J. Syncope. *Pediatr Rev.* 2000:21(6):201-204.

Item 153	Preferred Response: A

Bacterial vaginosis (BV) is the most common cause of vaginal discharge. The girl in this vignette gives a classic history for BV, which is often associated with a fishy-smelling, malodorous, thin, white-grayish discharge.

Bacterial vaginosis is caused by a shift in vaginal flora due to decreased levels of lactobacilli. Lactobacilli are hydrogen peroxide–producing organisms that keep the vaginal environment more acidic, with a pH between 3.8 and 4.5. When the levels of lactobacilli are decreased, the pH of the vaginal environment is increased, which allows for the overgrowth of bacteria, such as *Gardnerella vaginalis* and other anaerobic species including *Bacteroides*, *Peptostreptococcus*, *Prevotella*, *Mobiluncus*, *Ureaplasma*, and *Mycoplasma*, which can produce amines that cause the fishy odor. Factors that influence a decrease in lactobacilli include sexual activity without condoms, douching, and use of sex toys. Bacterial vaginosis has also been found in women who have sex with women.

A diagnosis of BV requires that 3 of the 4 Amsel criteria are met:

- A thin, white, homogenous vaginal discharge that coats the vaginal walls
- Vaginal pH greater than 4.5
- Positive whiff (amine) test result: a fishy odor is produced when 10% potassium hydroxide is added to a sample of discharge.
- Presence of at least 20% clue cells on wet mount slides. Clue cells usually have shaggy borders due to studding from coccobacilli (Item C153).

If the patient does not want a pelvic examination to evaluate the discharge, a blind swab of the vagina with a cotton swab can be performed by the provider or self-collected by the patient.

This patient is less likely to have *Candida* because itching and burning are not her main symptoms, and her symptoms did not improve with a course of an intravaginal antifungal. Although this patient is at risk for sexually transmitted infections, such as *Neisseria gonorrhoeae* and *Chlamydia trachomatis,* most cases are asymptomatic, and this patient

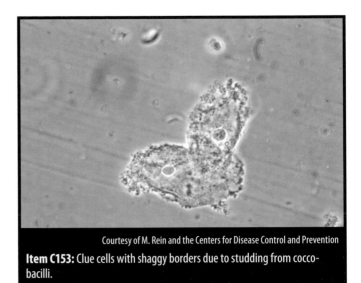

Courtesy of M. Rein and the Centers for Disease Control and Prevention

Item C153: Clue cells with shaggy borders due to studding from coccobacilli.

does not report dysuria, dyspareunia, or mucopurulent discharge. However, she would benefit from vaginal or urine-based nucleic acid amplification testing for *N gonorrhoeae* and *C trachomatis.*

PREP Pearls

- Bacterial vaginosis is caused by a shift in vaginal flora that results in decreased levels of lactobacilli.
- Fishy-smelling discharge is a hallmark of bacterial vaginosis.
- The most common cause of vaginal discharge is bacterial vaginosis.

American Board of Pediatrics Content Specification(s)/Content Area

- Recognize the clinical findings associated with bacterial vaginosis

Suggested Readings

Berlan ED, Emans SJ, O'Brien RF. Vulvovaginal complaints in the adolescent. In: Emans SJH, Laufer MR, eds. *Emans, Laufer, and Goldstein's Pediatric and Adolescent Gynecology.* 6th ed. Philadelphia, PA: Wolters Kluwer; 2012:305-324.

Kaskowitz A, Quint E. A practical overview of managing adolescent gynecology conditions in the pediatric office. *Pediatr Rev.* 2014;35(9):371-381.

Loveless M, Myint O. Vulvovaginitis–presentation of common problems in pediatric and adolescent gynecology. *Best Pract Res Clin Obstet Gynaecol.* 2018;48:14-27.

O'Brien G. Bacterial vaginosis. *Pediatr Rev.* 2008;29(6):209-211.

Item 154	Preferred Response: B

The girl in the vignette, who takes aspirin and warfarin daily, has been prescribed oral fluconazole for vulvovaginal candidiasis. Because fluconazole decreases the metabolism of warfarin, the most likely adverse effect is bleeding.

A drug interaction can be defined as 1 drug affecting the activity and/or side effect profile of another drug when they are coadministered. The interaction results in a change in the metabolism (pharmacokinetic properties) or distribution (pharmacodynamic properties) of 1 or more of the drugs. Critical illness with organ dysfunction may increase the risk for drug interaction, because of concomitant hepatic or renal dysfunction, polypharmacy, and/or metabolic disturbances. Administration of oral medications in relation to the intake of food and other medications can affect absorption and bioavailability. For example, medications that alter the gastrointestinal pH, such as histamine-2 antagonists or proton pump inhibitors, can affect the ratio of ionized to nonionized drug and the rate of absorption. Medications and other patient-related factors that either increase or slow gastric emptying can also affect the rate of absorption of some oral medications.

The distribution of drugs to body compartments, tissues, and cells is affected by binding to circulating plasma proteins, most importantly, albumin and α1-glycoprotein. Conditions that decrease serum protein levels such as nephrotic syndrome, protein-losing enteropathy, and malnutrition, can increase serum levels of protein-bound drugs. Concomitant administration of drugs with a higher affinity for serum proteins can displace other protein-bound drugs, thereby increasing their serum concentrations. These effects can be dangerous for patients treated with drugs that have a narrow therapeutic index. Consultation with a pharmacist and/or using resources such as the *Pediatric Dosage Handbook*, Trissel's *Handbook on Injectable Drugs*, or *Micromedex* can aid the clinician in prescribing safely for patients with polypharmacy or organ dysfunction.

Another important factor in drug metabolism is the cytochrome P450 (CYP) system, which consists of several hepatic enzymes responsible for the oxidation of 75% of all drugs. Hepatic function and drugs can affect the activity of CYP enzymes. Drugs such as rifampin, glucocorticoids, and some anticonvulsants can induce the activity of CYP enzymes, leading to subtherapeutic concentrations of some coadministered drugs. In contrast, a drug can inhibit the metabolism of another drug if they are both substrates of the same CYP enzyme.

Warfarin is an oral anticoagulant used as treatment or prophylaxis in patients with venous thrombosis or thromboembolism, end-stage congestive heart failure, atrial fibrillation, and prosthetic heart valves. Warfarin is metabolized by the cytochrome P450 2C9 isoenzyme (CYP2C9). Several medications can either induce or inhibit CYP2C9, altering warfarin levels. Fluconazole, the antifungal medication prescribed for the girl in the vignette, inhibits warfarin metabolism via the CYP system, thereby increasing warfarin levels in the blood. The mechanism of action of warfarin is to decrease the reduced form of vitamin K, which decreases the activity of the vitamin K–dependent clotting factors II, VII, IX, and

X. Increased warfarin levels can result in supratherapeutic anticoagulation caused by the inhibition of CYP2C9, leading to an increased risk of bleeding, not thromboembolic stroke. Although warfarin is metabolized in the liver, increased warfarin levels do not cause fulminant hepatic failure. Although fluconazole is nephrotoxic, its interaction with warfarin is not severe enough to cause renal failure.

PREP Pearls

- Consultation with a pharmacist and/or using resources such as the *Pediatric Dosage Handbook*, Trissel's *Handbook on Injectable Drugs*, or *Micromedex* can aid the clinician in prescribing for patients with polypharmacy or organ dysfunction.
- The cytochrome P450 system consists of several hepatic enzymes responsible for the oxidation of 75% of all drugs; its inducement or inhibition can alter drug metabolism.
- Warfarin is an anticoagulant that decreases the activity of the vitamin K–dependent clotting factors II, VII, IX, and X; its effect can be increased or decreased by the activity of the cytochrome P450 system.

American Board of Pediatrics Content Specification(s)/ Content Area

- Understand that concomitant administration of certain drugs can alter the serum concentrations of other drugs
- Recognize potential interactions between drugs and complementary therapies

Suggested Readings

Bungard TJ, Yakiwchuk E, Foisy M, Brocklebank C. Drug interactions involving warfarin: practice tool and practical management tips. *Can Pharmacists J.* 2011;144(1).

Tom-Revzon C. Drug interactions. *Pediatr Rev.* 2006;27:315.

Wilkinson GR. Drug metabolism and variability among patients in drug response. *N Engl J Med.* 2005;352(21):2211-2221.

Item 155   Preferred Response: D

The boy in this vignette, with a personal and family history of joint hypermobility, is at increased risk for joint dislocation. This diagnosis does not confer an increased risk for fracture, concussion, or hyperthermia.

Joint hypermobility syndrome (JHS) is a hereditary connective tissue disorder characterized by generalized joint hypermobility and chronic pain (Item C155). It is clinically indistinguishable from the hypermobility subtype of Ehlers-Danlos syndrome and may in fact be the same disorder.

Item C155. Clinical Symptoms of Joint Hypermobility Syndrome.

Musculoskeletal	Dermatologic	Gastrointestinal/Genitourinary	Other
Joint pain, ligament, and tendon injuries	Hyperextensible skin	Gastroesophageal reflux	Chronic widespread pain, chronic fatigue
Joint subluxations and dislocations	Easy bruising	Constipation alternating with diarrhea, bloating, early satiety	Anxiety, depression, phobias
Marfanoid habitus	Stretch marks		Palpitations, chest pain, postural tachycardia and hypotension, syncope
Difficulties with proprioception		Pelvic floor weakness, bladder dysfunction, stress incontinence	Drooping eyelids, myopia

Courtesy of I. Larson.

There is no known genetic defect or biologic marker in JHS, and the underlying pathophysiology is not well understood. Genetic studies suggest a dominant inheritance pattern with variable phenotypic penetrance.

Treatment of JHS is targeted to presenting symptoms, with an emphasis on physical therapy, multimodal pain control, and treatment of any associated anxiety or depression.

PREP Pearls

- Clinical features of joint hypermobility syndrome include musculoskeletal abnormalities (ligament and tendon injuries, joint dislocations, problems with proprioception) and dermatologic features (hyperextensible skin, easy bruising, and stretch marks) and may also include gastrointestinal dysmotility, chronic pain, chronic fatigue, autonomic dysfunction, and/or anxiety and depression.
- Joint hypermobility syndrome is a hereditary connective tissue disorder characterized by generalized joint hypermobility and chronic pain. It is clinically indistinguishable from the hypermobility subtype of Ehlers-Danlos syndrome and may in fact be the same disorder.

American Board of Pediatrics Content Specification(s)/ Content Area

- Recognize the clinical findings associated with hypermobility syndrome and manage appropriately

Suggested Readings

Fikree A, Aziz Q, Grahame R. Joint hypermobility syndrome. *Rheum Dis Clin North Am.* 2013;39(2):419-430.

Scheper MC, Nicholson LL, Adams RD, Tofts L, Pacey V. The natural history of children with joint hypermobility syndrome and Ehlers-Danlos hypermobility type: a longitudinal cohort study. *Rheumatology (Oxford).* 2017;56(12):2073-2083.

Item 156   Preferred Response: B

The asymptomatic, term neonate described in the vignette was born via vaginal delivery to a mother with an ulcerative genital lesion that is strongly suspicious for herpes simplex virus (HSV). There is no history of maternal HSV infection preceding the pregnancy. In this setting, performing a diagnostic evaluation of the neonate at approximately 24 hours of age and then starting empiric intravenous (IV) acyclovir is the most appropriate next step in the management.

Maternal classification of HSV infection determines the risk of intrapartum HSV transmission (Item C156A). The risk of herpes transmission is highest (25%-60%) in neonates born to mothers with primary genital HSV infection compared with mothers with recurrent genital HSV infection (<2%). The American Academy of Pediatrics (AAP) has published guidance on the management of asymptomatic neonates after vaginal or cesarean delivery to women with active genital HSV lesions (Item C156B and Item C156C). However, these guidelines may not be useful in settings with limited or no access to HSV polymerase chain reaction (PCR) assay and type-specific, maternal serologic tests.

Item C156A. Maternal Infection Classification by Genital HSV Viral Type and Maternal Serology[a].

Classification of Maternal Infection	PCR/Culture From Genital Lesion	Maternal HSV-1 and HSV-2 IgG Antibody Status
Documented first-episode primary infection	Positive, either virus	Both negative
Documented first-episode nonprimary infection	Positive for HSV-1 Positive for HSV-2	Positive for HSV-2 AND negative for HSV-1 Positive for HSV-1 AND negative for HSV-2
Assume first-episode (primary or nonprimary) infection	Positive for HSV-1 OR HSV-2 Negative OR not available[b]	Not available Negative for HSV-1 and/or HSV-2 OR not available
Recurrent infection	Positive for HSV-1 Positive for HSV-2	Positive for HSV-1 Positive for HSV-2

[a] To be used for women without a clinical history of genital herpes.

[b] When a genital lesion is strongly suspicious for HSV, clinical judgment should supersede the virological test results for the conservative purposes of this neonatal management algorithm. Conversely, if in retrospect, the genital lesion was not likely to be caused by HSV and the PCR assay result or culture is negative, departure from the evaluation and management in this conservative algorithm may be warranted.

Reference: Kimberlin DW, Baley J. American Academy of Pediatrics. Committee on Infectious Diseases, Guidance on management of asymptomatic neonates born to women with active genital herpes lesions. *Pediatrics.* 2013;131(2):e641.

For asymptomatic neonates born by vaginal or cesarean delivery to women with active genital lesions, performing a diagnostic evaluation and starting empiric IV acyclovir before 24 hours of age is not recommended; positive surface cultures before this time may represent contamination from intrapartum exposure and not viral replication suggestive of infection. In contrast, if the neonate becomes symptomatic at any time before 24 hours of age, immediate diagnostic evaluation and initiation of IV acyclovir are indicated. Immediate evaluation and treatment should also be considered in premature infants (<37 weeks of gestation) and when there is a maternal history of prolonged rupture of membranes. Close observation for signs of neonatal HSV infection (such as skin vesicles, signs of sepsis) with no diagnostic evaluation or empiric acyclovir therapy is an appropriate management for neonates born to mothers with a history of genital HSV, but no active genital lesions at delivery. In addition, parents and caregivers should be counseled to watch for these signs for a period of 6 weeks.

The incidence of neonatal herpes in the United States is between 1 in 3,000 and 1 in 20,000 live births. Approximately 70% of neonates with perinatal HSV infection are born to mothers with asymptomatic genital herpes infection near the time of delivery. Neonatal herpes can be caused by HSV1 or HSV2; approximately 75% of cases are caused by HSV2. Approximately 85% of neonatal HSV infection is acquired at delivery by fetal exposure to the virus in the maternal genital tract. Herpes simplex virus may also be acquired via ascending infection, both with membrane rupture or apparently intact membranes. In 5% of cases, HSV transmission occurs

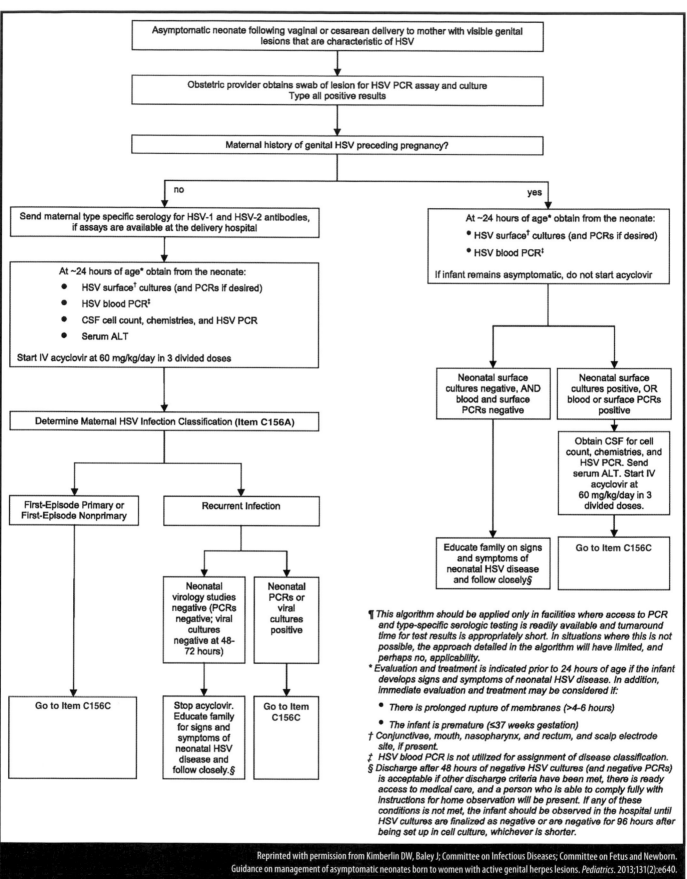

Item C156B: Management of asymptomatic newborns born to mothers with active genital HSV lesions. Abbreviations: ALT, alanine aminotransferase; D/C, discontinue.

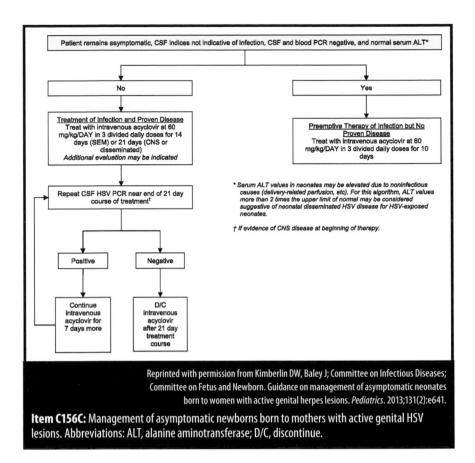

Reprinted with permission from Kimberlin DW, Baley J; Committee on Infectious Diseases; Committee on Fetus and Newborn. Guidance on management of asymptomatic neonates born to women with active genital herpes lesions. *Pediatrics*. 2013;131(2):e641.

Item C156C: Management of asymptomatic newborns born to mothers with active genital HSV lesions. Abbreviations: ALT, alanine aminotransferase; D/C, discontinue.

during pregnancy. Postnatal transmission, from a parent or other caregiver (often from non-genital infection), occurs in 10% of cases.

Neonatal herpes manifests as skin, eye, and mouth disease in 45% of cases; disseminated disease in 25% of cases; and central nervous system (CNS) disease, with or without skin lesions, in 30% of cases. Disseminated disease, which often presents around 10 to 12 days after birth, is the most severe form of neonatal HSV infection; it affects many organ systems, especially the lung, liver, and brain. The clinical presentation is often characterized by sepsis syndrome with pneumonitis, hepatitis, severe coagulopathy, and encephalitis. Skin lesions may be absent at disease onset, but approximately 66% of cases of disseminated disease have cutaneous vesicles.

Neonatal HSV disease may be diagnosed by detection of virus, by culture or PCR, from vesicles (if present) or surface swabs (conjunctivae, mouth, nasopharynx, or anus). Lumbar puncture should be performed in all cases of suspected neonatal herpes to evaluate for CNS involvement. The diagnostic evaluation of neonatal HSV infection should also include HSV PCR assays of cerebrospinal fluid and whole blood, cerebrospinal fluid cell count and chemistries, and serum alanine transferase levels. Neuroimaging and ophthalmologic evaluation are also recommended. In asymptomatic neonates born (via vaginal delivery or cesarean section) to women with active genital HSV lesions, a positive PCR test result or viral culture from surface swabs collected approximately 24 hours after delivery are indicative of neonatal HSV infection.

All neonates with suspected or confirmed HSV infection must receive IV acyclovir (60 mg/kg per day in 3 divided doses). The recommended duration of acyclovir therapy is 21 days for CNS or disseminated disease or 14 days for skin, eye, and mouth disease. For infants with CNS disease, a repeat lumbar puncture is recommended at the completion of the 3-week acyclovir course to demonstrate negative cerebrospinal fluid HSV PCR test results. If the results remain positive, intravenous acyclovir is continued for 1 additional week, followed by repeated cerebrospinal fluid testing. In such cases, pediatric infectious disease consultation is recommended. With appropriate and timely IV acyclovir therapy, the risk of mortality in disseminated neonatal HSV infection has decreased from 85% to 30%, and neurologic development is normal in 85% of survivors.

Following completion of intravenous acyclovir therapy, all infants with neonatal HSV infection (disseminated; skin, eye, and mouth; or CNS) must receive oral acyclovir suppressive therapy for 6 months. Improvement in neurodevelopmental outcomes in neonates with CNS disease and prevention of cutaneous recurrences in all 3 forms of HSV disease have been reported with oral acyclovir suppressive therapy. Infants must be closely monitored for neutropenia, with serial complete blood cell counts, while receiving this treatment.

PREP Pearls

- For asymptomatic neonates born to women with active genital lesions suggestive for herpes simplex virus, with no maternal history of genital herpes, performing a diagnostic evaluation in the neonate and starting empiric intravenous acyclovir at approximately 24 hours of age is recommended.

- Neonatal herpes simplex virus (HSV) disease may be diagnosed by virus detection, by culture or polymerase chain reaction (PCR), from vesicles or surface swabs. Additional evaluation should include HSV PCR assays of cerebrospinal fluid and whole blood, cerebrospinal fluid cell count and chemistries, and serum alanine transferase levels.

- The risk of herpes transmission is higher (25%-60%) among neonates of mothers with primary genital herpes simplex virus (HSV) infection compared with neonates of mothers with recurrent genital HSV infection (<2%).

American Board of Pediatrics Content Specification(s)/ Content Area

- Understand the epidemiology of herpes simplex virus
- Understand the risk of maternal transmission of herpes simplex virus infection to newborn infants

Suggested Readings

American Academy of Pediatrics. Herpes simplex. In: Kimberlin DW, Brady MT, Jackson MA, Long SS, eds. *Red Book: 2018 Report of the Committee on Infectious Diseases*. 31st ed. Itasca, IL: American Academy of Pediatrics; 2018:437-449.

Kimberlin DW, Baley J. American Academy of Pediatrics. Committee on Infectious Diseases, Guidance on management of asymptomatic neonates born to women with active genital herpes lesions. *Pediatrics*. 2013;131(2):e635-e646.

Kimberlin DW, Lin CY, Jacobs RF, et al. Natural history of neonatal herpes simplex virus infections in the acyclovir era. *Pediatrics*. 2001;108(2):223-229.

Item 157   Preferred Response: D

For a given diagnostic test, the ability to detect disease varies. Positive predictive value (PPV) and negative predictive value (NPV) quantify the proportion of patients with disease whose test results are positive and negative. Of note, positive predictive values and negative predictive values differ based on the prevalence of disease in a particular population. Therefore, a diagnostic test will have different PPVs and NPVs depending on the patient population in question.

For the study described in the vignette, the population is neonates admitted to the neonatal intensive care unit with concern for infection. C-reactive protein (CRP) is the diagnostic test being evaluated for its ability to detect infection. Positive predictive value is defined as the number of true positives out of all the positives detected by the test, in this case an elevated CRP. Negative predictive value is the number of true negatives out of all the negatives detected by the test, that is, a CRP less than 1 mg/dL.

	Bacteremia	No bacteremia
CRP >1 mg/dL	TP	FP
CRP <1 mg/dL	FN	TN

Positive predictive value: TP/TP+FP
Negative predictive value: TN/FN+TN

In this case, the negative predictive value is the number of true negatives (79) divided by the number of true negatives plus false negatives (79+3) which equals 96%.

Sensitivity and specificity detect the ability of the test to identify disease. These attributes are defined by the test itself, independent of the patient population. Sensitivity describes how many neonates with infection are identified by a CRP less than 1 mg/dL (95 nmol/L). Specificity is how many neonates without bacteremia have a low CRP.

Sensitivity = TP/TP + FN = 3/3+3 = 50%
Specificity = TN/FP + TN = 84%

PREP Pearls

- Both positive and negative predictive value vary with the prevalence of disease in the population in question and are not intrinsic to the test.

- Negative predictive value is the fraction of patients with a negative test value who do not have the disease.

- Positive predictive value is the fraction of patients with a positive test value who have the disease.

American Board of Pediatrics Content Specification(s)/ Content Area

- Understand positive and negative predictive values
- Understand sensitivity and specificity and how to apply them to test results

Suggested Readings

Carvajal DN, Rowe PC. Research and statistics: sensitivity, specificity, predictive values, and Likelihood Ratios. *Pediatr Rev*. 2010;31;511.

Lo S. Sensitivity, accuracy and analytic testing. In: Kliegman RM, Stanton BF, St Geme JW, Schor NF, eds. *Nelson Textbook of Pediatrics*. 20th ed. Philadelphia, PA: Saunders Elsevier; 2016:3460-3464.

Item 158   Preferred Response: D

The patient in this vignette has exercise-related dyspnea that most likely is caused by bronchospasm. Onset of symptoms after several minutes of aerobic exercise in the context of a family history of asthma is strongly suggestive of exercise-induced asthma. In the face of normal baseline spirometry and no symptoms from other triggers, the appropriate therapy is pretreatment with inhaled bronchodilator. At least a therapeutic trial of albuterol is needed, with formal exercise testing recommended if he does not get adequate prevention of symptoms from albuterol administered before running. Because there is a clear association of symptoms with exercise and a reported response to albuterol, a lack of drug therapy would be inappropriate.

The patient does not appear to have persistent asthma as he has no symptoms other than with exercise and a normal baseline spirogram. Without a diagnosis or suspicion of persistent asthma, daily controller therapy is unnecessary at this point. However, because he appears to have allergies based on his perennial nasal symptoms superimposed on seasonal allergies, he is at risk for having persistent asthma and that should be an ongoing consideration.

It is not appropriate to use inhaled long-acting β-agonists as sole therapy for asthma. The only accepted use for long-acting β-agonists in the pediatric population is in combination with inhaled corticosteroids as step-up therapy for moderate or severe persistent asthma.

PREP Pearls

- Exercise may be one of many triggers in the child predisposed to asthma.
- Exercise may be the only trigger for wheezing in some children.

American Board of Pediatrics Content Specification(s)/ Content Area

- Recognize the clinical features associated with exercise-induced asthma

Suggested Readings

Boulet L-P, O'Byrne PM. Asthma and exercise-induced bronchoconstriction in athletes. *N Engl J Med*. 2015;372(7):641-648.

Tilles SA. Exercise-induced respiratory symptoms: an epidemic among adolescents. *Ann Allergy Asthma Immunol*. 2010;104(5):361-367.

Wood PR, Hill VL. Practical management of asthma. *Pediatr Rev*. 2009;30(10):375-385.

Item 159 — Preferred Response: A

The boy in this vignette has a painful rash around the anus that is intensely erythematous and has a well-defined border; there is maceration and some exudate. These findings are typical of perianal bacterial dermatitis (formerly termed perianal streptococcal dermatitis or perianal cellulitis). Accordingly, treatment with oral cephalexin is appropriate. Other common forms of diaper rash (irritant contact, candidiasis, seborrheic dermatitis, psoriasis) are not limited to the perianal area and, therefore, treatment with topical hydrocortisone or clotrimazole or oral nystatin is not warranted.

Perianal bacterial dermatitis is a superficial cellulitis caused by *Streptococcus pyogenes* or *Staphylococcus aureus*. The peak incidence is between 3 and 4 years of age, and boys are affected more often than girls. Most patients are well but some may have a concomitant streptococcal pharyngitis. Other family members may be affected, especially if there has been co-bathing with the index case.

Perianal bacterial dermatitis is characterized by intense perianal erythema with a well-defined border. Pruritus or discomfort usually is present, and a foul odor may be noted. Children may experience pain with defecation, stool withholding, or passage of blood-tinged stools. Occasional patients have associated balanoposthitis or vulvovaginitis. Less commonly, the neck folds, axillae, or inguinal creases may be involved as part of streptococcal intertrigo (Item C159).

The diagnosis usually is made clinically but may be confirmed with bacterial skin culture. If a culture is performed it is prudent to inform the laboratory because routine processing of perianal swabs may involve the use of inhibitors to the growth of *S pyogenes*.

Treatment with a 10-day course of oral penicillin or amoxicillin often is advised. However, because *S aureus* appears to be an increasingly common cause of perianal bacterial der-

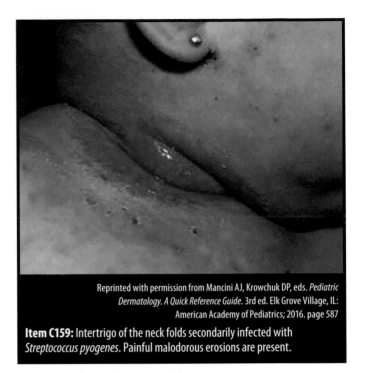

Reprinted with permission from Mancini AJ, Krowchuk DP, eds. Pediatric Dermatology. A Quick Reference Guide. 3rd ed. Elk Grove Village, IL: American Academy of Pediatrics; 2016. page 587

Item C159: Intertrigo of the neck folds secondarily infected with *Streptococcus pyogenes*. Painful malodorous erosions are present.

matitis, some clinicians prefer oral cephalexin (or another antibiotic that also possesses antistaphylococcal activity based on local resistance patterns or the results of bacterial culture and sensitivity).

PREP Pearls

- Because perianal bacterial dermatitis may be caused by *Streptococcus pyogenes* or *Staphylococcus aureus*, empiric treatment is with oral cephalexin or another antistaphylococcal antibiotic based on local sensitivity patterns.
- Perianal bacterial dermatitis is characterized by intense, well-defined perianal erythema, often with maceration and exudate.

American Board of Pediatrics Content Specification(s)/ Content Area

- Plan the appropriate management of cellulitis of the skin of various etiologies

Suggested Readings

American Academy of Pediatrics Section on Dermatology. Perianal bacterial dermatitis. In: Mancini AJ, Krowchuk DP, eds. *Pediatric Dermatology: A Quick Reference Guide*. 3rd ed. Elk Grove Village, IL: American Academy of Pediatrics; 2016:187-189.

Stevens DL, Bisno AL, Chambers HF, et al. Practice guidelines for the diagnosis and management of skin and soft tissue infections: 2014 update by the Infectious Disease Society of America. *Clin Infect Dis*. 2014;59(2):147-159.

Item 160 — Preferred Response: D

The girl in this vignette has ketotic hypoglycemia. It is the most common cause of childhood hypoglycemia and is a diagnosis of exclusion. The girl's age, presentation, laboratory results at the time of hypoglycemia ("critical sample"), and rapid recovery after treatment with intravenous glucose are consistent with ketotic hypoglycemia.

The typical age range for ketotic hypoglycemia is 18 months to 5 years with resolution by age 7 years. These children have a decreased tolerance for fasting. Hypoglycemic episodes often occur in the morning after a fast of approximately 10 to 16 hours and may be precipitated by an acute illness. The etiology is unclear but seems to be caused by a lack of substrate availability. Children with ketotic hypoglycemia are often thin and have decreased lean body mass. Fasting levels of alanine, a substrate for gluconeogenesis, are reportedly lower than in normal controls. Long-term management consists of avoidance of fasting and ensuring adequate sugar-containing fluids when ill.

A critical sample, drawn at the time of hypoglycemia, is helpful in determining the underlying diagnosis. Recommended tests to be drawn prior to treatment include: glucose, lactate, insulin, C-peptide, β-hydroxybutyrate, free fatty acids, cortisol, and growth hormone. Urine ketones and urine organic acids can be assessed with the first voided urine after an episode of hypoglycemia. Tests that can be drawn after correction of the hypoglycemia may include: acylcarnitines, plasma amino acids, ammonia, electrolytes, and liver function tests.

The critical sample for the girl in this vignette shows a normal physiologic response to hypoglycemia. Elevated serum and urine ketone levels are characteristic of ketotic hypoglycemia and represent activation of fat metabolism as an alternative fuel source. Similarly, the elevated fatty acids are additional markers of activated fat metabolism. Cortisol and growth hormone are counterregulatory hormones and are normally elevated in response to hypoglycemia. Although not given for the girl in this vignette, an insulin level is useful at the time of hypoglycemia to help evaluate for hyperinsulinism. Insulin is normally undetectable in the context of hypoglycemia.

The presence of high ketone levels (β-hydroxybutyric acid) in the girl's critical sample is not consistent with hyperinsulinism or a fatty acid oxidation disorder. Insulin suppresses fat breakdown and ketone body formation. Thus, in the context of hyperinsulinism, fatty acid and ketone levels are low at the time of hypoglycemia. A detectable insulin level at the time of hypoglycemia is also consistent with hyperinsulinism. A child with glycogen storage disease would likely have hepatomegaly and an elevated lactate level in the critical sample.

Other potential causes of hypoglycemia in children include metabolic disorders and alcohol ingestion. Alcohol causes hypoglycemia by inhibiting gluconeogenesis. After fasting overnight, a young child who ingests alcohol that was inadvertently left out can easily become hypoglycemic.

PREP Pearls

- A critical sample, drawn at the time of hypoglycemia, is helpful in the evaluation of hypoglycemia. Recommended tests to be drawn prior to treatment include: glucose, lactate, insulin, C-peptide, β-hydroxybutyrate, free fatty acids, cortisol, and growth hormone.
- Ketotic hypoglycemia is the most common cause of childhood hypoglycemia and is a diagnosis of exclusion.

American Board of Pediatrics Content Specification(s)/ Content Area
- Recognize the clinical features associated with ketotic hypoglycemia in children of various ages

Suggested Readings

Ghosh A, Banerjee I, Morris AA. Recognition, assessment and management of hypoglycaemia in childhood. *Arch Dis Child*. 2016;101(6):575-80.

Sperling MA. Hypoglycemia. In: Kliegman RM, Stanton BF, St. Geme JW, and Schor NF, eds. *Nelson Textbook of Pediatrics*. 20th ed. Philadelphia, PA: Elsevier; 2016:773-788.

Thornton PS, Stanley CA, De Leon DD, et al; Pediatric Endocrine Society. Recommendations from the Pediatric Endocrine Society for evaluation and management of persistent hypoglycemia in neonates, infants, and children. *J Pediatr*. 2015;167(2):238-245.

Item 161   Preferred Response: C

47,XYY syndrome is a sex chromosomal disorder that occurs in approximately 1 in 1,000 male newborns, though it is largely underdiagnosed because of the lack of unusual physical features or facial dysmorphology. Most boys with 47,XYY syndrome will have normal sexual development and fertility, though testicular failure has been reported. Classic features include taller than normal stature, speech and language delay, cystic acne in adolescence, and learning disabilities. Normal intelligence is typical; however, affected children have IQs that are on average 10 to 15 points lower than those of their siblings. Behavioral problems are common, including impulsivity and hyperactivity.

A normal complement of chromosomes within each human cell includes 46 chromosomes; the X and Y chromosomes are called sex chromosomes. A female will have 2 X chromosomes (46,XX) and a male will have 1 X and 1 Y chromosome (46,XY). In 47,XYY syndrome there is an extra copy of the Y chromosome within each cell. This is not an inherited condition; it occurs as a random cell division error during sperm cell formation.

A sex chromosomal disorder seen in girls is 47,XXX syndrome, also known as triple X syndrome, which has an additional X chromosome in each of a female's cells. These girls can have tall stature, learning disabilities, and speech/language delays. They have no unusual dysmorphology or physical features and normal sexual development and fertility.

Macroorchidism is a common postpubertal finding in boys with fragile X syndrome. Precocious puberty is not a typical presentation in children with fragile X. Precocious puberty is commonly seen in neurofibromatosis type 1 and McCune Albright syndrome, both of which have distinctive cutaneous features on examination.

American Board of Pediatrics Content Specification(s)/ Content Area

- Recognize the clinical features associated with a 47,XXX chromosome abnormality
- Recognize the clinical features associated with a 47,XYY chromosome abnormality

Suggested Readings

National Center for Advancing Translational Sciences, National Institutes of Health. 47,XYY syndrome. https://rarediseases.info.nih.gov/diseases/5674/47-xyy-syndrome.

Otter M, Schrander-Stumpel CTRM, Curfs LMG. Triple X syndrome: a review of the literature. *Eur J Hum Genet*. 2010;18(3): 265-271.

Genetics Home Reference, National Institutes of Health. 47,XYY syndrome. https://ghr.nlm.nih.gov/condition/47xyy-syndrome.

Item 162   Preferred Response: A

For the child in this vignette, deferring allergy testing, but reconsidering if he has further reactions to specific foods, reduces the risk of an incorrect diagnosis of food allergy, as compared to initiating allergy testing now. The child's clinical presentation is mild and self-resolving, and both the rash and vomiting are nonspecific. The child ate a range of foods, thereby offering no useful information to direct testing for reaction to specific foods. Therefore, refraining from allergy testing at this juncture represents a prudent use of resources and recognition of the limits of allergy testing.

If the child in this vignette had a history that was more suggestive of a systemic IgE-mediated reaction (eg, urticaria or angioedema; respiratory manifestations, such as stridor or wheezing; and gastrointestinal manifestations, such as nausea, vomiting, cramping, or diarrhea), or if the child had a reaction that consistently occurred with repeated exposure, then allergy testing would be appropriate. Dietary avoidance, which is the mainstay of management for food allergies, can have implications on social, financial, emotional, and nutritional aspects of family life. Therefore, over-diagnosis should be avoided.

Although many foods have been associated with allergic reactions, milk, soy, wheat, eggs, peanuts, tree nuts, and shellfish are the most common in children. It is recommended that allergy testing be directed to specific foods whenever possible. The use of broad allergy panels is not recommended. Initial allergy testing can be done 2 ways:

- Skin-prick testing, whereby a small amount of allergen is introduced into the surface of the skin, resulting, if positive, in a wheal-and-flare response
- Serum allergen-specific IgE (sIgE) levels, which quantify IgE levels to specific foods

Skin-prick testing is traditionally administered by an allergist and requires intact skin. Therefore, patients with skin abnormalities such as severe eczema and younger patients may not be candidates for this testing. Skin-prick testing also requires patients to forego antihistamine medications prior to testing. Skin-prick testing is less expensive than serum sIgE levels; however, sIgE levels can be ordered by the primary care pediatrician without referral to an allergist and are not affected by exposure to antihistamine. Both approaches have high false-positive rates, and selection and interpretation of these tests should be done with the clinical presentation in mind. However, very elevated sIgE levels, combined with a convincing history of food allergy, indicates a high likelihood of a food allergy. Skin-prick testing results and sIgE levels generally correlate with each other, so performing both tests for a specific food is not helpful. If needed, an oral food challenge administered in an allergist's office can confirm a suspected food allergy.

Respiratory allergens can also be detected with skin-prick testing or serum sIgE levels. Testing for reaction to indoor allergens (eg, dust mite, animal dander) is recommended for children with persistent asthma to optimize symptom control, in combination with appropriate medications. As with food allergy, selecting which tests are appropriate is based on known environmental exposures and suspected triggers. Identification of which allergens are most likely triggers of their child's asthma can help caregivers prioritize avoidance measures most likely to be effective. However, as with food allergy testing, results should be interpreted in a clinical context before expecting a family to take drastic measures to avoid certain allergens.

American Board of Pediatrics Content Specification(s)/ Content Area

- Understand the limitations of allergy testing in children
- Understand the indications for serum-specific IgE testing and that results correlate closely with results of allergy skin testing
- Know the indications for allergy skin testing, and what medications can alter the results

Suggested Readings

Link HW. Pediatric asthma in a nutshell. *Pediatr Rev.* 2014;35(7):287-298.

Sicherer SH, Wood RA; American Academy of Pediatrics Section on Allergy and Immunology. Allergy testing in childhood: using allergen-specific IgE tests. *Pediatrics.* 2012;129(1):193-197.

Item 163   Preferred Response: B

The most appropriate antibiotic to use as monotherapy for the neonate in this vignette is meropenem. A urinary tract infection caused by *Escherichia coli* is present but the neonate has not had evaluation of cerebrospinal fluid to rule out meningitis. The most appropriate antibiotic given the antimicrobial susceptibility pattern of the organism and incomplete evaluation for invasive infection is meropenem.

While *E coli* are normal inhabitants of the human gastrointestinal tract, virulent strains have the potential to cause clinical syndromes including diarrheal illness, urinary tract infections, bacteremia, and meningitis. Diarrheagenic strains are typically acquired via contaminated food and water. The maternal genital tract is the usual source of infection in neonates that develop disease in the first few days after birth, although colonization can occur in the hospital setting via medical personnel, devices, or procedures.

The organism is susceptible to gentamicin. This antibiotic would be an appropriate and more narrow therapy if the *E coli* infection were limited to the urinary tract. However, until meningitis is excluded, gentamicin monotherapy should not be used because aminoglycoside antibiotics have poor cerebrospinal fluid penetration.

Nitrofurantoin should not be used in febrile urinary tract infections in young children. Nitrofurantoin does not have adequate kidney tissue penetration. In young children with febrile urinary tract infections, it is very difficult to discern cystitis from pyelonephritis. Therefore, antibiotics with good tissue penetration should be used given the possibility of renal parenchymal involvement.

Trimethoprim-sulfamethoxazole is contraindicated in infants less than 2 months of age, per the manufacturer's labeling. Sulfonamides displace bilirubin from their albumin-binding sites, leading to increases in bilirubin plasma levels. Additionally, trimethoprim-sulfamethoxazole has limited usefulness in the setting of meningitis, which has not been excluded in the patient in this vignette.

PREP Pearls

- Although *Escherichia coli* are normal inhabitants of the human gastrointestinal tract, virulent strains may cause clinical syndromes including diarrheal illness, urinary tract infections, bacteremia, and meningitis.
- Aminoglycoside monotherapy should not be used for treatment of gram-negative meningitis because this antibiotic class has poor cerebrospinal fluid penetration.
- Nitrofurantoin should not be used in febrile urinary tract infections in young children because it does not have adequate kidney tissue penetration.

American Board of Pediatrics Content Specification(s)/ Content Area

- Plan appropriate management for a patient with *Escherichia coli* infection
- Understand the epidemiology of *Escherichia coli* infection

Suggested Readings

American Academy of Pediatrics. Serious bacterial infections caused by *Enterobacteriaceae* (with emphasis on septicemia and meningitis in neonates). In: Kimberlin DW, Brady MT, Jackson MA, Long SS, eds. *Red Book: 2018 Report of the Committee on Infectious Diseases.* 31st ed. Itasca, IL: American Academy of Pediatrics; 2018:328-331.

Makvana S, Krilov l. *Escherichia coli* infections. *Pediatr Rev.* 2015;36(4):167-171.

Item 164   Preferred Response: C

The boy in the vignette has calf muscle pain and difficulty walking after an acute illness. His history and physical examination are suggestive of acute myositis following influenza infection.

Benign acute childhood myositis (BACM) most commonly occurs after an influenza B infection, and typically affects preschool and early school-aged children. Influenza A, coxsackievirus, adenovirus, parainfluenza virus, and other viruses have also been associated with BACM. Affected children generally present with calf pain and a stiff-legged gait. Creatine kinase levels are usually highly elevated, but decrease within 2 to 3 weeks of onset. Treatment is primarily supportive care. In a recent study of patients at 2 large pediatric hospitals, all affected patients fully recovered without sequelae.

Juvenile dermatomyositis (JDM) and juvenile polymyositis (JMP) should be included in the differential diagnosis of BACM. The boy in the vignette has a history of recent viral infection and does not exhibit characteristic signs and symptoms of inflammatory myositis (eg, systemic symptoms), the diffuse muscle involvement seen with JMP, or the characteristic rashes seen with JDM. Heliotrope rash, a red-violet discoloration of the eyelids, and/or Gottron papules, a papular rash over the dorsal surface of the finger joints, are found in most children with JDM.

Given that the boy in the vignette does not have joint pain or swelling, and his complete blood cell count and erythrocyte sedimentation rate are normal, juvenile idiopathic arthritis is unlikely to be the cause of his symptoms.

Both hyperkalemia and severe hypokalemia can cause an ascending muscle weakness. Hypokalemia is a rare adverse effect of albuterol but would not be expected to occur with short term use.

Arthritis can be a late manifestation of Lyme disease. Calf pain occurring 1 week after an upper respiratory infection would not be consistent with *Borrelia burgdorferi* infection. Leg pain can be an early symptom in children with Duchenne muscular dystrophy (DMD). Although DMD does not explain this boy's recent viral infection, this diagnosis should be considered if his condition does not improve within several weeks.

PREP Pearls

- Benign acute childhood myositis causes calf pain and stiff-legged gait; it most commonly occurs after an influenza B infection.
- Benign acute childhood myositis is treated with supportive care and resolves without sequelae.

American Board of Pediatrics Content Specification(s)/Content Area

- Plan the appropriate evaluation and management of myositis
- Identify the etiology of myositis

Suggested Readings

Rider L, Lindsley C, Miller F. Juvenile Dermatomyositis. In: Petty R, Laxer R, Lindsley C, ed. *Textbook of Pediatric Rheumatology, 7th edition.* Philadelphia: Elsevier; 2016:351-383.

Rosenberg T, Heitner S, Scolnik D, Levin Ben-Adiva E, Rimon A, Glatstein M. Outcome of benign acute childhood myositis: the experience of 2 large tertiary care pediatric hospitals. *Pediatr Emerg Care.* 2018; 34(6):400-402.

Item 165   Preferred Response: B

The girl in the vignette has the characteristic physical examination findings of enthesitis of the Achilles tendon. The best initial management step for her is the use of a non-steroidal anti-inflammatory drug (NSAID). Enthesitis is defined as inflammation at the site of insertion of ligaments, tendons, joint capsule, or fascia to bone. Her recent history of *Chlamydia trachomatis* infection followed by acute onset of localized heel pain and swelling, in light of being otherwise well and afebrile, suggests reactive or postinfectious arthritis as the most likely cause of her symptoms. Children with reactive arthritis typically present with mono- or asymmetric oligoarthritis 1 to 4 weeks after infection. As in this case, laboratory results usually reveal a mild elevation in inflammatory markers and white blood cell count without a significant left shift. No microorganisms are present in the joint fluid.

Reactive or postinfectious arthritis is a clinical diagnosis most commonly associated with genitourinary or gastrointestinal infections. Other types of arthritis must be excluded. Management is supportive; NSAIDs, rest, and ice are the mainstays of initial treatment. Continuous use of maximal anti-inflammatory doses of NSAIDs for at least 2 weeks is recommended to control pain and inflammation. If the girl's gonorrhea or chlamydia test results are positive, she would also require appropriate antimicrobial treatment. If the inciting infection is enteric, antimicrobial treatment is usually not necessary. Intra-articular glucocorticoids may be administered in children with persistent symptoms, despite maximized NSAID use. Systemic glucocorticoids may be used in children with several joints involved, or those who do not respond to intra-articular therapy. If the arthritis fails to resolve after 6 months, a rheumatology referral is recommended for the management of chronic reactive arthritis. Physical therapy may be an appropriate adjunct treatment.

PREP Pearls

- For patients with persistent symptoms despite maximized nonsteroidal anti-inflammatory drug use, intra-articular glucocorticoids may be administered.
- Reactive or postinfectious arthritis is a clinical diagnosis most commonly associated with genitourinary or gastrointestinal infections.
- The initial management of reactive arthritis is supportive: nonsteroidal anti-inflammatory drugs, rest, and ice are the mainstays of treatment.

American Board of Pediatrics Content Specification(s)/Content Area

- Plan the appropriate management of postinfectious arthritis

Suggested Readings

Bernard R. Approach to the child with joint inflammation. *Pediatr Clin North Am.* 2012;59:245-262.

John J, Chandran L. Arthritis in children and adolescents. *Pediatr Rev.* 2011;32(11):470-480.

Siegel DM, Marston B. Joint pain. In: McInerny TK, Adam HM, Campbell DE, DeWitt TG, Foy JM, Kamat DM, eds. *American Academy of Pediatrics Textbook of Pediatric Care.* 2nd ed. Elk Grove Village, IL: American Academy of Pediatrics; 2017:1480-1484.

Item 166   Preferred Response: C

The adolescent girl in this vignette has Crohn disease, a subset of inflammatory bowel disease (IBD), with a combination of intestinal and extraintestinal manifestations. Inflammatory bowel disease is an immune-mediated disorder resulting in chronic gastrointestinal inflammation. Generally, IBD presents with intestinal symptoms including abdominal pain, vomiting, diarrhea, and weight loss, however (as in this vignette), extraintestinal manifestations can predominate and be the presenting sign or symptom. While this patient's primary concern was joint pain, other signs and symptoms, particularly the constellation of gastrointestinal symptoms and findings suggestive of perianal disease, raise the suspicion of IBD. In addition, her laboratory results, including the microcytic anemia, elevated C-reactive protein level, and increased erythrocyte sedimentation rate, are consistent with IBD. A diagnosis of IBD is established based on endoscopic evaluation with biopsies, thus a colonoscopy is most likely to establish this patient's diagnosis.

The 2 major subtypes of IBD are Crohn disease and ulcerative colitis. Crohn disease is characterized by transmural involvement that may be patchy but can affect any part of the intestinal tract from the mouth to the anus. Ulcerative colitis affects the superficial mucosa and its involvement of the intestinal tract is limited to the colon, generally beginning in the distal colon and extending proximally in a continuous fashion.

Both ulcerative colitis and Crohn disease can present with extraintestinal manifestations including growth failure, arthritis and arthralgias, autoimmune hepatitis, primary sclerosing cholangitis, pancreatitis, uveitis, erythema nodosum, pyoderma gangrenosum, hypercoagulability, reactive airway disease, and nephrolithiasis.

Antinuclear antibody testing is not helpful for the diagnosis of inflammatory bowel disease, however antinuclear antibody levels could be elevated in autoimmune hepatitis, an extraintestinal manifestation of IBD. Bone marrow biopsy is not used for diagnosis of IBD. This patient has a low hemoglobin level, but her white blood cell count and platelet count are normal/elevated, making bone marrow disease unlikely. Radiographs of the ankle and knee would not diagnose inflammatory bowel disease.

PREP Pearls

- Although inflammatory bowel disease usually presents with gastrointestinal symptoms, including diarrhea and abdominal pain, the initial presentation may be with extraintestinal manifestations, including arthritis or arthralgias.
- Crohn disease is characterized by transmural involvement that may be patchy but can affect any part of the intestinal tract.
- Diagnosis of inflammatory bowel disease is made following endoscopic evaluation with biopsies.
- The 2 major subtypes of inflammatory bowel disease are Crohn disease and ulcerative colitis.
- Ulcerative colitis affects the superficial mucosa, and its involvement of the intestinal tract is limited to the colon.

American Board of Pediatrics Content Specification(s)/Content Area

- Formulate a differential diagnosis of acute colitis
- Plan the initial evaluation of inflammatory bowel disease
- Distinguish the clinical features associated with Crohn disease from those of ulcerative colitis
- Recognize the association of arthritis with inflammatory bowel disease
- Plan appropriate management of severe colitis
- Recognize the clinical features associated with inflammatory bowel disease (eg, Crohn disease, ulcerative colitis)

Suggested Readings

Rufo PA, Denson LA, Sylvester FA, et al. Health supervision in the management of children and adolescents with IBD: NASPGHAN recommendations. *J Pediatr Gastroenterol Nutr.* 2012;55(1):93-108.

Shapiro JM, Subedi S, LeLeiko NS. Inflammatory bowel disease. *Pediatr Rev.* 2016;37(8):337-347.

| Item 167 | Preferred Response: A |

The boy in this vignette has oppositional defiant disorder (ODD) for which psychosocial intervention via parent behavioral training is indicated. Behavioral management principles include applying consequences for challenging behaviors, providing immediate (not delayed) responses to the unwanted behaviors, decreasing (not increasing) positive reinforcement of disruptive behaviors, and providing a consistent (not varied) response to the behaviors. Punishments such as time-out, which removes the child from attention, interaction, and activities, or loss of privileges can also be used to decrease undesired behaviors. Positive reinforcement of desired compliant behavior through praise is generally preferred over negative consequences.

Typically developing children may tantrum as toddlers and may exhibit defiance in adolescence. Children with temperamental characteristics of low frustration tolerance, high reactivity, and high emotional intensity are generally more easily annoyed, less compliant, and more likely to respond negatively than children with comparatively "easy" temperaments. However, children with "difficult" temperaments should not be diagnosed with ODD unless they demonstrate behaviors of irritability, anger, resentfulness, defiance, and vindictiveness that are developmentally inappropriate, persistent, intense, frequent, and/or functionally impairing. A diagnosis of conduct disorder (CD) would not be warranted unless there is aggression towards people or animals, destruction of property, theft, deceit, and/or disregard for societal rules.

When evaluating a child for possible ODD or CD, input from the child, parents, and other adults (eg, teachers, coaches, other caregivers) should be considered. The specific behaviors, their triggers and duration, and resultant functional impairment should be ascertained. Standardized tools (eg, Child Behavior Checklist, Behavior Assessment System for Children, Youth Self-Report, Conners 3) can be used to determine when behaviors exceed developmental expectations and which mental health diagnoses may be present. Since ODD and CD commonly coexist with other mental health diagnoses, particularly attention-deficit/hyperactivity disorder, these conditions (eg, anxiety, depression, learning disorder, substance use disorder) should be considered during the initial evaluation.

Evidence-based treatment of ODD and CD includes individual approaches (eg, problem-solving skills training) and family approaches (eg, parent management training in effective discipline and supervision). Parent training is emphasized in younger children whereas individual approaches are more often employed in adolescents. More than one mode of treatment may be used. When behavioral strategies are insufficient, treating coexisting conditions such as attention-deficit/hyperactivity disorder or anxiety with medication may lessen the oppositional behaviors.

PREP Pearls

- For disruptive behavior disorders (eg, oppositional defiant disorder, conduct disorder) parent training on behavior management including applying consequences for challenging behaviors is emphasized in younger children whereas individual approaches (eg, problem-solving skills training) are more often used in adolescents.
- Since oppositional defiant disorder and conduct disorder commonly coexist with other mental health diagnoses, particularly attention-deficit/hyperactivity disorder, these conditions (eg, anxiety, depression, learning disorder, substance use disorder) should be considered during the initial evaluation.
- When behavioral strategies are insufficient, treating coexisting conditions, such as attention-deficit/hyperactivity disorder or anxiety, with medication may lessen the oppositional behaviors.

American Board of Pediatrics Content Specification(s)/ Content Area

- Plan the appropriate management of oppositional defiant or conduct disorder
- Plan the appropriate evaluation of oppositional defiant or conduct disorder
- Differentiate the findings associated with oppositional defiant or conduct disorder from those of temperamental variations

Suggested Readings

Blair RJ, Leibenluft E, Pine DS. Conduct disorder and callous-unemotional traits in youth. *N Engl J Med.* 2014;371(23):2207-2216.

Steiner H, Remsing L; Work Group on Quality Issues. Practice parameter for the assessment and treatment of children and adolescents with oppositional defiant disorder. *J Am Acad Child Adolesc Psychiatry.* 2007;46(1):126-141.

Zahrt DM, Melzer-Lange MD. Aggressive behavior in children and adolescents. *Pediatr Rev.* 2011;32(8):325-331.

Item 168   Preferred Response: B

The boy in the vignette has benign sleep myoclonus of infancy. This is characterized by jerking movements of the limb(s) that only occur when the infant is asleep. Arousing the infant stops the movements. The limb jerking occurs for variable intervals, from a few seconds or minutes up to 30 minutes. It may move from 1 limb to another and then back to the first limb. There is no alteration in breathing. This is a benign disorder that typically starts in early infancy and resolves over 2 to 3 months.

Benign infantile myoclonic epilepsy is an epileptic syndrome. Myoclonic seizures begin around 6 months of age and are characterized by brief head nodding and eye rolling; sometimes they are associated with myoclonic jerks of the arms. The movements occur during both sleep and wakefulness. Electroencephalography will show epileptiform discharges associated with the clinical symptoms. The infant in the vignette is much younger than the typical child with benign infantile myoclonic epilepsy, and his clinical appearance of limb jerking that migrates from limb to limb is not characteristic of myoclonic seizures.

Motor stereotypies are repetitive, nonepileptic movements that can start in infancy. These can include shuddering attacks, which look like a sudden shiver or 'chill', limb stiffening or trembling, or hand flapping. They occur when the child is awake, and often when the child is excited or overstimulated. The limb jerking of the infant in the vignette only occurs during sleep.

Motor tics are a type of movement disorder that typically starts around age 5 years and almost never before 2 years. These present as a brief motor movement, often involving the face, head, neck, or upper extremities, though the lower extremities may be involved. Examples are forceful blinking, shoulder shrugging, or head nodding. Tics have an associated premonitory urge, a sense of needing to perform the movement, which can differentiate them from motor stereotypies. Tics can wax and wane or change, whereas motor stereotypies typically stay the same. Tics only occur during wakefulness. The infant in the vignette is too young to be having motor tics, and his limb jerking only occurs during sleep.

PREP Pearls

- Benign sleep myoclonus of infancy is characterized by jerking movements of the limb that only occur when the infant is asleep. The jerking may move from 1 limb to another and then back to the first limb. There is no alteration in breathing.
- Motor tics typically start around age 5 years and almost never before 2 years.
- Tics have an associated premonitory urge which can differentiate them from motor stereotypies.

American Board of Pediatrics Content Specification(s)/ Content Area

- Differentiate between normal and abnormal repetitive movements during infancy

Suggested Readings

International League Against Epilepsy. https://www.epilepsydiagnosis.org/index.html.

Kruer MC. Pediatric movement disorders. *Pediatr Rev.* 2015;36(3):104-116.

Item 169   Preferred Response: D

The infant in this vignette has pseudostrabismus. Although the right eye in the image appears to be turned in, the symmetric corneal reflex and normal cover/uncover test results rule out true strabismus. In reality, the epicanthal folds result in a wide nasal bridge that covers the white part of the eye creating the illusion of esotropia.

Early detection of ocular disorders is essential to prevent vision-threatening conditions such as amblyopia, or "lazy eye." Amblyopia is caused by inadequate development of central vision resulting in decreased visual acuity due to strabismus, refractive disorders, or anisometropia (different visual acuity of each eye) in infancy. The American Academy of Pediatrics recommends visual assessment of all infants, children, and adolescents at each health supervision visit. In infants, evaluation consists of an ocular history, external inspection of the eyelids and eyes, red reflex examination, pupillary examination, and visual acuity fixate and follow response; infants 6 months and older should also undergo ocular motility assessment. Children aged 1 year and older should undergo instrument-based assessment when available and visual acuity age-appropriate optotype assessment.

The red reflex is an essential component of the visual evaluation that begins with newborns. Patients should be examined for a red reflex in a darkened room with an ophthalmoscope. First, each eye should be examined individually from a distance of 1 to 2 feet, followed by the Bruckner reflex, during which both eyes are examined simultaneously from 2 to 3 feet. Referral to an ophthalmologist should be initiated for findings such as an asymmetric, absent, dulled, or opaque red reflex; dark spots in the red reflex; or leukocoria (white reflex). After 3 months of age, poor tracking, lack of fixation, head tilt, nystagmus, or squinting warrant a referral.

To evaluate for ocular misalignment, the cover and Hirschberg tests are used. The cover test involves the child fixating on a nearby object. A cover is placed briefly over 1 eye and then removed while observing both eyes for movement; the misaligned eye will move inward or outward. The process is repeated for both eyes and then again with the child focusing on a distant object. The unilateral cover test involves fixation on an object, covering the fixating eye, and removing the cover while observing the other eye for motion. Alternate cover testing involves the examiner moving the cover from 1 eye to the other without allowing binocular viewing while the patient is fixating on an object. The 2 primary types of ocular misalignment are the tropia, which is a deviation of the 2 eyes when a patient is looking with both eyes uncovered (constant misalignment) and the phoria, which appears when binocular viewing is interrupted and both eyes are no longer looking at the same object (latent deviation).

The Hirschberg test, during which a penlight is directed at both pupils and the light reflex (corneal reflex) is assessed to determine if asymmetry is present, is performed when there is constant misalignment. Normally, the light reflex should be in the center of both pupils when the patient is fixating on the light. A nasal displacement of the light reflex indicates an exotropia, while a temporal displacement indicates an esotropia.

PREP Pearls

- Early detection of ocular misalignment is crucial to prevent and/or treat amblyopia.
- True strabismus may be ruled out with normal examination findings of the red reflex, corneal light reflex (Hirschberg test), and cover test.

American Board of Pediatrics Content Specification(s)/Content Area

- Plan the appropriate evaluation of strabismus, including timing of evaluation to prevent complications
- Differentiate the clinical findings associated with strabismus from those of pseudostrabismus
- Evaluate a patient for ocular tropias and phorias

Suggested Readings

Donahue SP, Baker CN; Committee on Practice and Ambulatory Medicine; Section on Ophthalmology; American Association of Certified Orthoptists; American Association for Pediatric Ophthalmology and Strabismus; American Academy of Ophthalmology. Procedures for the evaluation of the visual system by pediatricians. *Pediatrics.* 2016;137(1):e20153597.

Jefferis JM, Connor AJ, Clarke MP. Amblyopia. *BMJ.* 2015;351:h5811.

Rogers GL, Jordan CO. Pediatric vision screening. *Pediatr Rev.* 2013;34(3):126-133.

Item 170   Preferred Response: C

Screening for a disease or complication is of value when that disease or complication is prevalent within a population, there is a test with a sufficiently high sensitivity and specificity to limit false-positive and false-negative results, and there is an intervention that can change the morbidity or mortality of the disease if it is identified early. A prime example of a setting in which screening is appropriate is in patients with genetic cancer predisposition syndromes.

The boy in this vignette has a history most consistent with the overgrowth syndrome Beckwith-Wiedemann syndrome (BWS). This epigenetic imprinting disorder is marked by abnormal methylation at locus 11p15.5. The abnormal methylation results in dysregulated overexpression of *IGF2* or underexpression of *KCNQ1OT1*, both of which can result in overgrowth. The presentation of BWS includes overgrowth (generalized macrosomia or hemihyperplasia), macroglossia, anterior abdominal wall defects, and neonatal hypoglycemia. Depending on the specific epigenetic change, up to 10% of patients with BWS develop embryonal tumors within the first 7 years. These tumors are most commonly nephroblastoma (Wilms tumor) or hepatoblastoma.

Because embryonal solid tumors have a higher rate of cure when identified at an earlier stage, screening in patients with BWS is appropriate. While screening recommendations vary slightly, surveillance guidelines published in 2017 recommend measuring serum α-fetoprotein every 3 months for the first 4 years to screen for hepatoblastoma and complete abdominal ultrasonography every 3 months for the first 7 years to screen for Wilms tumor.

Hypogammaglobulinemia, coagulopathies or liver failure, or elevated urine ketones are not associated with BWS. Measurement of IgG levels is an appropriate screening test for immunodeficiencies such as agammaglobulinemia, severe combined immune deficiency, or common variable immunodeficiency. The prothrombin time and partial thromboplastin time would be appropriate screening tests for factor deficiency–associated coagulopathies. Urine ketones would be an appropriate screening test for diabetic ketoacidosis.

PREP Pearls

- Beckwith-Wiedemann syndrome presents with overgrowth (generalized macrosomia or hemihyperplasia), macroglossia, anterior abdominal wall defects, and neonatal hypoglycemia.
- Screening for a disease or complication is of value when that disease or complication is prevalent within a population, there is a test with a sufficiently high sensitivity and specificity to limit false-positive and false-negative results, and there is an intervention that can change the morbidity or mortality of the disease if it is identified early.
- Up to 10% of patients with Beckwith-Wiedemann syndrome develop embryonal tumors within the first 7 years (mostly nephroblastoma [Wilms tumor] or hepatoblastoma).

American Board of Pediatrics Content Specification(s)/Content Area

- Recognize clinical findings associated with embryonal tumors
- Recognize the laboratory findings associated with a germ cell tumor
- Recognize the laboratory findings associated with hepatoblastoma

Suggested Readings

Carvajal DN, Rowe PC. Sensitivity, specificity, predictive values, and likelihood ratios. *Pediatr Rev.* 2010;31(12):511-513.

Kalish JM, Doros L, Helman LJ, et al. Surveillance recommendations for children with overgrowth syndromes and predisposition to wilms tumors and hepatoblastoma. *Clin Cancer Res.* 2017;23(13):e115-e122.

Puumala SE, Hoyme HE. Epigenetics in pediatrics. *Pediatr Rev.* 2015;36(1):14-21.

The 2-year-old girl in the vignette has had a plastic object lodged in her left naris for several hours. She is not in any respiratory distress. The most appropriate next step in her management is application of topical neosynephrine to her left naris to help facilitate removal of the object.

Because of their developmentally normal exploratory behaviors, it is not at all uncommon for young children to place foreign bodies in their noses, mouths, and ears. The diagnosis of nasal foreign body should be suspected in children with persistent purulent and/or foul-smelling nasal discharge (especially when it is unilateral) and malodorous breath. Children may also have epistaxis or blood-tinged nasal discharge. The diagnosis is characteristically confirmed through direct visualization of a foreign object in the naris. Diagnostic imaging, such as plain radiography, is generally *not* indicated unless there is a specific concern for a radio-opaque foreign object that cannot be visualized on physical examination.

Various approaches can be used for nasal foreign body removal; the recommended technique will depend on the type of foreign body and its location. In some cases, a child can simply be instructed to blow his or her nose to remove the foreign body. In cases in which this strategy is not possible or successful, the lodged object must be removed under direct visualization.

Preparation of the child and his/her caregiver to minimize anxiety and discomfort, minimize patient movement, and maximize visualization of the foreign body is paramount to successful object removal. Use of a topical vasoconstricting agent, such as neosynephrine or oxymetazoline, is generally recommended a few minutes (~10 minutes) before any attempt is made to remove a nasal foreign body. These agents decrease localized swelling (which improves the chances of successful foreign body removal) and decrease bleeding. Nasal secretions should be cleared using a suction tip or catheter until the foreign body can be seen; the suctioning itself is sometimes effective in removing the foreign body. In children who are cooperative and/or can be safely immobilized, tools such as alligator forceps or a hook can be used to grasp and remove foreign objects from the nose. Alternative techniques include insertion of a small French foley catheter or commercially available extractor device beyond the object followed by gentle retraction of the catheter with its balloon inflated to dislodge the object. Techniques such as bonding a wooden stick to the foreign body with adhesive such as cyanoacrylate have been tried successfully, but must be used cautiously; if not performed correctly, this technique could result in bonding of the stick to the nasal mucosa instead of the foreign body, further compounding the problem.

Insertion of a nasogastric tube into the left naris would not be the best technique for foreign body removal in this patient. Attempts to push a nasal foreign body into a child's posterior nasopharynx are not recommended, given the risk that the foreign body could either be lodged more firmly into the naris or aspirated.

Irrigation of the girl's left naris with sterile nasal saline spray would not be recommended. The use of irrigation to manage nasal foreign bodies is not recommended because this could cause the foreign body to slide posteriorly and be aspirated. Furthermore, foreign bodies that absorb water (ie, food/organic matter, sponges, and foam) may swell and become even more difficult to remove when irrigated.

Urgent referral of this girl to a pediatric otolaryngologist is not recommended at this point. Consultation is generally required for removal of foreign bodies that have been lodged for a prolonged period (especially those with surrounding granulation tissue or resulting in obstructive sinusitis); foreign bodies that may be caustic/destructive to the nasal structures (particularly button batteries); those causing significant respiratory difficulty and/or bleeding; and those that cannot be successfully removed by a trained provider.

PREP Pearls

- Nasal foreign body should be suspected in children with persistent purulent and/or foul-smelling nasal discharge (especially when unilateral) and malodorous breath.
- The diagnosis of nasal foreign body is characteristically made though direct visualization of a foreign object. Diagnostic imaging is generally *not* indicated.
- Use of a topical vasoconstricting agent, such as neosynephrine or oxymetazoline, is generally recommended before any attempt is made to remove a nasal foreign body. These agents decrease localized swelling (which improves the chances of successful foreign body removal) and decrease bleeding.

American Board of Pediatrics Content Specification(s)/Content Area

- Recognize the clinical findings associated with a nasal foreign body, and manage appropriately

Suggested Readings

King C, Henretig FN, eds. *Textbook of Pediatric Emergency Procedures.* 2nd ed. Philadelphia, PA: Lippincott Williams & Wilkins; 2008.

Mittiga MR, Ruddy RM. Procedures. In: Shaw K, Bachur RG, eds. *Fleisher and Ludwig's Textbook of Pediatric Emergency Medicine.* 7th ed. Philadelphia, PA: Lippincott Williams & Wilkins; 2015:chap 141.

Niescierenko ML, Lee GS. ENT trauma. In: Shaw K, Bachur RG, eds. *Fleisher and Ludwig's Textbook of Pediatric Emergency Medicine.* 7th ed. Philadelphia, PA: Lippincott Williams & Wilkins; 2015;chap 114.

Of the response choices, the most common extrarenal manifestation seen in children with autosomal dominant polycystic kidney disease (ADPKD) is cerebral aneurysm. Autosomal dominant polycystic kidney disease is the most common genetic renal disorder, occurring in 1 in every 400 to 1,000 live births. It is characterized by the replacement of normal renal parenchyma with cysts, which gradually increase in size, leading to loss of renal function and eventual renal failure.

Children with ADPKD are usually asymptomatic; they are generally diagnosed when renal cysts are detected incidentally during imaging studies or when screening children with a positive family history. Disease manifestations in children are similar to those seen in adults, including persistent microscopic hematuria, hypertension, flank pain (associated with renal cyst hemorrhage), or urinary tract infection. Serum creatinine is not usually elevated in children with ADPKD, because renal function remains normal until the fourth decade of life.

Renal ultrasonography is the preferred imaging modality for children suspected of having ADPKD. The presence of 3 unilateral or bilateral kidney cysts has a specificity and positive predictive value of 100%, and a sensitivity of 82% to 96%, for the diagnosis of ADPKD in children aged 15 to 39 years. The presence of 2 cysts in each kidney has a specificity and positive predictive value of 100% and a sensitivity of 90% for the diagnosis of ADPKD in the 40- to 60-year-old age group. Computed tomography (CT) and magnetic resonance imaging (MRI) have a higher sensitivity than ultrasonography for detecting renal cysts associated with ADPKD. However, in view of the increased cost (MRI) and radiation exposure (CT) with these modalities, renal ultrasonography is the preferred imaging study. In patients with equivocal results on renal ultrasonography, CT or MRI may be indicated if there is a strong suspicion for ADPKD.

Extrarenal manifestations reported in association with ADPKD include cerebral aneurysm; hepatic, pancreatic, and seminal vesicle cyst; cardiac valve disease; colonic diverticula; and abdominal wall hernia. These reflect defective epithelial cell differentiation or extracellular matrix function associated with the genetic abnormality in ADPKD.

Intracranial bleeding resulting from ruptured cerebral aneurysms is the most serious complication of ADPKD. Prevalence of cerebral aneurysms is lower in younger patients (around 5%) and increases up to 20% in older patients. Larger aneurysms (>7 mm), poorly controlled hypertension, and age less than 50 years is associated with increased risk for aneurysm rupture. Hypertension is present in 50% to 70% of patients with ADPKD by age 30 years, developing before the deterioration of kidney function. The role of routine radiological screening for cerebral aneurysms in asymptomatic patients with ADPKD is unclear. Patients with (1) a history of previous aneurysm rupture, (2) a positive family history of intracerebral bleeding or intracranial aneurysm, (3) an occupation in which loss of consciousness would place them or others at extreme risk, and (4) marked hemodynamic instability and hypertension associated with surgeries are considered at high risk for intracerebral hemorrhage. Routine screening for cerebral aneurysm is indicated in these high-risk populations.

Children with ADPKD have an increased incidence of cardiac involvement such as valvular abnormalities (mitral valve prolapse and aortic regurgitation), asymptomatic pericardial effusions, coronary aneurysms, and cardiomyopathies. Because most affected children are asymptomatic, echocardiographic evaluation is suggested for patients with ADPKD with audible murmurs or symptoms of cardiac dysfunction.

Genetic testing for ADPKD can be conducted by DNA linkage or sequence analysis. Linkage analysis identifies known mutations in a family, and therefore requires an adequate number of known family members with the genetic disorder for accuracy. Therefore, this method cannot identify all ADPKD cases, especially those suspected of having a spontaneous mutation. Direct DNA analysis for ADPKD is not routinely performed because of the large size, complexity, and heterogeneity of the associated PKD genes.

Abnormalities of the liver are the most commonly seen extrarenal manifestations of autosomal recessive polycystic kidney disease (ARPKD), which is usually detected with antenatal ultrasonography after 24 weeks of gestation, and confirmed with postnatal ultrasonography. In patients with ARPKD, ultrasonography demonstrates large, echogenic kidneys with decreased corticomedullary differentiation. Macrocysts are typically not seen in ARPKD in contrast to ADPKD. Congenital hepatic fibrosis and associated extrahepatic portal hypertension is characterized by periportal and perilobular fibrosis surrounding dysplastic (hyperplastic, ectatic) biliary ducts with normal-appearing hepatocytes. Some children may also have macroscopic dilations of the intrahepatic bile ducts, referred to as "Caroli syndrome." In neonates with ARPKD, abnormalities of the lungs (pulmonary hypoplasia) or limbs (as in Potter sequence) may occur secondary to severe renal dysfunction resulting in oligohydramnios.

Alport syndrome (AS) is an inherited disorder of basement membrane collagen IV characterized by involvement of the kidneys (always), ears (often), and eyes (occasionally). Anterior lenticonus is the conical protrusion of the lens and is pathognomonic of AS. Present in 20% to 30% of males with X-linked AS, anterior lenticonus may be associated with subcapsular cataracts affecting visual acuity.

PREP Pearls

- Children with autosomal dominant polycystic kidney disease are usually asymptomatic; they are usually diagnosed when renal cysts are detected incidentally during imaging studies for nonrenal abdominal symptoms or when screening children with positive family history.

- Disease manifestations in children are similar to adults; common presentations include persistent microscopic hematuria, hypertension, flank pain (associated with renal cyst hemorrhage), or urinary tract infection. Serum creatinine is not usually elevated in children with autosomal dominant polycystic kidney disease because renal function remains normal until the fourth decade of life.

- Extrarenal manifestations associated with autosomal dominant polycystic kidney disease include cerebral aneurysms; hepatic, pancreatic, and seminal vesicle cysts; cardiac valve diseases; colonic diverticula; and abdominal wall hernia.

American Board of Pediatrics Content Specification(s)/Content Area

- Recognize the clinical findings associated with autosomal-dominant polycystic kidney disease in patients of various ages
- Plan the appropriate diagnostic evaluation for a patient in whom autosomal-dominant polycystic kidney disease is suspected

Suggested Readings

Benun J, Lewis C. Polycystic kidney disease. *Pediatr Rev.* 2009;30(10):e78-e79.

National Human Genome Research Institute, National Institutes of Health. Learning about autosomal dominant polycystic kidney disease. https://www.genome.gov/20019622/learning-about-autosomal-polycystic-kidney-disease/#al-1.

Torres VE, Harris PC, Pirson Y. Autosomal dominant polycystic kidney disease. *Lancet.* 2007;369(9569):1287.

Item 173   Preferred Response: D

The infant in this vignette has symptoms and physical examination findings that are consistent with myocardial dysfunction and congestive heart failure (CHF). Echocardiography should be the next step in evaluation and management to assess myocardial function and to evaluate for structural cardiac defects.

The etiologies of CHF can be divided into causes that occur with structural heart disease (Item C173A) and causes that occur with a structurally normal heart (Item C173B).

Item C173A. Cardiac Malformations Leading to Heart Failure.

Shunt Lesions
- Ventricular septal defect
- Patent ductus arteriosus
- Aortopulmonary window
- Atrioventricular septal defect
- Single ventricle without pulmonary stenosis
- Atrial septal defect (rare)

Total/Partial Anomalous Pulmonary Venous Connection

Valvular Regurgitation
- Mitral regurgitation
- Aortic regurgitation

Inflow Obstruction
- Cor triatriatum
- Pulmonary vein stenosis
- Mitral stenosis

Outflow Obstruction
- Aortic valve stenosis/subaortic stenosis/supravalvular aortic stenosis
- Aortic coarctation

Reprinted with permission from Madriago E, Silberbach M. Heart failure in infants and children. *Pediatr Rev*. 2010;31(1):6.

Item C173B. Sources of Heart Failure With a Structurally Normal Heart.

Primary Cardiac
- Cardiomyopathy
- Myocarditis
- Myocardial infarction
- Acquired valve disorders
- Hypertension
- Kawasaki syndrome
- Arrhythmia (bradycardia or tachycardia)

Noncardiac
- Anemia
- Sepsis
- Hypoglycemia
- Diabetic ketoacidosis
- Hypothyroidism
- Other endocrinopathies
- Arteriovenous fistula
- Renal failure
- Muscular dystrophies

Reprinted with permission from Madriago E, Silberbach M. Heart failure in infants and children. *Pediatr Rev*. 2010;31(1):6.

The clinical manifestations of CHF depend somewhat on the age of the patient and their level of activities. Infants, for example, "exercise" when eating. Heart failure in infancy frequently presents with feeding difficulties, distress with eating, or refusal to eat. Infants and young children often present with failure to thrive and can also have respiratory symptoms such as tachypnea, retractions, and grunting. Tachycardia, a murmur or gallop, and hepatomegaly are often seen. In older children, CHF can often present with exercise intolerance, manifest typically by difficulty keeping up with their peers. Respiratory symptoms and vomiting, which is reflective of decreased gut perfusion, are also common in this age group.

The other response choices would not be appropriate next steps in the management of this patient. Hypertonic saline nebulizer treatments are often used in the context of airway clearance of secretions. The infant in this vignette is not noted to have an important secretion burden. Although an infant or child with CHF may be dehydrated from vomiting or decreased oral intake, fluid must be given judiciously because these patients are in a volume-overloaded state. Thus, giving a 20-mL/kg normal saline bolus could be harmful. The hepatomegaly in this infant is caused by the CHF from volume overload of the right ventricle; thus, liver ultrasonography is unlikely to prove useful.

PREP Pearls
- Exercise intolerance, vomiting, and respiratory signs and symptoms are common presentations of heart failure.
- Heart failure can be caused by structural heart disease or occur with a normally structured heart.

American Board of Pediatrics Content Specification(s)/Content Area
- Identify the causes of congestive heart failure in children of various ages
- Recognize the clinical findings associated with congestive heart failure in children of various ages

Suggested Readings

Madriago E, Silberbach M. Heart failure in infants and children. *Pediatr Rev*. 2010:31(1):4-12.

Subramaniam S, Rutman M. Cardiogenic shock. *Pediatr Rev*. 2015:36(5):225-226.

Item 174 — Preferred Response: D

This sexually active adolescent female has dysuria and frequency, which are classic symptoms of bacterial cystitis. The first step to establishing a diagnosis is to obtain a clean-catch urine sample for a urine test strip analysis and culture prior to the start of antibiotics. The urine test strip analysis can help guide the direction of management.

Dysuria is a burning sensation associated with urination that can be caused by infectious or noninfectious causes. It is important to determine if the patient has other symptoms, such as fever, abdominal/back pain, vaginal discharge, rashes, or ulcerations. In a sexually active adolescent, the most common cause of dysuria is a lower urinary tract infection (UTI).

Females have a higher incidence of UTIs because of a shorter urethra and its proximity to the vagina and rectum, which allows for increased exposure to enteric organisms. The most common pathogen associated with acute UTI is *Escherichia coli* (75%-95%). *Staphylococcus saprophyticus* is often associated with cystitis in sexually active adolescent females; however, gram-negative organisms such as *Klebsiella* and *Proteus* species are more prevalent.

Dysuria can be caused by genitourinary infections, systemic illness, and other conditions, making the history and physical examination key to aiding the diagnosis. The age and sex of a patient must also be considered in the differential diagnosis and diagnostic evaluation. In a prepubertal boy older than 2 years with dysuria, a UTI should be considered. If ulcers, vesicles, or penile discharge are present, sexually transmitted infections such as herpes simplex virus, *Chlamydia trachomatis*, and *Neisseria gonorrhoeae* would be in the differential diagnosis. Sexual abuse should be considered, although herpes simplex virus could be spread via autoinoculation. If there is a positive urine culture result and fever, cystitis and pyelonephritis are more likely. Other causes of pain with urination include balanitis, urethral strictures, viral cystitis, and trauma. Hypercalciuria and renal stones should be considered in a patient with dysuria and hematuria. Varicella may cause dysuria if the rash spreads to the genital region. Lower UTIs may also be related to dysfunctional voiding caused by constipation.

In a prepubertal girl older than 2 years, many of the etiologies for prepubertal boys should be considered, with the addition of vaginal discharge that may be caused by a foreign body or labial adhesions.

For adolescents, consider infections caused by *C trachomatis* and *N gonorrhoeae*, which can cause urethritis in males and females, as well as vaginitis, cervicitis, and pelvic inflammatory disease in females.

Regardless of age, obtaining a urine test strip analysis (or urinalysis) and urine culture would be the first step in the evaluation of dysuria. A complete blood cell count and blood culture would not be warranted in an immunocompetent adolescent without fever. Although the patient in this vignette should be tested for *C trachomatis* and *N gonorrhoeae* as part of routine screening in a sexually active adolescent, this testing will not address the acute symptoms that are most consistent with a lower UTI. Performing a potassium-hydroxide wet mount via microscopy is not likely to provide additional information in a patient without vaginal discharge.

PREP Pearls

- A urine test strip analysis and culture are essential in the evaluation of dysuria.
- The most common pathogen associated with lower urinary tract infections is *Escherichia coli*.

American Board of Pediatrics Content Specification(s)/ Content Area

- Recognize the etiology of dysuria in patients of various ages
- Plan the appropriate diagnostic evaluation of dysuria in patients of various ages

Suggested Readings

D'Angelo LJ, Tuchman S. Renal and genitourinary tract infections in adolescents and young adults. In: Neinstein LS, Katzman DK, Callahan ST, Gordon CM, Joffe A, Rickert VI, eds. *Neinstein's Adolescent and Young Adult Health Care: A Practical Guide.* 6th ed. Philadelphia, PA: Wolters Kluwer; 2016:249-251.

Jackson EC. Urinary tract infections in children: knowledge updates and a salute to the future. *Pediatr Rev.* 2015;36(4):153-166.

Peters CA, Campbell FG. Pediatric urology. In: Emans SJH, Laufer MR. *Emans, Laufer, and Goldstein's Pediatric and Adolescent Gynecology.* 6th ed. Philadelphia, PA: Wolters Kluwer; 2012:278-282.

Item 175	Preferred Response: D

Evidenced by her clinical deterioration, signs of low cardiac output, rales, and hepatomegaly, the infant in this vignette has cardiogenic shock, likely from acute myocarditis. Of the choices, the predominant mechanism of compensation for cardiogenic shock in children is increased heart rate.

Shock is a condition of insufficient cardiac output to meet the metabolic demands of end organs. When the primary cause of shock is failure of forward flow from the heart, it is further classified as cardiogenic shock. Cardiac output is the product of stroke volume and heart rate. Children have a limited capacity to increase stroke volume in response to shock, but the sinoatrial node is particularly sensitive to stimulation, thus increased chronotropy (tachycardia) is the most likely early compensatory mechanism to improve cardiac output for the child in the vignette. It is important for the clinician to recognize tachycardia as an important clinical indicator of early shock, maintaining a high index of suspicion for heart failure and cardiogenic shock. These life-threatening conditions are sometimes missed, because they can masquerade as other, less severe conditions. Other than tachycardia, the most common early signs and symptoms of heart disease in children are nonspecific; they include respiratory distress, cough, feeding difficulty, and fatigue. The more specific indicators of heart failure, such as chest pain, orthopnea, and edema, are typically present in adults and often absent in children.

In children, although tachycardia is the most effective compensatory mechanism for improving cardiac output, stroke volume can be increased by elevated circulating endogenous catecholamines as well as with therapeutic interventions. Stroke volume is determined by the relationships among preload, afterload, and contractility.

Preload is defined as the degree to which cardiac myocytes are stretched, and can be practically conceptualized by ventricular end-diastolic volume. The Frank-Starling relationship of the heart describes an optimum preload that maximizes cardiac output. An underfilled ventricle contains less blood to eject and the contractile elements will overlap, whereas an overstretched ventricle will have insufficient interaction of contractile elements and will thus eject a smaller fraction of the blood. A failing heart is especially

Item C175. Cardiovascular Medications for the Treatment of Shock.

Medication	Site of Action	Clinical Effects	Uses in Shock
Dopamine	β < α (at higher doses), D_1, D_2	↑ inotropy, ↑ HR, ↑ SVR, ↑ PVR	• Hypovolemic shock (temporizing measure only during volume expansion) • Septic shock (all forms) • Cardiogenic shock
Dobutamine	$β_1 >> β_2$	↑ inotropy, ↑ HR, ↓ SVR, ↓ PVR	• Cardiogenic shock • Septic shock with ↓ CO, ↑ SVR
Epinephrine	β > α	↑ inotropy, ↑ HR, ↑ SVR	• Septic shock with ↓ CO, ↓ SVR • Cardiogenic shock • Anaphylactic shock
Norepinephrine	α >> β	↑ SVR, ↑ inotropy, ↑ HR	• Hypovolemic shock (temporizing measure only during volume expansion) • Distributive shock • Septic shock with ↑ CO, ↓ SVR
Milrinone	PDE III inhibitor	↑ inotropy, ↓ SVR, ↓ PVR, ↑ lusitropy	• Cardiogenic shock with stable BP • Septic shock with ↓ CO, ↑ SVR
Phenylephrine	$α_1 > α_2$	↑ SVR	• Septic shock with ↑ CO, ↓ SVR
Vasopressin	V_1, V_2	↑ SVR	• Distributive shock • Septic shock with ↑ CO, ↓ SVR
Prostaglandin E1	PGE1	Dilation of ductus arteriosus	• Cardiogenic shock in neonate with suspected ductus-dependent lesion
Nitroprusside	arteries > veins	↓ SVR, ↑ coronary perfusion	• Cardiogenic shock
Inhaled nitric oxide	pulmonary vessels	↓ PVR	• Cardiogenic shock with PHTN, RV failure
Levosimendan, enoximone	cardiac troponin C, ATP-dependent potassium channels in cardiac myocytes	↑ inotropy, ?cardioprotection	• Experimental use in cardiogenic shock

Abbreviations: ATP, adenosine triphosphate; BP, blood pressure; CO, cardiac output; HR, heart rate; PDE, phosphodiesterase; PGE, prostaglandin E; PHTN, pulmonary hypertension; PVR, pulmonary vascular resistance; RV, right ventricle; SVR, systemic vascular resistance

Reprinted with permission from Yager P, Noviski N. Shock. *Pediatr Rev*. 2010; 31(8):316.

sensitive to suboptimal preload. Children with cardiogenic shock may be intravascularly depleted because of poor oral intake and increased insensible losses from tachypnea, and may benefit from very judicious fluid boluses. The clinician should frequently assess the child for pulmonary edema, hepatomegaly, and clinical improvement or deterioration and tailor therapy accordingly. Long-term, or sometimes even early in the presentation, diuretics will decrease the work required for the failing heart, and restore an optimal status on the Frank-Starling curve.

Afterload is the resistance against which the ventricle contracts. Left ventricular afterload is increased by mechanical obstruction to its outflow, negative intrathoracic pressure, and systemic vascular resistance. Thus, positive pressure ventilation and medications that cause vasodilation can decrease left ventricular afterload.

Lastly, contractility determines the fraction of blood ejected from the ventricle. Catecholamines such as epinephrine, norepinephrine, and dopamine, and the phosphodiesterase inhibitor milrinone, can all increase contractility. It should be noted that some medications can have opposing effects on cardiac output (Item C175). For example, while epinephrine increases contractility, blood pressure, and coronary perfusion, it can also increase myocardial oxygen demand and afterload.

Decreasing afterload, decreasing cardiac myocyte stretch with diuretics, and increasing actin-myosin interactions by optimizing preload may improve stroke volume in some children with cardiogenic shock. All can be goals of therapeutic interventions at the bedside. However, they are not common compensatory mechanisms.

PREP Pearls

- Clinicians should maintain a high index of suspicion for heart failure in children; the typical indicators of heart failure seen in adults are often absent in children.
- Tachycardia, poor feeding, fatigue, cough, and difficulty breathing are important early indicators of heart failure in children.
- The determinants of stroke volume are preload, afterload, and contractility.

- Plan appropriate management of cardiogenic shock in children of various ages

Suggested Readings

Mtaweh H, Trakas EV, Su E, Carcillo JA, Aneja RK. Advances in monitoring and management of shock. *Pediatr Clin North Am.* 2013;60(3):641-654.

Subramaniam S, Rutman M. Cardiogenic shock. *Pediatr Rev.* 2015;36:225.

Yager P, Noviski N. Shock. *Pediatr Rev.* 2010; 31:311-319.

Item 176   Preferred Response: D

The adolescent in this vignette has examination findings highly suggestive of a peritonsillar abscess, which should be drained by needle aspiration. Although antibiotics may be used as adjunctive treatment for a peritonsillar abscess after drainage and would be the appropriate treatment for peritonsillar cellulitis, needle aspiration is the most appropriate next step in this case. Needle aspiration is also used to differentiate between a peritonsillar abscess (in which a collection of pus would be present between the capsule of the palatine tonsil and the pharyngeal muscles) and peritonsillar cellulitis (in which no collection of pus would be present), and it is therapeutic if an abscess is present. Imaging is not necessary to establish the diagnosis, and neither lateral neck radiograph nor magnetic resonance imaging would be the best imaging modality.

Peritonsillar abscesses are the most common deep neck infection in pediatric patients. They present most often in adolescents and young adults, and are typically polymicrobial, with *Streptococcus pyogenes* (group A *Streptococcus*), *Streptococcus anginosus, Staphylococcus aureus,* and respiratory anaerobes representing the organisms most commonly found on culture. A peritonsillar abscess in a child may present with a severe sore throat (sometimes unilateral), fever, muffled or "hot potato" voice, and trismus. Patients may have drooling and decreased oral intake because of odynophagia. Children typically have a swollen tonsil or swelling of the adjacent soft palate, as well as deviation of the uvula to the opposite side. The diagnosis can be made clinically and does not necessitate laboratory or radiologic evaluation. It is sometimes difficult to distinguish between peritonsillar abscess and peritonsillar cellulitis. In these cases, ultrasonography may be helpful if it identifies a clear fluid collection. Magnetic resonance imaging is not often used because it takes longer, may require sedation, and requires a patient with difficulty swallowing and potential airway compromise to lay supine.

In the stable patient with a probable peritonsillar abscess, needle aspiration is both diagnostic and therapeutic. In the stable patient with probable peritonsillar cellulitis without abscess, a trial of empiric antibiotics is reasonable. If physical examination findings are equivocal, ultrasonography, a therapeutic trial of antibiotics, or needle aspiration can each be considered to differentiate between a peritonsillar abscess and peritonsillar cellulitis. Appropriate empiric antibiotics include ampicillin-sulbactam or clindamycin. Therapy should be expanded to include vancomycin or linezolid for coverage of methicillin-resistant *S aureus* in unstable patients or patients who do not respond to initial antimicrobial treatment.

PREP Pearls

- Appropriate empiric antibiotics for treatment of peritonsillar infections include ampicillin-sulbactam or clindamycin. Therapy should be expanded to include methicillin-resistant *Staphylococcus aureus* coverage in unstable patients or patients who do not respond to initial antimicrobials.
- Children with a peritonsillar abscess present with a severe sore throat (sometimes unilateral), fever, a muffled or "hot potato" voice, trismus, and odynophagia. They typically have a swollen tonsil or swelling of the adjacent soft palate as well as deviation of the uvula to the opposite side.
- Needle aspiration of a peritonsillar abscess is both diagnostic and therapeutic.

**American Board of Pediatrics Content Specification(s)/
Content Area**

- Plan the appropriate management of a peritonsillar abscess
- Plan the appropriate diagnostic evaluation of a peritonsillar abscess, considering commonly associated pathogens

Suggested Readings

Bochner RE, Gangar M, Belamarich PF. A clinical approach to tonsillitis, tonsillar hypertrophy, and peritonsillar and retropharyngeal abscesses. *Pediatr Rev.* 2017;38(2):81-92.

Galioto NJ. Peritonsillar abscess. *Am Fam Physician.* 2008;77(2):199-202.

Item 177   Preferred Response: C

The diagnosis of coccidioidomycosis must be suspected in the adolescent patient described in the vignette. He has a potential exposure (residence in the San Joaquin Valley of California); systemic symptoms of fever, cough, night sweats, and weight loss; and radiographic abnormalities including pulmonary consolidation, paratracheal and hilar adenopathy, and lytic lesion in the spine concerning for disseminated disease. Coccidioidomycosis is a systemic fungal infection caused by 2 species of the dimorphic soil-dwelling fungus, *Coccidioides immitis* and *Coccidioides posadasii*. Although several diagnostic tests may be useful, serology would be the preferred initial test for confirming the diagnosis of coccidioidomycosis in the patient in the vignette. If serology is inconclusive but disseminated coccidioidomycosis is suspected, additional testing such as CT, urine antigen testing, and tissue biopsy may aid in the diagnosis.

Coccidioidomycosis is limited to the western hemisphere. In the United States, the disease is endemic to the southwestern region, including parts of west and south Texas, Arizona, New Mexico, and much of central and southern California. The geographic distribution of *C immitis* is limited primarily to the San Joaquin Valley of California, whereas *C posadasii* is endemic to the southwestern United States, northern Mexico, and areas of Central and South America. Arizona and California account for 97% of reported cases. Since

2010, the incidence of coccidioidomycosis has been increasing in California from annual incidence rates ranging from 1.9 to 8.4 per 100,000 in 2009 to 13.7 per 100,000 in 2016 (5,372 reported cases). Climatic and environmental factors related to proliferation and airborne release of *Coccidioides* are believed to contribute to the increased incidence in California.

Human infection occurs after inhalation of arthroconidia (spores) of *Coccidioides* species in dry desert soil in endemic areas. The spores germinate into spherules that later rupture to release endospores. The incubation period ranges from 1 to 3 weeks. Acute primary infection in the lung is asymptomatic in more than 60% of cases, but may manifest as a self-limited influenza-like illness or community-acquired pneumonia. Radiographic findings of lobar consolidation, interstitial or reticulonodular infiltrates, hilar adenopathy, and pleural effusions may be present in symptomatic pneumonia. In 5% to 10% of cases, chronic pulmonary sequelae such as thin-walled cavitation or nodules may occur.

Disseminated disease due to lymphohematogenous spread occurs in less than 1% of cases. Associated systemic complaints include fever, cough, night sweats, and prolonged fatigue; any organ system may be involved, but the skin and skin structure, skeletal system, and central nervous system are the most frequently affected. A history of primary pulmonary infection many months before the onset of disseminated disease is present in approximately 50% of patients. Risk factors for disseminated disease include immunocompromised status, pregnancy, and African American, Filipino, or Native American descent.

The differential diagnosis for pulmonary coccidioidomycosis includes tuberculosis, nontuberculous mycobacterial infection, and hematologic malignancy. The diagnosis of coccidioidomycosis may be established by serology, tissue culture, or histopathology. Immunodiffusion, enzyme immunoassay (EIA), or complement fixation (CF) are the most widely used serologic tests for the diagnosis of coccidioidomycosis (Item C177).

Serologic assays for coccidioidomycosis can detect immunoglobulin M (IgM) or immunoglobulin G (IgG). The highly sensitive qualitative EIA or immunodiffusion methods can detect IgM within the 1st week (in ~50%) and 3rd week (in ~90%) after symptom onset. Enzyme immunoassay is often the initial screening test recommended, but false-positive results may occur. Therefore, positive EIA results need confirmation with more specific immunodiffusion and/or CF tests. If the qualitative immunodiffusion test is positive for IgG antibodies, additional testing with the conventional CF test or a quantitative immunodiffusion test for IgG antibodies should be performed.

The highly specific quantitative immunodiffusion and CF tests can detect IgG anticoccidioidal antibodies between 2 and 28 weeks after symptom onset, and generally correlate with disease severity. Patients with mild disease have low serum titers, whereas persistently high (>1:16) titers are typically observed in disseminated disease. Antibodies in cerebrospinal fluid can also be detected with the CF or immunodiffusion methods. Quantitative serologic tests are helpful in monitoring therapeutic response. However, serology may yield false-negative results early in the disease course and among immunocompromised individuals.

Isolation of the organism via tissue culture is the gold standard for diagnosis. The presence of mature thick-walled spherules in tissue biopsy specimens, large in size (10-80 µm), containing endospores is considered pathognomonic of infection. In severe disease, the *Coccidioides* antigen may be detected in the urine and other specimens (eg, serum, plasma, or bronchoalveolar lavage fluid) with EIA, but this assay is not widely available, and cross-reactivity may occur in patients with other endemic mycosis such as blastomycosis and histoplasmosis. In complicated pulmonary infection or disseminated disease, additional imaging modalities may be considered.

Uncomplicated pneumonia may be managed without antifungal therapy; close monitoring of clinical status in conjunction with periodic serologic and radiographic evaluation is required. Oral azole antifungal therapy, such as fluconazole and itraconazole, is frequently used for mild to moderate disease with good outcomes. Amphotericin B is recommended for severe or life-threatening infections (eg, diffuse pneumonia), followed by an oral azole, for a total of 12 months; treatment may be longer for bone lesions. Treatment with fluconazole for life is recommended for coccidioidomycosis meningitis. Relapses are common, and mortality rates up to 28% have been reported in disseminated disease.

Item C177. Commonly Used Serologic Tests for Coccidioidomycosis.

Test	Antibody Detected	Sensitivity/Specificity	Comments
Qualitative EIA	IgM and IgG	High sensitivity	Often used for initial screening; false positive results may occur; positive results need confirmation by ID tests
Qualitative ID	IgM and IgG	Less sensitive, more specific than EIA	Positive results may need additional testing by quantitative ID or CF tests
Quantitative ID	IgG	High specificity	Correlates to disease severity; can also detect antibody in CSF
Quantitative CF	IgG	High specificity	Correlates to disease severity; useful in monitoring response to treatment; can also detect antibody in CSF.

Abbreviations: CF, complement fixation; CSF, cerebrospinal fluid; EIA, enzyme immunoassay; ID, immunodiffusion; IgG, immunoglobulin G; IgM, immunoglobulin M.

Courtesy of A. Shetty.

American Board of Pediatrics Content Specification(s)/ Content Area

- Recognize the clinical features associated with *Coccidioides* infection

- Understand the epidemiology of *Coccidioides*

Suggested Readings

Cooksey GS, Nguyen A, Knutson K, et al. Notes from the field: increase in coccidioidomycosis - California, 2016.*MMWR Morb Mortal Wkly Rep.* 2017;66(31):833-834.

Galgiani JN, Ampel NM, Blair JE, et al. 2016 Infectious Diseases Society of America (IDSA) clinical practice guideline for the treatment of coccidioidomycosis. *Clin Infect Dis.* 2016;63:e112-146.

McCarty JM, Demetral LC, Dabrowski L, Kahal AK, Bowser AM, Hahn JE. Pediatric coccidioidomycosis in central California: a retrospective case series. *Clin Infect Dis.* 2013;56(11):1579-1585.

Item 178   Preferred Response: C

The neonate in the vignette, delivered with vacuum assistance, has an increase in head circumference likely because of a subgaleal hemorrhage. Bleeding occurs under the aponeurosis from damage to emissary veins that drain the dural sinus. Bleeding may extend into the nape of the neck. Large amounts of blood can quickly accumulate in this space and present as a boggy mass at the occiput. When there is a large volume of blood loss, the effective cardiac stroke volume is reduced. Neonates are unable to increase stroke volume. Instead, to maintain cardiac output, the heart rate increases, as seen in the neonate in the vignette. When tachycardia cannot compensate for reduced stroke volume to maintain cardiac output, peripheral perfusion is diminished, resulting in reduced oxygen delivery to peripheral tissues. Cells then switch to anaerobic metabolism and produce lactic acid as a byproduct. The increased serum lactic acid causes acidemia. To maintain a normal pH, the body then increases the respiratory rate, as seen in this neonate. In contrast, adults and older children can increase stroke volume to maintain their cardiac output in the setting of hypovolemia or blood loss.

Hypoglycemia in neonates may not result in clinical signs. Hypoglycemic neonates may have tremors or jitteriness. Less commonly, hypoglycemia may present with shrill cry, lethargy, cyanosis, apnea, or poor feeding. Tachypnea is not typically seen with hypoglycemia.

Risk factors for pneumothorax include meconium aspiration syndrome, respiratory distress syndrome, renal anomalies, prematurity, and a history of positive pressure ventilation. On physical examination, neonates with pneumothorax may have asymmetric breath sounds and increased work of breathing.

There may be asymmetric chest rise. An asymptomatic pneumothorax may be seen in up to 2% of term neonates after birth.

Transient tachypnea of the newborn is caused by delayed resorption of amniotic fluid. Neonates present with tachypnea, grunting, and typically a barrel-shaped chest. Chest radiography shows increased markings with good lung expansion. Symptoms typically resolve within 24 hours after birth.

American Board of Pediatrics Content Specification(s)/ Content Area

- Understand the metabolic consequences of continued poor perfusion in a newborn infant

Suggested Readings

Carlo WA, Maheshwari A. Respiratory tract disorders. In: Kliegman RM, Stanton BF, St Geme JW, Schor NF, eds. *Nelson Textbook of Pediatrics.* 20th ed. Philadelphia, PA: Saunders Elsevier; 2016:848-867.

Reuter S, Moser C, Baack M. Respiratory distress in the newborn. *Pediatr Rev.* 2014;35:417.

Item 179   Preferred Response: D

The infant in this vignette has had an episode of apnea that is most likely related to a viral bronchiolitis. In addition to oxygen supplementation for the low oxygen saturation and respiratory symptoms, cardiorespiratory monitoring to detect any further episodes of apnea is appropriate while she is acutely ill.

There is nothing in the history to suggest that the apnea was caused by aspiration or that she has a swallowing dysfunction; therefore, a barium swallow study will offer little to her management. Lack of fever and the presence of wheezing rather than rales make pneumonia very unlikely. The most likely underlying diagnosis is bronchiolitis, for which treatment with ceftriaxone or any other antibiotic is not indicated.

The wheezing associated with bronchiolitis is not responsive to albuterol. Treatment of bronchiolitis with albuterol is outside the guidelines for management of bronchiolitis from the American Academy of Pediatrics.

Lack of fever suggests that even in this age group a full sepsis evaluation is not indicated. The presence of fever in a premature infant less than 2 months old would trigger evaluation for sepsis as a cause of the fever and apnea.

The infant in this vignette had duskiness and lack of breathing, 2 of the 4 criteria for a brief resolved unexplained event (BRUE). If she had lost tone or been unresponsive, a BRUE would be a consideration. However, she has wheezing and signs to suggest bronchiolitis, which is a reasonable explanation for her apnea, and a BRUE is not under consideration. Her admission is for supplemental oxygen, supportive treatment of bronchiolitis, and close monitoring while she is hospitalized. There is no indication for an extensive evaluation or home apnea monitoring (after hospitalization).

American Board of Pediatrics Content Specification(s)/ Content Area

- Plan the appropriate clinical and diagnostic evaluation of apnea of various etiologies
- Plan appropriate management for apnea of various etiologies

Suggested Readings

Matiz A, Roman EA. Apnea. *Pediatr Rev.* 2003;24(1):32-34

Schroeder AR, Mansbach JM, Stevenson M, et al. Apnea in children hospitalized with bronchiolitis. *Pediatrics.* 2013;132(5):e1194-e1201.

Tieder JS, Bonkowsky JL, Etzel RA, et al. Brief resolved unexplained events (formerly apparent life-threatening events) and evaluation of lower-risk infants: executive summary. *Pediatrics.* 2016;137(5):e20160591.

Item 180 **Preferred Response: B**

The boy in this vignette has unique facial features, including thin, lightly pigmented scalp hair; a prominent frontal bone; periorbital hyperpigmentation; and a retruded (moved backward) midface. In addition, he has hypodontia (reduced number of teeth) and teeth that have a conical appearance. These findings are consistent with hypohidrotic ectodermal dysplasia (HED).

The key features of HED are:

- Hypotrichosis: Sparse, lightly pigmented, slow-growing scalp and body hair that also has increased fragility
- Hypohidrosis: Reduced ability to sweat, which may lead to episodes of hyperthermia that often begin during infancy
- Hypodontia: Eruption is delayed; teeth are reduced in number and often are smaller than expected and abnormally shaped (ie, the anterior teeth often have a conical shape)

Hypohidrotic ectodermal dysplasia is estimated to occur in 1 in 5,000 to 10,000 newborns. The most common form is inherited in an X-linked fashion and results from pathogenic variants of *EDA*. Carriers may have abnormalities of sweat gland number and function, and most carriers have some degree of hypodontia. In addition to the key features of HED, patients have characteristic facial features, as exhibited by the boy in this vignette. The diagnosis is made clinically but can be confirmed with molecular genetic testing. Clinical suspicion is raised when teeth fail to erupt as expected or when teeth that erupt have a conical shape. The management of HED addresses the key features of the disease. Gentle hair care practices are encouraged (to avoid breaking fragile hairs) and wigs may be appropriate for some individuals. In hot weather, patients should have access to measures that facilitate body cooling (eg, a spray water bottle, a wet T-shirt, air conditioning, or a fan). Evaluation by an experienced dentist is important to determine the extent of hypodontia and the need for restorations, dentures, or dental implants. A medical genetics consultation is appropriate to confirm the diagnosis and counsel and educate families. Information and support is available at the National Foundation for Ectodermal Dysplasias (https://www.nfed.org/).

Several inherited disorders have both dermatologic and dental abnormalities. Their clinical features help distinguish them from HED. Severe forms of epidermolysis bullosa (eg, the recessive dystrophic type), a group of disorders characterized by spontaneous blister formation, are associated with dental enamel hypoplasia and severe caries. Incontinentia pigmenti affects the skin, hair, teeth, nails, eyes, and central nervous system. Children have swirling macular hyperpigmentation (Item C180A) and teeth that are reduced in number or absent, small, or abnormally shaped (Item C180B). The cutaneous abnormalities in tuberous sclerosis complex include hypomelanotic macules, facial angiofibromas,

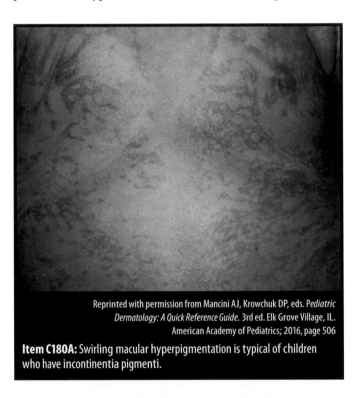

Reprinted with permission from Mancini AJ, Krowchuk DP, eds. *Pediatric Dermatology: A Quick Reference Guide.* 3rd ed. Elk Grove Village, IL. American Academy of Pediatrics; 2016, page 506

Item C180A: Swirling macular hyperpigmentation is typical of children who have incontinentia pigmenti.

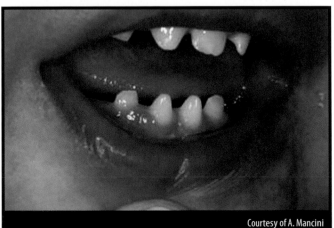

Courtesy of A. Mancini

Item C180B: The teeth in incontinentia pigmenti may be abnormally shaped. In this patient, the mandibular central incisors have a conical appearance.

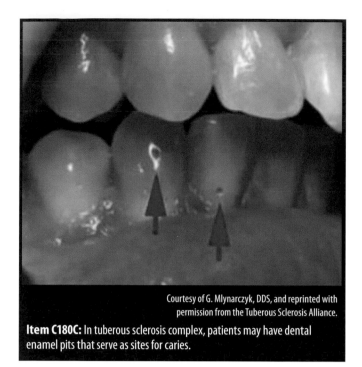

Courtesy of G. Mlynarczyk, DDS, and reprinted with permission from the Tuberous Sclerosis Alliance.

Item C180C: In tuberous sclerosis complex, patients may have dental enamel pits that serve as sites for caries.

shagreen patches, and ungual fibromas. Dental enamel pits (≥ 3) (Item C180C) are 1 of the minor diagnostic criteria.

PREP Pearls

- Hypohidrotic ectodermal dysplasia is characterized by hypotrichosis, hypohidrosis, and hypodontia.
- Individuals with hypohidrotic ectodermal dysplasia have characteristic facial features, including thin, lightly pigmented scalp hair; a prominent frontal bone; periorbital hyperpigmentation; and a retruded (moved backward) midface.

American Board of Pediatrics Content Specification(s)/ Content Area

- Recognize the clinical findings associated with ectodermal dysplasia

Suggested Readings

Northrup H, Koenig MK, Pearson DA, Au KS. Tuberous sclerosis complex. *GeneReviews*. https://www.ncbi.nlm.nih.gov/books/NBK1220/.

Scheuerle AE, Ursini MV. Incontinentia pigmenti. *GeneReviews*. https://www.ncbi.nlm.nih.gov/books/NBK1472/. https://www.ncbi.nlm.nih.gov/books/NBK1472/.

Wright JT, Grange DK, Fete M. Hypohidrotic ectodermal dysplasia. *GeneReviews*. https://www.ncbi.nlm.nih.gov/books/NBK1112/.

Item 181 **Preferred Response: C**

This vignette describes a situation that represents a conflict of interest for the program director. The program director was asked to score an abstract submitted by his trainee, and he played a role in the project. These factors could introduce bias into how the abstract is scored. The program director has a personal interest in how well the abstract does in the competition. To resolve this conflict of interest, the best option is to discuss the situation with the organizers and abstain from scoring this abstract.

The option to ask a colleague to score the abstract is not preferred because it keeps the organizers of the competition unaware of the conflict of interest and leaves them out of the decision. The option for him to decline participation as an abstract scorer and ask the organizers to replace him is not preferred because there is no reason why the program director cannot score other abstracts. Program directors were specifically asked to participate. The option to score the abstract using the rubric provided to ensure optimal objectivity is not preferred because it does not resolve the conflict of interest.

The Institute of Medicine defines conflicts of interest as "circumstances that create a risk that professional judgments or actions regarding a primary interest will be unduly influenced by a secondary interest." Conflicts of interest can occur in research, education, and clinical practice. They are commonly financial in nature but may also relate to academic promotion or doing favors for others. Examples of financial conflicts of interest may include accepting gifts from pharmaceutical companies, receiving outside funding for educational programs, and having relationships with industry. Disclosure of any potential conflicts of interest is an important step in mitigating them.

PREP Pearls

- Disclosure of any potential conflicts of interest is an important step in mitigating them.
- The Institute of Medicine defines conflicts of interest as "circumstances that create a risk that professional judgments or actions regarding a primary interest will be unduly influenced by a secondary interest."

American Board of Pediatrics Content Specification(s)/ Content Area

- Recognize and apply ethical principles regarding conflicts of interest

Suggested Readings

Harari DY, Macauley RC. Session 18: conflict of interest. In: Adam MB, Diekema DS, Mercurio MR, eds. *American Academy of Pediatrics Bioethics Resident Curriculum: Case-Based Teaching Guides*. 2017. https://www.aap.org/en-us/about-the-aap/Committees-Councils-Sections/Section-on-Bioethics/Pages/Bioethics-Case-Based-Teaching-Guides-for-Resident-Training.aspx.

Institute of Medicine. Summary. In: Lo B, Field MJ, eds. *Conflict of Interest in Medical Research, Education, and Practice*. Washington, DC: National Academies Press; 2009.

Tonelli MR. Conflict of interest in clinical practice. *Chest*. 2007;132(2):664-670.

Item 182 **Preferred Response: C**

The girl in the vignette has familial lipoprotein lipase (LPL) deficiency, which presents in childhood with severe hypertriglyceridemia, intermittent abdominal pain, recurrent acute pancreatitis, hepatosplenomegaly, and a distinctive rash known as eruptive cutaneous xanthomata (Item C182). It is an autosomal recessive disorder requiring

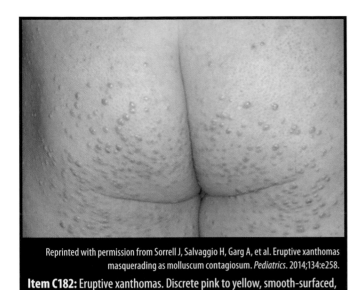

Reprinted with permission from Sorrell J, Salvaggio H, Garg A, et al. Eruptive xanthomas masquerading as molluscum contagiosum. *Pediatrics*. 2014;134:e258.

Item C182: Eruptive xanthomas. Discrete pink to yellow, smooth-surfaced, firm, monomorphous papules on the buttocks.

biallelic pathogenic gene mutation in *LPL,* thus there is not always a family history of disease. Children with this disorder have impaired chylomicron clearance, which results in triglyceride accumulation in the plasma, giving it a milky or lipemic appearance. The symptoms will abate with strict nutrition therapy; a total dietary restriction of fat to less than or equal to 20 g/day or 15% of total energy intake is required. The goal is to achieve a triglyceride concentration below 1,000 mg/dL (11.3 mmol/L). Although other genetic dyslipidemias are commonly treated with a low-fat diet, increased exercise, and lipid-lowering medications, these medications are ineffective in treating familial LPL deficiency. Fish oil supplementation is contraindicated because it will further elevate chylomicron levels. Plasma triglyceride levels should be followed routinely.

Other lipoprotein disorders that could present similarly include familial combined hyperlipidemia and monogenic familial hypertriglyceridemia. When evaluating a child with hypertriglyceridemia, one must always consider secondary causes including diabetes mellitus, lymphoproliferative disorders, alcohol abuse, and certain drug therapies such as isotretinoin, selective serotonin reuptake inhibitors, estrogen, β-blockers, and glucocorticoids. Glucocorticoids can lead to hypertriglyceridemia but are not used to treat this disorder.

A low-protein diet would be recommended for children with specific inborn errors of metabolism such as urea cycle defects, phenylketonuria, or maple syrup urine disease.

Current guidelines by the National Heart, Lung, and Blood Institute and American Academy of Pediatrics recommend lipid screening as a part of the routine health supervision visit at least once between 9 and 11 years of age and again between 17 and 21 years of age. Lipid screening is recommended at a younger age if there is a family history of early cardiovascular disease, if a parent has dyslipidemia, or if the child has other risk factors.

PREP Pearls

- Familial lipoprotein lipase deficiency presents in childhood with severe hypertriglyceridemia, intermittent abdominal pain, recurrent acute pancreatitis, hepatosplenomegaly, and a distinctive rash known as eruptive cutaneous xanthomata.
- Substances that can worsen or cause hypertriglyceridemia include fish oil supplementation, isotretinoin, selective serotonin reuptake inhibitors, estrogen, beta-blockers, and glucocorticoids.
- Treatment of familial lipoprotein lipase deficiency is with strict nutrition therapy, with a total dietary restriction of fat to less than or equal to 20 g/day or 15% of total energy intake. The goal is to achieve a triglyceride concentration below 1,000 mg/dL (11.3 mmol/L).

American Board of Pediatrics Content Specification(s)/ Content Area

- Recognize the clinical features associated with lipoprotein disorders
- Plan the appropriate immediate and long-term management of lipoprotein disorders, while considering the long-term prognosis

Suggested Readings

Burnett JR, Hooper AJ, Hegele RA. Familial lipoprotein lipase deficiency. *GeneReviews.* https://www.ncbi.nlm.nih.gov/books/NBK1308/.

Expert Panel on Integrated Guidelines for Cardiovascular Health and Risk Reduction in Children and Adolescents; National Heart, Lung, and Blood Institute. Expert panel on integrated guidelines for cardiovascular health and risk reduction in children and adolescents: summary report. *Pediatrics.* 2011;128(suppl 5):S213-S256.

Item 183 **Preferred Response: C**

The bruise on the chest wall in this nonambulatory infant may represent a sentinel injury suspicious for child physical abuse and warrants further investigation. A good starting point is a skeletal survey, as well as consultation with the child protection specialist if the clinician is uncertain whether a referral to the state child welfare agency should be initiated. Children who are not yet mobile should not have any bruising, and, if found on routine examination, should prompt the clinician to consider physical abuse.

Of 700,000 substantiated annual cases of child maltreatment, about 17% are attributable to physical abuse. Infants in the first year of age are at higher risk for physical abuse compared to older children. Other risk factors include parental substance abuse, mental illness, interpersonal violence, single parent, young parent, and having an unrelated adult in the home. Also, parental social isolation, poverty, and lower levels of education are associated with physical abuse. Prematurity, low birthweight, and developmental and physical disabilities place an infant or child at greater risk for abuse.

A history of unexplained or concerning injuries documented by medical professionals is common among children ultimately suffering from severe forms of physical abuse. Therefore, it is incumbent upon the pediatric community to identify these early injuries and report concerns to appropriate authorities. Bruises on the torso, ear, or neck of a young child (ie, under 5 years of age) are highly suspicious for abuse, as is any bruising in a child less than 4 months of age.

Furthermore, oral injuries in nonambulatory infants, multiple injuries of different ages and/or involving different organ systems, burns to genitalia or in stocking/glove distribution, implausible explanation for the injury, or lack of caregiver concern about the injury despite an unclear etiology are concerning signs for child physical abuse.

Children younger than 2 years with a suspicious injury or with a sibling who was found to be abused should undergo a skeletal survey in accordance with practice standards established by the American College of Radiology. Because very recent rib and long bone fractures are more evident with the passage of time, a repeat skeletal survey 10 to 14 days later may be indicated. In addition, laboratory studies for bone health may be helpful, including measurements of calcium, magnesium, phosphorus, and alkaline phosphatase. The patient should be evaluated for vitamin D deficiency if suspected. For bruising suspicious for abuse, a diagnostic evaluation for a bleeding disorder may be useful. Head computed tomography or magnetic resonance imaging can be used to investigate concerns for abusive head trauma. For patients with suspected traumatic injuries, particularly abdominal injuries, a complete blood cell count, complete metabolic panel, pancreatic enzyme levels, and urinalysis should be obtained.

Primary care clinicians are mandated reporters of suspected child abuse. Consultation with a colleague with expertise in child abuse can be valuable when a clinician is uncertain about whether a clinical presentation warrants a report. Many children's hospitals have child protection teams in place to answer inquiries from primary care clinicians. Other specialists (eg, neurologists, radiologists, and orthopedists) can also be helpful, depending on the injury. The clinician should err on the side of reporting if uncertain and no expert is available; for the child in this vignette, reporting would be appropriate. It is good practice to inform the caretaker prior to making a report of suspected child abuse and continue open communication regarding any testing and procedures ordered for the evaluation.

Chest radiography alone is not sensitive enough to detect fractures common in child abuse, although many occult fractures are detected on chest radiographs obtained for another reason. Clinicians should document suspicious findings with photographs in the medical record whenever possible, along with the size of the lesion and location on the body. However, there is no way to accurately determine the age of a bruise, so referral to a dermatologist would not be helpful for the patient in this vignette.

PREP Pearls

- A skeletal survey is indicated in any child under 2 years of age when physical abuse of any kind is suspected.
- Any bruising on a nonmobile infant should raise concern for child physical abuse.
- Pediatric clinicians with expertise in child abuse and child protection teams at tertiary centers can be valuable resources when a clinician is uncertain whether a clinical presentation is suspicious for abuse.

American Board of Pediatrics Content Specification(s)/ Content Area

- Understand the common trigger events (eg, incessant crying) for physical abuse
- Understand the epidemiology of and the psychosocial and environmental risk factors for physical abuse

Suggested Readings

Brodie N, McColgan MD, Spector ND, Turchi RM. Child abuse in children and youth with special health care needs. *Pediatr Rev.* 2017;38(10):463-470.

Christian CW; Committee on Child Abuse and Neglect. The evaluation of suspected child physical abuse. *Pediatrics.* 2015;135(5):e1337-e1354.

Glick JC, Lorand MA, Bilka KR. Physical abuse of children. *Pediatr Rev.* 2016;37(4):146-158.

Item 184   Preferred Response: C

Standard pediatric care is recommended for the neonate in this vignette. The mother of the neonate lived in a country with endemic transmission of Zika virus, and during the first trimester she developed an illness that could be consistent with Zika virus infection. However, she was not tested for Zika virus infection. Because the neonate in this vignette does not have abnormalities consistent with congenital Zika virus infection and there is no laboratory evidence of infection in his mother, he should receive standard care.

Women can acquire Zika virus through the bite of an infected mosquito or via sexual contact. The fetus becomes infected via the transplacental route. Abnormalities associated with congenital Zika syndrome include microcephaly, intracranial calcifications (typically subcortical), other brain malformations, and eye anomalies, including abnormalities of the retinal and optic nerves. Fetal brain disruption sequence, characterized by severe microcephaly, overlapping of cranial sutures, prominent occipital bone, and redundant scalp skin, has been described in infants with congenital Zika syndrome. Neurologic examination can reveal problems with tone, spasticity, and hyperreflexia. Clubfoot and arthrogryposis have also been associated with congenital Zika syndrome.

An evaluation for congenital Zika virus infection should be pursued in neonates with clinical findings consistent with congenital Zika virus infection or if there is laboratory evidence of possible maternal Zika virus infection during pregnancy. The evaluation should include Zika virus testing in the neonate (ideally in the first few days after birth) in addition to head ultrasonography, comprehensive ophthalmologic evaluation, and hearing testing via automated auditory brainstem response methodology, all by 1 month of age.

Lumbar puncture is not specifically warranted in the evaluation of congenital Zika virus infection. However, if a lumbar puncture is being performed for other reasons, such as evaluation of other congenital infections, cerebrospinal fluid can be evaluated for Zika virus RNA by polymerase chain reaction and testing for anti–Zika virus IgM.

American Board of Pediatrics Content Specification(s)/ Content Area

- Evaluate patient for mosquito-borne infections

Suggested Readings

Adebanjo T, Godfred-Cato S, Viens L, et al. Update: interim guidance for the diagnosis, evaluation, and management of infants with possible congenital Zika virus infection—United States, October 2017. *MMWR Morb Mortal Wkly Rep*. 2017;66(41):1089-1099.

American Academy of Pediatrics. Zika virus. In: Kimberlin DW, Brady MT, Jackson MA, Long SS, eds. *Red Book: 2018 Report of the Committee on Infectious Diseases*. 31st ed. Itasca, IL: American Academy of Pediatrics; 2018:894-902.

Moore C, Staples J, Dobyns W, et al. Characterizing the pattern anomalies in congenital Zika syndrome for pediatric clinicians. *JAMA Pediatr*. 2017;171(3):288-295.

Item 185   Preferred Response: B

The boy in this vignette has ascariasis that was most likely acquired via ingestion of soil-contaminated food. The eggs of *Ascaris lumbricoides* become infectious only after incubating in soil for a few weeks, thus infections result from direct ingestion of soil or consumption of a soil-contaminated product.

Helminth infections are common in developing countries and areas with poor sanitation. It is recommended that immigrants from developing countries be screened for parasites upon arrival to the United States. *Ascaris lumbricoides* is the most common human nematode or roundworm infection. Humans become infected with *A lumbricoides* after they ingest embryonated eggs. Larvae hatch from the eggs in the small intestine, penetrate the mucosa, and travel to the lungs where they penetrate into the airways. They then travel up to the pharynx, are swallowed, and eventually mature into adults in the small intestine.

Many infections with *A lumbricoides* are silent. When manifestations are present, they can vary widely in severity and can include abdominal pain, abdominal distention, intestinal obstruction, intestinal perforation, and peritonitis. Occasionally, adult worms are passed by rectum or through the nose or mouth after vomiting. Pneumonitis can be observed during the larval migratory phase. Some patients become malnourished with heavy infections and can have associated stunting of growth and cognitive deficits. Ascariasis can be treated with antiparasitic drugs including albendazole, mebendazole, ivermectin, and nitazoxanide.

Helminths vary in how they are acquired and their clinical manifestations. Infection with *Enterobius vermicularis* (pinworms) typically occurs via contact with a contaminated fomite. Anal pruritus is the most common manifestation of pinworm infection. *Necator americanus* (hookworm) infection results from skin penetration by larvae in soil. While abdominal pain can occur in the setting of hookworm infection, adult worms are rarely observed in this infection. Moderate to severe anemia can result from hookworm infection. Trichinellosis occurs by ingesting undercooked meat, most typically pork. While abdominal pain can occur in trichinosis, the key clinical manifestation is pain as larvae migrate to skeletal muscle.

American Board of Pediatrics Content Specification(s)/ Content Area

- Recognize the clinical features associated with ascariasis, and manage appropriately
- Understand the epidemiology of ascariasis

Suggested Readings

American Academy of Pediatrics. *Ascaris lumbricoides* infections. In: Kimberlin DW, Brady MT, Jackson MA, Long SS, eds. *Red Book: 2018 Report of the Committee on Infectious Diseases*. 31st ed. Itasca, IL: American Academy of Pediatrics; 2018:228-229.

Weatherhead J, Hotez P. Worm infections in children. *Pediatr Rev*. 2015;36(8):341-354.

Item 186   Preferred Response: B

The girl in the vignette was hit in the thigh with a hard projectile object. She has pain, swelling, and tenderness involving the quadriceps muscle belly and decreased flexion of the right knee; these signs and symptoms are consistent with a quadriceps contusion. Quadriceps contusion is caused by a direct blow to the muscle belly resulting in bleeding into the muscle. Most affected individuals will have decreased knee flexion after the injury. Early treatment consists of icing, muscle compression, and very light stretching to a degree that does not cause pain. Individuals with severe pain should use crutches to avoid weight-bearing. Once pain subsides, in the first 3 to 7 days after injury, the child can progress with stretching and strengthening. Excessive stretching, massage, and heat should be avoided in the first few days after injury because these can increase bleeding into the muscle. In rare cases, bleeding can lead to a compartment syndrome involving the thigh. Unlike most types of compartment syndrome, athletes with thigh compartment syndrome typically do not require surgical intervention.

Myositis ossificans traumatica is a late complication of muscle contusion. Calcifications begin to form in the muscle 2 to 3 weeks after injury. Myositis ossificans should be suspected in an athlete with initial recovery after muscle contusion, who in the weeks after an injury, develops increased pain with activity. In some cases, the calcified tissue can be detected with palpation. Radiography can be used to detect and quantify myositis ossificans. Typically, the body resorbs the calcifications very slowly over time.

Quadriceps tendon rupture mainly affects middle-aged adults; it is very uncommon in children and adolescents. Affected individuals often experience chronic pain above the knee, and subsequently experience an acute increase in pain. Quadriceps tendon rupture results in the inability to actively straighten the knee.

A stress fracture is a gradual weakening of the bone from overuse. A stress fracture involving the midshaft of the femur could produce pain similar to that seen with a muscle contusion. However, most athletes with stress fracture report a history of insidious-onset, gradually worsening pain with activity.

PREP Pearls

- In rare cases, bleeding after a quadriceps contusion can lead to compartment syndrome involving the thigh.
- Myositis ossificans traumatica is a late complication of muscle contusion. Calcifications begin to form in the muscle 2 to 3 weeks after contusion.
- Quadriceps contusions are caused by a direct blow to the muscle belly resulting in bleeding into the muscle. Most affected individuals will have decreased knee flexion after the injury.

American Board of Pediatrics Content Specification(s)/ Content Area

- Identify complications associated with a deep hematoma of the thigh
- Plan the appropriate management of bruises and hematomas

Suggested Readings

Lamplot JD, Matava MJ. Thigh injuries in American football. *Am J Orthop (Belle Mead NJ)*. 2016;45(6):e308-e318.

Item 187   **Preferred Response: A**

The girl in this vignette has allergic rhinitis. First-line pharmacologic treatment for allergic rhinitis includes an intranasal corticosteroid spray or a second-generation oral antihistamine. First-generation sedating oral antihistamines, oral steroids, and intranasal decongestants should not be used.

Allergic rhinitis is an IgE-mediated hypersensitivity reaction that causes inflammation of the nasal passages and manifests as nasal congestion, rhinorrhea, sneezing, nasal itching, and/or postnasal discharge. Patients may also note itching of the eyes or throat, headaches, difficulty concentrating, nighttime cough, and disrupted sleep. Allergic rhinitis occurs in sensitized individuals in response to a specific allergen. Depending on the triggering allergen(s), it may have a seasonal or perennial pattern. Allergic rhinitis is common and the incidence in the United States is rising; one study found that more than 40% of children are diagnosed with allergic rhinitis before the age of 6 years. Allergic rhinitis is most common in children with a personal or family history of atopy (eg, asthma, atopic dermatitis, or allergy).

Children with allergic rhinitis often have pale, bluish nasal mucosa, boggy and erythematous nasal turbinates, pharyngeal cobblestoning, nasal obstruction, or clear nasal discharge. Allergic shiners and a transverse nasal crease may accompany these findings. The differential diagnosis for allergic rhinitis includes infectious rhinitis, sinusitis, nasal foreign body, and structural abnormalities of the nasal passage.

Treatment of allergic rhinitis begins with the avoidance or reduction of allergen exposure. Nasal saline irrigation or spray may alleviate mild symptoms. Intranasal corticosteroid sprays are effective at reducing symptoms of allergic rhinitis with limited adverse effects and are therefore recommended as first-line treatment, although some children do not tolerate intranasal administration because of fear or discomfort. Oral antihistamines are also efficacious. First-generation antihistamines (eg, diphenhydramine) should be avoided because of their sedating adverse effects. Second-generation antihistamines (eg, loratadine, cetirizine) lack these adverse effects and are therefore the preferred oral agent. Intranasal antihistamines (eg, azelastine or olopatadine) and intranasal cromolyn have minimal adverse effect profiles, but are less effective than intranasal steroids; these drugs are preferred over steroids by some families.

Intranasal decongestants work by vasoconstricting the nasal mucosa and can quickly reduce symptoms of allergic rhinitis. They are not recommended, however, because they lead to downregulation of α-adrenergic receptors and can cause rebound nasal congestion. Although oral corticosteroids usually eliminate symptoms of allergic rhinitis, they have significant adverse effects and are not recommended except in extremely severe and refractory cases.

PREP Pearls

- Allergic rhinitis is an IgE-mediated hypersensitivity reaction that causes inflammation of the nasal passages and manifests as nasal congestion, rhinorrhea, sneezing, nasal itching, and/or postnasal discharge. Patients may also note itching of the eyes or throat, headaches, difficulty concentrating, nighttime cough, and disrupted sleep.
- Treatment of allergic rhinitis begins with avoidance or reduction of allergen exposures. First-line pharmacologic treatment includes intranasal corticosteroid sprays and/or second-generation oral antihistamines.

American Board of Pediatrics Content Specification(s)/ Content Area

- Recognize the common characteristics of allergic rhinitis, and manage appropriately
- Formulate a differential diagnosis of chronic rhinitis

Suggested Readings

Mahr TA, Sheth K. Update on allergic rhinitis. *Pediatr Rev.* 2005;26(8):284-289.

Seidman MD, Gurgel RK, Lin SY, et al. Clinical practice guideline: allergic rhinitis. *Otolaryngol Head Neck Surg.* 2015;152(1 suppl):S1-S43.

Wallace DV, Dykewicz MS, Bernstein DI, et al. The diagnosis and management of rhinitis: an updated practice parameter. *J Allergy Clin Immunol.* 2008;122(2 suppl):S1-S84.

The boy in this vignette requires long-term enteral nutritional supplementation to improve his nutritional status. A gastrostomy tube is the most appropriate method to deliver his nutrition. A gastrostomy tube is indicated because there is no significant history of vomiting or feeding intolerance to suggest that postpyloric feedings (or jejunal feedings) would be needed.

Enteral nutritional supplementation, which can be delivered by a variety of methods, is recommended in children with an intact gastrointestinal tract and insufficient oral intake to improve nutritional status.

Nasogastric feeding tubes may be used for intermittent or short-term nutritional support (generally considered less than 3 months). Nasogastric feeding tubes can be replaced at the bedside, or caregivers and even older patients can be educated to replace the tubes at home. There are some conditions, such as Crohn disease, for which it is appropriate to place a nasogastric tube at bedtime, administer enteral nutrition overnight, and then remove the tube in the morning. Nasogastric tubes also allow flexibility to administer bolus feedings directly into the stomach. Long-term, continuous, nasogastric tube use is often difficult because of nasal irritation and general discomfort.

Nasojejunal tubes are also used for short-term nutritional support. Because the formula is administered past the pylorus, continuous feedings must be used. Radiology or endoscopy is required for placement and replacement (if needed). Complications of nasojejunal tubes include nasal irritation and displacement of the distal end of the tube (it may become dislodged from the small intestine and coil in the stomach).

Gastrostomy tubes are indicated for more long-term nutritional support needs. A gastrostomy tube is a surgically placed feeding tube with direct access to the stomach. It may be placed endoscopically, surgically, or with interventional radiology procedures. Like nasogastric tubes, nutritional supplementation may be administered as a bolus or as continuous feeds. Continuous feedings via a gastrostomy tube are generally considered with overnight feedings or in children who cannot tolerate bolus enteral feedings. Complications of gastrostomy tubes include infection, granulation tissue, and inadvertent removal. Older patients and caregivers can be educated to replace the gastrostomy tube. Gastrostomy tubes are generally changed every 3 to 6 months and can be easily removed if nutritional supplementation is no longer required.

Jejunostomy tubes are surgically placed feeding tubes with direct access to the small intestine. Their use requires continuous enteral feedings. Risks of jejunostomy tubes are similar to gastrostomy tubes, however dislodgement can be problematic and may require fluoroscopic guidance for replacement. A gastrojejunostomy tube can also be placed, which can offer the flexibility of both gastric and jejunal feeding options; however, the risk of dislodgement and need for fluoroscopic guidance for replacement is similar to jejunostomy tubes.

A central venous catheter is not appropriate in this scenario, as parenteral nutrition is not indicated for initial nutritional rehabilitation given the boy's intact gastrointestinal tract. Jejunostomy tube placement is not indicated because there are no clinical indications that he requires postpyloric feedings (specifically there is no significant history of vomiting or feeding intolerance). While a nasogastric tube could be a reasonable short-term solution to improve his nutritional status, his care team is anticipating prolonged enteral nutritional support.

PREP Pearls

- Continuous feedings are required if enteral nutrition is delivered past the stomach.
- Longer term nutritional supplementation should prompt consideration of gastrostomy tube placement.
- Nasogastric tube placement is recommended for short-term or intermittent nutritional support needs.

American Board of Pediatrics Content Specification(s)/ Content Area

- Know when to prescribe intermittent (bolus) feeding rather than continuous tube feeding
- Recognize the complications associated with tube feeding

Suggested Readings

Braegger C, Decsi T, Dias JA, et al; ESPGHAN Committee on Nutrition. Practical approach to paediatric enteral nutrition: a comment by the ESPGHAN Committee on Nutrition. *J Pediatr Gastroenterol Nutr.* 2010;51:110-122.

Seres DS, Valcarcel M, Guillaume A. Advantages of enteral nutrition over parenteral nutrition. *Therap Adv Gastroenterol.* 2013;6(2):157-167.

Singhal S, Baker SS, Bojczuk GA, Baker RD. Tube feeding in children. *Pediatr Rev.* 2017;38(1)23-34.

Although various communication methods can be used for the boy in this vignette, the oral communication method maximizes the use of his residual hearing to develop speech. This method emphasizes listening skills and speech articulation and uses hearing, speech, and lipreading to develop spoken language.

In typical development, language understanding (ie, receptive language) is ahead of language production (ie, expressive language). Speech is the articulation of sounds. Receptive language milestones include recognition of one's name around 6 months of age and single words around 8 to 10 months and the ability to follow 1-step commands by 1 year, 2-step commands by 2 years, and 3-step commands by 3 years. Expressive language milestones include babbling around 3 to 6 months, first words and jargoning (ie, babbling with intonation and inflection) around 12 months, combining 2 words by 2 years, and combining 3 words by 3 years. Speech should be 50% intelligible to strangers by 2 years, 75% by 3 years, and 100% by 4 years. Clear articulation of certain speech sounds may not be present until 8 years. Of note, language rapidly develops in the preschool years and word repetitions (ie, developmental dysfluency) may occur and then resolve by 4 to 5 years.

Language development is influenced by genetics and the environment. Expressive language delay is associated with a family history of language or reading problems. Bilingualism and male sex do not result in significantly delayed language. Children who are exposed to more language and language that is child-directed rather than overheard have advanced language skills compared to children with more limited language exposure. Low socioeconomic environments tend to be lower in language exposure and access to books. Enhancing the child's language environment through reading to the child and engaging verbally with the child can stimulate language development.

Language disorders, or persistent difficulties in learning language with resultant impairment, occur in 2% to 3% of school-aged children. Speech disorders occur in 3% to 6% of school-aged children and include problems with articulation and with fluency (eg, stuttering). When a child has delayed or atypical language development, a formal audiology evaluation should be done to determine if hearing loss is a cause or contributor. A child with mild to moderate, progressive, or acquired hearing loss may have had a normal newborn hearing screen but be identified in a later audiology evaluation.

For children with hearing loss, 3 educational/communication methods are commonly used. The oral communication method uses the child's residual hearing, speech, and lipreading to develop spoken language and thus facilitate participation in mainstream environments. The manual communication method uses signing and fingerspelling. This method is helpful for children who have greater difficulty taking in auditory information. It can facilitate earlier communication as children can use sign language prior to spoken language. American Sign Language is a rich language that uses hand and body movements and facial expressions to fully express ideas. Manual English uses traditional American Sign Language signs with English grammar conventions to facilitate reading and writing in English. Total language communication allows communication with the child by any means available (eg, speech, sign, gestures, writing, pictures). Children with hearing loss may receive instruction across different settings, such as a mainstream classroom using an interpreter or assistive listening device, a deaf education classroom, or a residential school for the deaf.

PREP Pearls

- A child with mild to moderate, progressive, or acquired hearing loss may have had a normal newborn hearing screen result but be identified in a later audiology evaluation.
- Children who are exposed to more language and language that is child-directed rather than overheard have advanced language skills compared to children with more limited language exposure.
- In typical development, language understanding (ie, receptive language) is ahead of language production (ie, expressive language).
- The oral communication method emphasizes listening skills and speech articulation and uses hearing, speech, and lip reading to develop spoken language.

American Board of Pediatrics Content Specification(s)/Content Area

- Understand the major approaches to education for hearing impaired children
- Recognize age-related normal and abnormal variations in speech and language
- Understand factors that influence language development

Suggested Readings

Coplan J. Language delays. In: Augustyn M, Zuckerman B, Caronna EB, eds. *The Zuckerman Parker Handbook of Developmental and Behavioral Pediatrics for Primary Care*. 3rd ed. Philadelphia, PA: Wolters Kluwer; 2011:258-262.

McQuiston S, Kloczko N. Speech and language development: monitoring process and problems. *Pediatr Rev*. 2011;32(6):230-239.

Wills LM, Wills KE. Hearing loss and deafness. In: Augustyn M, Zuckerman B, Caronna EB, eds. *The Zuckerman Parker Handbook of Developmental and Behavioral Pediatrics for Primary Care*. 3rd ed. Philadelphia, PA: Wolters Kluwer; 2011:242-249.

Item 190	Preferred Response: A

The boy in the vignette most likely has pseudotumor cerebri due to doxycycline. The brief episodes of blurry, gray vision are called transient visual obscurations and are associated with increased intracranial pressure. The clinician should recognize this and stop doxycycline immediately, because of the high likelihood that it has caused pseudotumor cerebri in this adolescent. The boy should also be referred to ophthalmology to confirm the presence of papillitis and assess for vision loss. The best next management step for this boy is brain imaging to evaluate for other causes of increased intracranial pressure, even though suspicion is high that doxycycline has caused pseudotumor cerebri. This typically includes magnetic resonance imaging of the brain and magnetic resonance venography of the head (to look for a cerebral sinovenous thrombosis). If these findings are normal, lumbar puncture should be performed to measure cerebrospinal fluid pressure. Even when suspicion for pseudotumor cerebri is high, brain imaging should be performed before the lumbar puncture, in case there is an intracranial mass that is causing increased intracranial pressure. Lumbar puncture in that situation can cause brain herniation. Clinicians should be aware that normal cerebrospinal fluid opening pressure in pediatric patients is between 10 and 28 cm H_2O (see Suggested reading 1 Avery et al).

Pseudotumor cerebri is characterized by elevated intracranial pressure that occurs in the absence of a primary cause such as intracranial mass, intracranial outflow obstruction, or encephalitis. Risk factors include obesity (especially with recent weight gain); female sex; and the use of certain medications, including tetracyclines (eg, doxycycline and minocycline), excess vitamin A ingestion (including medications that are vitamin A derivatives such as isotretinoin), and growth hormone. The clinical presentation of pseudotumor cerebri can be similar to migraine headaches; children may have severe headaches with associated phonophobia, photophobia, nausea, and vomiting. Patients can also experience transient visual obscurations, as did the boy in the vignette, pulse-synchronous tinnitus, and diplopia (resulting from cranial nerve VI palsy), none of which are expected in migraine headaches.

The first step in treatment of pseudotumor cerebri is to stop any medication that may be causing it. A medication to decrease cerebrospinal fluid production should be prescribed, as well as a weight loss program, if appropriate. Acetazolamide and topiramate are most commonly prescribed in this situation, though these are off-label uses. Untreated pseudotumor cerebri can result in permanent vision loss, so prompt diagnosis and treatment are essential. For the boy in the vignette, starting a migraine prophylaxis medication is not the best next step because he most likely has pseudotumor cerebri. Similarly, stopping creatine supplements would not address the underlying diagnosis.

PREP Pearls

- Normal cerebrospinal fluid opening pressure in pediatric patients is 10 to 28 cm H_2O.
- Pseudotumor cerebri can present with symptoms similar to migraines, with additional symptoms of transient visual obscurations, pulse synchronous tinnitus, and diplopia.
- Risk factors for pseudotumor cerebri include obesity (especially with recent weight gain), female sex, and certain medications (eg, doxycycline, minocycline, isotretinoin, and growth hormone).

American Board of Pediatrics Content Specification(s)/ Content Area

- Plan the appropriate diagnostic evaluation of increased intracranial pressure, and manage appropriately
- Know the common causes of pseudotumor cerebri
- Understand the indications and contraindications for examination of the cerebrospinal fluid in a patient who has increased intracranial pressure
- Recognize the clinical findings associated with increased intracranial pressure in patients of various ages

Suggested Readings

Avery RA, Licht DJ, Shah SS, et al. CSF opening pressure in children with optic nerve edema. *Neurology.* 2011;76(19):1658-1661.

Blume HK. Pediatric headache: a review. *Pediatr Rev.* 2012;33:562.

Item 191   **Preferred Response: C**

The girl in this vignette has tonsillar hypertrophy, as indicated by her history and physical examination findings. Her tonsils meet in the midline, which is sometimes called "kissing tonsils." Chronic or recurrent tonsillitis, rare neoplastic processes, or some lysosomal storage diseases may lead to tonsillar and adenoidal hypertrophy. Tonsillar and/ or adenoidal hypertrophy, in addition to overweight or obesity, may lead to upper airway obstruction and result in sleep-disordered breathing (obstructive sleep apnea). The American Academy of Pediatrics recommends that patients be screened at health supervision visits for snoring and other signs/symptoms of sleep-disordered breathing. For patients with positive screening results, polysomnography (a sleep study) or referral to a specialist is recommended.

Additional conditions associated with tonsillar/adenoidal hypertrophy include: feeding difficulty, dysphagia, and/or failure to thrive in young children; upper airway obstruction (noisy breathing, mouth breathing); sleep-disordered breathing (loud snoring, restless sleep, hypersomnolence, morning headaches); secondary enuresis; and night terrors. Long-term tonsillar/adenoidal hypertrophy may lead to pulmonary hypertension because of prolonged hypoxemia, which causes vasoconstriction of the pulmonary vasculature and increased pulmonary vascular resistance. Protracted pulmonary hypertension may result in cor pulmonale and heart failure.

The girl in this vignette is a social girl who performs well cognitively on school testing, indicating that she does not have a learning disability. Therefore, psychoeducational testing would not be helpful. She is inattentive at school and irritable at home, which may suggest attention-deficit/ hyperactivity disorder (ADHD) or a hearing problem. However, upon further questioning, she screens positive for sleep-disordered breathing. Therefore, administration of an ADHD-specific rating scale, such as the Vanderbilt questionnaire, would not be appropriate, and an audiology evaluation would be normal. Consequences of sleep-disordered breathing include behavioral and neurocognitive dysfunction, such as hyperactivity, inattention, reduced scholastic achievement, and aggressive behaviors. Because many of the symptoms of ADHD and sleep-disordered breathing are remarkably similar, assessment of sleep-disordered breathing begins with a detailed history, including questions about sleep onset, nighttime awakenings, daytime sleepiness, duration of sleep, patterns of sleep, and additional symptoms such as snoring or leg movements. Polysomnography is the gold standard in diagnosing sleep-related breathing disorders in children.

PREP Pearls

- Adenoidal and tonsillar hypertrophy are associated with pediatric sleep apnea.
- Evaluation of academic or behavioral concerns should include a thorough history and review for sleep issues.
- If sleep-disordered breathing is suspected, polysomnography (a sleep study) is indicated.

American Board of Pediatrics Content Specification(s)/ Content Area

- Recognize conditions associated with tonsillar and/or adenoidal hypertrophy

Suggested Readings

Bochner RE, Gangar M, Belamarich PF. A Clinical approach to tonsillitis, tonsillar hypertrophy, and peritonsillar and retropharyngeal abscesses. *Pediatr Rev.* 2017;38(2):81-92.

Capdevila OS, Kheirandish-Gozal L, Dayyat E, Gozal D. Pediatric obstructive sleep apnea: complications, management, and long-term outcomes. *Proc Am Thorac Soc.* 2008;5(2):274-282.

Gross CW, Harrison SE. Tonsils and adenoids. *Pediatr Rev.* 2000;21(3):75-78.

Marcus CL, Brooks LJ, Draper KA, et al. Diagnosis and management of childhood obstructive sleep apnea syndrome. *Pediatrics.* 2012;130(3):e714-e755.

Item 192

Preferred Response: A

Retinoblastoma is a tumor of the retinal cells that occurs in young children, with two-thirds of the cases diagnosed by 2 years of age and 95% diagnosed by 5 years of age. The development of retinoblastoma requires the inactivation of both copies of *RB1* on band 13q14 through mutation, deletion, or epigenetic silencing. Hereditary retinoblastoma occurs when there is a germline mutation of one of the *RB1* alleles and a somatic event silencing the other. Nonhereditary or sporadic retinoblastoma occurs when there are 2 independent somatic events silencing both *RB1* loci. Despite having a pathophysiology resembling an autosomal recessive disease (the development of retinoblastoma requires the inactivation of both copies of *RB1*), most germline *RB1* mutations have a penetrance of approximately 90%, meaning that hereditary retinoblastoma behaves in a manner approximating an autosomal dominant Mendelian disease. Approximately 40% of cases are hereditary. Of these, 80% arise from de novo mutations in the father's germ cells with no known family history.

The mother of the neonate in this vignette is a carrier of an abnormal *RB1* allele. There is therefore a 50% chance that the neonate inherited this abnormal allele. As germline mutations are approximately 90% penetrant, his chance of developing retinoblastoma is calculated as: (chance of inheriting the abnormal allele) × penetrance

$$= 0.5 \times 0.9$$
$$= 0.45$$

Therefore, the chance that this neonate will develop retinoblastoma is less than 50% but more than 25%. If it was certain that the neonate had inherited the abnormal *RB1* allele from his mother, then his chances of developing retinoblastoma would be 75% to 100%. However, it is not known if he inherited the mutated gene. Retinoblastoma as a whole is very rare with a prevalence of 11 cases per million children under 5 years, and 80% of heritable retinoblastoma is caused by de novo mutations; therefore, it is reasonable to assume that the father does not carry a germline *RB1* mutation.

PREP Pearls

- Approximately 40% of cases of retinoblastoma are hereditary, of which approximately 80% arise from de novo mutations in the father's germ cells with no known family history.
- Retinoblastoma can be heritable or nonheritable. Heritable retinoblastoma has a penetrance of approximately 90%.
- The development of retinoblastoma requires the inactivation of both copies of *RB1* on band 13q14 through mutation, deletion, or epigenetic silencing.

American Board of Pediatrics Content Specification(s)/Content Area

- Recognize the clinical and laboratory findings associated with retinoblastoma
- Recognize the inheritance pattern associated with retinoblastoma and the significance of the family history in planning management
- Differentiate the historical and clinical findings associated with hereditary retinoblastoma from those of sporadic retinoblastoma

Suggested Readings

Gill J. Inherited hematologic and oncologic syndromes. *Pediatr Rev.* 2011;32(9):401-404.

PDQ Pediatric Treatment Editorial Board, National Cancer Institute. PDQ cancer information summaries: retinoblastoma treatment. https://www.ncbi.nlm.nih.gov/books/NBK66006/.

Wilson WG. Retinoblastoma. *Pediatr Rev.* 2007;28(1):37-38.

Item 193

Preferred Response: C

The girl in the vignette presents after having a generalized seizure, preceded by acute onset of "clumsiness," vomiting, and abnormal respirations. Given the rapid onset of symptoms, severe metabolic acidosis, and presence of urine calcium oxalate crystals, the most likely cause of the girl's symptoms is ethylene glycol toxicity.

Ethylene glycol is an odorless, sweet-tasting substance found most commonly in antifreeze products. Ingestion of even very small quantities can be lethal to children. This toxic alcohol is absorbed rapidly from the gastrointestinal tract; initial signs of intoxication may be observed within 30 minutes after ingestion. Ethylene glycol is metabolized in the liver by alcohol dehydrogenase to form toxic metabolites that bind with calcium and are excreted in the urine in the form of calcium oxalate crystals.

Characteristic features of ethylene glycol poisoning include an elevated anion gap metabolic acidosis, hypocalcemia, and renal failure. Renal failure results from the precipitation of calcium oxalate crystals in the kidney; calcium oxalate crystals also precipitate in other body organs. The diagnosis should be considered in any child with a metabolic acidosis of unknown etiology.

The clinical effects of ethylene glycol toxicity are often grouped into 3 stages:

Stage 1 (typically within 12 hours after ingestion): Central nervous system effects, including ataxia, slurred speech, nystagmus, headache, lethargy, coma, and seizures. Nausea and vomiting occurs in many patients. Urine calcium oxalate crystals are found in about one-third of cases.

Stage 2 (12-36 hours after ingestion): Children may develop tachypnea, cyanosis, pulmonary edema, respiratory distress, tachycardia or bradycardia, cardiomegaly, and congestive heart failure. Cardiac dysrhythmias may occur because of hypocalcemia, and circulatory shock may develop. Death is most common during this stage.

Stage 3 (2-3 days after ingestion): Manifestations may include flank pain, decreased urine output (or complete anuria), proteinuria, hematuria, and acute renal failure.

Although ethylene glycol poisoning is confirmed by an elevated serum ethylene glycol level, this test may not be rapidly available in many institutions. Treatment should not be delayed to await the result of a patient's serum ethylene glycol concentration. Other laboratory studies that should be obtained in children with suspected ethylene glycol poisoning include an arterial blood gas (which typically reveals an elevated anion gap metabolic acidosis); complete blood cell count; serum electrolytes including calcium, blood glucose, blood urea nitrogen, serum creatinine, serum osmolarity, and creatine kinase; and urinalysis for crystals, protein, and blood. Both the anion gap and osmolar gaps should be calculated (typically elevated with ethylene glycol toxicity). Because significant cardiopulmonary toxicity can result from ethylene glycol toxicity, chest radiography and electrocardiography are also recommended.

For children with ethylene glycol poisoning, the management focus should be on support of the airway, breathing, and circulation. Fomepizole, an agent that blocks the conversion of ethylene glycol to its toxic metabolites, is the antidote of choice for managing ethylene glycol poisoning. Because ethylene glycol is absorbed so rapidly from the gastrointestinal tract and is poorly bound by activated charcoal, administration of activated charcoal is not indicated after ingestion. Hemodialysis may be required for children with severe renal toxicity.

All children with altered mental status, metabolic acidosis, elevated serum ethylene glycol concentration, or any indication of renal pathology because of ethylene glycol poisoning require admission to a pediatric intensive care setting. Children who are completely asymptomatic, do not have metabolic acidosis, and have an ethylene glycol serum concentration that is less than 20 mg/mL can be safely discharged from the hospital.

Acute intracranial hemorrhage could explain the sudden onset of altered mental status and seizures seen in the girl in the vignette, but she has no reported history of trauma and no signs of traumatic injury on physical examination. Although intracranial injury resulting from child abuse is possible, this would not explain the girl's laboratory findings of profound metabolic acidosis, hematuria, and urine calcium oxalate crystals.

Children with carbon monoxide poisoning may display various progressive central nervous system (CNS) symptoms ranging from headache and confusion to seizures and coma. However, urinary calcium oxalate crystals are not seen in patients with this diagnosis.

Although ingestion of a hydrocarbon substance could cause CNS symptoms, the girl in the vignette had no history of coughing or gagging before the onset of her symptoms (which would suggest hydrocarbon aspiration). She also lacks the manifestations of cough, tachypnea, wheezing, and increased work of breathing that would typically be seen with hydrocarbon aspiration.

PREP Pearls

- Characteristic features of ethylene glycol poisoning include an elevated anion gap metabolic acidosis, hypocalcemia, and renal failure (because of precipitation of calcium oxalate crystals).
- Fomepizole, an agent that blocks the conversion of ethylene glycol to its toxic metabolites, is the antidote of choice in the management of ethylene glycol poisoning.
- Management of children with ethylene glycol poisoning should focus on aggressive support of the airway, breathing, and circulation.

American Board of Pediatrics Content Specification(s)/ Content Area

- Recognize the signs and symptoms of ingestion of ethylene glycol, and manage appropriately

Suggested Readings

Erickson TB, Nelson ME. Alcohols. In: Schafermeyer R, Tenenbein M, Macias CG, Sharieff GQ, Yamamoto LG, eds. *Strange and Schafermeyer's Pediatric Emergency Medicine*. 4th ed. New York, NY: McGraw Hill; 2015;chap 124

Kruse JA. Methanol and ethylene glycol intoxication. *Crit Care Clin* 2012;28:661-711.

O'Donnell KA, Osterhoudt KC, Burns MM, Calello DP, Henretig FM. Chapter 110: Toxicologic Emergencies. In: Shaw K, Bachur R, ed. *Textbook of Pediatric Emergency Medicine*. 7th ed. Philadelphia, PA: Lippincott, Williams & Wilkins; 2016

Item 194	Preferred Response: D

The most likely cause of hypertension for the boy in the vignette is Liddle syndrome. Secondary hypertension in children can be renal, cardiac, or endocrine in origin, with renal disease and renovascular anomalies reported in about 80% to 90% of affected children. Evaluation of all patients with hypertension should include blood urea nitrogen, creatinine, electrolytes, and fasting glucose levels; urinalysis; complete blood cell count; fasting lipid profile; renal ultrasonography; and echocardiography. A fasting lipid profile and glucose level are also recommended in overweight and prehypertensive patients, as well as patients with diabetes, chronic kidney disease, or a family history of hypertension or cardiovascular disease. Hypertensive children who are very young, have stage 2 hypertension (blood pressure >99th percentile + 5 mm Hg), and children and adolescents with clinical signs suggestive of a systemic condition are at higher risk for having secondary hypertension; these children require detailed investigation for a cause of their hypertension. In these cases, additional studies such as plasma renin activity, renovascular imaging (renal scan, duplex Doppler renal ultrasonography, arteriography), plasma and urine steroid, or catecholamine levels are indicated.

Liddle syndrome (pseudoaldosteronism) and Gordon syndrome (pseudohypoaldosteronism) are rare genetic disorders associated with abnormalities in the renal tubules, leading to hypertension. Liddle syndrome is an autosomal dominant condition in which there is a primary increase in collecting tubule sodium reabsorption and potassium secretion. Children with mineralocorticoid excess, such as primary aldosteronism, Liddle syndrome, apparent mineralocorticoid excess syndrome, or licorice ingestion (glycyrrhizic acid) typically present with hypertension, hypokalemia, and metabolic alkalosis (with high urinary chloride).

Gordon syndrome is characterized by hypertension, hyperkalemia, metabolic acidosis, and normal renal function. Renal tubular anomalies lead to increased sodium chloride reabsorption in the distal tubule, causing volume expansion and hypertension in association with diminished renin secretion. This also leads to reduced potassium and hydrogen excretion, which accounts for the hyperkalemia and acidosis seen in these children.

Renal tubular disorders with sodium chloride wasting present with metabolic alkalosis in association with high urinary chloride levels (>20-40 mEq/L). Both Bartter syndrome and Gitelman syndrome are characterized by hypokalemia and metabolic alkalosis. Bartter syndrome results from a primary defect in sodium chloride reabsorption in the medullary thick ascending limb of the loop of Henle, similar to the effect of chronic furosemide therapy. Bartter syndrome often presents in childhood with growth restriction, hypokalemia, metabolic alkalosis, and polyuria or polydipsia. Gitelman syndrome results from mutations in the gene coding for the thiazide-sensitive Na-Cl transporter in the distal tubule. Gitelman syndrome generally presents in late childhood or adulthood with muscle cramps (hypokalemia), and polyuria or polydipsia. In contrast to Bartter syndrome, children with Gitelman syndrome have reduced urinary calcium and hypomagnesemia (more common). Children with either Bartter or Gitelman syndrome will be volume depleted because of excessive salt and water losses secondary to the underlying renal tubular defects. Thus, hypertension is not present on initial diagnosis in either Bartter or Gitelman syndrome.

PREP Pearls

- Bartter syndrome and Gitelman syndrome are characterized by hypokalemia and metabolic alkalosis; they are not associated with hypertension at initial diagnosis.
- Patients with mineralocorticoid excess, such as primary aldosteronism, Liddle syndrome, apparent mineralocorticoid excess syndrome, or licorice ingestion, (glycyrrhizic acid) typically present with hypertension, hypokalemia, and metabolic alkalosis (with high urinary chloride).
- Renal disease and renovascular anomalies are the most common reported causes of hypertension in children.

American Board of Pediatrics Content Specification(s)/ Content Area

- Recognize the causes of renal hypertension
- Recognize the signs and symptoms of a renal hypertensive emergency, and manage appropriately

Suggested Readings

Flynn JT, Kaelber DC, Baker-Smith CM, et al. Clinical practice guideline for screening and management of high blood pressure in children and adolescents. *Pediatrics.* 2017;140(3). pii: e20171904.

Jaffe AC. Failure to thrive: current clinical concepts. *Pediatr Rev.* 2011;32:100-108.

Item 195   Preferred Response: A

The number needed to treat (NNT) analysis helps providers determine the risk-benefit ratio for an individual patient for a specific therapy. The paired t test, power, and sample size do not specifically address this concept.

The NNT is the number of patients that need to be treated to prevent 1 additional adverse event. The formula used to calculate NNT is:

$$NNT = 1 \div Absolute\ Risk\ Reduction$$

Absolute risk reduction is the difference in the risk of adverse outcomes between the study population and a control group. The solution to this formula should be rounded to a whole number.

Data from studies can lead an investigator to an incorrect conclusion, whether due to a random sample not actually being reflective of the general population or the presence of bias. When the sample is not representative of the general population, type 1 or type 2 errors can occur. A type 1 error or false-positive occurs when an investigator rejects the null hypothesis when it is actually true. A type 2 error, or false-negative, occurs when an investigator fails to reject the null hypothesis that is actually false. Type 2 error is inversely related to the power of a study. The larger the sample size, the less likely type 1 or type 2 errors will occur.

PREP Pearls

- The number needed to treat analysis helps providers determine the risk-benefit ratio for an individual patient for a specific therapy.
- The number needed to treat, which is calculated as 1 ÷ Absolute Risk Reduction, is the number of patients needed to be treated to prevent 1 additional adverse event.

American Board of Pediatrics Content Specification(s)/ Content Area

- Understand the concept of number-needed-to-treat when utilized to describe therapeutic interventions
- Distinguish between type I and type II statistical errors

Suggested Readings

Banerjee A, Chitnis UB, Jadhav SL, Bhawalkar JS, Chaudhury S. Hypothesis testing, type 1 and type 2 errors. *Ind Psychiatry J.* 2009;18(2):127-131.

Nuovo J, Melnikow J, Chang D. Reporting number needed to treat and absolute risk reduction in randomized controlled trials. *JAMA.* 2002:287(21):2813-2814

Tschudy MM, Rowe PC. Research and statistics: Number needed to treat and intention to treat analysis. *Pediatr Rev.* 2010;31(9):380-382.

Item 196   Preferred Response: C

The patient in this vignette is a sexually active heterosexual adolescent male with dysuria, a common symptom of urethritis. Urethritis is an inflammation of the urethra that is usually caused by an infectious etiology. Other symptoms include urethral pruritus and discharge that may be mucoid or purulent.

Urethritis in males can be divided into gonococcal or nongonococcal. Gonococcal urethritis is usually associated with purulent discharge. Nongonococcal urethritis, which may not have discharge, is most frequently caused by *Chlamydia trachomatis* (most common), *Mycoplasma genitalium*, and *Trichomonas vaginalis*. Enteric organisms may play a role in urethritis in men who have sex with men and engage in insertive anal sex. A few viral pathogens have been associated with urethritis and include herpes simplex virus and adenovirus.

The diagnosis of urethritis is established by demonstrating urethral inflammation by one of the following criteria according to the Centers for Disease Control and Prevention:
- Evidence of discharge from the meatus during physical examination
- A Gram stain of the urethral discharge with 5 or more white blood cells (WBCs) per hpf. This used to be the primary test for diagnosis, however, most medical offices are not designed to perform Gram stains and microscopy. Gram staining can also be useful in identifying gram-negative

intracellular diplococci, which is consistent with *Neisseria gonorrhoeae.*

- Positive leukocyte esterase on urine test strip analysis
- First void urine with 10 or more WBCs per hpf

If urethritis is suspected, urine-based nucleic acid amplification testing from a first void urine should be obtained for gonorrhea and chlamydia. Urine-based testing is the most cost- and time-efficient method of identifying an etiology and causes less discomfort than urethral swabs. Testing for other pathogens may be warranted depending on clinical findings (eg, an ulcer suspect for herpes simplex virus).

Treatment for uncomplicated gonococcal urethritis includes a single dose of ceftriaxone 250 mg intramuscularly plus a single dose of azithromycin 1 g orally. An alternative regimen, if ceftriaxone is not available, is a single dose of cefixime 400 mg orally plus a single dose of azithromycin 1 g orally. Treatment of nongonococcal urethritis would include a single dose of azithromycin 1 g orally or doxycycline 100 mg orally twice daily for 7 days. Alternative regimens include erythromycin 500 mg orally 4 times daily for 7 days, or levofloxacin 500 mg orally daily for 7 days, or ofloxacin 300 mg orally twice daily for 7 days.

The adolescent boy in this vignette has a presumed diagnosis of urethritis and should have urine nucleic acid amplification testing for gonorrhea and chlamydia to identify an etiology. If the test result is positive, a discussion is needed regarding partner notification and treatment; education on acquiring sexually transmitted infections and prevention by using condoms consistently; refraining from sexual activity for one week after treatment in an effort to stop spread of infection to other partners and prevent reinfection; and the need for follow-up testing (test of reinfection). This patient would also benefit from screening for other sexually transmitted infections.

A blood culture and complete blood cell count are not likely to identify a pathogen associated with urethritis in an afebrile, nonseptic adolescent. A comprehensive metabolic panel would not be useful in identifying any infectious etiologies associated with dysuria. A urinalysis may be helpful in identifying positive leukocyte esterase and increased WBCs on microscopy, but a routine urine culture will not identify *C trachomatis* or *N gonorrhoeae*, which are the 2 most well-established pathogens associated with urethritis.

PREP Pearls

- Consistent condom use will help prevent sexually transmitted infections associated with urethritis.
- Male adolescents with dysuria or urethral discharge should have urine nucleic acid amplification testing to evaluate for gonorrhea and chlamydia.

American Board of Pediatrics Content Specification(s)/ Content Area

- Recognize the clinical findings associated with urethritis in male adolescents
- Formulate a differential diagnosis of urethritis in male adolescents
- Plan the appropriate evaluation and management of urethritis in male adolescents

Suggested Readings

Bachman LH, Manhart LE, Martin DH, et al. Advances in the understanding and treatment of male urethritis. *Clin Infect Dis.* 2015;61(suppl 8):S763-S769.

Centers for Disease Control and Prevention. 2015 Sexually transmitted diseases treatment guidelines: diseases characterized by urethritis and cervicitis. https://www.cdc.gov/std/tg2015/urethritis-and-cervicitis.htm.

Item 197	Preferred Response: A

The boy in the vignette has failure to thrive, vomiting, dehydration, and hyponatremia with hypochloremic metabolic alkalosis. The most likely diagnosis is hypertrophic pyloric stenosis, and the best diagnostic test is abdominal ultrasonography.

In large part, the equilibrium among carbon dioxide (CO_2), carbonic acid (H_2CO_3), and bicarbonate (HCO_3^-) anion determine the acid-base balance of the body.

$$CO_2 + H_2O <-> H_2CO_3 <-> H^+ + HCO_3^-$$

Thus, the respiratory system's modulation of the amount of dissolved CO_2 in the blood, and the metabolic system's regulation of HCO_3 levels, are the main determinants of acid-base balance. A blood gas specimen and an electrolyte panel are important in determining acid-base status. pH values above and below the reference range represent alkalosis and acidosis, respectively (Item C197). It is important to determine the degree to which the respiratory and metabolic systems are contributing to acid-base disturbances. Metabolic acidosis is present if the pH and the serum bicarbonate levels are both low. Two broad categories of metabolic acidosis include elevated anion gap metabolic acidosis and normal anion gap acidosis; the formula for anion gap calculation is (Na^+ – HCO_3^- – Cl^-). Normal anion gap (≤12) metabolic acidosis is caused by loss of bicarbonate from the urine, for example, in renal tubular acidosis, or from the stool, as in severe diarrhea. The causes of elevated anion gap metabolic acidosis (>12) can be remembered by the mnemonic MUDPILES (methanol, uremia, diabetic ketoacidosis, paraldehyde, isoniazid, lactic acidosis, ethylene glycol, salicylates). The presence of these unmeasured anions contributes to the elevated anion gap.

Item C197. General Reference Ranges for Arterial and Venous Blood Gases.

	Arterial	Venous
pH	7.38 - 7.42	7.36 - 7.38
P_{O_2} (mm Hg)	80 - 100	30 - 50
P_{CO_2} (mm Hg)	38 - 42	43 - 48
$H_{CO_3}^-$ (mm Hg)	22 - 24	25 - 26

$H_{CO_3}^-$=bicarbonate, P_{CO_2}=partial pressure of carbon dioxide, P_{O_2}=partial pressure of oxygen. Reference normal values are laboratory-dependent and may vary due to differing techniques.

Reprinted with permission from Hsu BS, Lakhani SA, Wilhelm M. Acid base disorders. *Pediatr Rev.* 2016;37(9):362.

Metabolic alkalosis is marked by an increase in serum HCO_3. This is often caused by either gastrointestinal or renal losses of chloride. In normal situations, to maintain serum electroneutrality, bicarbonate is reabsorbed in the kidney and the buffering equilibrium in the body shifts toward increasing bicarbonate concentration. Common causes of chloride losses include diuretic use, vomiting, or diarrhea. Hypertrophic pyloric stenosis is a common cause of "contraction alkalosis," in which the hydrochloric acid secreted from the stomach is lost due to profuse vomiting caused by the gastric obstruction. The physiologic bicarbonate secretion from the pancreas is also decreased, because acidic stomach contents are not presented to the duodenum, further increasing serum HCO_3 concentration. The central nervous system respiratory center relies on slight decreases in cerebrospinal fluid pH as a stimulus to breathe; therefore, hypoventilation occurs as a compensatory mechanism for metabolic alkalosis. Thus, preoperative management to correct electrolytes and restore intravascular volume is important to prevent postoperative apnea. Severe hyponatremia can be present in this condition, as seen in the child in this vignette. However, unless encephalopathy or hyponatremic seizures are present, sodium should be slowly corrected to prevent myelinolysis.

Although urine pH measurement can be helpful in the diagnosis of acid-base disturbances, it is usually not specific enough to diagnose the cause. An upper gastrointestinal radiography series can be helpful in identifying obstruction, but it is not sensitive enough to detect hypertrophic pyloric stenosis. A plasma aldosterone/renin activity ratio is helpful in differentiating the causes of hyperaldosteronism, but is not helpful in acid-base disturbances.

PREP Pearls

- A blood gas specimen and an electrolyte panel are important in determining acid-base status.
- Normal anion gap metabolic acidosis is caused by the loss of bicarbonate from the urine (eg, renal tubular acidosis), or from the stool, as in severe diarrhea.
- Preoperative management to correct electrolytes and restore intravascular volume in hypertrophic pyloric stenosis is important to prevent postoperative apnea.

American Board of Pediatrics Content Specification(s)/Content Area

- Recognize the clinical and laboratory features associated with metabolic acidosis, and manage appropriately
- Identify factors contributing to metabolic alkalosis
- Identify the renal compensatory changes associated with primary respiratory alkalosis

Suggested Readings

Eberly MD, Eide MB, Thompson JL, Nylund CM. Azithromycin in early infancy and pyloric stenosis. *Pediatrics*. 2015;135(3):483-488.

Hsu BS, Lakhani SA, Wilhelm M. Acid base disorders. *Pediatr Rev*. 2016;37:361.

Kamata M, Cartabuke RS, Tobias JD. Perioperative care of infants with pyloric stenosis. *Paediatr Anaesth*. 2015;25(12):1193-1206.

Item 198	Preferred Response: A

The boy in this vignette has evidence of weakness, which should be evaluated further. It would not be appropriate to reassure his mother that the boy's development is normal. Without evidence of language, fine motor, or social delays, referral for evaluation of global developmental delay is not indicated. Although the boy may benefit from physical therapy, he should first be evaluated for causes of muscle weakness.

The boy cannot skip, has difficulty balancing on 1 foot and climbing the stairs, and has a Gower sign (ie, he uses hand support to push himself upright when arising from the ground). Although the classic finding of calf pseudohypertrophy is absent in this case, his findings are worrisome and warrant evaluation for muscular dystrophy or other progressive myopathy. A creatine kinase level can be used to screen for myopathy; an elevated level is indicative of muscle inflammation.

The remainder of this boy's development is normal (Item C198); he draws pictures of people and animals with at least 6 to 7 details, can use scissors, tells stories and jokes, and will follow a 3- to 4-step command. It is not concerning that he cannot yet read.

Item C198. Developmental Milestones for a 5-Year-Old Child.

Gross Motor	Fine Motor	Social-Emotional	Receptive Language	Expressive Language
• Walks down stairs with alternating feet	• Copies triangle	• Has friends	• Recalls parts of a story	• Tells a story
• Balances on 1 foot for > 8 seconds	• Cuts with scissors	• Apologizes for mistakes	• Understands number concepts	• Knows 2,000 or more words
• Hops on 1 foot 15 times	• Writes first name		• Follows 3-part commands	• Responds to "why" questions
• Skips	• Draws person with at least 6 parts		• Appreciates jokes	• Uses future tense
• Jumps backwards				• Produces rhymes
• Walks backwards heel-toe				

Courtesy of I Larson.

PREP Pearls

- At age 5 years, children should be able to balance on 1 foot for more than 8 seconds, skip, cut with scissors, draw a person with at least 6 parts, follow a 3-part command, appreciate jokes and rhymes, use future tense, and tell a story.

- Measurement of serum creatine kinase is the best first step in laboratory testing to evaluate for congenital or acquired muscle diseases.

American Board of Pediatrics Content Specification(s)/ Content Area

- Evaluate the motor developmental progress/status of a child at 5 years of age
- Evaluate the cognitive and behavioral developmental progress/status of a child at 5 years of age

Suggested Readings

Emery AE. The muscular dystrophies. *Lancet*. 2002;359(9307):687-695.

Gerber RJ, Wilks T, Erdie-Lalena C. Developmental milestones: motor development. *Pediatr Rev*. 2010;31(7):267-277.

Noritz GH, Murphy NA; Neuromotor Screening Expert Panel. Motor delays: early identification and evaluation. *Pediatrics*. 2013;131(6):e2016-e2027.

Tsao C-Y. Muscle disease. *Pediatr Rev*. 2014;35(2):49-61.

Item 199   Preferred Response: C

In the cross-sectional study design described in the vignette, which is aimed at investigating the burden of chronic fatigue and the related psychosocial exposures among young women in Nicaragua, it is feasible to estimate the prevalence of chronic fatigue among women in the community. Because chronic fatigue was determined at a point in time, it is not possible to describe the trends in chronic fatigue among women in this study. Cross-sectional studies may indicate possible risk factors for a disease (eg, intimate partner violence and anxiety associated with chronic fatigue in the current vignette), but do not estimate the disease incidence or establish a cause.

Determination of prevalence, incidence, etiology, prognosis, and treatment effect remain a top priority for many clinical studies. Descriptive studies include correlation (ecologic) studies, case reports and case series, and cross-sectional surveys, which describe the general characteristics of the disease distribution, especially in the context of person, place, and time. A cross-sectional survey may describe current health status or condition, and exposures in a population, at 1 point in time or over a brief period. Cross-sectional studies are ideal for measuring prevalence, and for identifying associations that can then be investigated further using experimental or analytic studies. Although cross-sectional studies may be used to explore causation, the associations must be interpreted with caution because selection bias may distort the exposure-outcome relationship. Cross-sectional studies are relatively less expensive and easy to perform over a brief period, but cannot distinguish cause and effect or sequence of events from simple association. Rare disorders cannot be reliably studied with cross-sectional methods.

Experimental or analytical studies investigate the association between an exposure and disease outcome (or disease) by testing a hypothesis using comparison groups. The exposure is controlled by the investigator, who systematically determines whether the risk of a health outcome (or disease) is different between persons exposed and not exposed to a particular factor of interest, risk factor, or intervention. Examples of analytic or experimental study designs include observational studies (eg, cohort and case-control) or randomized clinical trials.

Cohort studies are used to determine incidence, natural history, or etiology, assess risk factors, and calculate relative risk. Because cohort studies determine the temporal sequence of events, distinguishing cause from effects is feasible. Compared with retrospective cohort studies, prospective cohort studies are expensive and may take longer to perform. Other limitations of cohort studies include confounding variables and bias due to subject selection and loss to follow-up.

Case control studies can retrospectively compare groups, study unusual diseases or outcomes, identify predictors of an outcome, and measure odds ratios that approximate the relative risks for each variable. Case control studies are helpful in generating hypotheses that can be studied further by more rigorous study designs (eg, prospective cohort or randomized clinical trials). Bias (sampling, observation, and recall) is a major issue with case control studies.

PREP Pearls

- A cross-sectional survey may describe current health status or condition and exposures in a population, at 1 point in time or over a brief period.

- Cross-sectional studies are ideal to measure prevalence, and identify associations, that can then be investigated further using experimental or analytic studies.

- Cross-sectional studies are relatively inexpensive and easy to perform in a brief period, but cannot distinguish between cause and effect.

American Board of Pediatrics Content Specification(s)/ Content Area

- Understand the uses and limitations of cross-sectional and longitudinal studies
- Understand the uses and limitations of case reports/series and anecdotal evidence
- Understand the uses and limitations of cohort studies
- Understand the uses and limitations of case-control studies

Suggested Readings

Johnson SL. Research and statistics: a question of time—cross-sectional versus longitudinal study designs. *Pediatr Rev*. 2010;31(6):250-251.

Mann CJ. Observational research methods: research design II: cohort, cross sectional, and case-control studies. *Emerg Med J*. 2003;20(1):54-60

Silverman SL. From randomized controlled trials to observational studies. *Am J Med*. 2009;122(2):114-120.

Item 200   Preferred Response: C

The most likely explanation for this neonate's jaundice, hypotonia, and poor suck is acute bilirubin encephalopathy, or kernicterus, which is diagnosed based on the serum bilirubin level. Acute bilirubin encephalopathy presents in the first 2 to 5 days after birth. Affected neonates may have decreased muscle tone, absent Moro reflex, and seizures. In the first week after birth, symptoms can progress to include fever, hypertonia, and opisthotonus. During the first year, infants with chronic bilirubin encephalopathy may develop extrapyramidal symptoms, hypotonia, hearing loss, and choreoathetosis. The symptoms of chronic bilirubin encephalopathy are irreversible. Though the incidence of kernicterus is low in the developed world, kernicterus causes significant morbidity and mortality in the developing world. Risk factors for kernicterus include prematurity, serum bilirubin level greater than 20 mg/dL (342 µmol/L), infection, asphyxia, breast milk feeding, and low serum albumin levels.

Hyperbilirubinemia affects as many as 85% of neonates for multiple reasons. Neonates have both increased bilirubin production and decreased activity of glucuronosyl transferase, the enzyme responsible for conjugating bilirubin into a water-soluble form for excretion. In the first days after birth, enteral intake is limited, resulting in decreased bile secretion and increased enterohepatic circulation. For most neonates, these acute issues resolve in the first 3 to 4 days after birth with concurrent reduction in serum bilirubin levels.

Even when hyperbilirubinemia lasts for only a short period, neonates remain at risk for neurologic injury from elevated serum bilirubin levels. They have an immature blood-brain barrier, allowing transit of bilirubin into the brain. In addition, clinical conditions such as infection and asphyxia increase the susceptibility of neurons to damage. Bilirubin preferentially damages the cerebellum, hippocampus, globus pallidus, subthalamic nuclei, and brainstem nuclei.

Neonatal hypoglycemia typically presents in the first 24 hours after birth. Most cases are asymptomatic. Symptomatic neonates may be jittery with mild hypotonia. Risk factors for symptomatic hypoglycemia include late preterm gestation and maternal diabetes.

Serum ammonia levels may be elevated in neonates with urea cycle defects and acute neonatal liver failure. Neonates with urea cycle defects present with metabolic alkalosis, poor feeding, and may have ammonia levels as high as the thousands (micromoles per liter). Neonates with acute liver failure would have other signs of liver dysfunction, including hepatomegaly and coagulopathy.

Early-onset sepsis in the late preterm neonate is most often caused by group B *Streptococcus* (GBS) after perinatal exposure to maternal GBS. Most neonates with early-onset sepsis due to GBS present with increased work of breathing, with chest radiography showing pneumonia.

PREP Pearls

- Acute bilirubin encephalopathy, kernicterus, presents in the first 5 days after birth with hypotonia, jaundice, and poor suck. Later in the first week after birth, neonates may develop fever, opisthotonos, and hypertonia.
- Chronic bilirubin encephalopathy, which develops during the first year after birth, is irreversible. Infants may exhibit hypotonia, extrapyramidal symptoms, hearing loss, or choreoathetosis.
- Risk factors for kernicterus include prematurity, breast milk feedings, infection, asphyxia, and hypoalbuminemia.

American Board of Pediatrics Content Specification(s)/ Content Area

- Recognize the clinical features and sequelae of acute bilirubin encephalopathy in newborn infants, and manage appropriately

Suggested Readings

American Academy of Pediatrics, Subcommittee on Hyperbilirubinemia. Clinical practice guideline: management of hyperbilirubinemia in the newborn infant 35 or more weeks of gestation. *Pediatrics*. 2004;114:297-316.

Lauer BJ, Spector ND. Hyperbilirubinemia in the newborn. *Pediatr Rev*. 2011;32:341.

Watchko JF, Tiribelli C. Bilirubin-induced neurologic damage-mechanisms and management approaches. *N Engl J Med*. 2013;369(21):20121-20130.

Item 201   Preferred Response: C

The boy in this vignette has recent onset of cough with focal pulmonary findings on the right side unassociated with signs of infection. Despite the lack of a history of choking or gagging, an unwitnessed foreign body aspiration must be considered. Of the choices available, inspiratory and expiratory chest radiographs will be the best tool for evaluation of localized hyperinflation and air trapping on the right side of the chest.

A barium swallow study might be helpful if there were concern for chronic aspiration of food or liquids, but will not help with evaluation for an acute aspiration event. Computed tomography of the chest would demonstrate focal hyperinflation or air trapping, but it is more invasive and costly than plain radiography. Magnetic resonance imaging is best for visualization of vascular structures and does have some benefit for lung parenchyma but is not commonly used for chest evaluation other than for cardiovascular anomalies.

Without a specific history to suggest aspiration and without focal findings on examination there would be little indication to get even a plain chest radiograph. Most 5-year-old children could give appropriate history that would lead to suspicion of aspiration. However, younger children or developmentally disabled children are often the subjects of concern for unwitnessed aspiration, especially if they have the habit of putting things in their mouths. In such situations, a careful examination to evaluate for differential airflow between the right and left sides and proceeding with plain chest radiographs are appropriate as baseline investigations. Reevaluation at intervals of days to even a week or more may be needed for comparison examinations. Children unable to fully cooperate to obtain good inspiratory and expiratory radiographs can be evaluated with bilateral decubitus images to evaluate for expected relative deflation of the dependent lung; if there is air trapping, the affected side will not deflate when dependent. Alternatively, fluoroscopy of the lungs and airways may show asynchrony of the diaphragms or poor inspiratory/expiratory change of one lung in the presence of a foreign body that is causing airway obstruction. Availability of a radiologist for the fluoroscopy may be problematic in some emergency departments.

Distally lodged foreign bodies can remain in the airway, undetected, for weeks or even months with only a chronic cough as the historic finding. Organic substances in the airway are usually very irritating, with local inflammation leading to cough and possibly to systemic findings such as fever. Inorganic substances, such as plastic or metal, may be retained and trigger only a cough. The possibility exists for secondary pneumonia beyond an obstructed airway as a complication of foreign body aspiration. Retained foreign bodies can also erode into the airway mucosa or even through the airway, producing a fistula accompanied by pneumothorax or pneumomediastinum and further pulmonary complications.

A high index of suspicion for foreign body as a cause of chronic cough and repeat evaluations including history review and careful physical examination may be necessary for a delayed diagnosis.

More proximally lodged foreign bodies, in the trachea or mainstem bronchi, are likely to cause enough obstruction to be potentially life threatening and respiratory distress will be obvious. Removal of these objects by rigid bronchoscopy may be a medical emergency. The sudden onset of moderate to severe respiratory distress with poor air movement throughout or differential breath sounds should lead to prompt evaluation including careful physical examination and plain chest radiography with or without inspiratory/expiratory radiographs or fluoroscopy.

Regardless of the timing, once the suspicion of foreign body aspiration is high, the appropriate management is rigid bronchoscopy for removal. Rigid bronchoscopy is done urgently in the setting of respiratory distress or airway compromise but can be done after repeat evaluation when the signs and symptoms are less specific and require reevaluation.

PREP Pearls

- Focal findings on chest examination in the context of cough without other signs of illness should raise suspicion for foreign body aspiration, especially in a child from whom a direct history is not available or not reliable.
- Foreign body aspiration may not be apparent from initial history and examination. Repeat evaluations may be needed.
- The more proximal the site of obstruction from a foreign body, the greater the level of respiratory distress and urgency of resolution.

American Board of Pediatrics Content Specification(s)/ Content Area

- Recognize long-term complications associated with foreign body aspiration
- Plan the appropriate evaluation of suspected foreign body aspiration, and manage appropriately
- Recognize the historical, clinical, and laboratory findings associated with foreign body aspiration

Suggested Readings

Green SS. Ingested and aspirated foreign bodies. *Pediatr Rev.* 2015;36(10):430-437.

Louie MC, Bradin S. Foreign body ingestion and aspiration. *Pediatr Rev.* 2009;30(8):295-301.

Orji FT, Akpeh JO. Tracheobronchial foreign body aspiration in children: how reliable are clinical and radiological signs in the diagnosis? *Clin Otolaryngol.* 2010;35(6):479-485.

Item 202   **Preferred Response: D**

The boy in this vignette has thyroid-binding globulin (TBG) deficiency, which is a benign condition that does not cause clinical manifestations and requires no treatment. He has no signs or symptoms of a thyroid problem. His thyroid-stimulating hormone (TSH) level is normal but his total thyroxine (T_4) level is low. A free T_4 level would be normal. A TBG level, if measured, would be low.

Most circulating thyroid hormone is bound to TBG. A TBG deficiency affects the bound concentration of thyroxine so that the total thyroxine (T_4) level is low, but not the free thyroid hormone level, which represents active hormone. Deficiency in TBG is inherited in an X-linked manner. It is most often detected on newborn screens that use a primary T_4 screening method. Central hypothyroidism is part of the differential diagnosis of a low T_4 level with normal TSH level and should be ruled out in an infant with these screening results. A normal free T_4 level would rule out central hypothyroidism. A TBG level can also be measured.

Central hypothyroidism is unlikely for the boy in this vignette. He has no symptoms of hypothyroidism and no predisposing factors for central hypothyroidism, such as multiple pituitary hormone deficiencies or a history of central nervous system disease. Hypothyroidism caused by Hashimoto thyroiditis or iodine deficiency is primary (originating in the thyroid), so it would be associated with a high TSH level.

PREP Pearls

- Thyroid-binding globulin deficiency is a benign condition that does not cause clinical manifestations and requires no treatment.
- Thyroid-binding globulin deficiency is associated with normal thyroid-stimulating hormone, low total thyroxine, low thyroid-binding globulin, and normal free T_4 levels.

American Board of Pediatrics Content Specification(s)/ Content Area

- Recognize the clinical and laboratory features associated with thyroid-binding globulin deficiency

Suggested Readings

Diaz A, Lipman Diaz EG. Hypothyroidism. *Pediatr Rev*. 2014;35(8):336-347.

LaFranchi SH, Huang SA. Defects in thyroxine-binding globulin. In: Kliegman RM, Stanton BF, St. Geme JW, Schor NF, eds. *Nelson Textbook of Pediatrics*. 20th ed. Philadelphia, PA: Elsevier; 2016:2665.

Item 203   Preferred Response: C

The neonate in the vignette has a classic presentation for trisomy 13 (Patau syndrome), a chromosomal disorder in which there are 3 sets, rather than 2, of all or part of chromosome 13 in the cells of the body. In some individuals, only a portion of the cells contain the extra 13th chromosome; this is called mosaicism. Children with mosaicism may have a slightly less severe phenotype depending on the percentage of affected cells. Most cases are not inherited, but rather result from a maternal meiotic nondisjunction error with failure of 2 members of a chromosome pair to separate from one another during meiosis. Both chromosomes then go to a single daughter cell, yielding an extra chromosome. Less commonly, some cases are due to an unbalanced translocation or a cellular division error after fertilization.

Trisomy 13 is diagnosed through a comprehensive physical examination, with laboratory confirmation via karyotype or fluorescent in situ hybridization (FISH) analysis for trisomies. The range and severity of the clinical findings vary among patients. It occurs in about 1 in 10,000 to 16,000 live births, and is slightly more common in girls. The combined total prevalence including elective terminations, miscarriages, stillbirths, and live births is 1 in 1,800 conceptions. The risk of bearing a child with trisomy 13 increases with maternal age.

Many affected children feed poorly and require nutrition via a nasogastric or gastrostomy tube. A high percentage of infants with trisomy 13 die in the first year after birth because of complex congenital malformations. Those who survive beyond infancy have severe intellectual disability.

Classic phenotypic and clinical features of trisomy 13 include:

- Intrauterine growth restriction
- Craniofacial malformations—microcephaly, cutis aplasia (missing skin on the scalp), micrognathia, microphthalmia, close-set eyes, colobomas, malformed/low-set ears, cleft lip and/or palate
- Holoprosencephaly or incomplete development of the brain
- Polydactyly
- Clenched hands
- Rocker-bottom feet
- Hypotonia
- Complex structural cardiac anomalies
- Renal malformations
- Severe intellectual disability
- Cryptorchidism

5p- deletion presents with a classic high-pitched cry; intellectual disability; microcephaly; low birthweight; hypotonia; and distinctive facial features including hypertelorism, micrognathia, rounded face, and low-set ears.

22q11.2 deletion presents with congenital heart anomalies, palatal abnormalities, characteristic facial features, learning problems, hypocalcemia, immune deficiency, kidney abnormalities, and hearing loss. The most common cardiac anomalies are conotruncal defects, such as tetralogy of Fallot or interrupted aortic arch. Facial features include "hooded" eyelids, bulbous nose with a bifid nasal tip, and hypoplastic alae nasae.

Trisomy 18 clinical features, many of which are similar to trisomy 13, include a clenched fist with overriding fingers, rocker-bottom feet, characteristic facial dysmorphology, prenatal and postnatal growth deficiency, renal and cardiac anomalies, severe intellectual disability, and hypotonia. Facial dysmorphology consists of dolichocephaly, external ear anomalies, micrognathia, short palpebral fissures, and a small face. Only 5% to 10% of affected infants survive beyond the first year. Features seen in this neonate that are more specific for a trisomy 13 diagnosis include the cleft lip and/or palate, polydactyly, holoprosencephaly, and cutis aplasia.

Of the response choices, all diagnoses could be detected via a high-resolution karyotype, FISH-specific analysis, or microarray.

PREP Pearls

- Most infants with trisomy 13 die in the first year after birth because of complex congenital malformations. Surviving infants will have severe intellectual disability.
- Trisomy 13 is typically diagnosed based on physical examination findings noted at birth; laboratory confirmation is via karyotype or fluorescent in situ hybridization analysis for trisomies.
- Trisomy 13 syndrome features include microcephaly, microphthalmia, low-set ears, cleft lip and/or palate, holoprosencephaly, cutis aplasia, polydactyly, clenched hands, rocker bottom feet, cryptorchidism, renal anomalies, and cardiac malformations.

American Board of Pediatrics Content Specification(s)/ Content Area

- Recognize the clinical features associated with trisomy 13

Suggested Readings

Josephsen JB, Armbrecht ES, Braddock SR, Cibulskis CC. Procedures in the 1st year of life for children with trisomy 13 and trisomy 18, a 25-year, single-center review. *Am J Med Genet*. 2016;172(3):264-271.

National Organization for Rare Disorders. Trisomy 13 syndrome. https://rarediseases.org/rare-diseases/trisomy-13-syndrome/

Rios A, Furdon SA, Adams D, Clark DA. Recognizing the clinical features of trisomy 13 syndrome. *Adv Neonatal Care*. 2004;4(6):332-343.

Item 204   Preferred Response: A

The boy in this vignette should be retested for egg allergy to see if it has resolved. Most infants and young children with egg, milk, soy, and wheat allergies will eventually tolerate these foods later in childhood. In one study, 26% of egg allergies resolved by 6 years of age, and 53% resolved by 10 years of age. Food allergies associated with other atopic conditions (eg, atopic dermatitis and asthma), such as with the child in this vignette, are more likely to persist. However, because eliminating these common ingredients from a child's diet can be inconvenient, expensive, and lead to nutritional deficiencies, it is important to evaluate for resolution as early as possible.

Although 12% of children in the United States self-report food allergies, the actual prevalence is likely much lower. This may be due to oversubscribing the term "allergy" to nonimmune-mediated food intolerances (eg, intolerance to milk because of lactase deficiency). A food allergy is an immune-mediated, reproducible reaction to a specific food. Peanuts, tree nuts, shellfish, milk, egg, wheat, and soy are among the most common foods causing allergic reactions in children. Eliminating the offending food from the child's diet is the recommended approach to managing food allergies. An anaphylaxis emergency action plan and an epinephrine auto-injector are recommended for children who have a history of food-induced anaphylaxis, in case of inadvertent exposure. Immunotherapy approaches that introduce the allergen in small doses to desensitize the immune system to that allergen have emerged in recent years and are offered in specialty settings for select patients.

Patient-reported outcomes studies have found that food allergy, with the anxiety regarding accidental exposure and the effort needed to avoid certain foods, has a negative effect on the quality of life of children and their parents. While allergies to milk, egg, wheat, and soy often resolve during childhood, allergies to peanuts, tree nuts, and shellfish are much more likely to persist. Whether and when to retest a child for the allergy to see if it has resolved depends on the specific food, history of exposure and subsequent reaction, and the effect of the allergy on the child's nutritional status and quality of life. A child with a recent reaction is probably not a good candidate for retesting; however, in the absence of a recent reaction, many allergists recommend annual retesting for milk, egg, wheat, and soy allergies, and less frequent retesting for allergies more likely to persist. Such testing can be initiated with a skin-prick test or allergen-specific IgE levels. If the results are negative or low, respectively, the child should proceed to an oral food challenge, which involves consuming the food in a controlled medical environment, to confirm that the allergy has resolved. Because skin-prick tests and allergen-specific IgE levels can be falsely negative or positive, they should not be used alone in determining the persistence or resolution of the food allergy.

Children with food allergy are 2- to 4-times more likely to have another atopic condition, and in children with asthma, having a food allergy is a risk factor for more severe asthma. There is evidence that dietary avoidance can improve atopic dermatitis; however, it is not clear that it improves asthma symptoms. While a history of exposure with lack of reaction can help identify children in whom the allergy has likely resolved, it is not a substitute for accurate, safe retesting by medical professionals.

Like food allergies, allergies to medications, namely penicillins, are often inaccurately and overly reported by families. Allergic reactions to penicillin are typically either type I, IgE-mediated hypersensitivity reactions, inducing anaphylaxis, urticaria, and/or edema within 1 hour of administration, or T-cell–mediated delayed cutaneous reactions, typically occurring several days after the drug has been started. For both types of reactions, the offending drug should be stopped. The T-cell–mediated reaction takes many forms (Item C204) and can be similar to an exanthem associated with a viral illness.

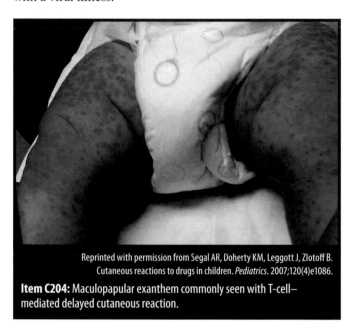

Reprinted with permission from Segal AR, Doherty KM, Leggott J, Zlotoff B. Cutaneous reactions to drugs in children. *Pediatrics*. 2007;120(4)e1086.

Item C204: Maculopapular exanthem commonly seen with T-cell–mediated delayed cutaneous reaction.

It is important to determine whether the child has a true penicillin allergy to reduce overuse of broader spectrum antibiotics. Referral to an allergist for skin-prick testing can help solidify the diagnosis of an allergy when the history is uncertain. For delayed cutaneous reactions, children with mild forms or uncertain histories can be referred to an allergist for a rechallenge. Clinicians in inpatient settings can also perform a penicillin challenge if a penicillin-based medication is clearly the most appropriate antibiotic for the infection being treated; this challenge is typically undertaken with hospital-wide, allergist-informed protocols to ensure that the patient is appropriate for the procedure and that the procedure is carried out in a safe environment.

PREP Pearls

- Children with allergies to wheat, egg, milk, and soy who have not had a reaction in several years should be considered for retesting because these allergies frequently resolve in childhood.
- Children with mild or questionable reactions to medications, particularly penicillins, can be referred to an allergist for rechallenge to guide future antibiotic use.
- Low allergen-specific IgE levels suggest resolution of the allergy, but this should be confirmed with an oral food challenge performed in a safe, prepared medical setting.

- Know the common foods that cause allergic reactions
- Recognize the relationship between eczema and food allergies, and how to evaluate a patient for both
- Understand the natural history of various food allergies
- Recognize the clinical features associated with a drug allergy or hypersensitivity, and manage appropriately

Suggested Readings

Burks AW, Jones SM, Boyce JA, et al. NIAID-sponsored 2010 guidelines for managing food allergy: applications in the pediatric population. *Pediatrics.* 2011;128(5):955-965.

Segal AR, Doherty KM, Leggott J, Zlotoff B. Cutaneous reactions to drugs in children. *Pediatrics.* 2007;120(4):e1082-e1096.

Sicherer SH, Wood RA; Section on Allergy and Immunology. Allergy testing in childhood: using allergen-specific IgE tests. *Pediatrics.* 2012;129(1):193-197.

Tatachar P, Kumar S. Food-induced anaphylaxis and oral allergy syndrome. *Pediatr Rev.* 2008;29(4):e23-e27.

Item 205   Preferred Response: D

The diagnostic test that will most influence the management of the infant in this vignette is viral polymerase chain reaction assay. The diagnosis of bronchiolitis can be made clinically. While viral testing is not routinely recommended in the setting of bronchiolitis, there are limited scenarios where a viral polymerase chain reaction assay can be useful. The 2015 American Academy of Pediatrics Clinical Practice Guideline for the Diagnosis, Management, and Prevention of Bronchiolitis recommends viral testing for infants that develop bronchiolitis while receiving palivizumab prophylaxis. If infection with respiratory syncytial virus (RSV) is confirmed, palivizumab prophylaxis for the season should be discontinued.

Similar to the infant in this vignette, infants with RSV infection most commonly display viral upper respiratory tract symptoms. Infants who develop bronchiolitis have lower tract symptomatology that can include cough, wheezing, tachypnea, and respiratory distress in the form of nasal flaring and retractions. Coarse rales are common.

There is a distinct seasonality to RSV infections. Although the pattern varies by region, outbreaks usually begin in November or December. The peak usually occurs 2 months into the season and ends by March or April.

For a select group of children with risk factors for severe RSV infection, palivizumab prophylaxis is recommended to start at the beginning of the RSV season in the patient's geographic location. In the first year of age, healthy infants with a gestational age less than or equal to 28 weeks and 6 days, infants with hemodynamically significant congenital heart disease, and infants with chronic lung disease of prematurity can receive a maximum of 5 monthly doses of palivizumab. Prophylaxis in the second year can be considered in children with chronic lung disease of prematurity who continue to require oxygen, corticosteroids, or diuretics within 6 months of the start of RSV season.

In children with bronchiolitis who are older than 30 days, serious bacterial and urinary tract infections are rare. Children with distinct viral syndromes have an estimated risk of bacteremia that is much less than 1% and a risk of urinary tract infection that is 1%. Therefore, blood and urine cultures are not routinely recommended in febrile infants older than 30 days with bronchiolitis.

Chest radiographs are also not routinely recommended in the setting of bronchiolitis. The aforementioned guidelines recommend limiting chest radiography to patients that warrant intensive care admission given the severity of their respiratory symptoms and for patients that are suspected of having an airway complication, such as a pneumothorax.

Management of RSV infections is mainly supportive. β-Agonists, epinephrine, and corticosteroids are not recommended. Although the literature is mixed, nebulized hypertonic saline may be considered in hospitalized children. Given the low risk of concomitant bacterial infections, antibiotics are not routinely recommended unless a bacterial infection is identified.

PREP Pearls

- If infection with respiratory syncytial virus is confirmed in a patient receiving palivizumab, prophylaxis for the season should be discontinued.
- In the first year of age, palivizumab prophylaxis is recommended for healthy infants with a gestational age of less than or equal to 28 weeks and 6 days, infants with hemodynamically significant congenital heart disease, and infants with chronic lung disease of prematurity.
- The diagnosis of bronchiolitis is based on history and physical examination; radiographs and diagnostic laboratory evaluations are not routinely recommended.

American Board of Pediatrics Content Specification(s)/ Content Area

- Identify and plan prophylaxis for patients at high risk of morbidity and mortality from respiratory syncytial virus infection
- Recognize the clinical features associated with respiratory syncytial virus infection, and manage appropriately
- Plan the appropriate diagnostic evaluation for respiratory syncytial virus infection
- Understand the epidemiology of respiratory syncytial virus

Suggested Readings

American Academy of Pediatrics. Respiratory syncytial virus. In: Kimberlin DW, Brady MT, Jackson MA, Long SS, eds. *Red Book: 2018 Report of the Committee on Infectious Diseases.* 31st ed. Itasca, IL: American Academy of Pediatrics; 2018:682-691.

Ralston S, Lieberthal A, Meissner H, et al. Clinical practice guideline: the diagnosis, management, and prevention of bronchiolitis. *Pediatrics.* 2014;134(5):e1474-e1502.

Item 206   Preferred Response: D

The girl in this vignette has a skin-colored ring (ie, annulus) with an elevated border and central clearing. The lesion has been treated unsuccessfully with a topical antifungal agent. Although the physical findings are reminiscent of tinea corporis (Item C206A), the absence of erythema and scale support a diagnosis of granuloma annulare (GA). As a result, no intervention is required. Clotrimazole is effective in the management of tinea corporis, and griseofulvin would

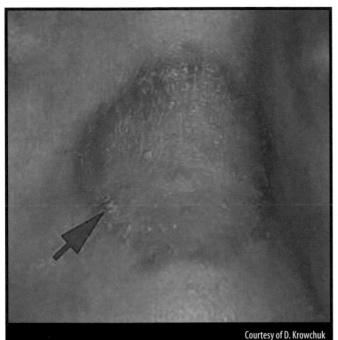

Courtesy of D. Krowchuk

Item C206A: Tinea corporis. This lesion on the nose exhibits an erythematous, scaling border (arrow) and some central clearing. (On the face, tinea corporis is sometimes called tinea faciei.)

feet. The lesions of GA may be skin-colored but often are erythematous (Item C206B) or violaceous (Item C206C). Most individuals have a single lesion but multiple lesions may occur (Item C206C). Because the pathology of GA occurs in the dermis, lesions have a "deeper" or "firmer" feel than the border of a tinea corporis lesion. A subcutaneous form of GA is characterized by multiple subcutaneous nodules with normal overlying skin. The diagnosis of GA is made clinically and may be confirmed with skin biopsy, although rarely required.

Granuloma annulare often is confused with tinea corporis as discussed previously. It also may mimic nummular eczema (Item C206D). However, nummular eczema does not exhibit

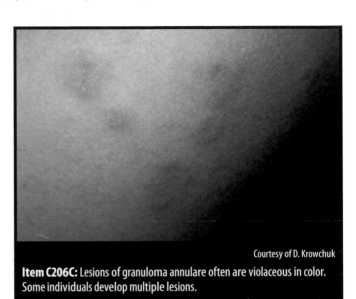

Courtesy of D. Krowchuk

Item C206C: Lesions of granuloma annulare often are violaceous in color. Some individuals develop multiple lesions.

be indicated in resistant infections or infections characterized by large or numerous lesions. An emollient and topical corticosteroid would be useful in managing nummular eczema.

Granuloma annulare is a relatively common disorder whose cause is unknown. It usually occurs in school-aged children and affects girls more often than boys. Although an association with diabetes mellitus has been suggested in adults, this is not the case in children.

Granuloma annulare is characterized by papules that form a ring; occasionally, the ring is incomplete (Item C206B). Lesions may occur at any body site but commonly involve areas that are prone to trauma like the dorsa of the hands or

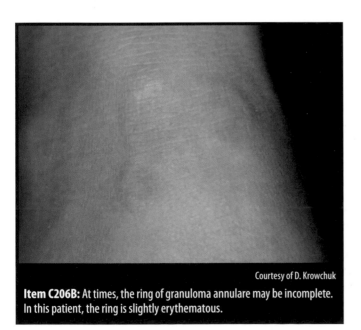

Reprinted with permission from Mancini AJ, Krowchuk DP, eds. *Pediatric Dermatology. A Quick Reference Guide.* 3rd ed. Elk Grove Village, IL; American Academy of Pediatrics: 2016, page 34

Item C206D: Nummular eczema is characterized by oval or round lesions that form crust (arrows).

Item C206B: At times, the ring of granuloma annulare may be incomplete. In this patient, the ring is slightly erythematous.

Courtesy of D. Krowchuk

border elevation or central clearing. In addition, a crust is present in nummular eczema. Subcutaneous GA may mimic a soft-tissue malignancy, rheumatoid nodules, or sarcoidosis.

The lesions of GA resolve in 2 to 4 years and, accordingly, no intervention is required. Occasionally, an intralesional or potent topical corticosteroid may be used to reduce inflammation. However, such treatments should be used with caution to avoid skin atrophy.

PREP Pearls

- Granuloma annulare may be differentiated from tinea corporis by the absence of scale, the firmness of the border, and tendency of lesions to have a violaceous color.
- Granuloma annulare results in rings that may mimic the lesions of tinea corporis.

American Board of Pediatrics Content Specification(s)/ Content Area

- Differentiate the clinical findings of tinea corporis from those of granuloma annulare, and manage appropriately

Suggested Readings

American Academy of Pediatrics Section on Dermatology. Granuloma annulare. In: Mancini AJ, Krowchuk DP, eds. *Pediatric Dermatology: A Quick Reference Guide*. 3rd ed. Elk Grove Village, IL: American Academy of Pediatrics; 2016:467-469

Piette EW, Rosenbach M. Granuloma annulare. Clinical and histologic variants, epidemiology, and genetics. *J Am Acad Dermatol*. 2016;75(3):457-465.

Item 207   Preferred Response: A

The boy in the vignette has chronic activity-related pain in both knees and both ankles. He does not have any joint swelling, malaise, fevers, or other symptoms that would suggest juvenile idiopathic arthritis. His ability to hyperextend his knees and ankles suggests joint hypermobility. "Generalized joint hypermobility" is the term used to describe diffuse ligamentous laxity leading to excess joint mobility. Joint hypermobility associated with joint pain is referred to as "joint hypermobility syndrome." The treatment of joint hypermobility is a physical therapy program to learn strengthening exercises that can be continued at home.

When evaluating a child with multiple joint complaints, providers should take a careful history to determine the cause of the child's pain. For example, a history of trauma may indicate that pain is a result of injury. Night pain that awakens a child, persistent limp, or refusal to bear weight or use a limb should prompt urgent evaluation for serious conditions, including infection and neoplasm. Symptoms such as fatigue, fever, and decreased appetite may indicate systemic illness, such as infection or an autoimmune condition. For a child with joint stiffness, swelling, and rashes, providers should pursue laboratory evaluation for juvenile idiopathic arthritis. Some medications can cause joint, muscle, or tendon pain. A history of recent infection is often present in children with reactive or postinfectious arthritis. When families travel, children may be exposed to pathogens not commonly seen in the area in which they reside. In addition to asking about travel, pediatricians should inquire about recent camping trips and tick or bug bites, because arthropods can transmit infections that lead to musculoskeletal complaints.

Many conditions that cause joint pain have a familial basis. For example, juvenile idiopathic arthritis is more common in children with a family history of rheumatologic disease and/or inflammatory bowel disease. The boy in the vignette exhibits joint hypermobility, which can be a component of genetic connective tissue disorders such as Marfan syndrome and Ehlers-Danlos syndrome.

Generalized hypermobility of the joints is common in children. The Beighton score can be used to assess the level of joint hypermobility. One point is assigned for each of the following abilities: hyperextending each knee and elbow more than 10 degrees, touching the thumb to the wrist while the wrist is flexed, extending the pinky metacarpal-phalangeal joint more than 90 degrees, and touching the palms to the floor without bending the knees. A Beighton score of 5 or more (out of 9 possible points) is considered positive for hypermobility. However, a large proportion of children have a positive Beighton score (in a study of Dutch school children, > one-third had a positive Beighton score), so the usefulness of this scoring system in children has been questioned.

The boy in the vignette does not have signs and symptoms of infection or inflammatory arthritis. Therefore, measurement of the complete blood cell count and C-reactive protein would not be indicated. Radiography in a child with diffuse chronic arthralgias without systemic symptoms is very unlikely to show any bony pathology. Children with joint hypermobility syndrome can participate in physical activities, such as gym class and sports, but should be cautioned to avoid excessive stretching at the joints.

PREP Pearls

- Generalized joint hypermobility is the term used to describe diffuse ligamentous laxity leading to excess joint mobility.
- Joint hypermobility associated with joint pain is referred to as "joint hypermobility syndrome."
- The treatment of joint hypermobility is a physical therapy program to learn strengthening exercises that can be continued at home.

American Board of Pediatrics Content Specification(s)/ Content Area

- Recognize the typical presentation of a patient with functional joint complaints

Suggested Readings

Lehman PJ, Carl RL. Growing pains. *Sports Health*. 2017;9(2):132-138

Sarwark JF, LaBella CR, ed *Pediatric Orthopaedics and Sports Injuries: A Quick Reference Guide*. 2nd ed. Elk Grove Village, IL: American Academy of Pediatrics; 2014

Smits-Engelsman B, Klerks M, Kirby A. Beighton score: a valid measure for generalized hypermobility in children. *J Pediatr*. 2011;158(1):119-123. e1-4.

Item 208 — Preferred Response: C

Providing positive praise and rewards after good behavior days is the best discipline technique parents can use to effectively change behaviors, particularly in preschool- and elementary school–aged children. Because this 4-year old just entered preschool and has no siblings, one should not assume he will automatically share well or follow rules. His occasional aggression to "get his way" likely reflects his limited understanding of how to be part of a group. By giving him specific and timely praise, he will learn desired actions and feel valued. Offering rewards after good behavior days through a graduated token economy strategy can help sustain behavior change.

Discipline is meant to teach and nurture correct behavior. It should involve the use of age- and developmentally appropriate methods that encourage progress toward independence, greater responsibility, and self-regulation. Effective discipline requires a positive, attentive, supportive, respectful, and consistent learning environment as a foundation. Good behaviors should be identified and recognized, along with intentional modeling of new skills, in an effort to teach and strengthen these behaviors. When undesirable behavior occurs, discipline strategies such as selectively ignoring the misbehavior, explaining limits, redirecting toward a correct behavior, allowing natural consequences, implementing time out, and withdrawing privileges may be used. These techniques are most successful when a positive relationship exists between the parent or caregiver and the child, and should be used in combination with strategies to stimulate more desirable behaviors. The child should not be encouraged to use alternative means to "get his way"; rather he should gain an understanding of group play and empathy for others.

Discipline does not equate to punishment. Punishment is the application of a negative stimulus, such as verbal reprimand or corporal punishment, to reduce or eliminate an undesirable behavior. The American Academy of Pediatrics "Guidance for Effective Discipline" policy statement notes that corporal punishment is ineffective, unnecessary, and potentially psychologically harmful. Pediatric health care providers can serve as valuable resources to parents in improving parenting skills by offering various discipline strategies.

PREP Pearls

- A graduated token economy strategy can help sustain behavior change.
- Discipline should be achieved through the use of age- and developmentally appropriate methods that nurture independence, progressive responsibility, and self-regulation.
- Through specific and timely praise, children will learn desired actions and feel valued.

American Board of Pediatrics Content Specification(s)/Content Area

- Advise parents regarding appropriate discipline and limit-setting for children of various ages

Suggested Readings

Committee on Psychosocial Aspects of Child and Family Health. Guidance for effective discipline. *Pediatrics*. 1998;101(4):723728

Lantos J. The patient-parent-pediatrician relationship: everyday ethics in the office. *Pediatr Rev*. 2015;36(1):22-30.

Pipan ME, Blum NJ. Basics of child behavior and primary care management of common behavioral problems. In: Voigt RG, Macias MM, Myers SM, eds. *American Academy of Pediatrics Developmental and Behavioral Pediatrics*. Elk Grove, IL: American Academy of Pediatrics; 2011:37-58

Schooler SJ. Parental monitoring and discipline in middle childhood. *Pediatr Rev*. 2009;30(9):366-367.

Item 209 — Preferred Response: C

The boy in this vignette most likely has hereditary pancreatitis. He currently has acute pancreatitis, confirmed by symptoms of epigastric pain coupled with an elevated lipase level. The calcifications seen on ultrasonography are consistent with chronic pancreatic damage. These calcifications along with his history of recurrent hospitalizations for epigastric abdominal pain provide evidence of chronic pancreatitis.

The diagnosis of acute pancreatitis is made when 2 of 3 criteria are met:

- Abdominal pain consistent with pancreatitis (acute onset of abdominal pain, particularly epigastric pain)
- Serum lipase level at least 3 times the upper limit of normal
- Imaging findings consistent with pancreatitis (edematous pancreas)

Causes of pancreatitis in children include systemic diseases, infections, medications, and trauma. Acute pancreatitis can also be seen in individuals with conditions causing recurrent or chronic pancreatitis.

Acute recurrent pancreatitis is defined as more than 1 episode of acute pancreatitis with either complete resolution of symptoms or complete normalization of lipase levels between episodes. Chronic pancreatitis is diagnosed when there is evidence of irreversible pancreatic damage with imaging consistent with chronic damage (eg, pancreatic calcifications, pancreatic ductal dilation) or evidence of exocrine or endocrine pancreatic insufficiency. Causes of acute recurrent pancreatitis and chronic pancreatitis are similar, including congenital anomalies of the pancreas or biliary tract, hereditary/genetic causes (*PRSS1*, *SPINK1*, or *CFTR* mutations), and autoimmune pancreatitis.

Gallstone pancreatitis is unlikely in this patient given the normal bilirubin and transaminase levels. In addition, no gallstones were detected by abdominal ultrasonography. Although hemolytic-uremic syndrome may be a relatively common cause of acute pancreatitis in young children, it does not cause chronic pancreatitis. Similarly, viral pancreatitis would not result in chronic pancreatitis.

Acute pancreatitis should be suspected in children with acute onset of pain, particularly in the epigastric region. Serum lipase level and/or imaging findings can confirm the diagnosis. If there are signs of pancreatic damage (pancreatic calcifications, pancreatic ductal dilation, or exocrine/endocrine pancreatic insufficiency), chronic pancreatitis should be considered. Causes of chronic pancreatitis can include anatomic abnormalities and hereditary pancreatitis.

American Board of Pediatrics Content Specification(s)/ Content Area

- Recognize the clinical and laboratory features associated with pancreatitis
- Formulate a differential diagnosis for a patient who has chronic or recurrent pancreatitis

Suggested Readings

Srinath AI, Lowe ME. Pediatric pancreatitis. *Pediatr Rev.* 2013;34(2):79-90.

Uc A, Fishman DS. Pancreatic disorders. *Pediatr Clin N Am.* 2017;64(3):685-706.

Item 210   **Preferred Response: A**

Intellectual disability (ID) is defined by significant limitations in intellectual functioning and in adaptive behavior with onset before age 18 years. It is essential to include a measure of adaptive function when assessing for possible ID. Adaptive skills are abilities that permit independence in self-care, health, home and community living, communication and relationships, recreation, and work.

The differential diagnosis of a child with academic difficulties includes learning disabilities (LDs) and ID. Learning disabilities occur in 5% to 13% of children, whereas ID has a prevalence of 1% to 2%. Learning disabilities are problems with understanding and acquiring knowledge that result in academic performance below expectations for the child's cognition. A child may qualify for special education services for a LD if there is a significant discrepancy (typically 1-2 standard deviations) between cognitive testing (eg, intelligence, aptitude, IQ) and achievement testing; low achievement in the setting of at least low average cognition; or lack of response to higher tiers of research-based instruction (ie, response to intervention). Learning disabilities may occur in reading (ie, dyslexia), written expression (ie, dysgraphia), or mathematics (ie, dyscalculia). Children with LDs typically have difficulties with specific subjects, unlike children with ID who have problems with general learning and for whom all subjects may be challenging. Unlike ID which requires deficits in both intellectual functioning and adaptive functioning, level of adaptive functioning is not a diagnostic criterion for LD. Although intelligence test scores are de-emphasized in the fifth edition of the *Diagnostic and Statistical Manual of Mental Disorders*, scores that are at least 2 standard deviations below the mean (< 70) on both mea-

sures of intellectual functioning and measures of adaptive functioning are in the intellectually disabled range.

To distinguish between LDs and ID, the evaluation of a child with learning difficulties should include administration of standardized measures of cognitive ability, achievement, and adaptive skills. The child's learning profile and areas of strength and weaknesses should also be identified. If the child meets special education eligibility criteria, results of this psychoeducational assessment should be used to develop an Individualized Education Program. The most appropriate setting, services, and accommodations to support the child's learning should be determined. The Individuals with Disabilities Education Act mandates that children should be educated in typical settings as much as possible; thus, the child with an LD is most likely to receive services within the general education classroom ("push in" services) or for a specific time during the school day outside the general classroom ("pull out" services). Placement in a special education classroom may be considered for a child with ID whose need for intensive instruction may not be met in the general education environment. However, the child with ID should be included in nonacademic activities with his typical peers when possible.

American Board of Pediatrics Content Specification(s)/ Content Area

- Recognize appropriate educational settings for patients with learning disabilities, and the various strategies utilized in those settings to circumvent weaknesses
- Distinguish the findings associated with learning disabilities from those of intellectual disabilities

Suggested Readings

Dworkin PH. School failure. In: Augustyn M, Zuckerman B, Caronna EB, eds. *The Zuckerman Parker Handbook of Developmental and Behavioral Pediatrics for Primary Care.* 3rd ed. Philadelphia, PA: Wolters Kluwer; 2011:317-321

Rimrodt SL, Lipkin PH. Learning disabilities and school failure. *Pediatr Rev.* 2011;32(8):315-324.

Shea SE. Intellectual disability (mental retardation). *Pediatr Rev.* 2012;33(3):110-121.

The girl in the vignette has migraine headaches. As the headaches have increased, she has been taking more and more ibuprofen, and at this point she is experiencing medication overuse headache in addition to the migraines. The best next step for her is to stop the ibuprofen.

Medication overuse headache occurs when a patient has been taking medications like ibuprofen, acetaminophen, caffeine, etc, more than 2 to 3 days a week for several months. The best treatment is to stop the overused medication immediately. The patient should be advised that headaches may worsen for 1 to 2 weeks, but then will improve. The clinician could consider starting a migraine prophylaxis medication to help decrease headaches overall. Opioids (eg, hydrocodone) are not recommended for pediatric migraines.

Migraines in pediatric patients are often frontal or bitemporal; they can also be retro-orbital, holocephalic, or occur just on 1 side of the head. Associated symptoms include nausea, vomiting, phonophobia, photophobia, and sometimes, an aura. Migraine aura is a transient sensory, visual, or speech abnormality that typically occurs at the beginning of the migraine. Examples include numbness and tingling, aphasia or dysarthria, or visual disturbances such as a scintillating scotoma or homonymous hemianopsia. Neuroimaging is not recommended in pediatric migraine when headaches have been recurrent, especially over 6 months or longer, and the patient's neurologic examination findings remain normal. It is even more reassuring when there is a family history of migraines. Neuroimaging can be considered in cases when: the neurologic findings are abnormal, migraines include hemiparesis, headaches occur on awakening with prominent associated vomiting, or a patient with migraines develops a new, different and severe headache.

The headache in pseudotumor cerebri may be similar to a migraine headache, with severe pain, nausea, vomiting, phonophobia, or photophobia. In addition, there can be pulse synchronous tinnitus or transient visual obscurations (brief, visual gray-outs lasting seconds). Examination of the fundi shows blurry optic disc margins, due to papillitis. When increased intracranial pressure due to pseudotumor cerebri is suspected, further diagnostic testing is needed. Magnetic resonance imaging of the brain will show any mass lesions that could be causing increased intracranial pressure, and magnetic resonance venography will show cerebral sinus venous thrombosis, which can have symptoms similar to pseudotumor cerebri and migraine. If these are both normal, then lumbar puncture should be performed to measure cerebrospinal fluid opening pressure. While the girl in the vignette is overweight, her headaches do not have the typical features of pseudotumor cerebri. She uses a topical retinoid, which is not a risk factor for pseudotumor cerebri, unlike systemic retinoids, which can be associated with pseudotumor cerebri. Her optic nerves have a normal appearance, so further evaluation for pseudotumor cerebri is not the best next step.

PREP Pearls

- In pediatric migraine, neuroimaging is not recommended when headaches are recurrent, especially over 6 months or longer, and the patient's neurologic examination findings remain normal. It is even more reassuring when there is a family history of migraines.
- Neuroimaging can be considered in cases of pediatric headache when: the neurologic findings are abnormal, there is an absence of a family history of migraines, migraines include hemiparesis or occur on awakening with prominent associated vomiting, or a patient with migraines develops a new, different and severe headache.

American Board of Pediatrics Content Specification(s)/Content Area

- Understand the appropriate use of neuroimaging in the evaluation of headache
- Recognize elements of history associated with headaches of various etiologies
- Recognize the clinical findings associated with headaches of various etiologies

Suggested Readings

IHS Classification ICHD-3. *International Classification of Headache Disorders*. 3rd ed. https://www.ichd-3.org/.

Lewis DW, Ashwal S, Dahl G, et al. Practice parameter: evaluation of children and adolescents with recurrent headaches—report of the Quality Standards Subcommittee of the American Academy of Neurology and the Practice Committee of the Child Neurology Society. *Neurology*. 2002;59(4):490-498.

Lewis DW. Pediatric migraine. *Pediatr Rev*. 2007;28:43.

The infant described in this vignette exhibits the cognitive/behavioral and motor milestones typically attained by 6 months of age. From a gross motor perspective, 6-month-old infants can sit momentarily when propped on hands, support weight with legs, and pivot in a prone position. The attainment of fine motor milestones at 6 months of age is demonstrated by banging and shaking toys, transferring objects from hand to hand, and raking small objects with hand. Socially, 6-month-old infants can recognize familiar persons, respond to others' emotions, and enjoy looking in a mirror. Language skills of 6-month-old infants include listening then vocalizing, recognizing own name, and stringing vowels together when babbling.

The infant described in this vignette has more advanced milestones than would be expected for a 4-month-old infant but has not yet achieved the developmental skills of a 9-month-old or a 12-month-old. At 4 months of age, an infant laughs, squeals, grasps objects voluntarily, and lifts both head and chest when prone. A 9-month-old infant may be afraid of strangers, copies sounds and gestures of others, uses thumb and index finger to grasp small objects, and pulls to stand. Twelve-month-old infants cry when their mother or father leaves, say "mama" and "dada," bang 2 objects together, and may take a few steps without holding on.

American Board of Pediatrics Content Specification(s)/ Content Area

- Evaluate the cognitive and behavioral developmental progress/status of an infant at 6 months of age
- Evaluate the motor developmental progress/status of an infant at 6 months of age, including recognition of abnormalities

Suggested Readings

Feigelman S. The first year. In: Kliegman RM, Stanton BF, St Geme JW III, Schor NF, Behrman RE, eds. *Nelson Textbook of Pediatrics.* 20th ed. Philadelphia, PA: Saunders Elsevier; 2015:65-69

Scharf RJ, Scharf GJ, Stroustrup A. Developmental milestones. *Pediatr Rev.* 2016;37(1):25-38.

Weitzman C, Wegner L; Section on Developmental and Behavioral Pediatrics; Committee on Psychosocial Aspects of Child and Family Health; Council on Early Childhood; Society for Developmental and Behavioral Pediatrics. Promoting optimal development: screening for behavioral and emotional problems. *Pediatrics.* 2015;135(2):384-395.

Item 213   Preferred Response: A

Lymphadenopathy is a common source of worry for parents and children that leads to visits to the pediatrician, urgent care center, and emergency department. Most lymphadenopathy is reactive or infectious. However, it is critical to recognize adenopathy that is out of the ordinary and needs further evaluation. Factors that should influence decisions about further evaluation of adenopathy include:

- Size greater than or equal to 2 cm
- Distribution (single vs multiple lymph nodes in single or multiple distinct chains)
- B symptoms (persistent fevers, weight loss greater than 10% of body weight, and drenching night sweats)
- Lack of resolution of the adenopathy with time and, if indicated, antibiotics

The adolescent girl in this vignette has multiple enlarged lymph nodes in a single lymph node chain, with the largest lymph node measuring 2 cm. She was followed without resolution of the adenopathy for over 4 weeks and treated with a course of antibiotics. A laboratory investigation revealed a mild normocytic anemia and markedly elevated erythrocyte sedimentation rate. The size, distribution, and lack of resolution of the adenopathy and the associated laboratory findings should raise concern for malignancy. The appropriate next steps include referring the patient to a pediatric oncologist, otolaryngologist, or surgeon for further evaluation as well as obtaining a chest radiograph to assess for adenopathy that is not evaluable by physical examination. It would not be appropriate to continue to provide reassurance to this patient without further action. Treatment with corticosteroids, including prednisone, is contraindicated in children in whom lymphoma or leukemia is suspected. Both leukemia

and lymphoma are very sensitive to corticosteroids, and their administration can delay diagnosis and lead to tumor lysis. Without fever or erythema overlying the marked adenopathy, further antibiotic therapy would not be indicated.

American Board of Pediatrics Content Specification(s)/ Content Area

- Plan the appropriate diagnostic evaluation of unexplained lymphadenopathy
- Recognize clinical findings associated with lymphoma

Suggested Readings

Friedmann A. Evaluation and management of lymphadenopathy in children. *Pediatr Rev.* 2008;29(2):53-60.

Rajasekaran K, Krakovitz P. Enlarged neck lymph nodes in children. *Pediatr Clin North Am.* 2013;60(4):923-936.

Sahai S. Lymphadenopathy. *Pediatr Rev.* 2013;34(5):216-227.

Item 214   Preferred Response: A

The adolescent girl in the vignette presents with a nondisplaced fracture involving the anterior wall of her right maxillary sinus after sustaining blunt trauma to her face while playing sports. Of the response choices, the most appropriate recommendation for her is treatment with a 1-week course of oral amoxicillin-clavulanate.

In children, fractures involving the paranasal sinuses can arise from injury to the nose or orbit. The pediatric nasal structure is composed of prominent soft cartilage, which tends to dissipate traumatic forces across the midface. However, the bony portions of the nose and nasal septum can be fractured and/or displaced when a child sustains blunt trauma to the nose and face. Ethmoid or anterior wall maxillary sinus fracture may arise from blunt trauma to the nose or cheek.

It is generally recommended that children with isolated sinus fractures be treated with a 1-week course of antibiotics. "Sinus precautions" (avoidance of nose blowing, swimming, straw use, and playing wind instruments) should be put in place. These patients should follow up with an otolaryngologist or plastic surgeon at 1 week; surgical intervention is rarely necessary.

Prescription of a 5-day course of oral prednisolone would not be indicated for the girl in the vignette, because there is no established role for corticosteroids for patients with isolated injuries to the paranasal sinuses. Recommending no medication or follow-up for the girl in the vignette would not be appropriate.

American Board of Pediatrics Content Specification(s)/ Content Area

- Plan the appropriate management of trauma to any of the paranasal sinuses

Suggested Readings

Munter DW. Head and facial trauma. In: Knoop KJ, Stack LB, Storrow AB, Thurman R, eds. *The Atlas of Emergency Medicine*. 4th ed. New York, NY: McGraw-Hill. http://accessmedicine.mhmedical.com/content.aspx?bookid=1763§ionid=125432768.

Niescierenko M, Lee GS. ENT trauma. In: Shaw KN, Bachur RG, eds. *Fleisher and Ludwig's Textbook of Pediatric Emergency Medicine*. 7th ed. Philadelphia, PA: Wolters Kluwer; 2016;chap 114

Item 215   **Preferred Response: A**

Of the response choices, this neonate's findings are most consistent with the diagnosis of posterior urethral valves (PUV). In most cases, PUV are initially suspected on prenatal ultrasonography. Bilateral hydronephrosis, dilated bladder, thickened bladder wall, and a dilated posterior urethra in male patients when noted on postnatal ultrasonography are highly suggestive of PUV. A voiding cystourethrogram will demonstrate the characteristic findings of a dilated and elongated posterior urethra during the voiding phase (after catheter removal). Direct visualization of the PUV using cystoscopy confirms the diagnosis.

Some infants with PUV present in the neonatal period with respiratory distress. After 16 weeks of gestation, decreased fetal urinary excretion due to severe bladder outlet obstruction may lead to maternal oligohydramnios, which leads to pulmonary hypoplasia; normal amniotic fluid levels are required for lung development between 16 and 28 weeks' gestation. The outcome for neonates with lung hypoplasia due to severe PUV is poor. Neonates with severe oligohydramnios may also present with the characteristic phenotypic features of Potter syndrome/Potter sequence. These include pulmonary hypoplasia (respiratory distress in the newborn), facial appearance (pseudoepicanthus, flattened ears and nose, recessed chin), skeletal abnormalities (hemivertebrae, sacral agenesis), ophthalmologic malformations, and limb abnormalities (club feet and hip dislocation)

Initial neonatal serum creatinine concentration (usually <1.0 mg/dL [88.4 µmol/L]) is reflective of the maternal serum level. In a full-term neonate, the serum creatinine concentration normalizes in 7 to 10 days, whereas in a preterm infant this may take up to 1 month. A serum creatinine concentration higher than 1.5 mg/dL (132.6 µmol/L) in a neonate usually indicates acute kidney injury; in the case of the neonate in the vignette, this is due to postrenal urinary obstruction

associated with PUV. Placement of a urinary catheter in these neonates is helpful in both evaluation and management; it bypasses the urethral/bladder outlet obstruction and also provides an accurate estimate of urine output. In some patients with severe obstruction, a urethral catheter cannot be placed; in such patients, urgent urology consultation for urinary drainage (vesicostomy or nephrostomy) is indicated.

Lack of prenatal care may delay the diagnosis of PUV. Urinary tract (more common) or respiratory problems (in neonates) may be the first indication of PUV in such cases. Postnatally, infants and young children with undiagnosed PUV usually present with urinary tract infection (UTI), failure to thrive, abdominal distention from enlarged bladder, poor urinary stream, or voiding difficulty. Older boys may present with UTIs or voiding dysfunction (urinary frequency, daytime and nocturnal enuresis, and poor urinary stream). Ablation of urethral valves during cystoscopy is the preferred initial surgical approach. Children with PUV may develop chronic renal failure due to associated renal dysplasia and/or acquired renal injury due to infection or poor bladder function. Affected children should have regular follow-up with a pediatric nephrologist for monitoring of their renal function, blood pressure, and growth.

In children, congenital or acquired ureteropelvic junction or ureterovesical junction obstruction generally present with unilateral hydronephrosis (dilation of the collecting system). Hydronephrosis without ureteral dilation is seen in ureteropelvic junction obstruction. Hydronephrosis with dilation of the distal ureter without bladder distention indicates ureterovesical obstruction.

Vesicoureteral reflux is the retrograde passage of urine from the bladder to the kidneys. Vesicoureteral reflux may be diagnosed prenatally as hydronephrosis on maternal screening ultrasonography or postnatally after an episode of UTI, usually before 6 to 7 years. Ureteropelvic junction, ureterovesical junction obstruction, and vesicoureteral reflux are not associated with a thickened bladder wall or a dilated posterior urethra.

American Board of Pediatrics Content Specification(s)/ Content Area

- Plan the appropriate long-term management of posterior urethral valves
- Recognize the clinical findings associated with posterior urethral valves in children of various ages

Suggested Readings

Elder JS. Obstruction of the urinary tract. In: Kliegman RM, Stanton BF, St. Geme J, Schor NF, eds. *Nelson Textbook of Pediatrics*. 20th ed. Philadelphia, PA: Elsevier Saunders; 2016:2567-2575

Nguyen HT. Obstructive uropathy and vesicoureteral reflux In: McInerny TK, Adam HM, Campbell DE, Kamat DM, Kelleher KJ, eds. *American Academy of Pediatrics Textbook of Pediatric Care*. 1st ed. Elk Grove Village, IL: American Academy of Pediatrics; 2009:2333-2343

Item 216   Preferred Response: A

The girl in this vignette has clinical evidence of acute rheumatic fever (ARF) and acute rheumatic heart disease. The Jones criteria were revised in 2015 and are the basis for guiding diagnosis in ARF. Evidence of a preceding group A streptococcal (GAS) infection is important in the diagnosis of ARF, given that other diseases and infections can appear similar to the presentation of ARF. Of the response choices listed, only the antistreptolysin O titer would give information regarding a preceding history of GAS infection.

In addition to an elevated (and especially a rising) antistreptolysin O titer, other evidence for a preceding GAS infection include a positive throat culture for GAS or a positive rapid streptococcal antigen test result in the clinical context of pharyngitis.

The revised Jones criteria are subdivided into major and minor criteria, and diagnosis is based on the risk spectrum of the population (see Gewitz et al). A low-risk population refers to an incidence of no more than 2 cases of ARF per 100,000 school-aged children or an all-age rheumatic heart disease prevalence of no more than 1 case per 1,000 population per year. Children not clearly from a low-risk population are in the moderate/high population. Major criteria include carditis, arthritis, chorea, erythema marginatum, and subcutaneous nodules. Minor criteria include prolonged PR interval, arthralgia, fever, and elevated erythrocyte sedimentation rate and C-reactive protein level.

The revised Jones criteria guidelines also discuss the use of echocardiographic data in the diagnosis of carditis. It is recommended that all patients with confirmed or suspected ARF undergo echocardiography with Doppler and that some patients undergo serial studies.

The molecular connection between GAS infection and ARF is still not fully understood, but molecular mimicry and autoimmunity are thought to be involved. Damage to the pericardium and myocardium can occur and, most relevant, is the damage to the valve tissue (most commonly the mitral valve). This damage results in the clinical picture of acute rheumatic heart disease. The incidence of ARF peaks between 5 and 15 years of age and is of higher prevalence in lower resourced countries as well as in indigenous populations in more affluent countries.

PREP Pearls

- Evidence of preceding group A streptococcal (GAS) infection is important to the diagnosis of acute rheumatic fever (an elevated antistreptolysin O titer, a positive throat culture for GAS, or a positive rapid streptococcal antigen test result in the clinical context of pharyngitis).
- The 2015 modified Jones criteria revise the major and minor criteria for acute rheumatic fever and base diagnosis on the risk stratification of the population.

American Board of Pediatrics Content Specification(s)/Content Area

- Recognize the clinical findings associated with rheumatic fever, including major and minor criteria
- Understand the natural history of rheumatic fever

Suggested Readings

Gewitz MH, Baltimore RS, Tani LY, et al. Revision of the Jones criteria for diagnosis of acute rheumatic fever in the era of Doppler echocardiography: a scientific statement from the American Heart Association. *Circulation*. 2015;131(20):1806-1818. doi: 10.1161/CIR.0000000000000205.

Zühlke LJ. Group A Streptococcus, acute rheumatic fever and rheumatic heart disease: epidemiology and clinical considerations. *Curr Treat Options Cardio Med*. 2017;19(2):15.

Item 217   Preferred Response: A

In medicine, screening tests are used to determine if people have a disease or if they are disease free. Instruments used for screening tests include scales, clinical laboratory tests, and questionnaires. Reliability and validity are used to determine if screening tests are accurate. Measuring tools can be used aside from determining if someone is at greater risk for developing a disease. They can be used in education and research to evaluate a variety of topics.

Reliability is the ability of a tool to give consistent results on repeated trials. For example, when investigating the reliability of a new scale, if you step on the scale 5 times in a row, it should give the same reading for weight. Test-retest reliability demonstrates if a screening tool yields the same results for the same sample under similar conditions. *Validity* is the ability of a tool to measure what was intended. For example, a personality test that scored an outgoing individual as an introvert would be a invalid test. *Internal validity* is when the tool used in a research study measured what was expected. *External validity* is when the results of a tool can be generalized outside of the initial study group. If an instrument is valid, it should be reliable. But, not all reliable instruments are valid.

In regard to the pre- and post-test in this vignette, there is not enough information to determine if the pre- and post-tests are reliable and valid. The differences in the pediatric residents' scores could be caused by systematic error based on confounding factors such as residents having additional experiences with eating disorder patients during the course of the academic year, the faculty having different teaching styles, and residents sharing prior tests and results.

PREP Pearls

- A valid instrument should also be reliable, but not all reliable instruments are valid.
- Reliability and validity help to determine if screening tools and other instruments are accurate.
- Reliability measures consistency, and validity assesses if a tool measures what it intended to measure.

American Board of Pediatrics Content Specification(s)/Content Area

- Understand reliability and how it might be compromised
- Understand generalizability and how it relates to validity
- Understand validity and how it might be compromised

Suggested Readings

Copeland-Linder N. Reliability and validity in pediatric practice. *Pediatr Rev.* 2009;30(7):278-279.

Friis RH, Sellers TA. Screening for disease in the community. In: *Epidemiology for Public Health Practice.* 5th ed. Burlington, MA: Jones & Bartlett Learning; 2014:461-490

Peeters MJ, Martin BA. Validation of learning assessments: a primer. *Curr Pharm Teach Learn.* 2017;9(5):925-933.

Item 218   **Preferred Response: A**

The neonate in the vignette has hypovolemic shock as evidenced by tachycardia, hypotension, and poor peripheral perfusion. The best initial step in management is a 20 mL/kg bolus of normal saline.

Shock is a clinical condition in which the cardiac output and oxygen delivery are insufficient to meet the metabolic demands of end organs. It is further classified as "hypovolemic shock," when the primary cause is decreased stroke volume because of insufficient intravascular volume. It is important for the clinician to distinguish hypovolemic shock from simple dehydration. The neonate in the vignette presents with several important signs and symptoms consistent with hypovolemic shock including severe tachycardia, delayed capillary refilling time, and altered mental status. She is also hypotensive, which implies a higher severity of shock. It is important to realize that hypotension is not always present in shock; compensatory mechanisms for shock that can prevent hypotension include elevated circulating catecholamines, tachycardia, vasoconstriction, and diversion of blood away from the skin and splanchnic circulation.

Cardiac output is the product of stroke volume and heart rate. Stroke volume is dependent on preload, afterload, and contractility. Children, compared with adults, are more likely to respond with an increased heart rate in case of shock rather than an increase in contractility. Thus, tachycardia is an important compensatory mechanism for shock. Fluid administration is an important early therapy in hypovolemic shock, as an underfilled ventricle contains less blood to eject. Also, contractile elements will overlap, leading to a lower fraction of the blood ejected. Early goal-directed resuscitation has been shown to improve outcomes in neonatal, pediatric, and adult shock (Item C218A). It begins with the

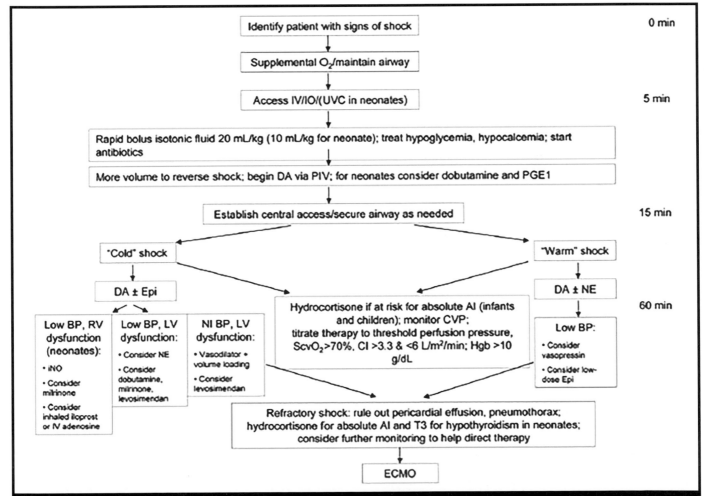

Reprinted with permission from Yager P, Noviski N. Shock. *Pediatr Rev.* 2010;31(8):315.

Item C218A: Algorithm for goal-directed management of hemodynamic support in septic shock. Adapted from the 2007 ACCM clinical practice parameters for hemodynamic support of pediatric and neonatal septic shock. Abbreviations: AI, adrenal insufficiency; BP, blood pressure; CI, cardiac index; CVP, central venous pressure; DA, dopamine; Dobut, dobutamine; ECMO, extracorporeal membrane oxygenation; Epi, epinephrine; IV, intravenous; iNO, inhaled nitric oxide; IO, intraosseous; LV, left ventricle; NL, normal; PGE1, prostaglandin E1; RV, right ventricle; ScvO2, mixed venous oxygen saturation; UVC, umbilical venous catheter.

recognition of decreased mental status and perfusion. Intravenous or intraosseous access should be established within the first few minutes, and starting within the first 15 minutes, isotonic fluid boluses of 20 mL/kg should be pushed up to and over 60 mL/kg, until perfusion improves or rales or hepatomegaly occur. Empiric antibiotics should also be administered early. Inotropes should be initiated for fluid-refractory shock, and corticosteroids should be considered for catecholamine-resistant shock. Neonates can be less able to handle the fluid load during resuscitation compared with older children. Thus, earlier initiation of inotropes may be warranted.

Other causes of shock should be considered in neonates (Item C218B). Septic shock can be caused by early-onset sepsis. Dissociative shock can be caused by an inborn error of metabolism or a mitochondrial disorder. Cardiogenic shock is caused by inadequate myocardial function or structural heart disease; the physical examination is notable for pulmonary edema, rales, and hepatomegaly. Ductal-dependent systemic blood flow lesions such as hypoplastic left heart syndrome, critical coarctation of the aorta, and critical aortic stenosis can present with shock within the first 48 hours after birth, when the ductus arteriosus closes. All neonates in shock should be started on a prostaglandin infusion unless a definitive noncardiac diagnosis has been made.

Item C218B. Etiology of Various Forms of Neonatal Shock.

Type	Etiology (Neonate)
Hypovolemic	Poor feeding, sepsis
Cardiogenic	Ductal dependent systemic blood flow lesions (HLHS, IAA, coarctation, critical AS), cardiomyopathy, SVT
Septic	Early-onset sepsis
Obstructive	Pericardial tamponade, IAA, coarctation, critical AS
Distributive	Sepsis, neurogenic shock
Dissociative	Methemoglobinemia, sepsis, inborn error of metabolism, mitochondrial disorder

Abbreviations: HLHS, hypoplastic left heart syndrome; IAA, interrupted aortic arch; AS, aortic stenosis; SVT, supraventricular tachycardia.

Courtesy of A. Sarnaik.

Offering formula or expressed breast milk by bottle or providing maintenance intravenous fluids are good management steps for simple dehydration, but would not be appropriate to treat a neonate in shock. Whole blood exchange transfusion has been effective in some forms of refractory septic shock, but it is not helpful in hypovolemic shock.

PREP Pearls

- All neonates in shock should be started on a prostaglandin infusion, unless a definitive noncardiac diagnosis has been made.
- Early goal-directed therapy aimed toward restoring cardiac output should be immediately initiated in all patients with shock.
- Hypotension is a late finding in pediatric shock; tachycardia is an early finding.

American Board of Pediatrics Content Specification(s)/Content Area

- Recognize the clinical signs of shock due to fluid loss, and manage appropriately

Suggested Readings

Bhat BV, Plakkal N. Management of shock in neonates. *Indian J Pediatr.* 2015;82(10):923-929.

Davis AL, Carcillo JA, Aneja RK, et al. American College of Critical Care Medicine clinical practice parameters for hemodynamic support of pediatric and neonatal septic shock. *Crit Care Med.* 2017;45(6):1061-1093.

Yager P, Noviski N. Shock. *Pediatr Rev.* 2010; 31:311-319.

Item 219 — Preferred Response: A

The boy in this vignette is obese, with a body mass index (BMI) greater than the 95th percentile for age and sex. Of the options provided, the most evidence-based intervention is to eliminate sugar-sweetened beverages from his diet. Pediatric obesity is a serious and growing public health concern. Currently, about one-third of children and adolescents in the United States are overweight or obese, and 5% are severely obese. Overweight and obesity are more prevalent in black, Native American, and Hispanic children as compared to non-Hispanic white children, and in children from low-income families. Parental obesity significantly increases the risk of childhood obesity. Obese children and adolescents are at high risk of becoming obese adults and have increased lifetime rates of cardiovascular disease and metabolic syndrome. There is good evidence that a substantial component of adolescent obesity is established before age 5 years; prevention and early treatment of childhood overweight and obesity, therefore, has the potential to make a significant impact on lifelong health.

Measuring an individual's BMI is the most appropriate means of assessing and categorizing weight. In adults, a BMI of 25 to 30 kg/m^2 is considered overweight, and a BMI of greater than or equal to 30 kg/m^2 is obese. In children, the average BMI varies with age and sex. Body mass index between the 85th and 95th percentile for age and sex is considered overweight, and BMI greater than or equal to the 95th percentile for age and sex is considered obese. Recently, an additional category of severe obesity was defined as a BMI greater than or equal to 120% of the 95th percentile for age and sex or greater than or equal to 35 kg/m^2, whichever is lower. At each health supervision visit, BMI should be calculated and compared to age- and sex-matched standards, and trends should be recorded.

Pediatric overweight and obesity is heavily influenced by environmental factors, including excess caloric intake and sedentary lifestyles. Specific factors that have been identified include the increased glycemic index of commonly consumed foods, prevalence of sugar-sweetened beverages, increasing portion sizes of prepared foods, availability of fast food, the rise of sedentary computer and television time, composition of school lunches, and the decreased occurrence of family meals, structured physical activity, and safe neighborhood environments for exercise. The best established environmental influence on the development and prevalence of childhood obesity is television watching—time spent watching television and the presence of a television in a child's room. Consumption of sugar-sweetened beverages is another well-established factor in the cause of obesity. In a study of school-aged children, each additional serving of a sugar-sweetened beverage accounted for an increase in BMI and in the prevalence of obesity. Genetic factors interact with environmental components leading to overweight and obesity, but the molecular mechanisms are not well understood. There is increasing evidence that environmental and nutritional influences during critical periods of development have a permanent effect on an individual's predisposition for obesity. Specifically, maternal body weight and nutrition during gestation, birth weight, early feeding practices, and rates of weight gain in early infancy affect a child's likelihood of becoming overweight or obese. Factors protective against the development of childhood obesity include breastfeeding, family-wide participation in physical activity, minimal television viewing, and having nonobese parents.

The results of studies examining prevention and treatment strategies for overweight and obesity in children are mixed. Many approaches require tremendous resources that are impractical for the clinical setting. The most evidence-based strategies include school-based programs with an emphasis on increased physical activity, nutritional education, good-quality school food, and family-based interventions focused on increasing activity and decreasing screen time. The most successful primary care–based programs for weight loss include motivational interviewing and setting goals for small, manageable changes. Decreasing sugar-sweetened beverage consumption and limiting screen time have been associated with success, although the effects are modest at best.

Commercial weight-loss programs have not been shown to have significant effects on BMI in pediatric populations. Although whole grain foods are part of a healthy diet, this change alone would not be expected to affect BMI. Participation in organized sports is certainly beneficial for many children, with positive effects on peer relationships, self-confidence, and physical activity, but participation alone has not been shown to decrease obesity.

PREP Pearls

- Although results are mixed and the effects are generally modest, strategies shown to prevent and treat childhood obesity include promoting breastfeeding, eliminating sugar-sweetened beverages, limiting computer and television screen time, encouraging family meals, and promoting family-wide participation in physical activity.
- Childhood obesity is defined as body mass index (BMI) greater than or equal to the 95th percentile for age and sex, and overweight is defined as BMI between the 85th and 95th percentiles for age and sex.
- Obese children and adolescents have a very high risk of being obese as adults and have an increased risk of lifetime cardiovascular disease and metabolic syndrome. Prevention and early treatment of childhood overweight and obesity can have effects on lifelong health.

American Board of Pediatrics Content Specification(s)/ Content Area

- Counsel a family with regard to obesity prevention and treatment
- Know which interventions have been effective and ineffective in caring for patients of various ages who are obese
- Understand the utility of the body mass index
- Identify the genetic and environmental risk factors for obesity, including lifestyle choices
- Understand the importance of body mass index (BMI) in identifying obesity and overweight

Suggested Readings

Rome ES. Obesity prevention and treatment. *Pediatr Rev.* 2011;32(9):363-373.

Styne DM, Arslanian SA, Connor EL, et al. Pediatric obesity—assessment, treatment, and prevention: an Endocrine Society clinical practice guideline. *J Clin Endocrinol Metab.* 2017;102(3):709-757.

Item 220	Preferred Response: C

In the vignette, the outbreak of diarrheal illness among children and adults after visiting a summer camp where there was contact with livestock, access to a swimming pool and lake, and consumption of meals from produce grown in the local garden is highly suggestive of *Cryptosporidium parvum* infection. *Bacillus cereus* is an important toxin-mediated foodborne illness and has been linked to outbreaks of diarrheal illness, but the incubation period ranges from 10 to 16 hours. Enteropathogenic *Escherichia coli* causes acute and chronic watery diarrhea, primarily in children younger than 2 years of age, living in low and middle-income countries. Although *Brucella melitensis*, the etiologic agent of brucellosis, may be transmitted to humans via exposure to livestock, patients usually present with high fever, night sweats, and other systemic symptoms with hepatomegaly, splenomegaly, and arthritis on physical examination.

Cryptosporidium species are coccidian protozoal organisms comprising 2 species (*Cryptosporidium hominis*, which typically affects humans, and *C parvum*, which infects humans and animals). The infection is transmitted by the fecal-oral route after ingestion of oocysts excreted by infected hosts. Major water-associated outbreaks of cryptosporidiosis, well described in the United States, have resulted from exposure to contaminated public drinking water and treated (eg, swimming pools) or untreated (eg, lakes) recreational water locations. Person-to-person transmission and outbreaks in daycare centers, with secondary spread, have been reported. Zoonotic transmission can occur in farmers and animal handlers, as well as children via exposure to pets and animals in petting zoos, especially preweaned calves.

Cryptosporidiosis is characterized by nonbloody, watery diarrhea with abdominal pain, emesis, fever, loss of appetite, and weight loss. The typical incubation period is 3 to 14 days. Infection can be asymptomatic. In immunocompetent hosts, gastroenteritis is usually self-limited, with symptoms resolving by 2 to 3 weeks. *Cryptosporidium* infection can also result in traveler's diarrhea. In immunocompromised individuals (eg, those with human immunodeficiency virus infection, solid organ transplant recipients), severe, chronic diarrhea may persist for weeks to months, associated with weight loss and extraintestinal disease.

Laboratory diagnosis of cryptosporidiosis can be made by detection of oocysts in stool by direct immunofluorescent antibody test or detection of antigen in stool by rapid point-of-care testing using enzyme immunoassay method. A modified Kinyoun acid-fast stain may detect the organism in a concentrated stool specimen. Because of the intermittent shedding of oocysts, a minimum of 3 stool specimens collected on separate days is recommended before excluding infection.

Antiparasitic therapy may not be necessary in immunocompetent people with mild disease. Oral nitazoxanide administered for 3 days is the recommended therapy for all immunocompetent individuals aged 1 year and older. Immunocompromised children may require nitazoxanide therapy for 14 days or longer. Contact precautions for the duration of illness are recommended for hospitalized patients or during institutional outbreak.

Other than *Cryptosporidium* species, frequently reported pathogens causing recreational water–associated outbreaks include *Shigella, Giardia*, norovirus, and *Escherichia coli* O157:H7. In 2011-2012, of 90 recreational water–associated outbreaks, 77% were linked to treated recreational water, with 52% due to *Cryptosporidium*. Twenty-three percent of outbreaks were linked to untreated recreational water, 33% of which were due to *E coli* O157:H7 or *E coli* O111. In the United States, there has been a rise in the incidence of cryptosporidiosis. Children aged 1 to 4 years are most commonly affected, followed by children aged 5 to 9 years. Seasonal peaks of cryptosporidiosis in late summer and early fall are related to the outdoor swimming season.

Prevention of recreational water–associated illness warrants epidemiologic surveillance and outbreak detection, environmental hygiene maintenance, appropriate disinfection, and water quality controls. The public and staff at recreational water venues must be educated about healthy swimming behaviors to prevent the spread of recreational water–associated illness including (1) avoidance of swimming during diarrheal illness; (2) not swallowing pool water, and (3) adherence to strict hygiene measures.

PREP Pearls

- *Cryptosporidium* typically is transmitted via the fecal-oral route, but exposure to contaminated water, livestock, and animals in petting zoos can also result in infection.
- Common pathogens causing recreational water–associated outbreaks include *Cryptosporidium, Shigella, Giardia*, norovirus, and *Escherichia coli* O157:H7.
- In immunocompetent hosts, the diarrheal illness caused by *Cryptosporidium* species is self-limited, whereas severe, chronic diarrhea associated with weight loss occurs in immunocompromised hosts.

American Board of Pediatrics Content Specification(s)/ Content Area

- Understand the epidemiology of *Cryptosporidium* infection
- Recognize the clinical features associated with *Cryptosporidium* infection, including *Cryptosporidium* diarrhea in an immunocompromised host

Suggested Readings

American Academy of Pediatrics. Cryptosporidiosis. In: Kimberlin DW, Brady MT, Jackson MA, Long SS, eds. *Red Book: 2018 Report of the Committee on Infectious Diseases*. 31st ed. Itasca, IL: American Academy of Pediatrics; 2018:304-307

Centers for Disease Control and Prevention. Cryptosporidiosis surveillance — United States, 2009-2010. *MMWR Surveill Summ.* 2012;61(SS-5):1-12.

Centers for Disease Control and Prevention. Recreational water-associated disease outbreaks —United States, 2009-2010. *MMWR Morb Mortal Wkly Rep.* 2014;63(1):6-10

Centers for Disease Control and Prevention. Steps of Healthy Swimming. https://www.cdc.gov/healthywater/swimming/swimmers/steps-healthy-swimming.html.

Item 221   Preferred Response: D

For the neonate in the vignette with extreme prematurity and bronchopulmonary dysplasia (BPD), pulmonary hypertension is the most likely complication. Neonates with extreme prematurity, born at less than 28 weeks of gestation, are at high risk for BPD. Their lung development is interrupted at birth, disrupting alveolar formation. Their lungs then receive exposures not encountered in utero, such as oxygen and pressure, which impair ongoing lung development. As a result, their lungs have fewer alveoli than normal, which function differently. Severe BPD is diagnosed clinically, based on a need for positive pressure ventilation or more than 30% oxygen beyond 36 weeks' postconceptional age. This was defined in a consensus statement from the National Institute of Infant and Child Health and Development published in 2004. Severe BPD is associated with poor neurodevelopmental outcomes, both because of intrinsic lung disease and the lack of developmentally appropriate interaction and stimulation, due to illness and invasive respiratory support. Pulmonary hypertension is also associated with severe BPD. Therefore, screening for pulmonary hypertension with echocardiography is recommended.

Spontaneous intestinal perforation (SIP) may be seen during the first week after birth. Affected neonates present with abdominal free air; they are often asymptomatic. The perforation may reseal without intervention or require surgical placement of an intra-abdominal drain. Neither neonates with SIP nor infants with BPD are at increased risk for protein-losing enteropathy.

Plagiocephaly is a common finding after prolonged hospitalization in the neonatal intensive care unit with invasive respiratory support. It is a positional deformity that occurs because of limited mobility and is not associated with craniosynostosis.

Posthemorrhagic hydrocephalus is a complication of severe intraventricular hemorrhage. Blood products in the ventricle may impair resorption of cerebrospinal fluid, resulting in hydrocephalus. It is typically associated with grade 3 or 4 intraventricular hemorrhage, not grade 2, as seen in the infant in the vignette.

American Board of Pediatrics Content Specification(s)/ Content Area

- Recognize the clinical features of bronchopulmonary dysplasia and its associated sequelae
- Recognize situations that may lead to bronchopulmonary dysplasia
- Plan appropriate inpatient and outpatient management of bronchopulmonary dysplasia

Suggested Readings

Kair LR, Leonard DT, Anderson JM. Bronchopulmonary dysplasia. *Pediatr Rev.* 2012;33;255.

Kelleher J, Salas AA, Bhat R, et al. Prophylactic indomethacin and intestinal perforation in extremely low birth weight infants. *Pediatrics.* 2014;134;e1369.

Walsh MC, Yao Q, Gettner P, et al. Impact of a physiologic definition on bronchopulmonary dysplasia rates. *Pediatrics.* 2004;114;1305.

Item 222   Preferred Response: D

The boy in this vignette has an exacerbation of persistent asthma triggered by a viral respiratory infection. The appropriate first intervention is short-acting β-adrenergic agonist by inhalation. His fever is the likely cause of tachycardia and tachypnea, although his airway reactivity may be contributing to the increased respiratory rate. β-Adrenergic agonists may cause tachycardia, but relief of bronchospasm may help to decrease his tachypnea and tachycardia also. The more selective β_2 agonists currently available as short-acting bronchodilators (albuterol, pirbuterol, and levalbuterol) have less cardiotoxicity than epinephrine, which has generalized β_1-, β_2-, and and α-adrenergic effects.

The long-acting β_2-agonists salmeterol and formoterol are not appropriate for use as rescue medications and are rarely indicated for a 2-year-old patient. They are slightly more β_2 selective than the short-acting β-agonist inhalants.

Although a subset of patients with acute exacerbation of asthma will respond to doubling or quadrupling their baseline inhaled steroid dose, there is no clear guidance for this as a standard intervention. Use of systemic steroids may be appropriate, but the first intervention is to escalate short-acting β-agonists.

β-Adrenergic agents may be associated with systemic adverse effects, especially when taken orally. Tachycardia and tremor are the most common adverse effects, even with inhaled medication. Irritability, agitation, and palpitations may all be associated with oral β-agonists and sometimes with frequent use of inhaled drug. The muscle tremor that is a pharmacologic effect of the drug is sometimes interpreted as nervousness or shakiness by patients or parents.

American Board of Pediatrics Content Specification(s)/ Content Area

- Understand the pharmacokinetics of short- and long-acting inhaled beta-adrenergic agonists and the risks associated with their excessive use

Suggested Readings

Kelly HW, Hendeles L. Bronchodilators. In: Light MJ, Blaisdell CJ, Homnick DN, Schechter MS, Weinberger MM, eds. *Pediatric Pulmonology.* Elk Grove Village, IL: American Academy of Pediatrics; 2011:933-951

Link HW. Pediatric asthma in a nutshell. *Pediatr Rev.* 2014;35(7):287-298.

Wood PR, Hill VL. Practical management of asthma. *Pediatr Rev.* 2009;30(10):375-385.

Item 223   Preferred Response: A

The adolescent girl in this vignette has obesity, with a body mass index (BMI) greater than the 95th percentile and elements of metabolic syndrome. Given her risk factors, screening for type 2 diabetes is indicated. A hemoglobin A1c level is an acceptable screening test for type 2 diabetes. The diagnostic cutoff of greater than or equal to 6.5% is established in adults, and it remains unclear if the same diagnostic value should be used for adolescents. However, hemoglobin A1c is commonly used as a screening test for adolescents because of its greater convenience, without the need for fasting, and stability compared to glucose-based testing.

Other options for diabetes screening include obtaining a:
- Fasting plasma glucose level (≥ 125 mg/dL [7 mmol/L] is diagnostic), or
- A 2-hour plasma glucose level during a 75-g oral glucose tolerance test (≥ 200 mg/dL [11.1 mmol/L] is diagnostic)

A random plasma glucose level of 200 mg/dL (11.1 mmol/L) or greater with classic symptoms of diabetes is also diagnostic. Unless there is unequivocal hyperglycemia, the testing should be repeated on a separate day before diabetes is diagnosed. The 2-hour plasma glucose level after a 75-g oral glucose load is the most sensitive screening method.

The American Diabetes Association recommends screening for type 2 diabetes in at-risk children and adolescents at least every 3 years. Screening is recommended in patients who are overweight (BMI > 85th percentile) and have at least 1 of the following risk factors:
- Family history of type 2 diabetes in a first- or second-degree relative
- Native American, African American, Latino, Asian American, or Pacific Islander race/ethnicity

- Signs of or conditions associated with insulin resistance, such as acanthosis nigricans, hypertension, dyslipidemia, polycystic ovary syndrome, or small-for–gestational age birth weight
- Maternal diabetes, including gestational diabetes while pregnant with the individual

Risk factors for the patient in this vignette include obesity, African American race, acanthosis nigricans, hypertension, and maternal history of gestational diabetes. Her associated oligomenorrhea and hirsutism are suggestive of polycystic ovary syndrome, another risk factor.

Metabolic syndrome is a constellation of risk factors for cardiovascular disease and type 2 diabetes. Components include obesity, hypertension, dyslipidemia, and glucose intolerance. Adults meet criteria for metabolic syndrome when 3 of the following are present:

- High waist circumference (> 35 inches for women, > 40 inches for men)
- High triglyceride level (≥ 150 mg/dL [1.7 mmol/L])
- Low high-density lipoprotein cholesterol level (< 40 mg/dL [1 mmol/L] in men, < 50 mg/dL [1.3 mmol/L] in women)
- High blood pressure (≥ 130 mm Hg systolic and/or ≥ 85 mm Hg diastolic)
- High fasting glucose level (≥ 100 mg/dL [5.6 mmol/L])

Although there is no consensus on the definition of metabolic syndrome in children and adolescents, attempts have been made to modify the adult criteria to reflect pediatric measurements. Obesity and insulin resistance play key roles in the pathogenesis of metabolic syndrome. In the pathogenesis of type 2 diabetes, there is both insulin resistance and relative pancreatic β-cell failure.

A 2017 Endocrine Society pediatric obesity guideline recommends that children and adolescents with a BMI at or above the 85th percentile be screened for complications and comorbidities of obesity. These complications include glucose intolerance, dyslipidemia, hypertension, nonalcoholic fatty liver disease, polycystic ovary syndrome, obstructive sleep apnea, and psychiatric comorbidities.

This guideline also recommends against measuring insulin levels as part of an evaluation for obesity because of a lack of diagnostic value. The guideline further recommends against routine testing for endocrine etiologies of obesity without other signs or symptoms, such as an abnormally low growth velocity. The patient in this vignette has no signs or symptoms of Cushing syndrome or hypothyroidism, so a midnight salivary cortisol level and thyroid-stimulating hormone level are not indicated.

PREP Pearls

- Metabolic syndrome is a constellation of risk factors for cardiovascular disease and type 2 diabetes. Components include obesity, hypertension, dyslipidemia, and glucose intolerance.
- Risk factors for type 2 diabetes include obesity, family history of type 2 diabetes, signs of insulin resistance or conditions associated with insulin resistance, and other elements of metabolic syndrome.

American Board of Pediatrics Content Specification(s)/ Content Area

- Understand the epidemiology of and risk factors associated with type 2 diabetes

Suggested Readings

American Diabetes Association. 2. Classification and diagnosis of diabetes: Standards of Medical Care in Diabetes—2018. *Diabetes Care.* 2018;41(suppl 1):S13-S27.

Styne DM, Arslanian SA, Connor EL, et al. Pediatric obesity—assessment, treatment, and prevention: an Endocrine Society clinical practice guideline. *J Clin Endocrinol Metab.* 2017;102(3):709-757.

Wittcopp C, Conroy R. Metabolic syndrome in children and adolescents. *Pediatr Rev.* 2016;37(5):193-202.

Item 224	Preferred Response: D

The boy in the vignette has neurofibromatosis type 2 (NF2), an autosomal dominant disorder, which presents with bilateral vestibular schwannomas that result in balance dysfunction, tinnitus, and hearing loss typically in the adolescent or early adult years. Affected individuals can also develop meningiomas, ependymomas, astrocytomas, and schwannomas of other cranial and peripheral nerves as seen in this boy's mother. The tumors associated with NF2 often lead to increased morbidity and mortality, with the average lifespan being 36 years. A unique ocular finding that can develop in childhood is posterior subcapsular lens opacity; this may be the first sign of NF2. It rarely will progress to a cataract. Mononeuropathy is another common finding in childhood, which can manifest as a hand/foot drop, strabismus, or a persistent facial palsy. The diagnosis of NF2 is based on specific clinical diagnostic criteria. Once a diagnosis has been established, the patient should undergo further evaluation including brain magnetic resonance imaging, hearing evaluation, full ophthalmologic examination, cutaneous examination, and a formal genetic consultation. Radiation therapy should be avoided if possible in children with NF2, because it can induce or accelerate the formation of tumors.

The only known gene to cause NF2 is the *NF2* gene. Because NF2 is an autosomal dominant disorder, an affected individual has a 50% chance of passing the disorder to his/ her children. Fifty percent of individuals have an affected parent, and 50% of individuals have the disorder as a result of a de novo or spontaneous pathogenic variant.

Neurocutaneous disorders are a broad group of disorders associated with brain, spine, and peripheral nerve tumors. Other neurocutaneous disorders include neurofibromatosis type 1 (NF1), tuberous sclerosis complex (TSC), schwannomatosis, and Sturge-Weber disease. NF1 and TSC are autosomal dominant disorders. Sturge-Weber disease is sporadic in nature, and the cause is unknown at this time.

Some ocular findings are unique to specific genetic disorders. Colobomas are commonly associated with CHARGE syndrome. Heterochromia iridis may occur in Waardenburg syndrome, Sturge-Weber syndrome, Parry-Romberg syndrome, and Horner syndrome. Iris Lisch nodules are specific to NF1.

PREP Pearls

- Neurofibromatosis type 2, an autosomal dominant disorder, typically presents in the adolescent or early adult years with bilateral vestibular schwannomas that result in balance dysfunction, tinnitus, and hearing loss. Other associated findings include meningiomas, ependymomas, astrocytomas, schwannomas of other cranial and peripheral nerves, mononeuropathy, and posterior subcapsular lens opacities.

- Neurofibromatosis type 2, neurofibromatosis type 1, and tuberous sclerosis are neurocutaneous disorders with autosomal dominant inheritance.

- Posterior subcapsular lens opacity is a unique ocular finding that can be the first sign of neurofibromatosis type 2 in childhood.

American Board of Pediatrics Content Specification(s)/Content Area

- Recognize the inheritance pattern of neurocutaneous hamartoses (eg, neurofibromatosis)

Suggested Readings

Baser ME, Friedman JM, Aeschliman D, et al. Predictors of the risk of mortality in neurofibromatosis 2. *Am J Hum Genet*. 2002;71:715-723

Evans DG. Neurofibromatosis 2. *Gene Reviews*. https://www.ncbi.nlm.nih.gov/books/NBK1201.

Hersh JH, American Academy of Pediatrics, Committee on Genetics. Health supervision for children with neurofibromatosis. *Pediatrics*. 2008;121(3):633-642.

Item 225   Preferred Response: A

Multiple elements of this child's history and physical examination findings suggest caregiver-fabricated illness in a child. In particular, the request for a procedure—central line placement—which does not seem to be indicated, raises concern. Discussing the patient with the child protection team at the children's hospital where she receives specialty care has many potential benefits. The child protection specialist can comprehensively review the child's medical record and offer an objective assessment of the likelihood of this condition. He or she can also help facilitate discussions with her specialists to see if the concerns regarding caregiver-fabricated illness are shared.

Caregiver-fabricated illness in a child was initially called Munchausen syndrome by proxy. The terminology has changed over time to include names such as factitious disorder by proxy, pediatric condition falsification, and child abuse in a medical setting. Currently, the 2 most widely accepted terms are:

- Caregiver-fabricated illness in a child, a term that centers on caregiver actions, based on a 2013 report from the American Academy of Pediatrics

- Medical child abuse, a term that centers on the harm inflicted on the child, based on a 2009 report from the American Academy of Pediatrics

Caregiver-fabricated illness in a child is a form of child maltreatment that occurs in medical settings, whereby a caregiver falsifies and/or induces a child's illness. This results in harm to the child through unnecessary procedures and treatments. Caregiver-fabricated illness has a mortality rate of 6% to 9%. Pediatric health care providers often delay or forego reporting suspicious cases because there is not absolute certainty of the diagnosis, which can increase morbidity and harm to the child by prolonging the child's unnecessary medical care. Even when a diagnostic evaluation is ongoing, as with the child in this vignette, it is better to consult the child protection team upon suspecting the diagnosis rather than waiting until the evaluation is complete.

There are several aspects of this child's care that, taken together, represent a pattern that raises suspicion for caregiver-fabricated illness. The mother is requesting equipment (a wheelchair) that does not seem to be needed based on the child's well appearance. Difficulty with previous intravenous line placement is not a medically valid reason for central venous line placement in an otherwise well-appearing child with no history of rapid decompensation with illnesses. The mother is requesting a change in specialty providers without a clear reason, which would likely result in additional tests, procedures, and treatment. Lastly, the parent-reported symptoms that have prompted hospitalizations are consistently unwitnessed and unverified by medical staff.

Studies of children with caregiver-fabricated illness indicate that common falsified conditions include food allergies, feeding difficulties, apnea, seizures, and rashes. Elements of the history that are common in caregiver-fabricated illness include the following:

- The patient has bizarre, physiologically improbable symptoms.
- The caregiver is not relieved by normal or reassuring test results.
- A sibling of the patient has an unexplained illness.
- The caregiver uses social media to solicit donations based on the child's illness.
- The caregiver has a history of somatization disorder.

The diagnosis of caregiver-fabricated illness is often aided by covert video surveillance (CVS) or separation of the child and the parent. Both approaches have their limitations. Some consider CVS to be an invasion of privacy, and it can be difficult in some cases to tell whether recorded events represent inducement of illness. In one case series, CVS provided evidence for abuse in about half of all patients. In some cases, it confirmed that the child had a true underlying medical condition. Separating the child from the parent and monitoring for resolution of symptoms can be traumatic for the child and often involves a prolonged stay in a monitored medical setting. The separation should be long enough to confirm that the resolution is due to the separation and not medical remission.

When child protection specialists are not available, the clinician should contact the child's specialists to discuss concerns for suspected caregiver-fabricated illness and report the caregiver to the state or local child welfare agency. Because many agencies are relatively unfamiliar with this type of maltreatment, a detailed summary of the reasons for suspicion, focusing on the detrimental effects on the child (eg, psychological harm, physical risk associated with unnecessary procedures, missed educational opportunities) should be submitted with the report. This information will help agency staff evaluate the need for intervention based on the harm, or risk of harm, to the child.

PREP Pearls

- A clinician who is concerned about caregiver-fabricated illness in a patient should promptly consult child protection specialists, communicate with the child's specialists, and/or submit a detailed report to the state child welfare agency, even when diagnostic evaluations are ongoing.
- Caregiver-fabricated illness in a child should be suspected with persistent or recurrent unexplained illness resulting in multiple procedures or treatments or in cases where the history, physical examination findings, and appearance of health are discrepant.

American Board of Pediatrics Content Specification(s)/ Content Area

- Recognize the clinical circumstances associated with caregiver-fabricated illness (eg, caregiver seeking unnecessary, duplicative, and/or harmful medical interventions; caregiver exaggerating, fabricating, or inducing a child's illness or symptoms)
- Understand the epidemiology of and the psychosocial and environmental risk factors for caregiver-fabricated illness

Suggested Readings

Bass C, Halligan P. Factitious disorders and malingering: challenges for clinical assessment and management. *Lancet.* 2014;383(9926):1422-1432.

Brown AN, Gonzalez GR, Wiester RT, Kelley MC, Feldman KW. Caretaker blogs in caregiver fabricated illness in a child: a window on the caretaker's thinking? *Child Abuse Negl.* 2014;38(3):488-497.

Flaherty EG, Macmillan HL; Committee on Child Abuse and Neglect. Caregiver-fabricated illness in a child: a manifestation of child maltreatment. *Pediatrics.* 2013;132(3):590-597.

Item 226   Preferred Response: B

The test most likely to determine the diagnosis for the boy in the vignette is serology. Serum antibodies to *Entamoeba histolytica* are detectable by commercially available enzyme immunoassay in 95% of individuals with invasive amebiasis.

Amebiasis is endemic in Central and South America, Africa, and Asia. Infection with *E histolytica* is transmitted by the fecal-oral route.

The majority of *E histolytica* infections are asymptomatic. However, the organism resides in the large intestine where it can produce gastrointestinal symptoms including abdominal pain, watery or bloody diarrhea, weight loss, amebomas, necrotizing colitis, and toxic megacolon. The organism can also invade the intestinal mucosa and produce extra-intestinal manifestations including abscesses in the liver, brain, and skin. Liver abscesses can present acutely or can have a more indolent presentation. Acute symptoms characteristic of liver abscesses include fever, abdominal pain, and hepatomegaly. Most abscesses are located in the right lobe of the liver.

Invasive disease requires treatment with metronidazole or tinidazole. Additionally, all patients with *E histolytica* infection should receive an amebicide to treat the intestinal

---

intraluminal infection. Intraluminal agents include paromomycin, iodoquinol, and diloxanide.

Stool microscopy has poor sensitivity for the cysts and trophozoites of *E histolytica*. Additionally, microscopy cannot distinguish between pathogenic *E histolytica* and nonpathogenic species such as *Entamoeba dispar*. Stool culture would be helpful in the setting of bacterial gastroenteritis but would not help with making the diagnosis of a parasitic gastrointestinal infection. Examination of the material aspirated from a liver abscess does not frequently reveal trophozoites or leukocytes. Trophozoites can be observed by tissue histopathology.

PREP Pearls

- Invasive *Entamoeba histolytica* infections require treatment with metronidazole or tinidazole in addition to an intraluminal amebicide.
- Serum antibodies to *Entamoeba histolytica* are detectable in 95% of individuals with invasive amebiasis.
- While the majority of *Entamoeba histolytica* infections are asymptomatic, manifestations of infection can include abdominal pain, diarrhea, weight loss, and abscesses, most commonly in the liver.

American Board of Pediatrics Content Specification(s)/ Content Area

- Recognize the clinical features associated with amoebiasis, and manage appropriately
- Understand the epidemiology of amoebiasis

Suggested Readings

American Academy of Pediatrics. Amebiasis. In: Kimberlin DW, Brady MT, Jackson MA, Long SS, eds. *Red Book: 2018 Report of the Committee on Infectious Diseases.* 31st ed. Itasca, IL: American Academy of Pediatrics; 2018:208-210

Custodio H. Protozoan parasites. *Pediatr Rev.* 2016;37(2):59-71.

Item 227   Preferred Response: C

In the vignette, a late preterm infant at 36 weeks' gestation was born to a mother who was group B *Streptococcus* (GBS)–positive and treated with 1 dose of penicillin. He should be evaluated with a complete blood cell count and blood culture and observed in the hospital for 48 hours because of premature gestation and inadequate intrapartum antibiotic prophylaxis during labor (<4 hours before delivery). Early-onset sepsis (EOS) continues to be a significant cause of morbidity and mortality for term neonates born in the United States, with a rate of 0.57 per 1,000 live births. Neonates are exposed to microorganisms from the maternal genital and anorectal tract during labor or via ascending spread after rupture of membranes. The primary organisms responsible for EOS are *Streptococcus agalactiae*, also known as GBS, and *Escherichia coli*. Most commonly, EOS due to GBS presents with respiratory distress secondary to GBS pneumonia. However, infected infants may also present with asymptomatic bacteremia.

Pregnant women should undergo vaginal-rectal screening for GBS colonization between 35 and 37 weeks of gestation.

Women who screen positive for GBS should receive prophylactic antibiotics during labor, at least 4 hours before delivery, to decrease transfer of GBS from the mother to infant. Since the advent of maternal screening and intrapartum prophylaxis against GBS, rates of EOS due to GBS have decreased. However, intrapartum antibiotic prophylaxis does not eliminate the risk of EOS infection. Other risk factors for EOS include prematurity, prolonged rupture of membranes, and maternal intrauterine infection. Inadequate intrapartum antibiotic prophylaxis in a high-risk group such as premature neonates, may result in partial treatment and delayed onset of symptoms.

Asymptomatic neonates of 37 or more weeks of gestation born to mothers with unknown or positive GBS status whose mothers receive inadequate intrapartum prophylaxis may be monitored without additional laboratory testing before discharge. Because of the increased risk of infection due to prematurity, asymptomatic neonates born before 37 weeks of gestation whose mothers received inadequate GBS prophylaxis should be evaluated with a complete blood cell count and blood culture. In addition, they should remain hospitalized and monitored for 48 hours before discharge.

Discharge from the hospital 24 hours after birth should be reserved for well-appearing term neonates born to mothers without GBS colonization or mothers with GBS colonization who receive adequate intrapartum antibiotic prophylaxis, provided adequate care and follow-up can be assured.

PREP Pearls

- Asymptomatic neonates born before 37 weeks of gestation whose mothers received inadequate group B *Streptococcus* prophylaxis may be evaluated with a complete blood cell count and blood culture, and should be monitored in the hospital for 48 hours before discharge.
- Inadequate intrapartum antibiotic prophylaxis in a high-risk group may result in partial treatment and delayed onset of symptoms.
- The primary organisms responsible for early-onset symptoms are *Streptococcus agalactiae*, also known as group B *Streptococcus*, and *Escherichia coli*.

American Board of Pediatrics Content Specification(s)/ Content Area

- Plan the appropriate management of an infant born to a mother with a positive culture for group B *Streptococcus*
- Recognize the major clinical features associated with group B streptococcal infection, and manage appropriately
- Understand the epidemiology of *Streptococcus agalactiae*

Suggested Readings

Stoll BJ, Hansen NI, Sanchez PJ et al. Early onset neonatal sepsis: the burden of group B Streptococcal and E. coli disease continues. *Pediatrics*. 2011;127(5):817-26.

Verani JR, McGee L, Schrag SJ; Division of Bacterial Diseases, National Center for Immunization and Respiratory Diseases, Centers for Disease Control and Prevention. Prevention of perinatal group B streptococcal disease revised guidelines from CDC, 2010. *MMWR Recomm Rep*. 2010;59(No. RR-10):1-36

For an athlete with type 1 diabetes mellitus (DM), decreasing the basal rate of insulin infusion is the best strategy to lower the risk of hypoglycemia after exercise. Exercise has important health benefits for children and adolescents. Children with DM have an increased risk of coronary artery disease, and routine physical activity is an important practice to mitigate this risk. In addition, regular physical activity may help improve blood glucose control.

In individuals without type 1 DM, exercise leads to increased glucose uptake and a subsequent decrease in insulin secretion. Because children with type 1 DM do not experience a physiologic drop in serum insulin with increased use of glucose, unless they strategically manage their use of exogenous insulin, they are at increased risk for hypoglycemia during and after exercise. The response to exercise varies among individuals with type 1 DM, so it can be very difficult to predict how each child's blood glucose levels will change with exercise. Blood glucose levels also depend on exercise duration and intensity, diet, and the type and amount of insulin administered.

When young athletes with type 1 DM begin a new sports season, they should introduce exercise gradually. Athletes using an insulin pump should decrease their basal insulin 1 to 2 hours before exercise. Individuals receiving multiple insulin injections throughout the day should decrease their pre-exercise doses. Athletes should have well-balanced meals 3 to 4 hours before intense exercise, and should have sugar (eg, sugar-sweetened drinks, glucose tablets) available at practices and games in case hypoglycemia occurs. Children and their families should keep a diary with details about the length and intensity of exercise, diet, and blood glucose levels so that their health care team members can make informed recommendations about changes to diet and insulin doses. Physicians should include in their counseling of patients with type 1 DM that athletic performance appears to be better in individuals with near-normal glucose and hemoglobin A1c levels. Performance improvements are often a better incentive for young athletes than future health benefits.

Exercise increases sensitivity to insulin. The timing of increased risk of postexercise hypoglycemia can vary, depending on the type of insulin given, but typically peaks about 3 to 4 hours after exercise. The increased risk persists for 12 or more hours after exercise, and is magnified with greater intensity and length of activity. Therefore, young athletes should always check their blood sugar after exercise, including shortly before bedtime. Serum cortisol levels are higher and insulin sensitivity is generally lower in the morning, so the risk of hypoglycemia appears to be lower with early morning exercise.

After intense physical activity, children with type 1 DM may need to consume snacks with a low-glycemic index to counter the risk of late hypoglycemia. Although a source of sugar should be available at sports practices and games in case an athlete experiences hypoglycemia, snacks before exercise are typically unnecessary if the basal rate of insulin is decreased. In addition, extra snacks before exercise may put an athlete at risk for hyperglycemia.

PREP Pearls

- Physicians should include in their counseling of patients with type 1 DM that athletic performance appears to be better in individuals with near-normal glucose and hemoglobin A1c levels. Performance improvements are often a better incentive for young athletes than future health benefits.
- The timing of increased risk of postexercise hypoglycemia can vary depending on the type of insulin given but typically peaks about 3 to 4 hours after exercise.
- Young athletes with type 1 diabetes mellitus should lower their pre-exercise insulin dose or decrease their basal infusion of insulin 1 to 2 hours before exercise.

American Board of Pediatrics Content Specification(s)/ Content Area

- Understand the guidelines for sports participation for patients who have type 1 diabetes

Suggested Readings

Draznin MB. Managing the adolescent athlete with type 1 diabetes mellitus. *Pediatr Clin North Am.* 2010;57(3):829-837.

Robertson K, Riddell MC, Guinhouya BC, Adolfsson P, Hanas R. ISPAD Clinical Practice Consensus Guidelines 2014: exercise in children and adolescents with diabetes. *Pediatr Diab.* 2014;15(suppl 20):203-223.

Sperling M. *Pediatric Endocrinology.* 4th ed. Philadelphia, PA: Elsevier/ Saunders; 2014

Item 229   Preferred Response: C

The 4-month-old infant in this vignette demonstrates frequent effortless regurgitation soon after feedings, is otherwise asymptomatic, continues to feed well, and has a normal growth trajectory. She most likely has uncomplicated gastroesophageal reflux (GER). Her parents can be reassured that this is a normal physiologic condition that usually resolves spontaneously by 12 months of age.

Gastroesophageal reflux is defined as the passage of gastric contents into the esophagus. It can occur several times per day in healthy individuals of all ages. Up to two-thirds of infants have GER. During the first 3 to 4 months of age, 50% of infants experience daily regurgitation, the effortless passage of gastric contents into the mouth, or vomiting, which is more forceful. By 12 months of age, only 5% of infants continue to experience episodes of spitting up. When associated with pathological consequences, this condition is known as gastroesophageal reflux disease (GERD). Common presenting signs or symptoms of GERD in infants include recurrent regurgitation or vomiting, poor weight gain, feeding refusal, dysphagia, irritability, arching of the back during feeds, sleep problems, and persistent respiratory complaints, such as cough, wheezing, or pneumonia.

Parents of infants with uncomplicated GER can be reassured that the prognosis is excellent. They should be educated on simple lifestyle modifications that may decrease the GER. Because large-volume feeds can promote regurgitation due to gastric distention, offering less volume per feeding while shortening the interval between feedings will often decrease the amount of spitting up, and still provide adequate caloric

nutrition. Other practical suggestions include frequent burping and holding the infant upright for 20 to 30 minutes after feedings. Offering rice cereal–thickened formula or breast milk, or a commercially thickened formula may be suggested as another strategy. Gastroesophageal reflux may be exacerbated by semi-supine positioning, as in an infant carrier or car seat, and should be avoided for the period immediately after feeding. Passive smoke exposure can worsen GER and should be discouraged. If the infant's condition does not improve with these suggestions, or progresses to GERD with feeding/swallowing problems or poor weight gain and undernutrition, further evaluation and treatment are warranted.

PREP Pearls

- Gastroesophageal reflux is defined as the passage of gastric contents into the esophagus; it can occur several times per day in healthy individuals of all ages.
- The prognosis of gastroesophageal reflux is excellent. Parents should be educated on simple dietary and positional modifications that may decrease gastroesophageal reflux in their infant.
- Up to two-thirds of infants have uncomplicated gastroesophageal reflux. By 12 months of age, only 5% of infants continue to experience episodes of regurgitation.

American Board of Pediatrics Content Specification(s)/ Content Area

- Understand the prognosis for patients who have gastroesophageal reflux

Suggested Readings

Lightdale JR, Gremse DA. Gastroesophageal reflux: management guidance for the pediatrician. *Pediatrics.* 2013;131(5):e1684-e1695.

Sullivan JS, Sundaram SS. Gastroesophageal reflux. *Pediatr Rev.* 2012;33(6):243-254.

Item 230   Preferred Response: B

The patient in this vignette has Wilson disease, an autosomal recessive neurologic disorder associated with chronic liver disease, resulting from abnormal copper deposition in tissue. Wilson disease may present with clinical features including acute hepatitis and/or chronic hepatitis or cirrhosis, neurologic symptoms (movement disorders, tremors, ataxia, seizures), psychiatric symptoms (dementia, depression, schizophrenia, bipolar disorder), and ocular findings (Kayser-Fleischer rings). Renal tubular dysfunction, hemolysis, cardiac arrhythmias, and endocrine disorders may also occur. The patient in this vignette has evidence of chronic liver disease and portal hypertension (scleral icterus, splenomegaly, ascites, palmar erythema, thrombocytopenia, elevated aminotransferase levels, elevated conjugated bilirubin level, and mild coagulopathy) with neurologic/psychiatric symptoms (ataxia and depression), consistent with Wilson disease. Wilson disease should be considered in any older child or adolescent with liver injury of any degree and should be highly suspected in individuals with liver injury and neurologic/psychiatric symptoms.

This patient has cholestasis, or conjugated hyperbilirubinemia. Causes of cholestasis in older children and adolescents include biliary tract obstruction (cholelithiasis, choledochal cyst), viral infections (eg, infectious hepatitis A, B, and C; Epstein-Barr virus; cytomegalovirus), autoimmune disease (primary sclerosing cholangitis, autoimmune hepatitis), drug-induced cholestasis, Wilson disease, and bile transport defects. In neonates, there are many more causes of cholestasis, including biliary atresia, congenital/acquired infections, genetic/metabolic diseases (eg, α_1-antitrypsin deficiency, cystic fibrosis), and endocrine disorders (eg, hypothyroidism, panhypopituitarism).

In patients with cholestasis, in addition to considering the etiology, careful attention should be paid to nutritional status. Cholestatic infants and children may be malnourished because of fat maldigestion and fat malabsorption resulting from poor bile flow from the liver to the small intestine. This maldigestion and malabsorption may result in greasy malodorous stools (steatorrhea), weight loss, poor growth, and fat-soluble vitamin deficiency. Nutritional management of these patients includes increasing caloric intake (through oral supplements or enteral supplementation with nasogastric feeding tubes; preferably with supplements that are high in medium-chain triglycerides) and using fat-soluble vitamin supplements.

Although α_1-antitrypsin deficiency is a cause of cholestasis, it most commonly presents early in life with prolonged jaundice. In addition, it is associated with emphysema in adults and is not associated with neurologic/psychiatric disease. Although chronic hepatitis C infection can result in significant chronic liver injury and portal hypertension, severe disease rarely occurs in children, and hepatitis C infection is not associated with neurologic/psychiatric disease. Partial thromboplastin time is used to assess bleeding disorders.

PREP Pearls

- A history of neuropsychiatric symptoms in combination with any degree of liver injury in an older child or adolescent should prompt evaluation for Wilson disease.

American Board of Pediatrics Content Specification(s)/ Content Area

- Understand the nutritional causes of growth failure associated with chronic cholestatic disease, including the effects of nutrient digestion and absorption
- Recognize the clinical features associated with α-1-antitrypsin deficiency
- Recognize the clinical features associated with Wilson disease

Suggested Readings

Brumbaugh D, Mack C. Conjugated hyperbilirubinemia in children. *Pediatr Rev.* 2012;33(7):291-302.

Perlmutter DH. Alpha-1 antitrypsin deficiency. In: Suchy FJ, Sokol RJ, Balistreri WF, eds. *Liver Disease in Children.* 4th ed. Cambridge, United Kingdom: Cambridge University Press; 2014:400-418.

Roberts EA, Schilsky ML. Diagnosis and treatment of Wilson disease: an update. *Hepatology.* 2008;47(6):2089-2111.

Sokol RJ. Copper metabolism and copper storage disorders. In: Suchy FJ, Sokol RJ, Balistreri WF, eds. *Liver Disease in Children.* 4th ed. Cambridge, United Kingdom: Cambridge University Press; 2014:465-492

Risk factors for suicide completion include the availability of a firearm in the home, use of lethal methods, male sex, history of prior suicide attempt, substance abuse, and history of a chronic mental health diagnosis such as depression or bipolar disorder. Completed suicide is most commonly accomplished by use of a firearm, which is the leading mechanism used by males. Suicide attempts are more frequent in girls whereas suicide completions are more common in boys. Decreasing access to firearms is an important component of addressing suicide risk. Attention-deficit/hyperactivity disorder and problems with academic achievement are risk factors for depression, not suicide completion. Poor social communication skills can cause difficulties in functioning but are not a risk factor for suicide completion.

When depression is suspected or diagnosed in a child or adolescent, risk factors for suicide must be determined. These risk factors include a previous suicide attempt, family history of suicide, mental health diagnosis (eg, depression, anxiety, bipolar disorder, psychosis), substance use, history of sexual abuse, being a sexual minority youth (eg, lesbian, gay, bisexual, transgender, questioning), bullying, access to lethal means (eg, firearms), and parental mental health disorder. Suicide attempts may be prompted by recent stressful experiences such as family loss, family conflict, academic difficulties, or end of a meaningful relationship. Clusters of suicide may occur when there has been a peer suicide, particularly when it has been accompanied by media coverage. Protective factors against suicidal behavior include family and peer support, school connectedness, religious involvement, and effective coping strategies.

In addition to interviewing the parents, the health care provider should also speak with the child or adolescent privately. Confidentiality should be reviewed and the patient should be asked about depressive symptoms; suicidal thoughts, plans, and behaviors; and substance use. Interviewing the child about these topics does not increase the chance of suicide. Concerning behaviors include revealing suicidal thoughts on social media, distributing possessions, and being preoccupied with death (eg, in drawings, play, music, or media). A history of self-harm or attempted suicide should be ascertained and recognized as a call for help. An emergent mental health evaluation (eg, same-day mental health professional appointment, emergency department transfer, hospitalization) is necessary if there is concern about the immediate safety of the child (eg, current suicidal intent or plan or unstable mental status such as psychosis), particularly when there is insufficient supervision or home support.

Outpatient treatment with appropriate mental health follow up may be considered for patients who are not acutely suicidal and who have adequate family and social supports. A safety plan should be developed and should include whom to contact and how to access care in case of crisis or worsening suicidality (eg, family and social supports, 911, crisis number, emergency department, on-call physician). Additional safety measures include removal of firearms, weapons, ropes, and poisons from the home and locking up medications. Identification and treatment of mental health conditions are important. Psychoeducation should be provided and evidence-based treatments discussed. Treatment of depression with psychotherapy (eg, cognitive behavioral therapy) and/or medication (eg, selective serotonin reuptake inhibitor) can reduce the risk of suicide. Families should be linked to local mental health resources. Ideally, the primary care physician and mental health professional should collaborate in the care of these at-risk patients.

PREP Pearls

- An emergent mental health evaluation (eg, same-day mental health professional appointment, emergency department transfer, hospitalization) is necessary if there is concern about the immediate safety of the child (eg, current suicidal intent or plan, unstable mental status such as psychosis), particularly when there is insufficient supervision or home support.
- Concerning behaviors for suicide include revealing suicidal thoughts on social media, distributing possessions, and being preoccupied with death (eg, in drawings, play, music, or media).
- Risk factors for suicide completion include the availability of a firearm in the home, use of lethal methods, male sex, history of prior suicide attempt, substance abuse, and history of chronic mental health diagnosis such as depression or bipolar disorder.

American Board of Pediatrics Content Specification(s)/ Content Area

- Understand risk factors associated with suicidal behavior/completed suicide
- Plan the appropriate assessment and management of suicidal ideation in patients of various ages
- Identify factors that are protective against suicidal behavior

Suggested Readings

Maslow GR, Dunlap K, Chung RJ. Depression and suicide in children and adolescents. *Pediatr Rev*. 2015;36(7):299-310.

Shain B; Committee on Adolescence. Suicide and suicide attempts in adolescents. *Pediatrics*. 2016;138(1):e1-e11.

Tang MH, Pinsky EG. Mood and affect disorders. *Pediatr Rev*. 2015;36(2):52-61.

Item 232   Preferred Response: D

The boy in the vignette had a simple febrile seizure. Age at onset of febrile seizures is a strong predictor of recurrence risk. In children younger than 1 year who have a simple febrile seizure, the recurrence risk is around 50%. In children older than 1 year, the recurrence risk is as low as 20%. Other risk factors for recurrent febrile seizure include febrile seizure in 1st degree relatives, low degree of fever in the emergency department, and brief duration between the onset of fever and the seizure. Compared with a simple febrile seizure, a complex febrile seizure (focal, duration >15 minutes, or recurrence within 24 hours), does not increase the risk of recurrence.

Immunizations can trigger febrile seizures. Diphtheria-tetanus-pertussis (DTaP) immunization is a risk factor for febrile seizure on the day of immunization only. Measles-mumps-rubella (MMR) immunization is a risk factor for febrile seizure on days 8 to 14 after immunization; in children 12 to 23 months of age, the MMR-varicella combination vaccine has a

slightly higher risk for febrile seizures 5 to 12 days after immunization. Occurrence of febrile seizure following DTaP and MMR immunizations is not associated with increased risk of epilepsy or adverse neurodevelopmental outcomes.

Electroencephalography has a limited value in predicting the risk for recurrent febrile seizure or later development of epilepsy, therefore it is not typically recommended after a febrile seizure.

PREP Pearls

- Compared with a simple febrile seizure, a complex febrile seizure does not have an increased risk of recurrence.
- Diphtheria-tetanus-pertussis immunization is a risk factor for febrile seizure on the day of immunization only. Measles-mumps-rubella immunization is a risk factor for febrile seizure 8 to 14 days after immunization. Occurrence of febrile seizure in these 2 situations is not associated with an increased risk of epilepsy or adverse neurodevelopmental outcomes.
- In children younger than 1 year who have a simple febrile seizure, the recurrence risk is around 50%. In children older than 1 year, the recurrence risk is as low as 20%.

American Board of Pediatrics Content Specification(s)/ Content Area

- Understand the risk factors associated with febrile seizures
- Understand the difference between simple and complex febrile seizures

Suggested Readings

Barlow WE, Davis RL, Glasser JW, et al; Centers for Disease Control and Prevention Vaccine Safety Datalink Working Group. The risk of seizures after receipt of whole-cell pertussis or measles, mumps, and rubella vaccine. *N Engl J Med*. 2001;345:656-661.

Berg AT, Shinnar S, Darefsky AS, Holford TR, Shapiro ED, Salomon ME, Crain EF, Hauser AW. Predictors of recurrent febrile seizures. a prospective cohort study. *Arch Pediatr Adolesc Med*. 1997;151(4):371–378.

Sidhu R, Velayudam K, Barnes G. Pediatric seizures. *Pediatr Rev*. 2013;34(8):333-342.

Subcommittee on Febrile Seizures; American Academy of Pediatrics. Neurodiagnostic evaluation of the child with a simple febrile seizure. *Pediatrics*. 2011;127(2):389-394.

Item 233   Preferred Response: A

The neonate in this vignette has proximal hypospadias located at the penoscrotal junction. Hypospadias is a congenital anomaly of the penis that results in abnormal ventral placement of the urethral meatus (Item C233). The urethral opening may be located distally (glandular, coronal, subcoronal), in the middle (distal shaft, midshaft, posterior penile), or proximally (penoscrotal, scrotal, perineal). Typically hypospadias develops as an isolated malformation, although it may also accompany chordee, ventral curvature of the penis, and other anomalies. While the etiology of hypospadias is unknown, studies suggest it is multifactorial, including genetic, maternal, fetal, and environmental factors. Any disruption in masculinization may result in hypospadias. The neonate in this vignette has proximal hypospadias in addition to bilateral cryptorchidism with a phallus length of 2 cm, which is considered microphallus (normal stretched length

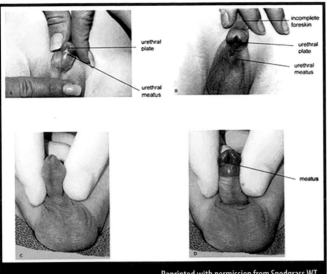

Reprinted with permission from Snodgrass WT. Consultation with the specialist: hypospadias. *Pediatr Rev.* 2004;25(2):64.

Item C233: Varieties of hypospadias. A. In most cases, the urethral opening is on or near the glans, and the tissue that should have completed tubularization extends distally as the "urethral plate." B. With proximal hypospadias, the urethral meatus is at the penoscrotal junction, with the urethral plate extending to the glans tips. Most cases of proximal hypospadias also have ventral curvature, commonly referred to as "chordee." C. Hypospadias variant with a completely developed foreskin concealing the defect. D. When the foreskin is retracted, the meatus is noted at the corona.

in full-term neonates is 2.5-3.5 cm). With this combination of findings, disorders of sexual development, such as XX virilization, XY undervirilization, mixed gonadal dysgenesis, and congenital adrenal hyperplasia, must be considered.

Hypospadias of the distal and middle penile shaft usually occurs as an isolated anomaly. However, it may be an associated feature in syndromes including aniridia associated with Wilms tumor, Opitz G/BBB syndrome, and Fraser syndrome. Cryptorchidism and inguinal hernia are the most common anomalies associated with the genital tract.

Initial management of typical hypospadias in which neither cryptorchidism nor other congenital anomalies are present is to delay circumcision. Because surgical management is often required for both cosmetic and functional purposes, preservation of the preputial skin may be necessary for urethroplasty. Surgical repair is often undertaken as an outpatient procedure between 3 and 18 months of age.

For proximal hypospadias associated with cryptorchidism or ambiguous genitalia, a more extensive evaluation should be performed. This includes pelvic ultrasonography to evaluate internal genitalia and a karyotype. Bilateral cryptorchidism warrants screening for salt-wasting forms of congenital adrenal hyperplasia by obtaining serum electrolytes and a 17a-hydroxyprogesterone level.

While vesicoureteral reflux and renal agenesis may occur in 5% of children who have proximal hypospadias, intersexuality is found in up to 50% of cases of proximal hypospadias associated with cryptorchidism, making it much more common. Rarely, imperforate anus is associated with hypospadias.

PREP Pearls

- Evaluation of proximal hypospadias and cryptorchidism includes pelvic ultrasonography for internal genitalia, karyotype, and serum electrolytes to screen for congenital adrenal hyperplasia.
- Infants with proximal hypospadias (penoscrotal, scrotal, perineal) and cryptorchidism should be evaluated for an intersex condition.
- Surgical management of hypospadias usually occurs between 3 and 18 months of age.

American Board of Pediatrics Content Specification(s)/ Content Area

- Plan the appropriate management of hypospadias
- Recognize disorders associated with hypospadias

Suggested Readings

Madhok N, Scarbach K, Shahid-Saless S. Hypospadias. *Pediatr Rev.* 2009;30(6):235-237.

McCann-Crosby B. Ambiguous genitalia: evaluation and management in the newborn. *NeoReviews.* 2016;17(3):e144-e153.

Snodgrass WT. Consultation with the specialist: hypospadias. *Pediatr Rev.* 2004;25(2):63-67.

Speiser PW, Azzis R, Baskin LS, et al. Congenital adrenal hyperplasia due to steroid 21-hydroxylase deficiency: an Endocrine Society clinical practice guideline. *J Clin Endocrinol Metab.* 2010;95(10):4133-4160.

Item 234	Preferred Response: C

The girl in this vignette has an unremarkable medical and developmental history, pallor and tachycardia, a severe, normocytic anemia, absolute reticulocytopenia, and a normal white blood cell count, differential, and platelet count. Although the differential diagnosis for childhood anemia is broad, it can quickly be narrowed with the use of a diagnostic algorithm (Item C234). A reasonable first step in narrowing the differential diagnosis is to assess whether the anemia is destructive or productive. The girl in this vignette has a very low reticulocyte count; thus, it is likely that her anemia is a result of failure of red blood cell production.

Following the algorithm, a next reasonable step is to ascertain whether the anemia is microcytic, normocytic, or macrocytic. The girl's mean corpuscular volume (MCV) is 75 fL. A general rule is that:

$$\text{Normal MCV (in a noninfant child)} = \text{approximately } 72 + \text{age in years}$$

Thus, the girl in this vignette has a normocytic anemia. The differential diagnosis for a normocytic anemia caused by a failure of red cell production is fairly small, and most commonly includes competition for marrow space (eg, leukemia), viral suppression, or transient erythroblastopenia of childhood (TEC). The girl's age, presentation, and laboratory evaluation are all consistent with TEC, which is an idiopathic, self-limited anemia. The white blood cell count and platelet count are typically normal. This condition usually affects children between 18 and 26 months of age. Patients with TEC should be followed with serial complete blood cell counts and reticulocyte counts to insure the expected full erythropoietic recovery.

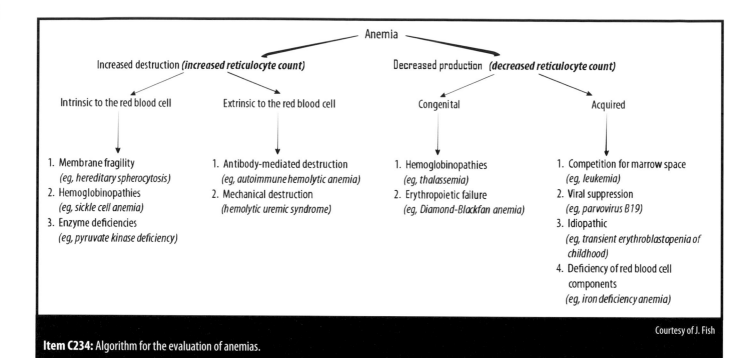

Item C234: Algorithm for the evaluation of anemias.

Anemia

Increased destruction (*increased reticulocyte count*)

Decreased production (*decreased reticulocyte count*)

Intrinsic to the red blood cell

1. Membrane fragility
   (*eg, hereditary spherocytosis*)
2. Hemoglobinopathies
   (*eg, sickle cell anemia*)
3. Enzyme deficiencies
   (*eg, pyruvate kinase deficiency*)

Extrinsic to the red blood cell

1. Antibody-mediated destruction
   (*eg, autoimmune hemolytic anemia*)
2. Mechanical destruction
   (*hemolytic uremic syndrome*)

Congenital

1. Hemoglobinopathies
   (*eg, thalassemia*)
2. Erythropoietic failure
   (*eg, Diamond-Blackfan anemia*)

Acquired

1. Competition for marrow space
   (*eg, leukemia*)
2. Viral suppression
   (*eg, parvovirus B19*)
3. Idiopathic
   (*eg, transient erythroblastopenia of childhood*)
4. Deficiency of red blood cell components
   (*eg, iron deficiency anemia*)

Courtesy of J. Fish

Flow cytometry is useful for evaluating the phenotype of the white blood cells and is the diagnostic test of choice for childhood acute leukemia. This child is very unlikely to have leukemia because her white blood cell count, differential, and platelet count are normal. If there were competition for bone marrow space, all 3 cell lines (white blood cells, red blood cells, and platelets) would be abnormal. Hemoglobin electrophoresis is the test of choice for assessing for hemoglobinopathies, such as thalassemia. This child does not have thalassemia because her MCV is normal. A Meckel scan would be useful to assess for occult blood loss. The low reticulocyte count, normal MCV (making iron deficiency unlikely), and generally well appearance of the child make an occult bleed unlikely.

PREP Pearls

- For failure of red cell production, the mean corpuscular volume can greatly narrow the differential diagnosis.
- The reticulocyte count distinguishes between anemia caused by a red cell destructive vs productive process.
- Transient erythroblastopenia of childhood is an idiopathic, self-limiting disease that should be followed by serial complete blood cell counts and reticulocyte counts.

American Board of Pediatrics Content Specification(s)/ Content Area

- Distinguish between the clinical characteristics of Diamond-Blackfan syndrome and transient erythroblastopenia of childhood
- Plan the appropriate management of transient erythroblastopenia of childhood
- Recognize the clinical and laboratory findings associated with transient erythroblastopenia of childhood
- Plan the appropriate management of severe anemia of various etiologies, while considering the risks associated with various therapies

Suggested Readings

Kelly N. Thalassemia. *Pediatr Rev.* 2012;33(9):434-435.

Segel GB, Hirsh MG, Feig SA. Managing anemia in a pediatric office practice: part 2. *Pediatr Rev.* 2002;23(4):111-122.

Segel GB, Hirsh MG, Feig SA. Managing anemia in pediatric office practice: part 1. *Pediatr Rev.* 2002;23(3):75-84.

Item 235   Preferred Response: A

The adolescent boy in the vignette presents with dyspnea, shallow respirations, and paradoxical chest wall movement after sustaining blunt chest wall trauma in a motor vehicle crash. Chest radiography reveals a sternal fracture as well as multiple rib fractures, resulting in flail chest. The best next step in management is endotracheal intubation and mechanical ventilation.

Significant thoracic trauma is relatively uncommon in children, accounting for approximately 4% to 6% of patients admitted to pediatric trauma centers; however, thoracic injuries can be life-threatening when they do occur. The pediatric chest wall is much more pliable than the adult chest wall, therefore providing less protection from blunt traumatic forces. In children, energy forces applied to the thorax are likely to be transferred through the chest wall to the underlying organs, resulting in internal injuries such as pulmonary contusions without evidence of external injuries (such as rib fractures).

The immediate priorities when stabilizing children with chest wall trauma are assessment and stabilization of the airway, breathing, and circulation, all of which may be affected because of the location of vital structures within the thorax and the critical role of an intact chest wall in normal respiratory function. In children with significant chest wall injuries, providers should be prepared to establish a definitive airway through emergent intubation or surgical airway maneuvers, initiate mechanical ventilation, administer intravenous fluids and/or blood products as indicated, and perform other life-saving procedures including needle decompression, placement of thoracostomy tubes, and pericardiocentesis.

Most chest wall injuries occur in the context of multisystem trauma in children; therefore, providers must also maintain a high suspicion for other injuries—including those to the head, neck, abdomen, and pelvis—when treating pediatric patients with thoracic trauma. The presence of rib, sternal, and scapular fractures should raise concern for significant associated intrathoracic injuries, given the pliability of the pediatric chest wall.

Fractures to segments of 2 or more ribs on the same side of the chest wall may cause a flail chest, with a chest wall segment that has lost continuity with the thoracic cage. Patients with this injury (such as the boy in the vignette) will have paradoxical movement of the chest wall, and may have impaired ventilation. Any patient with flail chest who is experiencing respiratory distress should undergo intubation and receive positive pressure ventilation to facilitate lung expansion and ensure adequate ventilation.

Immediate operative management by a cardiothoracic surgeon is not required at this time for the boy in the vignette. In patients sustaining blunt thoracic trauma, supportive measures and close clinical observation are most commonly indicated; in contrast, patients who sustain penetrating chest wall trauma often require surgical intervention, because of the high potential for injury to vital structures within the thoracic cavity.

Placement of an external splint device to stabilize the chest wall is not indicated in this patient. In children with rib fractures, splinting or binding the chest wall is contraindicated, as this may interfere with the child's ability to adequately ventilate.

Although the boy in the vignette has sustained significant chest wall injuries, his breath sounds are equal and his chest radiograph does not reveal a hemothorax or pneumothorax. Therefore, placement of chest tubes is not indicated at this time.

PREP Pearls

- Any patient with flail chest who is in respiratory distress should undergo intubation and be managed with positive pressure ventilation to facilitate lung expansion and ensure adequate ventilation.
- Immediate priorities when stabilizing children with chest wall trauma are assessment and stabilization of the airway, breathing, and circulation—all of which may be affected due to the location of vital structures within the thorax and the critical role of an intact chest wall in normal respiratory function.
- Most chest wall injuries occur in the context of multisystem trauma in children; therefore, providers must also maintain a high suspicion for other injuries, including those to the head, neck, abdomen, and pelvis.

American Board of Pediatrics Content Specification(s)/Content Area

- Plan the appropriate stabilization procedures for a child who has experienced chest wall trauma

Suggested Readings

American College of Surgeons Committee on Trauma. Thoracic trauma. In: *Advanced Trauma Life Support (ATLS) Student Course Manual*. 9th ed. Chicago, IL: American College of Surgeons; 2012;chap 4.

Eisenberg M, Mooney DP. Thoracic trauma. In: Shaw KN, Bachur RG, eds. *Fleisher and Ludwig's Textbook of Pediatric Emergency Medicine*. 7th ed. Philadelphia, PA: Lippincott Williams & Wilkins; 2016;chap 123.

Item 236   **Preferred Response: D**

The most likely diagnosis for the neonate in the vignette is multicystic dysplastic kidney (MCDK). Multicystic dysplastic kidney is the most common form of renal cystic disease in children. It is usually suspected prenatally based on renal abnormalities detected on ultrasonography or in neonates with an abdominal mass on physical examination. Multicystic dysplastic kidney usually involves the whole kidney, but segmental renal involvement is also seen. The classic findings on renal ultrasonography include unilateral multiple noncommunicating cysts of varying sizes with intervening dysplastic renal tissue. The affected MCDK is nonfunctional; the prognosis is dependent on the contralateral kidney function. There is an increased incidence of congenital renal anomalies such as vesicoureteral reflux, renal agenesis, or ureteropelvic junction obstruction in the contralateral "normal" kidney. In most cases, the MCDK will undergo spontaneous involution. There is a small risk for malignant transformation in the MCDK; thus, observation with serial ultrasonography is important to confirm involution, and is preferred over nephrectomy. Most patients with MCDK have normal renal function associated with compensatory hypertrophy of the contralateral kidney, with a favorable long-term prognosis. These patients with single functioning kidneys should be monitored for hypertension, proteinuria, and serum creatinine (glomerular filtration rate) to identify renal injury. Rare cases with bilateral MCDK or contralateral renal agenesis/severe hypoplasia generally present with severe oligohydramnios leading to Potter syndrome/sequence due to nonfunctioning kidneys. Such cases are usually lethal because of severe pulmonary hypoplasia and renal failure.

The neonate in the vignette has normal serum chemistry values. However, early on, the neonate's serum creatinine concentration (usually <1.0 mg/dL [88.4 μmol/L]) is reflective of maternal serum creatinine concentration. Subsequent serum creatinine levels will become reflective of the neonate's renal function. In a full-term neonate, the serum creatinine concentration normalizes in 7 to 10 days, whereas in a preterm infant, it may take up to 1 month to normalize.

Autosomal dominant polycystic kidney disease (ADPKD) is considered to be an adult-onset disease. Patients with ADPKD have renal macrocysts that are visible on renal ultrasonography. However, with recent improvements in ultrasonographic techniques, ADPKD is increasingly being reported in the pediatric population, including fetuses and neonates. Children with ADPKD are usually asymptomatic, and are diagnosed when renal cysts are detected during imaging studies for nonrenal abdominal symptoms or upon screening in those with a positive family history. Disease manifestations in children are similar to those seen in adults.

Common presentations include persistent microscopic hematuria, hypertension, flank pain (associated with renal cyst hemorrhage), or urinary tract infection. Serum creatinine is not usually elevated in children with ADPKD; renal function remains normal until the fourth decade of life.

Autosomal recessive polycystic kidney disease (ARPKD) is usually detected on antenatal ultrasonography after 24 weeks of gestation. Ultrasonography demonstrates large, echogenic kidneys with decreased corticomedullary differentiation. Macrocysts are typically not seen. Hepatomegaly and increased hepatic echogenicity are usually seen in severe cases of ARPKD, indicating the development of congenital hepatic fibrosis. Age at presentation is relatively evenly divided into one-third each before 1 year, between 1 and 20 years, and after age 20 years. Earlier presentation is associated with more severe renal involvement. Adolescents and adults commonly present with symptoms related to hepatomegaly and portal hypertension (secondary to congenital hepatic fibrosis). Occasionally, neonates with ARPKD may present with Potter syndrome (severe renal dysfunction and associated oligohydramnios) and associated ventilation problems immediately after birth, because of pulmonary hypoplasia. Renal failure develops in most patients with ARPKD, the progression of which is dependent on the severity of disease, with greater impairment reported in patients presenting in the neonatal period or infancy.

Autosomal dominant tubulointerstitial kidney disease (previously called "medullary cystic kidney disease") is slowly progressive, with onset in the teenage years and end-stage renal disease requiring renal replacement therapy between ages 20 and 70 years. Medullary renal cysts are not usually seen on renal ultrasonography. Early-onset gout, unexplained renal failure with an unremarkable urinalysis (minimal to no proteinuria, no hematuria), and a strong family history of gout or chronic kidney disease is suggestive of underlying tubulointerstitial kidney disease.

PREP Pearls

- Children with single functioning kidneys should be monitored for hypertension, proteinuria, and serum creatinine (glomerular filtration rate) to identify renal injury.
- Most patients with multicystic dysplastic kidney have normal renal function associated with compensatory hypertrophy of the contralateral kidney, with a favorable long-term prognosis.
- Multicystic dysplastic kidney, the most common form of renal cystic disease in children, is suspected based on renal abnormalities detected on antenatal ultrasonography or in neonates with abdominal mass on physical examination.

American Board of Pediatrics Content Specification(s)/ Content Area

- Recognize the clinical findings associated with multicystic dysplastic kidney in patients of various ages
- Recognize the clinical findings associated with autosomal-recessive polycystic kidney disease in patients of various ages

Suggested Readings

Elder JS. Congenital anomalies and dysgenesis of the kidney. In: Kliegman RM, Stanton BF, St Geme J, Schor NF, eds. *Nelson Textbook of Pediatrics*. 20th ed. Philadelphia, PA: Elsevier Saunders; 2016:2554-2556.

Fong KW, Kfouri JE, Weind Matthews KL. The fetal urogenital tract. In: Kliegman RM, Stanton BMD, St Geme J, Schor NF, eds. *Nelson Textbook of Pediatrics*. 20th ed. Philadelphia, PA: Elsevier Saunders; 2016:1336-1375.

Porter CC, Avner ED. Anatomic abnormalities associated with hematuria. In: Kliegman RM, Stanton BF, St Geme J, Schor NF, eds. *Nelson Textbook of Pediatrics*. 20th ed. Philadelphia, PA: Elsevier Saunders; 2016:2512-2517.

Item 237 Preferred Response: C

A medical home refers to the partnership of a primary health care provider with families to provide primary care that is "accessible, family-centered, coordinated, comprehensive, continuous, compassionate, and culturally effective" (see Sia et al). This is thought to be the standard for all pediatric patients but specifically so for those children with special health care needs. Limited evidence is available to suggest that medical homes may improve outcomes for medically complex patients, and studies have demonstrated mixed results in regards to decreasing costs of care for medically complex patients.

The purpose of the medical home is to improve the quality of care provided to each patient and the communication across specialties, especially for medically complex patients. There are data that support this outcome. Thus, improving the overall quality of care is the correct answer. The other answer choices are not supported by current evidence. Simon et al have demonstrated improved coordination of providers and improved efficiency and quality of health care (see Simon et al).

The concept of the medical home is endorsed as the optimal model for primary care delivery by medical societies including the American Academy of Pediatrics, as well as federal government agencies. The National Committee for Quality Assurance has published standards for implementation of the medical home practice (www.ncqa.org).

PREP Pearls

- The purpose of the medical home is to provide primary care that is accessible, family centered, coordinated, comprehensive, continuous, compassionate, and culturally effective.

American Board of Pediatrics Content Specification(s)/ Content Area

- Understand the importance of a medical home for children with chronic or handicapping conditions

Suggested Readings

Long WE, Garg A. A comparison of individual- versus practice-level measures of the medical home. *Pediatrics*. 2015;135(3):489-494.

Sia C, Tonniges TF, Osterhus E, Toba S. History of the medical home concept. *Pediatrics*. 2004;113(5):1473-1478. http://pediatrics.aappublications.org/content/pediatrics/113/Supplement_4/1473.full.pdf.

Simon TD, Whitlock KB, Haaland W, et al. Effectiveness of a comprehensive case management service for children with medical complexity. *Pediatrics*. 2017;140(6):1-13.

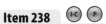

The adolescent in this vignette is conflicted because she feels attracted to males and females and has fostered a relationship with another female, but she believes she will be misunderstood by her parents. She would benefit from having a therapist to explore her feelings and identify how best to communicate with her parents. She is not having suicidal thoughts and does not endorse symptoms of depression, therefore antidepressant medication would not be recommended. Advising her to stop seeing her female partner will most likely alienate her from the provider and make her distrustful of the medical system. Although a discussion about birth control options and safe sex would provide her with accurate information, it is unlikely to be a priority for this adolescent at this time.

Sexuality is defined as the state of being sexual and is influenced by physical, psychological, social, and spiritual elements. During adolescence, one's sexuality develops in terms of the preferred gender of partners, sexual orientation, and preferences. Adolescents need to be educated about becoming sexually healthy adults. This knowledge can come from sex education classes at school, but it is helpful to receive truthful information from parents, medical providers, and other trusted individuals to prevent unwanted pregnancies, sexually transmitted infections (STIs), abusive relationships, and emotional harm. Studies have shown that adolescents of parents who communicate early on about decision making and sexual behavior often have a delay in sexual debut, use a contraceptive method when they do become sexually active, and have fewer sexual partners. Many parents, however, do not feel comfortable having detailed conversations about sexual behaviors with their teenager. Instead of having frank open discussions, many parents have brief discussions about puberty, such as getting a period; provide books that discuss sex; or highlight negative consequences, such as pregnancy. Some parents may be dismissive, avoid the conversation, or set strict rules (eg, "Do not have sex"). These approaches do not foster open lines of communication, and adolescents often turn to their friends or the internet and may not receive accurate information. Adolescents would benefit from their parents discussing topics such as masturbation, how to use a condom, and orgasm, topics that adolescents often have questions about or feel uncomfortable with.

Adolescence is a time of experimentation. It is common during early adolescence (10-13 years of age) to be attracted to individuals of the same sex. This attraction does not define an individual as homosexual or heterosexual. Studies have shown that gay and lesbian youth often have opposite-sex attractions prior to same-sex attractions. Youth in early adolescence are going through puberty and getting accustomed to their new bodies. It is normal to develop interests and attraction towards others. Middle adolescence (14-16 years of age) is a time when sexual identity and orientation are established, and many adolescents will become sexually active. Middle adolescence is often associated with increased risk-taking behaviors caused by feelings of invincibility. These youth are developing abstract thought but do not always consider consequences of being sexually active, such as pregnancy and STIs. Late adolescence (17-21 years of age) is characterized by abstract thought and planning for future goals. These youth are usually comfortable with their bodies and sexual orientation. However, older adolescents can also be impulsive regarding their sexual behavior. The highest incidence rates for acquiring new STIs occur in 15- to 19-year-olds. According to the 2015 Youth Risk Behavior Survey data, 41.2% of high school students nationwide (9th-12th grade) have had sexual intercourse. Thirty percent of the these students have had sex with at least 1 partner in the 3 months prior to the survey, and only 56.9% reported that they or their partner used a condom.

Adolescent sexual behavior incorporates many different facets. It includes sexual thoughts and fantasy, masturbation, use of sex toys, and intercourse (oral, vaginal, and anal). It also encompasses phone sex, sexting, and sex in chat rooms or virtual sex via webcams.

Providers need to address sexuality in a nonjudgmental unbiased manner and be aware of different terminology so that an adolescent does not feel offended. There is a difference between *sexual orientation* and gender identity. Sexual orientation is defined by whom an individual feels emotionally and physically attracted. This can be fluid, as a person may be primarily attracted to the opposite sex, same sex, or both sexes. *Gender identity* is an individual's perception of themself. This may be the same or different from their birth sex. *Transgender* is used to describe an individual whose gender identity is different from who he or she is expected to be based on their birth sex. It is completely separate from sexual orientation—to whom one is attracted. *Gender expression* is how one presents themself to the world in terms of clothing, hair style, and behavior. An individual may be described as being masculine or feminine. *Gender transition* is how some individuals align their internal sense of self to be more congruent with their appearance. This can be a social transition, such as a name change, identifying pronouns of preference to be called, and style of dress. Or, it can be a physical transition, which involves medical interventions such as hormonal therapy and surgery. *Gender dysphoria* is the diagnosis that replaced gender *identity disorder* in the fifth edition of the *Diagnostic and Statistical Manual of Mental Illness*. It refers to an individual who is significantly distressed that their birth sex is not consistent with how they identify themself.

PREP Pearls

- Adolescent sexual behavior encompasses many facets: thoughts, masturbation, physical acts of sex (oral, vaginal, anal), sexting, and virtual sex.
- Become familiar with sexual orientation and gender identity definitions to foster open communication with all adolescents.
- Encourage parents to play an active role in educating their adolescent about sexual behavior.

American Board of Pediatrics Content Specification(s)/
Content Area

- Identify common sources of information sought by adolescents regarding sexuality
- Recognize the common patterns of sexual behavior and experimentation in adolescents of various ages
- Plan appropriate parental counseling regarding adolescent sexuality

Suggested Readings

Akers AY, Holland CL, Bost J. Interventions to improve parental communication about sex: a systematic review. *Pediatrics.* 2011;127(3):494-510.

Martino SC, Elliott MN, Corona R, Kanouse DE, Schuster MA. Beyond the "Big Talk": the roles of breadth and repetition in parent-adolescent communication about sexual topics. *Pediatrics.* 2008;121(3):e612-e618.

Tulloch T, Kaufman M. Adolescent sexuality. *Pediatr Rev.* 2013;34(1):29-37.

Item 239   Preferred Response: D

The infant in the vignette is receiving mechanical ventilation for respiratory failure from bronchiolitis. He still requires moderate ventilator settings, so an unplanned extubation would be an adverse event. Of the choices, the best way to prevent this is to ensure a 1:1 nurse-to-patient ratio.

Harm occurs frequently in hospitalized patients. In a 1999 report, the Institute of Medicine (now National Academy of Medicine) reported that medical errors cause 98,000 patient deaths annually. They defined safety as the absence of clinical error either by commission (doing the wrong thing) or by omission (not doing the right thing). The World Health Organization defined safety as the reduction of risk of unnecessary harm to an acceptable minimum. An "adverse event" is a negative occurrence in a patient that is not a natural consequence of the course of illness or treatment. A "sentinel event," as defined by the Joint Commission, is a patient safety event that reaches the patient and leads to death, permanent harm, or severe temporary harm (Item C239A).

Reduction in harm can be achieved by implementing quality improvement initiatives and high-reliability organization principles that have been used in other safety-intensive industries, such as automotive and air-traffic control. Improving the knowledge, skills, and attitudes of hospital personnel to establish a culture of safety improvement is critical. Establishing error-prevention behaviors, identifying patient safety champions, implementing root cause analyses, and increasing patient-family involvement have all been shown to reduce errors. Reducible sources of medical harm include adverse drug events, catheter-related urinary tract infections, central line–associated bloodstream infections (CLABSI), falls, pressure ulcers, and ventilator-associated pneumonia (Item C239B). The likelihood of harm can be increased by patient-specific factors. For example, if an immunocompromised patient requires a central line for several weeks, a CLABSI may seem inevitable. However, many practices can reduce the risk of CLABSI, such as the implementation of insertion bundles to ensure sterile technique, catheter access bundles, reduction of instances of catheter entry, and emphasis on early catheter removal. A healthy culture of safety also facilitates and supports institution-specific quality assurance data collection and scientific study.

Item C239A. Definition of Sentinel Events.

A sentinel event is a patient safety event (not primarily related to the natural course of the patient's illness or underlying condition) that reaches the patient and results in any of the following:

1. Death

2. Permanent harm

3. Severe temporary harm

AN EVENT IS ALSO CONSIDERED SENTINEL IF IT IS ONE OF THE FOLLOWING:

4. Suicide of any patient receiving care, treatment, and services in a 24/7 care setting or within 72 hours of discharge

5. Unanticipated death of a full-term infant

6. Discharge of an infant to the wrong family

7. Abduction of any patient receiving care, treatment, and services

8. Any elopement (ie, unauthorized departure) of a patient from a 24/7 care setting (including the emergency department) leading to death, permanent harm, or severe temporary harm

9. Hemolytic transfusion reaction due to major blood group incompatibilities

10. Rape, assault (leading to death, permanent harm, or severe temporary harm), or homicide of any patient receiving care, treatment, and services or any staff member or visitor while on site at the hospital

11. Invasive procedures on the wrong patient, at the wrong site, or that is the wrong (unintended) procedure

12. Unintended retention of a foreign object after an invasive procedure

13. Neonatal hyperbilirubinemia exceeding 30 mg/dL

14. Fluoroscopic procedures in which the cumulative radiation dose exceeds 1,500 rads to a single field or any radiotherapy to the wrong body region or a dose greater than 25% above the planned radiotherapy dose

15. Fire, flame or unintended smoke, heat, or flashes occurring during an episode of patient care

16. Any intrapartum maternal death or severe maternal morbidity

Adapted and reprinted with permission from The Joint Commission Sentinel Event Policy and Procedures. Available at: http://www.jointcommission.org/sentinel_event_policy_and_procedures/. © The Joint Commission, 2016. Reprinted with permission.

The boy in the vignette still requires moderate ventilator settings, and did not tolerate a recent attempt to decrease his amount of ventilator support. Thus, it is likely that he would fail a planned extubation, and an unplanned extubation would cause him harm. Several patient factors can increase the risk of unplanned extubation, such as agitation and secretions. However, preventive measures can mitigate this risk, including an optimized level of sedation, effective security device or taping procedure, surveillance of endotracheal tube placement depth, higher nursing ratio, and restraints. Of the response choices, a 1:1 nurse-to-patient ratio is the most appropriate. A nurse who is always available at the bedside can effectively assess level of sedation, administer sedatives, provide nonpharmacologic mechanisms of calming/sedation, and physically restrain a patient who is about to dislodge the tube. The level of sedation for the boy in the vignette is appropriate; episodes of agitation during care is developmentally normal and manageable with occasional additional doses of sedatives and other nonpharmacologic mechanisms. Excessive sedation and neuromuscular blockade can lead to long-term weakness, decreased brain

Harm Type	Measurement	Notes
Adverse drug events	No. of adverse drug events per 1000 patient days	Preventable F-I events on NCC MERP scale
CAUTIs	No. of urinary tract infections per 1000 urinary catheter days	Operational definition per NHSN
Central line-associated blood stream infections	No. of blood stream infections per 1000 central line days	Operational definition per NHSN
Falls, moderate or greater harm	No. of falls of moderate or greater severity per 1000 patient days	Fall severity defined by NDNQI
Obstetric adverse events	No. of obstetric adverse events per 100 births	Per CMS
Surgical site infections	No. of surgical site infections per 100 surgical procedures	Cardiothoracic, spinal fusion, ventriculoperitoneal shunt procedures; operational definition per NHSN
Pressure ulcers	No. of pressure ulcers per 1000 patient days	Includes stages 3, 4, and unstageable; operational definition per NDNQI
Ventilator-associated pneumonia	No. of ventilator-associated pneumonia infections per 1000 ventilator days	Operational definition per NHSN
SSER 12-mo rolling average	No. of SSEs per 10 000 adjusted patient days in previous 12 mo	SSEs are harms that result in death, severe permanent harm, moderate permanent harm, or severe or moderate temporary harm resulting from deviations in standards of care
SSE monthly rate	No. of SSEs divided by 10 000 adjusted patient days in a given month	—
VTE events	No. of VTE events per 1000 patient days	—

Abbreviations: CAUTIs, catheter-associated urinary tract infections; CMS, Center for Medicare and Medicaid Services; NCC MERP, National Coordinating Council for Medication Error Reporting and Prevention; NDNQI, National Database of Nursing Quality Indicators; NHSN, National Healthcare Safety Network; SSE, serious safety events; SSER, serious safety event rate; VTE, venous thromboembolism; —, not applicable.

Reprinted with permission from Lyren A, Brilli RJ, Zieker MS, et al. Children's hospitals' solutions for patient safety collaborative impact on hospital-acquired harm. *Pediatrics*. 2017;140(3):e20163494.

volume, and pharmacologic addiction. Although end-tidal carbon dioxide monitoring can detect dislodgement of the endotracheal tube, it is not an effective preventive measure. Lastly, it is not appropriate to depend on parents for endotracheal tube security.

PREP Pearls

- Families should be involved in the culture of safety, but it is not appropriate to depend on them for medical care in the inpatient setting.
- Harm frequently occurs in hospitalized patients; improving the knowledge, skills, and attitudes of hospital personnel to establish a culture of safety improvement is critical to the prevention of harm.
- Preventive measures can mitigate the risk of unplanned extubation, including an optimized level of sedation, effective security device or taping procedure, surveillance of endotracheal tube placement depth, higher nursing ratio, and restraints.

American Board of Pediatrics Content Specification(s)/ Content Area

- Understand the role of patients and their families in reducing adverse events
- Understand the contribution of patient factors to adverse events

Suggested Readings

Lyren A, Brilli RJ, Zieker MS, et al. Children's hospitals' solutions for patient safety collaborative impact on hospital-acquired harm. *Pediatrics*. 2017;140(3):e20163494.

McClead RE, Brady M. Sentinel events/patient safety events. *Pediatr Rev*. 2016;37(10):448-450.

Muething SE, Goudie A, Schoettker PJ, et al. Quality improvement initiative to reduce serious safety events and improve patient safety culture. *Pediatrics*. 2012;130(2):e423-e431.

Sanchez JA, Lobdell KW, Moffatt-Bruce SD, et al. Investigating the causes of adverse events. *Ann Thorac Surg*. 2017;103:1693-1699.

Item 240   Preferred Response: C

The adolescent boy in the vignette has the classic clinical findings of a varicocele: painless asymmetry of scrotal size with a mass described as feeling like a "bag of worms" that can be palpated around the spermatic cord structures above the testicle. A varicocele is an abnormal collection of tortuous veins in the pampiniform plexus surrounding the spermatic cord in the scrotum. Varicoceles may result from increased venous pressure and/or valvular incompetence. Because the left spermatic vein enters the left renal vein at a 90-degree angle, while the right spermatic vein enters obtusely into the inferior vena cava, varicoceles occur more commonly on the left side.

About 10% to 25% of all adolescent boys have a varicocele; only 10% to 20% of boys with varicoceles will have fertility problems. Although most patients with varicoceles are asymptomatic, some may present with a sensation of heaviness, a dull ache, or scrotal pain, especially when standing. The physical examination for varicocele should be performed with the patient standing, followed by the addition of a Valsalva maneuver. A grade 1 varicocele is not visible and is palpable only with a Valsalva maneuver. Grade 2 varicoceles are not visible, but are palpable without Valsalva. A grade 3 varicocele is found on visual inspection. Although it is commonly proposed that the higher the varicocele grade, the greater the risk for poor outcomes, evidence shows that a higher varicocele grade does not correlate well with abnormal semen analysis, the risk for infertility in adult males, or with testicular size in adolescents.

To differentiate idiopathic varicoceles from those that occur secondary to obstructive venous processes (ie, thromboses or masses that compress the veins), it is important that patients with varicoceles be examined in the supine position. Idiopathic varicoceles are usually more prominent in the upright position and disappear when supine; however, secondary varicoceles will not vary much in size based on patient position. It is important to remember that 85% to 95% of idiopathic varicoceles occur on the left side, so further investigation may be warranted for unilateral right-sided varicoceles. The diagnosis of varicocele is most often made clinically. Additional studies are needed when there is concern for an underlying cause for the varicocele, there is significant discrepancy in testicular size, or the patient has marked discomfort, making the examination difficult. Significant loss of testicular volume, abnormal semen analysis, very large varicoceles, and pain are indications for surgical repair; otherwise, no treatment is needed.

PREP Pearls

- A varicocele is an abnormal collection of tortuous veins in the pampiniform plexus surrounding the spermatic cord in the scrotum.
- Idiopathic varicoceles are usually more prominent when the patient is standing and disappear when supine; 85% to 95% occur on the left side.
- Varicoceles are most often diagnosed clinically and are typically described as feeling like a "bag of worms" when palpated.

American Board of Pediatrics Content Specification(s)/Content Area

- Recognize the clinical findings associated with a varicocele, and manage appropriately

Suggested Readings

Blair RJ. Testicular and scrotal masses. *Pediatr Rev.* 2014;35(10):450-451.

Cavanaugh RM. Screening for genitourinary abnormalities in adolescent males. *Pediatr Rev.* 2009;30(11):431-438.

Palmer LS. Scrotal swelling and pain. In: McInerny TK, Adam HM, Campbell DE, DeWitt TG, Foy JM, Kamat DM, eds. *American Academy of Pediatrics Textbook of Pediatric Care.* 2nd ed. Elk Grove Village, IL: American Academy of Pediatrics; 2017:1571-1577

Item 241   Preferred Response: C

The girl described in the vignette presents with fever of unknown origin (FUO), abdominal pain, hepatosplenomegaly, elevated erythrocyte sedimentation rate, and abdominal ultrasound findings of hepatosplenic hypoechoic lesions. In the setting of contact with cats, this presentation is highly suggestive of hepatosplenic cat scratch disease (CSD). Thus,

serology is the most likely test to confirm the diagnosis of disseminated CSD in this case. The etiologic agent of CSD is *Bartonella henselae*, a fastidious, slow-growing gram-negative bacillus. Domestic cats, especially kittens, are the primary reservoir and vector for transmission of CSD. More than 40% of cats have sustained, asymptomatic, *B henselae* bacteremia. The horizontal transmission of the disease from cat to cat is maintained by cat fleas, and on occasion, arthropod vectors (fleas or ticks) may transmit the disease to humans. Most cases of CSD are reported in the autumn and winter seasons. More than 90% of patients with CSD report a history of contact with cats.

The typical clinical presentation of CSD is regional lymphadenopathy/lymphadenitis, often in the absence of systemic symptoms. A primary papule may be noted at the presumed inoculation site approximately 7 to 12 days after a cat scratch, followed 7 to 50 days later (average 12-14 days) by lymphadenopathy in the drainage region for the inoculation site. Axillary nodes are most frequently affected, but other regional nodes in the cervical, submental, epitrochlear, or inguinal areas may be involved. The skin overlying the lymph nodes is often warm, tender, and erythematous. The lymphadenopathy regresses over 2 to 4 months; approximately 25% of nodes may suppurate spontaneously. Low-grade fever, malaise, anorexia, and headache may accompany regional adenopathy.

Less common manifestations of CSD include prolonged fever/FUO because of disseminated disease, hepatosplenic abscesses, vertebral osteomyelitis, encephalopathy/encephalitis, conjunctivitis with preauricular adenopathy (Parinaud oculoglandular syndrome) and neuroretinitis. Immunocompromised patients may present with serious manifestations, such as bacillary angiomatosis and peliosis. Hepatosplenic CSD results from hematogenous spread of *B henselae*. Prolonged fever or FUO following contact with a cat or kitten is the most frequent manifestation. Other associated symptoms may include chills, malaise, headaches, myalgias, weight loss, and abdominal pain. Physical examination may reveal hepatomegaly and/or splenomegaly. Lymphadenopathy may be seen in some patients. Laboratory studies are significant for elevated acute-phase reactants and inflammatory markers, but liver enzymes are often normal. Abdominal imaging with ultrasonography or contrast-enhanced computed tomography may demonstrate multiple microabscesses in the liver and/or spleen similar to the case in the vignette. The diagnosis of CSD is best established with a serologic test, via indirect immunofluorescent assay performed at a reputed commercial laboratory or the CDC. High titers (>1:256) of immunoglobulin G antibody to *B henselae* are highly suggestive of CSD. In rare instances, fine-needle aspirate or tissue biopsy of an affected lymph node may reveal the organism via polymerase chain reaction. Detection of *B henselae* in tissue specimens using special stains, such as Warthin-Starry silver stain, is unusual. Tissue biopsy may demonstrate necrotizing granulomas similar to other granulomatous infections (eg, tuberculosis, brucellosis, tularemia).

Invasive diagnostic procedures, such as liver biopsy and bone marrow biopsy, may be indicated in some cases of FUO to establish the diagnosis of unusual zoonotic infections (eg, brucellosis given exposure to livestock) or neoplastic disease. Cat scratch disease must be included in the differential diagnosis of FUO and hepatosplenic disease with a history of cat contact. The history and physical examination findings of the child in the vignette are consistent with the diagnosis of CSD, thus, serology is the most likely test to confirm the diagnosis. Her clinical presentation and abdominal imaging findings are not consistent with a parasitic disease.

Most patients with CSD do not require antimicrobial therapy because the illness is self-limited in the majority of cases. Needle aspiration may be indicated to relieve pressure in painful suppurative nodes. Many oral antimicrobial agents (such as azithromycin, rifampin, trimethoprim-sulfamethoxazole, doxycycline, and parenteral gentamicin) have been used in patients with CSD with anecdotal reports of success. One randomized controlled trial found a significantly greater decrease in lymph node size in azithromycin-treated patients at 1 month compared with placebo, but there was no significant difference thereafter. Antimicrobial therapy may be considered to speed recovery in immunocompetent patients with severe manifestations of CSD, such as FUO associated with granulomatous hepatitis/hepatosplenic disease, vertebral osteomyelitis, and neuroretinitis. Antimicrobial therapy is always recommended for the treatment of CSD in immunocompromised patients.

PREP Pearls

- Hepatosplenic CSD is an atypical manifestation commonly presenting as persistent fever or fever of unknown origin following cat or kitten contact.
- The laboratory diagnosis of CSD is best established with a serologic test via indirect immunofluorescent assay.
- The typical clinical presentation of cat scratch disease (CSD) is regional lymphadenopathy/lymphadenitis, often in the absence of systemic symptoms.

American Board of Pediatrics Content Specification(s)/ Content Area

- Recognize the clinical features associated with cat-scratch disease
- Understand the epidemiology of cat-scratch disease
- Plan appropriate management for a patient with cat-scratch disease

Suggested Readings

American Academy of Pediatrics. *Bartonella henselae* (cat-scratch disease). In: Kimberlin DW, Brady MT, Jackson MA, Long SS, eds. *Red Book: 2018 Report of the Committee on Infectious Diseases.* 31st ed. Itasca, IL: American Academy of Pediatrics; 2018:244-247

Arisoy ES, Correa AG, Wagner ML, Kaplan SL. Hepatosplenic cat-scratch disease in children: selected clinical features and treatment. *Clin Infect Dis.* 1999;28(4):778-784.

Florin TA, Zaoutis TE, Zaoutis LB. Beyond cat scratch disease: widening spectrum of *Bartonella henselae* infection. *Pediatrics.* 2008;121(5):e1413-e1425.

The neonate in the vignette has gastroschisis, which is associated with necrotizing enterocolitis. The incidence of gastroschisis has been rising over the past 20 years; it is currently estimated to be 4.9 per 10,000 live births in the United States. Risk factors for gastroschisis include low maternal age, low maternal body mass index, genitourinary infection, illicit drug use, cigarette smoking, and over-the-counter analgesia use. Cases occur in geographic clusters, suggesting that environmental exposures may contribute to its pathogenesis. The etiology of gastroschisis remains unclear, but may involve vascular disruption of normal intestinal development.

On physical examination, gastroschisis presents with abdominal contents herniated to the right of the umbilical cord without a covering membrane. The defect usually involves only intestines; rarely the stomach, ovaries, and colon may also be involved. After delivery, neonates with gastroschisis should be placed in a sterile bag up to the axilla and positioned with the right side down. The bowel should be supported to prevent compromise of blood flow. Affected neonates are at risk for hypothermia and insensible fluid loss. Gastroschisis typically occurs in isolation without other congenital anomalies. Postoperative complications include dysmotility and a 15% to 20% risk of necrotizing enterocolitis.

In comparison, omphalocele is the herniation of abdominal contents through the base of the umbilical cord. On physical examination, the defect is covered by a thin membrane. The midline defect potentially involves bowel, liver, and less often, the stomach. Omphalocele commonly occurs with other anomalies. In 75% of cases, omphalocele is associated with a genetic abnormality.

Neonates with Beckwith Wiedemann syndrome have macroglossia, hypoglycemia from pancreatic islet cell hyperplasia, and may present with omphalocele. They have an increased risk of childhood neoplasms, including Wilms tumor, hepatoblastoma, neuroblastoma, and adrenocortical carcinoma.

Neonates with cloacal exstrophy present with bladder exstrophy and omphalocele. Cloacal exstrophy is associated with upper urinary tract anomaly (50%) and spina bifida (50%). Despite surgical revision, neonates with cloacal exstrophy will not achieve urinary continence.

PREP Pearls

- Gastroschisis is an abdominal wall defect located to the right of the umbilicus, usually involving herniation of only the intestine.
- Necrotizing enterocolitis is seen in 15% to 20% of neonates with gastroschisis after surgical repair.
- The pathogenesis of gastroschisis is unclear; it has been associated with low maternal age, low maternal body mass index, illicit drug use, cigarette smoking, and over-the-counter analgesia use.

American Board of Pediatrics Content Specification(s)/ Content Area

- Plan the appropriate evaluation and management of a newborn infant who has abdominal-intestinal wall defect

Karr C. Addressing environmental contaminants in pediatric practice. *Pediatr Rev.* 2011;32(5):190-200.

National Center for Chronic Disease Prevention and Health Promotion, (US) Office on Smoking and Health. *The Health Consequences of Smoking—50 Years of Progress: A Report of the Surgeon General.* Atlanta, GA: Centers for Disease Control and Prevention; 2014.

Rigotti NA. Strategies to help a smoker who is struggling to quit. *JAMA.* 2012;308(15):1573-1580.

Suggested Readings

Carlo WA, Maheshwari A. The umbilicus. In: Kliegman RM, Stanton BF, St Geme JW, Schor NF, eds. *Nelson Textbook of Pediatrics.* 20th ed. Philadelphia, PA: Saunders Elsevier; 2016:890-891

D'Antonio F, Virgone C, Rizzo G, et al. Prenatal risk factors and outcomes in gastroschisis: a meta-analysis. *Pediatrics.* 2015;136(1):e159-169.

Item 243 Preferred Response: C

Environmental tobacco smoke exposure is the most common indoor pollutant and involuntary in-home toxic exposure for children. The girl in this vignette is having recurrent respiratory illnesses in the context of second- and third-hand tobacco smoke exposure. Counseling this child's mother regarding the adverse effects of indoor tobacco smoke exposure is the action that will have the greatest potential benefit among the response choices offered. Chronic cough and chronic or recurrent respiratory infections are the most common adverse effects of indoor tobacco smoke exposure in children.

Initiation of antihistamines may have some benefit for her nasal congestion and runny nose, but will not address the underlying cause of the symptoms. There is a family history of allergy and this child may be at risk for development of allergies, but avoidance of tobacco smoke exposure will have a greater impact on her health than will taking daily antihistamines. House dust mite antigen avoidance measures, including impermeable zip covers on mattress and pillows, may be appropriate if she is determined to be atopic, but that is not the most effective first approach for this particular patient in the context of tobacco smoke exposure. Good ventilation in homes will help to minimize a variety of indoor air pollutants; but, again, elimination of tobacco smoke as the most prevalent of those pollutants will be more effective than improving ventilation.

There are other indoor air pollutants that may have an effect on respiratory health for children. Natural gas, propane, and kerosene as heating agents may have very small emissions that have been implicated in some cases of poor respiratory health when the exposure is high.

PREP Pearls

- Chronic cough and chronic or recurrent respiratory infections are the most common adverse effects of indoor tobacco smoke exposure in children.
- Environmental tobacco smoke exposure is the most common indoor pollutant and involuntary in-home toxic exposure for children.

American Board of Pediatrics Content Specification(s)/ Content Area

- Recognize the possible side effects of environmental tobacco smoke exposure
- Identify the common environmental irritants present in the home that can contribute to respiratory disease in children

Suggested Readings

Farber HJ, Nelson KE, Grener JA, Walley SC; Section on Tobacco Control. Public policy to protect children from tobacco, nicotine, and tobacco smoke. *Pediatrics.* 2015;136(5):998-1007.

Galvez MP, Balk SJ. Environmental risks to children: prioritizing health messages in pediatric practice. *Pediatr Rev.* 2017;38(6):263-279.

Item 244 Preferred Response: C

The most likely cause of hypoglycemia for the neonate in this vignette is hypopituitarism. The neonate has evidence of gonadotropin deficiency with a small penis and cryptorchidism. For a term infant, a stretched phallic length of less than 2 to 2.5 cm meets the definition for micropenis. These findings associated with hypoglycemia make other anterior pituitary hormone deficiencies likely. Hypoglycemia is the predominant presenting symptom of congenital hypopituitarism. The neonate's history of breech position is another clue that anterior pituitary hormone deficiencies might be present.

A fatty acid oxidation disorder is less likely given the physical findings and does not typically present in the neonatal period. Similarly, hyperinsulinism is not associated with hypogonadism. Hyperinsulinism is often associated with maternal diabetes, large-for–gestational age birth weight, or significant perinatal stress, none of which apply to the neonate in this vignette. Transitional hypoglycemia is not typically as severe as the hypoglycemia described in this vignette and usually resolves by 48 hours after birth.

Other clinical features of congenital hypopituitarism caused by the effects of anterior pituitary hormone deficiencies may include postdates gestation, poor feeding, hypotonia, and prolonged jaundice with direct hyperbilirubinemia. There may also be associated midline defects. Wandering nystagmus suggests septo-optic dysplasia. If the posterior pituitary hormone vasopressin is deficient, diabetes insipidus results. In addition to hypoglycemia, laboratory evaluation may reveal hyponatremia caused by central adrenal insufficiency, or hypernatremia if diabetes insipidus is present. Central adrenal insufficiency also results in a low serum cortisol level. Relative thyroid-stimulating hormone deficiency results in a low free thyroxine level with a low or inappropriately normal thyroid-stimulating hormone level. A random growth hormone level is a useful measure of growth hormone status in the first week after birth. After this time period, insulin-like growth factor-1 and insulin-like growth factor binding protein-3 are more appropriate measures of growth hormone status and will be low in individuals with hypopituitarism. Magnetic resonance imaging of the brain is indicated in children with hypopituitarism. An anatomic abnormality is likely with congenital hypopituitarism. Potential anatomic findings include pituitary stalk interruption syndrome, the triad of hypoplastic anterior pituitary, absent pituitary stalk, and ectopic posterior pituitary, or evidence of septo-optic dysplasia with optic nerve hypoplasia and absent corpus callosum or septum pellucidum.

PREP Pearls

- Consider hypopituitarism in male neonates with a small penis. A stretched phallic length of less than 2 to 2.5 cm meets the definition for micropenis.
- Hypoglycemia is the predominant presenting symptom of congenital hypopituitarism.

American Board of Pediatrics Content Specification(s)/ Content Area

- Recognize the clinical and laboratory features associated with hypopituitarism

Suggested Readings

Parks KS, Felner EI. Hypopituitarism. In: Kliegman RM, Stanton BF, St. Geme JW, Schor NF, eds. *Nelson Textbook of Pediatrics*. 20th ed. Philadelphia, PA: Elsevier; 2016:2637-2644.

Pierce M, Madison L. Evaluation and initial management of hypopituitarism. *Pediatr Rev*. 2016;37(9):370-376.

Thompson-Branch A, Havranek T. Neonatal hypoglycemia. *Pediatr Rev*. 2017;38(4):147-157.

Thornton PS, Stanley CA, De Leon DD, et al; Pediatric Endocrine Society. Recommendations from the Pediatric Endocrine Society for evaluation and management of persistent hypoglycemia in neonates, infants, and children. *J Pediatr*. 2015;167(2):238-245.

Item 245	Preferred Response: B

The neonate in the vignette has Apert syndrome, which is a disorder of the *FGFR*-related craniosynostosis spectrum that also includes Pfeiffer syndrome, Crouzon syndrome, Jackson-Weiss syndrome, and Muenke syndrome. Craniosynostosis is premature fusion of the skull bone sutures, which can interfere with brain growth. In *FGFR*-related disorders, affected individuals present with unicoronal or bicoronal craniosynostosis, or cloverleaf skull; characteristic facial features; and varying foot and hand findings, including mitten-deformity, which is most common in Apert syndrome. Coronal craniosynostosis causes the skull to acquire a tower-shaped or turribrachycephalic appearance. Cloverleaf skull is caused by synostoses of the sagittal, metopic, lambdoid, and coronal sutures leading to a trilobar deformity. Individuals with Apert syndrome have varying degrees of intellectual disability, while individuals with Crouzon syndrome have normal intellect. Apert syndrome is caused by *FGFR2* pathogenic gene mutations.

Molecular genetic panel testing for *FGFR1, FGFR2,* and *FGFR3* gene mutations is available to establish a specific diagnosis, though the clinical presentation alone may be sufficient. *FGFR*-related craniosynostosis syndromes are of autosomal dominant inheritance, thus yielding a 50% chance of the affected individual passing the disorder to their children.

Abnormal head growth or shape could indicate a medical or developmental problem, thus mandating further evaluation by the health care provider. For all children, head circumference should be measured serially and followed over time with a growth chart at each health supervision visit up until 36 months of age. If concern arises, obtaining a detailed perinatal and family history, careful attention to developmental progress, and a comprehensive physical and neurologic examination are warranted. Imaging, such as brain magnetic resonance imaging or head ultrasonography, may also be indicated.

Microcephaly is defined as a head circumference greater than 2 standard deviations (SDs) below normal or below the 2nd percentile. Microcephaly can be classified as primary or acquired. Primary microcephaly presents at birth, and can be due to an autosomal dominant or recessive disorder, inborn error of metabolism, Smith-Lemli-Opitz syndrome, a trisomy, or perinatal infection, such as cytomegalovirus or Zika virus. Acquired microcephaly presents with a normal head circumference at birth, followed by a deceleration of head growth to microcephalic parameters, typically because of a brain abnormality or insult. Causes can include meningitis, encephalitis, stroke, Rett syndrome, in utero teratogen exposure, hypoxic-ischemic encephalopathy, inborn errors of metabolism, severe malnutrition, and infections during pregnancy. Magnetic resonance imaging of the brain is preferred over head ultrasonography in the evaluation of microcephaly because of the greater degree of detail, such as myelination or calcifications that can be identified. This type of imaging is generally not ordered emergently. Genetic testing may be ordered if a specific disorder is suspected.

Macrocephaly is defined as a head circumference greater than 2 SDs above normal or above the 98th percentile. The differential diagnosis for macrocephaly can include benign enlargement of the subarachnoid space in infancy, normal familial variant, intracranial mass (tumor or cyst), subdural hemorrhage, hydrocephalus, or megalencephaly due to a genetic disorder such as skeletal dysplasias or mucopolysaccharidoses (MPS). In the case of a suspected normal familial variant, the parents' head circumferences should be measured and a thorough developmental history obtained; if the infant is otherwise healthy, no other workup is indicated. If features of a skeletal dysplasia or MPS disorder are present, further testing such as a bone survey or urine mucopolysaccharide screen may be indicated. If the history is significant for vomiting, lethargy, decreased level of consciousness, poor feeding, increased irritability, or rapid head growth, emergent imaging such as head ultrasonography (if the anterior fontanelle is still open) or computed tomography of the brain would be recommended to exclude hydrocephalus or intracranial mass. Physical examination should focus on any suggestion of a particular disorder, such as hypertonia, hyperreflexia, seizure activity, cranial bruits, or skeletal dysplasias or an emergent situation such as "sunsetting" eyes or impaired upward gaze, a bulging fontanelle, or splayed sutures. Computed tomography of the brain would yield greater detail and can be obtained quickly, but would expose the infant to radiation so one must determine if it is necessary.

Plagiocephaly is a very common disorder that occurs when an infant's head acquires a flattened appearance, typically in the occipital region, because of repeated pressure on 1 part of the infant's head. This can occur when an infant always sleeps in the same position. It is generally treatable by varying the infant's sleeping position. It is important to exclude craniosynostosis in an infant with suspected plagiocephaly.

Amniotic band sequence is a condition in which bands form from the inner lining of the amniotic sac and attach to different parts of the fetus' developing body, affecting the formation of the particular body part. This can cause constriction of the affected region and even amputation. Physical findings can include shortened or missing digits or limbs, abdominal wall defects, facial clefts, and brain protrusions such as an encephalocele.

Holt-Oram syndrome presents with a combination of upper extremity malformations and the presence or family history of congenital heart malformation, most commonly an atrial septal defect or ventricular septal defect. Cardiac conduction disease may also be present. An abnormal carpal bone is noted in all affected individuals. Holt-Oram syndrome is inherited as an autosomal dominant disorder due to *TBX5* gene mutations.

Shprintzen-Goldberg syndrome presents with coronal, sagittal, or lambdoid craniosynostosis; dolichocephaly; marfanoid skeletal features; intellectual disability; brain anomalies; and classic facial features. Craniofacial features include a tall/prominent forehead, ocular proptosis, hypertelorism, downslanting palpebral fissures, malar flattening, high arched palate, micrognathia, and low-set ears. Brain anomalies include hydrocephalus, lateral ventricular dilatation, and Chiari 1 malformation. Shprintzen-Goldberg syndrome is inherited as an autosomal dominant disorder due to mutations in the *SKI* gene.

PREP Pearls

- In *FGFR*-related disorders, such as Apert syndrome, affected individuals present with unicoronal or bicoronal craniosynostosis or cloverleaf skull, characteristic facial features, and varying foot and hand findings.
- Macrocephaly is defined as a head circumference greater than 2 standard deviations above normal or above the 98th percentile.
- Microcephaly is defined as a head circumference greater than 2 standard deviations below normal or below the 2nd percentile.

American Board of Pediatrics Content Specification(s)/ Content Area

- Differentiate between normal and abnormal variations in head shape and/or growth (eg, craniosynostosis, plagiocephaly, microcephaly, macrocephaly)
- Plan the management of a patient with an abnormal head shape and/or growth (eg, craniosynostosis, plagiocephaly, microcephaly, macrocephaly)
- Differentiate among the possible causes of abnormal head shape and/or growth (eg, craniosynostosis, plagiocephaly, microcephaly, macrocephaly)

Suggested Readings

Liptak GS, Serletti JM. Consultation with the specialist: pediatric approach to craniosynostosis. *Pediatr Rev.* 1998;19(10):352-359.

Puruggagan OH. Abnormalities in head size. *Pediatr Rev.* 2006;27(12):473-476.

Robin NH, Falk MJ, Haldeman-Englert CR. FGFR-related craniosynostosis syndromes. *GeneReviews.* https://www.ncbi.nlm.nih.gov/books/NBK1455/.

The child in this vignette most likely has benign paroxysmal vertigo of childhood (BPVC), as suggested by the brief, episodic nature of her symptoms, lack of trauma and otological findings, age, and normal neurological examination findings. Watchful waiting is recommended for BPVC, which is typically a self-limited condition. Referral to a neurologist for medication management and further diagnostic evaluation is recommended only if symptoms worsen or impact functioning. The cause of BPVC is unknown, but children with BPVC often have a family history of migraines, and some will develop migraines later in childhood.

Young children can have difficulty describing vertigo, but this symptom is defined as having the perception of rotational movement and involves the vestibular system. Other types of dizziness can include lightheadedness caused by orthostatic hypotension or unsteadiness caused by ataxia, but these conditions are distinct from vertigo.

The vestibular system has both peripheral (located in the inner ear) and central (brainstem, cerebellum, and eighth cranial nerve) components, and a lesion along any part of this system can cause vertigo.

The history and physical examination findings provide important clues as to etiology. Concurrent migraine or viral symptoms and a history of head trauma are important to elicit. A careful and complete examination of the tympanic membranes is essential, and referral to an otolaryngologist may be indicated in difficult or equivocal examinations if symptoms are severe. A detailed neurological examination, including evaluation for nystagmus, is important.

In infants and younger children, otitis media and related middle ear conditions are the most common causes of vertigo. An absence of fever, ear pain, or a recent history of otitis media, and normal findings on examination, including pneumotoscopy, make this condition less likely for the child in this vignette. Otological complications of otitis media, including cholesteatoma, can cause vertigo as well. Benign paroxysmal vertigo of childhood is the next most common etiology in younger children. Episodes often occur in clusters and can be associated with nausea and vomiting. The neurological examination findings are normal between episodes. A vestibular migraine can also cause vertigo, and children with this condition will have a history of migraine but may not consistently have a headache along with episodes of vertigo. Minor head trauma resulting in a temporal bone fracture can damage the peripheral vestibular system and cause vertigo.

In older children, Meniere disease can be a cause of vertigo; it is often associated with tinnitus and hearing loss. Benign paroxysmal positional vertigo (BPPV) is caused by calcium debris in the posterior semicircular canal. Symptoms often appear upon sitting on the edge of the bed after waking from sleep. Vertigo can be elicited by the Dix-Hallpike maneuver, whereby the patient's neck is extended and turned to one side, and then the patient is quickly placed in a supine position. Treatment involves particle repositioning maneuvers that can be done in the outpatient setting. Self-treatment maneuvers have also been developed. Cases of BPPV are rare in young children and much more common in adults, making this unlikely in the girl in the vignette. Vestibular neuritis can be a complication of infections due to viruses, such as herpes simplex virus and influenza. However, it is typically more severe and persistent than BPVC. Cerebellar and brainstem tumors can cause vertigo and if suspected, brain magnetic resonance imaging should be obtained; however, these tumors are rare and associated with other symptoms, such as headache, nystagmus, emesis, and gait changes, findings not seen in the girl in the vignette. While antiemetic medications such as promethazine and diazepam can be used for vertigo, this child's episodes are too brief to warrant treatment. Additionally, oseltamivir is not indicated in this child whose symptoms of influenza have resolved.

PREP Pearls

- Benign paroxysmal vertigo of childhood is associated with brief episodic symptoms of vertigo with a normal neurologic examination in between episodes. It is typically a self-limited condition, and watchful waiting is recommended.
- Benign paroxysmal vertigo of childhood is distinct from benign paroxysmal positional vertigo, a common cause of vertigo in adults.
- Otitis media and other middle ear conditions are the most common cause of vertigo in young children.

American Board of Pediatrics Content Specification(s)/ Content Area

- Recognize the clinical findings associated with benign paroxysmal vertigo
- Formulate a differential diagnosis of balance disturbance in patients of various ages
- Recognize the etiology of inner ear infections

Suggested Readings

Benun J. Balance and vertigo in children. *Pediatr Rev*. 2011;32(2):84-85.

Kim JS, Zee DS. Clinical practice. Benign paroxysmal positional vertigo. *N Engl J Med*. 2014;370(12):1138-1147.

Malhotra A, Manganas L, Downs T, Chang S, Chandran L. Case 1: vertigo and episodes of slurred speech in a 5-year-old girl. *Pediatr Rev*. 2017;38(4):182.

Item 247   **Preferred Response: B**

The most likely etiology for this neonate's illness is *Chlamydia trachomatis*. Neonatal conjunctivitis caused by *C trachomatis* typically presents between days 5 and 14 after birth. It begins as a watery discharge that then becomes purulent.

Chlamydia trachomatis causes 3 distinct clinical syndromes in children: ocular infections, pneumonia, and urogenital infections. In the pediatric population, ocular infections are typically observed during the neonatal period, after acquiring the organism via vertical transmission. Pneumonia is also a result of vertical transmission, although symptoms usually begin in the late neonatal period, up to several months of age. Symptoms of chlamydia pneumonia include rhinorrhea, congestion, tachypnea, and a staccato cough. Urogenital infections typically occur in sexually active adolescents and can include cervicitis, pelvic inflammatory disease, urethritis, and proctitis. *Chlamydia trachomatis* is the most prevalent sexually transmitted infection in the United States.

In the United States, ocular infections are typically limited to conjunctivitis, whereas in developing countries, trachoma can be observed. Trachoma results from repeated ocular infections with *C trachomatis* associated with scarring and inflammation that can ultimately lead to blindness.

Nucleic acid amplification tests are the most sensitive assays available for the diagnosis of *C trachomatis* infection, although they are only Food and Drug Administration approved for testing of genital sites and urine. Less sensitive culture is used to detect ocular or respiratory infection.

Infants with conjunctivitis or pneumonia are treated with erythromycin for 14 days or azithromycin for 3 days. An additional course of therapy may be needed in patients who do not respond to the initial treatment. Infants younger than 6 weeks should be monitored for the development of hypertrophic pyloric stenosis, which has been associated with the use of macrolides in this age group.

In suspected urogenital infections, empiric therapy should target both *C trachomatis* and *Neisseria gonorrhoeae*. Uncomplicated urogenital infections confirmed to be caused by *C trachomatis* can be treated with a single dose of azithromycin. Complicated infections, such as pelvic inflammatory disease, are treated with doxycycline for 7 to 14 days and may require additional antimicrobials.

Adenovirus conjunctivitis is more commonly observed in older children and can have associated pharyngitis and cervical adenitis. Herpes simplex eye infection caused by vertical transmission usually presents in the first 2 weeks after birth. Symptoms of herpes simplex eye infection include excessive tearing, conjunctival injection, and periorbital vesicular lesions. Excessive purulent drainage would not be typical of herpes simplex infection. In contrast to chlamydial conjunctivitis, ocular infection caused by *N gonorrhoeae* typically manifests within 2 to 5 days after birth and has a more fulminant presentation. Topical eye prophylaxis provided to newborns is directed against *N gonorrhoeae* and does not prevent infections caused by *C trachomatis*.

PREP Pearls

- *Chlamydia trachomatis* causes 3 distinct clinical syndromes in children: ocular infections, pneumonia, and urogenital infections.
- Neonatal conjunctivitis caused by *Chlamydia trachomatis* typically presents between 5 and 14 days after birth as a watery discharge that then becomes purulent.
- Topical eye prophylaxis provided to newborns is directed against *Neisseria gonorrhoeae* and does not prevent infections caused by *Chlamydia trachomatis*.

American Board of Pediatrics Content Specification(s)/ Content Area

- Plan appropriate diagnostic evaluation for chlamydial infection depending on the site of infection (eg, genital, respiratory)
- Recognize the clinical features associated with chlamydial infection in patients of various ages
- Understand the epidemiology of *Chlamydia trachomatis*
- Plan the management of chlamydial infection in patients of various ages

Suggested Readings

American Academy of Pediatrics. *Chlamydia trachomatis.* In: Kimberlin DW, Brady MT, Jackson MA, Long SS, eds. *Red Book: 2018 Report of the Committee on Infectious Diseases.* 31st ed. Itasca, IL: American Academy of Pediatrics; 2018:276-283

Siqueira L. *Chlamydia* infections in children and adolescents. *Pediatr Rev.* 2014;35(4):145 154.

Item 248   Preferred Response: D

The infant in this vignette has multiple café au lait macules (CALMs). The presence of 6 or more macules measuring more than 5 mm in a child is one of the diagnostic criteria for neurofibromatosis type 1 (NF1). An ophthalmology consultation is warranted to evaluate for Lisch nodules and optic glioma. These are other diagnostic criteria which, if present, would secure a definite diagnosis for this infant. If she has NF1, she would be at increased risk for central nervous system tumors, but imaging is not indicated in the absence of concerning symptoms or signs. Learning disabilities are common in children who have NF1 but referral to a developmental specialist at this age is not warranted.

Neurofibromatosis type 1 is a multisystem disease that primarily affects the skin and central nervous system. It is inherited in an autosomal dominant fashion but half of all cases result from a de novo mutation in *NF1*. Two or more of the following criteria are required for diagnosis of NF1:

- Six or more CALMs measuring more than 5 mm in a pre-pubertal individual or more than 1.5 cm in a postpubertal individual
  - Multiple CALMs are observed in nearly all individuals with NF1; they often are present at birth and increase in number during the first years of age.
  - Frequently they are the first sign of NF1.
  - The presence of 1 or 2 CALMs is common in normal individuals, but in 1 study, 76% of children with 6 or more CALMs were ultimately diagnosed as having NF1.
- Axillary or inguinal freckling often appears in children aged 3 to 5 years (Item C248A).
- Optic glioma occurs in approximately 15% of children; it usually presents before age 6 years and may cause reduced visual acuity or proptosis.
- Two or more Lisch nodules (iris hamartomas, Item C248B) are present in 25% of patients with NF1 by age 5 years, 50% by age 10 years, and 95% by age 20 years.
- Two or more neurofibromas (Item C248C) or 1 or more plexiform neurofibroma (Item C248D): neurofibromas are common in adults but rare before late childhood; plexiform neurofibromas occur in about 50% of persons.
- Characteristic osseous lesion (sphenoid dysplasia, anterolateral bowing of the tibia and fibula [Item C248E])
- First-degree relative who has NF1

Other important clinical features of NF1 include:
- Neurocognitive deficits: These are the most commonly reported complications of NF1 and include specific learning disabilities, attention-deficit/hyperactivity disorder, autism spectrum disorder, and behavioral difficulties.

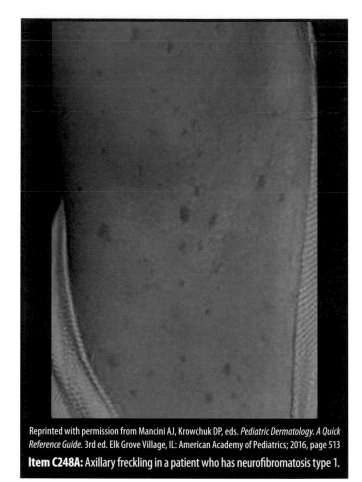

Reprinted with permission from Mancini AJ, Krowchuk DP, eds. *Pediatric Dermatology. A Quick Reference Guide.* 3rd ed. Elk Grove Village, IL: American Academy of Pediatrics; 2016, page 513

Item C248A: Axillary freckling in a patient who has neurofibromatosis type 1.

- Musculoskeletal abnormalities: In addition to the osseous lesions described before, patients are at increased risk for scoliosis.
- Hypertension: Common in NF1 and may develop at any age. Although usually primary, hypertension may result from renal artery stenosis or coarctation of the aorta.

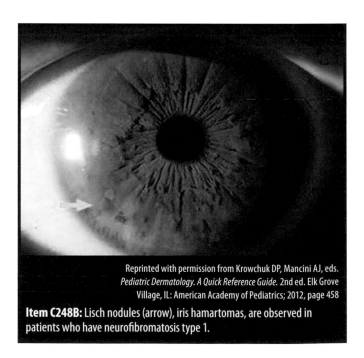

Reprinted with permission from Krowchuk DP, Mancini AJ, eds. *Pediatric Dermatology. A Quick Reference Guide.* 2nd ed. Elk Grove Village, IL: American Academy of Pediatrics; 2012, page 458

Item C248B: Lisch nodules (arrow), iris hamartomas, are observed in patients who have neurofibromatosis type 1.

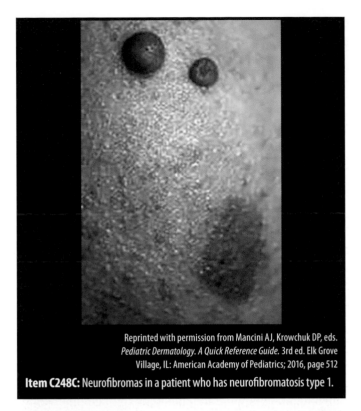

Reprinted with permission from Mancini AJ, Krowchuk DP, eds. *Pediatric Dermatology. A Quick Reference Guide.* 3rd ed. Elk Grove Village, IL: American Academy of Pediatrics; 2016, page 512

Item C248C: Neurofibromas in a patient who has neurofibromatosis type 1.

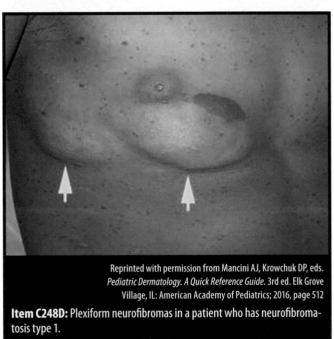

Reprinted with permission from Mancini AJ, Krowchuk DP, eds. *Pediatric Dermatology. A Quick Reference Guide.* 3rd ed. Elk Grove Village, IL: American Academy of Pediatrics; 2016, page 512

Item C248D: Plexiform neurofibromas in a patient who has neurofibromatosis type 1.

Many disorders are characterized by multiple CALMs but rarely are these confused with NF1. Three disorders that may mimic NF1 include:

- Legius syndrome: a dominantly inherited condition characterized by multiple CALMs, axillary freckling, and macrocephaly
- Familial CALMs without other signs of NF1
- Lynch syndrome: this may be clinically indistinguishable from NF1

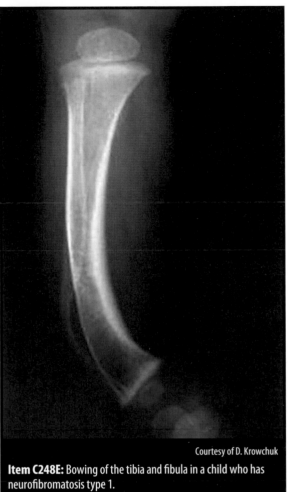

Courtesy of D. Krowchuk

Item C248E: Bowing of the tibia and fibula in a child who has neurofibromatosis type 1.

If a child has 6 or more CALMs without other features of NF1, an annual ophthalmology evaluation and monitoring for the appearance of other features of NF1 are indicated. If a child meets 2 or more diagnostic criteria (ie, meets the definition of NF1) then the following are indicated: medical genetics consultation, annual pediatric ophthalmology evaluation, regular developmental assessment, and regular blood pressure monitoring.

PREP Pearls

- Most children who have more than 6 café au lait macules ultimately will be diagnosed as having neurofibromatosis type 1.
- Six or more café au lait macules measuring more than 5 mm in a prepubertal individual or more than 1.5 cm in a postpubertal individual are among the diagnostic criteria for neurofibromatosis type 1.

American Board of Pediatrics Content Specification(s)/ Content Area

- Recognize the clinical findings associated with neurofibromatosis in patients of various ages

Suggested Readings

Friedman JM. Neurofibromatosis 1. *GeneReviews*. https://www.ncbi.nlm. nih.gov/books/NBK1109/.

Hersh JH; Committee on Genetics. Health supervision for children with neurofibromatosis. *Pediatrics*. 2008;121(3):633-642.

Korf BR. Neurocutaneous disorders in children. *Pediatr Rev*. 2017;38(3):119-127.

Williams VC, Lucas J, Babcock MA, Gutmann DH, Korf B, Maria BL. Neurofibromatosis type 1 revisited. *Pediatrics*. 2009;123(1):124-133.

Item 249   Preferred Response: A

The girl in the vignette has lateral ankle pain and swelling after an inversion injury. The ankle is tender to palpation over the anterior tibiofibular ligament (ATFL) including the ligament attachment site on the fibula. Her history and physical examination suggest a sprain of the ATFL. Ankle sprains are common injuries in children and adults. Inversion injuries leading to lateral ankle ligament sprains are the most common. Children typically present with acute-onset pain and swelling following ankle inversion, often with landing from a jump, twisting, or changing direction. On physical examination, affected individuals often have swelling, bruising, and tenderness over the lateral ankle ligaments. Ligamentous testing may reveal laxity for higher-grade injuries.

Radiography of the ankle may be indicated to rule out associated fractures. The Ottawa Ankle Rules (OAR) were developed to determine whether ankle radiography is indicated after an injury. The OAR note that ankle radiographs should be obtained for individuals with bony tenderness over the posterior aspect of the lateral or medial malleolus, and in patients who are unable to bear weight after their injury and in the clinic or emergency department. Although these rules were developed for adults, subsequent research has shown that they are a valid, reliable tool when applied to children.

Initial management of an ankle injury should include rest, ice, compression, and elevation. Full immobilization, for example, with a cast or walking boot, may delay return to activity. Therefore, a stirrup type of ankle brace that allows dorsiflexion and plantarflexion, but limits eversion and inversion is preferred for children who can walk in this type of brace with minimal discomfort. Subsequent treatment involves rehabilitation exercises to improve movement, followed by strength and balance exercises. Children with good range of motion, strength, and stability can be gradually advanced back to sports activities. Soft ankle support braces have been shown to decrease the rate of ankle injuries and should be considered for children who engage in sports with repetitive jumping and landing, particularly if they have a history of 1 or more ankle sprains.

Conventional wisdom has historically included the idea that many young athletes with apparent ankle sprains actually have Salter-Harris I growth plate injuries involving the distal fibula. Salter-Harris I injuries affect only the growth plate, not the surrounding bone and often go undetected on radiography. Recent studies using magnetic resonance imaging have demonstrated that Salter-Harris I injuries represent a small minority of radiography-negative ankle injuries in children. However, children are more likely than adults to have a bony avulsion injury associated with an ankle sprain.

Deltoid ligament sprains cause medial ankle tenderness. Some children with inversion ankle injuries have pain over the lateral ankle due to stretching of the ligaments and medial pain due to an impaction of the deltoid ligament. Peroneus brevis tendon injuries are less common than lateral ligament sprains. Individuals with peroneus brevis tendon injuries generally exhibit tenderness along the tendon's course posterior and inferior to the lateral malleolus.

PREP Pearls

- Although the Ottawa Ankle Rules were developed to determine whether ankle radiography is indicated for adult patients after an injury, subsequent research has shown they are a valid, reliable tool when applied to children.
- Inversion injuries leading to lateral ankle ligament sprains are the most common ankle injuries in children and adolescents.
- Recent studies using magnetic resonance imaging have demonstrated that Salter-Harris I represents a small minority of radiograph-negative ankle injuries in children.

American Board of Pediatrics Content Specification(s)/ Content Area

- Formulate a differential diagnosis of ankle sprain in patients of various ages
- Recognize possible complications associated with an ankle sprain in a young athlete whose growth plates have not closed
- Plan the appropriate management of an uncomplicated sports-related ankle injury

Suggested Readings

Boutis K, Plint A, Stimec J, et al. Radiograph-negative lateral ankle injuries in children: occult growth plate fracture or sprain? *JAMA Pediatr*. 2016;170(1):e154114.

Dowling S, Spooner CH, Liang Y, et al. Accuracy of Ottawa Ankle Rules to exclude fractures of the ankle and midfoot in children: a meta-analysis. *Acad Emerg Med*. 2009;16(4):277-287

McGuine TA, Brooks A, Hetzel S. The effect of lace-up ankle braces on injury rates in high school basketball players. *Am J Sports Med*. 2011;39(9):1840-1848.

Sarwark JF, LaBella CR, eds. *Pediatric Orthopaedics and Sports Injuries: A Quick Reference Guide*. 2nd ed. Elk Grove Village, IL: American Academy of Pediatrics; 2014.

Item 250   Preferred Response: C

Sharing evidence-based recommendations with parents regarding the introduction of complementary solid foods into an infant's diet is an important piece of routine anticipatory guidance offered by pediatric health care providers. The possible association of risk of food allergies and the timing of introduction of potential food allergens has been debated over the years. In 2008, the American Academy of Pediatrics modified its previous recommendation to delay the introduction of certain highly allergenic foods in high-risk children, stating that the evidence was insufficient to support this practice. To the contrary, the latest evidence shows that delaying the introduction of solid foods beyond 4 to 6 months of age may increase the risk of allergy, while early introduction of certain foods (between 4 and 6 months of age) may, in fact, decrease the risk of allergy to that specific food.

Although adding cereal to the bedtime bottle may be a common practice among parents hoping to promote longer sleep duration in their infants, there is no evidence to support this belief. Adding cereal to the bottle will increase calories, providing more caloric intake than may be needed. Fruit juice provides no nutritional benefit for infants, and may have adverse consequences; based on the 2017 AAP policy statement, juice is not recommended for children younger than 12 months unless medically indicated (see Heyman et al). For infants between 6 and 12 months, mashed or puréed whole fruit should be offered to meet the daily requirements of vitamin C. If parents choose to offer juice to their infants, or it is medically necessary, consumption of 100% fruit juice should be limited to 4 ounces (120 mL) or less per day and should be offered in a cup, not a bottle, when developmentally appropriate. The texture of complementary foods should be advanced based on the oral motor skills of the infant, not solely following an age-based schedule. The advancement of textures and flavors is important to promote the acceptance by children of variety in foods.

PREP Pearls

- Adding cereal to the bedtime bottle does not promote longer sleep duration in infants.
- Delaying the introduction of complementary solid foods beyond 4 to 6 months of age has not been shown to prevent the development of food allergies. The texture of complementary foods should be advanced based on the oral motor skills of the infant.
- Fruit juice is not recommended for children younger than 12 months of age.

American Board of Pediatrics Content Specification(s)/Content Area

- Identify the age-related changes in the ability to absorb and digest different nutrients relevant to infant feeding
- Understand the consequences of introducing solid food prematurely
- Know the appropriate age and sequence for introducing solid food into an infant's diet

Suggested Readings

American Academy of Pediatrics Committee on Nutrition. Complementary feeding. In: Kleinman RE, Greer FR, eds. *American Academy of Pediatrics Pediatric Nutrition*. 7th ed. Elk Grove Village, IL: American Academy of Pediatrics; 2014:123-140.

Greer FR. Healthy nutrition. In: McInerny TK, Adam HM, Campbell DE, DeWitt TG, Foy JM, Kamat DM, eds. *American Academy of Pediatrics Textbook of Pediatric Care*. 2nd ed. Elk Grove Village, IL: American Academy of Pediatrics; 2017:265-273.

Heyman MB, Abrams SA, Section on Gastroenterology, Hepatology, and Nutrition, Committee on Nutrition. Fruit juice in infants, children, and adolescents: current recommendations. *Pediatrics*. 2017;139(6):pii: e20170967.

Item 251   Preferred Response: B

The boy in this vignette has hypopigmented scaling macules on his face. The borders of the lesions are not sharply demarcated; rather, there is a gradual transition from normal to abnormal pigmentation. These features are most consistent with pityriasis alba and, accordingly, treatment with an

emollient is appropriate. Some clinicians treat with a low-potency topical corticosteroid (eg, hydrocortisone 1% or 2.5%) for 7 days, but using a midpotency preparation like triamcinolone is not advisable because of the potential for skin atrophy. Tinea versicolor may cause hypopigmented macules that occasionally may involve the face. However, it is an uncommon infection in children, and the borders of lesions are well defined (Item C251A). Localized infection may be treated with clotrimazole. The lesions of vitiligo are depigmented macules or patches that have well-defined borders (Item C251B); scaling is not present. First-line treatment usually is with a topical corticosteroid or a topical calcineurin inhibitor. Other options include narrowband ultraviolet B phototherapy, photochemotherapy using psoralen and ultraviolet A, and excimer laser.

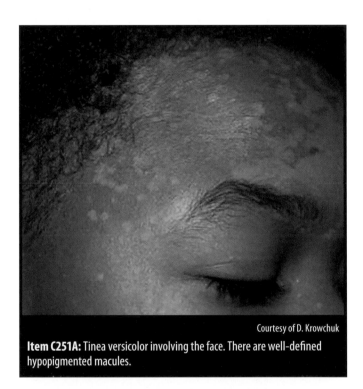

Courtesy of D. Krowchuk

Item C251A: Tinea versicolor involving the face. There are well-defined hypopigmented macules.

Courtesy of D. Krowchuk

Item C251B: In vitiligo, lesions are well-defined depigmented macules or patches. In this patient, some areas have begun repigmenting.

Pityriasis alba is a form of postinflammatory hypopigmentation that often occurs in children who have a history of atopic dermatitis. Lesions commonly involve the face but may occur on the trunk and extremities. Pityriasis alba often becomes apparent after sun exposure because normal skin tans but affected areas do not. The diagnosis is made clinically based on the characteristic appearance of lesions. Regardless of the treatment selected, the patient and family should be counseled that the return of normal pigmentation takes months. In addition, they should be instructed to treat new lesions (pink, scaling macules) with a low-potency topical corticosteroid to prevent new areas of hypopigmentation.

PREP Pearls

- Pityriasis alba is a form of postinflammatory hypopigmentation that often occurs in children who have a history of atopic dermatitis.
- Pityriasis alba is characterized by hypopigmented macules that may have associated scale. The borders of lesions are indistinct, with a gradual transition from normal to abnormal pigmentation.
- Treatment of pityriasis alba is with an emollient or a short course (7 days) of a low-potency topical corticosteroid.

American Board of Pediatrics Content Specification(s)/ Content Area

- Recognize the clinical features of pityriasis alba
- Recognize the clinical manifestations of vitiligo

Suggested Readings

American Academy of Pediatrics Section on Dermatology. Pityriasis alba. In: Mancini AJ, Krowchuk DP, eds. *Pediatric Dermatology: A Quick Reference Guide*. 3rd ed. Elk Grove Village, IL: American Academy of Pediatrics; 2016:405-407.

Item 252   Preferred Response: A

The patient in this vignette has evidence of an active gastrointestinal bleed with hemodynamic instability in the context of significant anemia; thus, the best next step in management is to stabilize the patient by the rapid administration of isotonic fluids and packed red blood cells. Patients with hemodynamic instability should be considered for intensive care management.

Gastrointestinal bleeding may manifest in various ways. Upper gastrointestinal tract bleeding (proximal to the ligament of Treitz) can present with hematemesis, melena, or even hematochezia if the bleeding is rapid. Lower gastrointestinal tract bleeding can present as melena or hematochezia. Although determining the source of the bleeding is necessary, regardless of the etiology, stabilization (with intravenous fluid, packed red blood cells, and/or other supportive measures) is the necessary first step. Confirming the presence of blood (in emesis or stool) is generally recommend with guaiac testing. Additional testing, including assessment of a complete blood cell count, coagulation studies, and liver function testing can help determine the bleeding severity and diagnosis.

If an upper gastrointestinal tract bleed is suspected (ie, hematemesis or melena), nasogastric lavage may help to confirm the presence of blood in the stomach. Causes of upper gastrointestinal tract bleeding include esophagitis, foreign body, Mallory-Weiss tear, esophageal varices, gastritis, gastric or duodenal ulcer, arteriovenous malformation, and portal hypertensive gastropathy. Endoscopy is generally recommended to diagnose the etiology of the upper gastrointestinal bleed and can be used therapeutically to provide hemostasis (through clips, coagulants, and other endoscopic tools).

Causes of lower gastrointestinal tract bleeding include anal fissure, infectious enteritis/colitis, eosinophilic gastrointestinal disease, intestinal polyp, arteriovenous malformation, Meckel diverticulum, intussusception, and inflammatory bowel disease. Colonoscopy is generally indicated if infection and surgical causes of bleeding (intussusception, Meckel diverticulum) are unlikely.

Although abdominal ultrasonography with Doppler, endoscopy, and a Meckel scan could be helpful diagnostic tests, stabilization of this hemodynamically unstable patient should occur prior to these studies. Given that blood was noted during the nasogastric lavage, a lower gastrointestinal bleed is unlikely and therefore a Meckel scan would not be initially recommended.

PREP Pearls

- Gastrointestinal bleeding can present with hematemesis, melena, and/or hematochezia.
- Initial assessment should include vital sign determination and laboratory testing to evaluate the severity of the gastrointestinal bleeding.
- Initial management of patients with gastrointestinal bleeding should include stabilization with intravenous fluids and packed red blood cells as necessary.

American Board of Pediatrics Content Specification(s)/ Content Area

- Plan the appropriate evaluation of blood in vomitus or stool, including in a patient who has hemodynamically significant blood loss
- Plan the appropriate evaluation of upper gastrointestinal bleeding

Suggested Readings

Neidich GA, Cole SR. Gastrointestinal bleeding. *Pediatr Rev*. 2014;35(6):243-254.

Sahn B, Mamula P, Friedlander J. Gastrointestinal hemorrhage. In: Wyllie R, Hyams JS, Kay M, eds. *Pediatric Gastrointestinal and Liver Diseases*. 5th ed. Philadelphia, PA: Elsevier; 2016:144-154.

Item 253   Preferred Response: A

For the boy in this vignette with attention-deficit/hyperactivity disorder (ADHD) and a possible learning disability, the symptoms of ADHD should be addressed regardless of the outcome of the school assessment. Classroom accommodations are indicated and can assist in optimizing the educational environment. These may include preferential seating, breaking assignments into smaller segments, extended time for tests, testing in a quiet environment, teaching organizational skills, and using positive reinforcement for desired behaviors. Although behavioral therapy is an evidence-based treatment for ADHD that involves parent training in behavioral therapy techniques to use with their child, cognitive behavioral therapy, which involves changing maladaptive thinking to change behavior, does not have sufficient evidence to be a standard treatment for ADHD in children. Extended school year services may be offered to some children with Individualized Education Programs but are not standard for children with ADHD, not all of whom qualify for special education services. Although results of the boy's current school assessment may have been affected by his ADHD symptoms (eg, they may be an underestimate of his abilities or function because of significant distractibility), re-evaluation may be more helpful after his ADHD symptoms are under control.

School-based assessments for possible learning disability typically include administration of measures of intelligence and achievement. Intelligence quotient tests are administered to assess a child's cognitive abilities. These cognitive abilities are influenced by factors including neurological conditions (eg, brain injury, brain disease), genetics, parental education and involvement, quality of home and educational environments, social support, and socioeconomic stability. Socioeconomic and cultural factors should be considered when interpreting IQ test results, as the test is valid only for the population for which it was standardized. In addition, many factors can affect a child's ability to perform at their best during test administration. The child's emotional well-being (eg, anxiety, depression), attention, motivation, interest, frustration tolerance, and rapport with the examiner can influence his performance. Health concerns, such as visual or hearing impairment and acute or chronic illness symptoms, can also affect the child's ability to do well on testing.

Standardized achievement tests typically evaluate learning in areas such as reading, written language, and mathematics. Specialized achievement tests measure specific areas of learning such as science, geography, and foreign language. A child's achievement test results can be compared to his same-age peers by reviewing his standard scores and percentiles. In addition, the child's performance in each category of learning can be compared; typically, performance between categories is within one standard deviation. A greater than one standard deviation difference between categories is typically significant and indicates relative strengths and weaknesses in learning.

Children with learning disabilities are educated in various environments, ranging from "push-in" assistance in a mainstream class to "pull-out" help outside of the mainstream class or placement in a special education class. The Individuals with Disabilities in Education Act mandates that education take place in the least restrictive environment (eg, "push-in" is preferred over "pull-out"). Strategies to assist with learning include presenting concepts using the child's preferred learning style (eg, visual demonstrations, using manipulative materials, auditory instruction), teaching and practicing skills in context instead of in isolation, consistent reinforcement of concepts and strategies across multiple settings, and providing instruction using topics of special interest to the student.

PREP Pearls

- A greater than one standard deviation difference between categories of learning is typically significant and indicates relative strengths and weaknesses in learning.
- Factors that can affect a child's performance on psychoeducational testing include the child's emotional well-being (eg, anxiety, depression), attention, motivation, interest, frustration tolerance, and rapport with the examiner.
- Socioeconomic and cultural factors should be considered when interpreting IQ test results, because the test is valid only for the population for which it was standardized.

American Board of Pediatrics Content Specification(s)/Content Area

- Interpret the results of specialized and standardized achievement tests, with emphasis on understanding the significance of discrepancies between categories
- Recognize appropriate educational settings for patients with learning disabilities, and the various strategies utilized in those settings to circumvent weaknesses
- Identify factors that can influence the results of intelligence quotient tests

Suggested Readings

Braaten EB, Norman D. Intelligence (IQ) testing. *Pediatr Rev*. 2006;27(11):403-408.

Dworkin PH. School failure. In: Augustyn M, Zuckerman B, Caronna EB, eds. *The Zuckerman Parker Handbook of Developmental and Behavioral Pediatrics for Primary Care*. 3rd ed. Philadelphia, PA: Wolters Kluwer; 2011:317-321

Rimrodt SL, Lipkin PH. Learning disabilities and school failure. *Pediatr Rev*. 2011;32(8):315-324.

Item 254	Preferred Response: C

The boy in the vignette has had symptoms of an upper respiratory illness for 2 weeks, presented to the emergency department with fever and headache, and then had a focal seizure. In this situation, intracranial complication of bacterial rhinosinusitis is high on the differential diagnosis. Therefore, of the responses, performing brain imaging is the best next step. Computed tomography of the head, with and without contrast, or magnetic resonance imaging of the brain, with and without contrast, should be considered to evaluate for epidural, subdural, or parenchymal abscess, or for cavernous sinus thrombosis. A brain abscess, as shown in the T1 axial magnetic resonance image with contrast (Item C254), could cause a focal seizure as in the boy in the vignette.

While awaiting brain imaging, other management steps should be initiated. Due to the high clinical suspicion for an intracranial infectious process, such as an abscess, a blood culture should be obtained and empiric antibiotics should be started.

In this setting, empiric antibiotics must cover pathogens associated with acute and chronic sinusitis such as *Staphylococcus aureus* (including methicillin-resistant *S aureus*), pneumococcus, nontypeable *Haemophilus influenzae*, *Moraxella catarrhalis*, group A *Streptococcus*, and anaerobes. Empiric antimicrobial choices include intravenous vancomycin plus

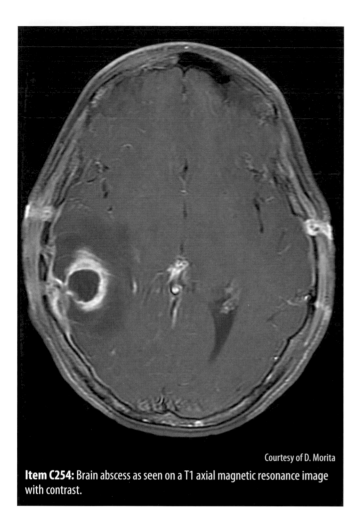

Item C254: Brain abscess as seen on a T1 axial magnetic resonance image with contrast.

Courtesy of D. Morita

American Board of Pediatrics Content Specification(s)/ Content Area

- Plan the appropriate diagnostic evaluation of a brain abscess
- Recognize the clinical findings associated with brain abscess
- Plan the appropriate management of a brain abscess

Suggested Readings

Lasley M. The role of antibiotics in the treatment of acute rhinosinusitis in children: a systematic review. *Pediatrics.* 2013;132(suppl 1):S31.

Teelin K. Case 2: New-onset seizures in a 14-year-old boy. *Pediatr Rev.* 2017;38(8):384.

Item 255   **Preferred Response: D**

ceftriaxone plus metronidazole. An alternative regimen includes intravenous vancomycin and meropenem.

If there is an intracranial abscess, seizure recurrence risk is high, so an anticonvulsant should be strongly considered. Neurosurgical consultation will be needed for further management if an abscess or other intracranial abnormality is identified on imaging.

Acetaminophen for analgesia and its antipyretic properties may increase patient comfort, but is not the best next step in this situation. The boy's seizure has stopped spontaneously, so intravenous lorazepam is not necessary. Because this presentation raises significant concern for an intracranial mass lesion, lumbar puncture is contraindicated due to the risk of precipitating brain herniation.

PREP Pearls

- Empiric antibiotics must cover pathogens associated with acute and chronic sinusitis such as *Staphylococcus aureus* (including methicillin-resistant *S aureus*), pneumococcus, nontypeable *Haemophilus influenzae, Moraxella catarrhalis*, group A *Streptococcus*, and anaerobes.
- When there is concern for an intracranial abscess, broad-spectrum antibiotics should be started empirically.
- When there is concern for an intracranial mass lesion, lumbar puncture is contraindicated because of the risk of precipitating brain herniation.

The infant in this vignette has a slightly elevated peanut-specific immunoglobulin E (IgE) level in the setting of severe eczema. In the 2017 addendum to the 2010 Guidelines for the Diagnosis and Management of Food Allergy in the United States (https://www.ncbi.nlm.nih.gov/pmc/articles/PMC5217343/), the expert pannel recommends that children with severe eczema, egg allergy, or both have introduction of age-appropriate peanut-containing food as early as 4 to 6 months to reduce the risk of peanut allergy. Prior to introducing peanut, the expert panel recommends evaluation with serum peanut-specific IgE (sIgE) measurement, which may be the preferred initial approach to prevent delays in peanut introduction, especially if skin-prick testing is not routine, or if referral for assessment by a specialist is not available in a timely manner. A peanut sIgE of less than 0.35 kU/L has a strong negative predictive value for the diagnosis of peanut allergy. However, the expert panel emphasizes that a peanut sIgE level of 0.35 kU/L or greater lacks adequate positive predictive value for the diagnosis of peanut allergy, and infants should be referred to a specialist for further evaluation during which a supervised oral challenge may be attempted.

Given the lack of positive predictive value of sIgE, an elevated level would not necessarily mean that an infant should avoid peanuts in the future. Skin-prick testing may be performed at any age. For patients under 2 years of age, skin prick test reactions to peanuts that have wheal diameters of 8 mm or greater are almost 95% predictive of clinical reactivity. The expert panel does not recommend food allergen panel testing or the addition of sIgE testing for foods other than peanut because of their poor positive predictive value, leading to misinterpretation, overdiagnosis, or unnecessary dietary restriction.

The risk of developing an atopic condition includes environmental and nonenvironmental factors. Atopy, encompassed by atopic dermatitis, allergic rhinitis, food allergy, and asthma, has a genetic predisposition. When both parents have an atopic disease, there is a 50% likelihood that their offspring will develop atopy, while only 13% of offspring whose parents do not have atopic disease will develop atopy. When 1 parent or sibling has atopy, the risk of atopic disease in another child is 29%. Having 1 component of atopy portends a 3-fold risk of developing another atopic condition. Males are more likely to develop atopic disease than females, with a ratio of approximately 1.8:1. As compared to whites, asthma is 2.5 times more prevalent among African Americans.

A number of variables influence the development of asthma and related atopic diseases. Child care exposure or having multiple siblings in the household increases the risk of lower respiratory infections but is protective against atopy. Infants exposed to maternal secondhand smoke have 1.4 to 2.8 times the risk of developing lower respiratory tract symptoms. Studies of breastfeeding suggest that it may postpone the onset of atopic disease in high-risk children but does not prevent its eventual development. Recent investigations of children's homes in the urban environment suggest that children exposed to high indoor levels of pet or pest allergens during infancy had a lower risk of developing asthma by age 7. The hygiene-microbiota hypothesis theorizes that increased infant gut microbiota diversity may reduce the risk of allergic disease. Evidence suggests that strategies such as promoting vaginal childbirth, breastfeeding, increased social exposure through sport, outdoor activities, less time spent indoors, pet exposure, and appropriate antibiotic use could help support a healthy gut microbiome and mature the immune system.

> ## PREP Pearls
>
> - Although a peanut immunoglobulin E blood level of less than 0.35 kU/L is associated with a low risk of reaction, an elevated level often occurs in individuals who tolerate peanut.
> - Based on the 2017 peanut allergy prevention guidelines, infants with severe eczema, egg allergy, or both should be evaluated for peanut reactivity by serum and/or skin-prick test, and if necessary, oral food challenge.

American Board of Pediatrics Content Specification(s)/Content Area

- Understand the role of the environment (eg, indoor pets, passive exposure to cigarette smoke) in the development and severity of allergic disease

- Recognize the non-environmental factors (eg, genetics, diet, infection) that influence the incidence and severity of atopy in infants and children

Suggested Readings

Du Toit G, Roberts G, Sayre PH, et al; LEAP Study Team. Randomized trial of peanut consumption in infants at risk for peanut allergy. *New Engl J Med*. 2015;372(9):803-813.

Nimmagadda SR, Evans R. Allergy: etiology and epidemiology. *Pediatr Rev*. 1999;20(4):110-116.

Tatachar P, Kumar S. Food-induced anaphylaxis and oral allergy syndrome. *Pediatr Rev*. 2008;29(4):e23-e27.

Togias A, Cooper SF, Acebal ML, et al. Addendum guidelines for the prevention of peanut allergy in the United States: report of the NIAID-sponsored expert panel. *J Allergy Clin Immunol*. 2017;139(1):29-44.

Item 256	Preferred Response: C

Nephroblastoma, also known as Wilms tumor, is the most common kidney tumor in children. There are approximately 500 cases of Wilms tumor diagnosed in the United States annually. Approximately 75% of cases arise in otherwise healthy children, while 25% arise as part of a genetic syndrome (Item C256). The mean age at diagnosis is 3 years for sporadic cases and 2 years for cases associated with underlying syndromes.

Nephroblastoma is treated with a combination of surgery, chemotherapy, and radiation that is dictated by its clinical and pathological features. These features include patient age, disease stage, tumor size and histology, and presence or absence of loss of heterozygosity at chromosome arm 1p and 16q. Nephroblastoma in children younger than 2 years with stage 1, favorable histology tumors that are small (< 550 g) can be managed with a nephrectomy alone; however, most children with nephroblastoma will require chemotherapy and some radiation therapy as well. While the overall cure rate for nephroblastoma is approximately 90%, it varies with the clinical and pathological features of the disease.

Table C256. Syndromes With ≥ 5% Chance of Wilms Tumor.

Syndrome	Chromosome Locus	Implicated Gene(s)	Phenotype	Estimated Wilms Tumor Risk (%)
WAGR	11p13	WT1	Aniridia, genitourinary anomalies, delayed-onset renal failure	30
Denys-Drash	11p13	WT1	Ambiguous genitalia, diffuse mesangial sclerosis	> 90
Frasier	11p13	WT1	Ambiguous genitalia, streak gonads, focal segmental glomerulosclerosis	8
Beckwith-Wiedemann isolated hemihypertrophy	11p15	IGF2, H19, KCNQ1 (KvLQT1), KCNQ1OT1 (LIT1), or CDKN1C (p57^{KIP2})	Organomegaly, large birth weight, macroglossia, omphalocele, hemihypertrophy, ear pits and creases, neonatal hypoglycemia	5
Perlman	2q37	DIS3L2	Prenatal overgrowth, facial dysmorphism, developmental delay, cryptorchidism, renal dysplasia	33
Mosaic variegated aneuploidy	15q15	BUB1B	Microcephaly, growth retardation, developmental delay, cataracts, heart defects	25
Fanconi anemia D1	13q12	BRCA2	Short stature, radial ray defects, bone marrow failure	20
Simpson-Golabi-Behmel	Xq26	GPC3	Overgrowth, coarse facial features	10

Reprinted with permission from Warwick AB, Dome JS. Renal tumors. In: Lanzkowsky P, Lipton JM, Fish JD, eds. *Lanzkowsky's Manual of Pediatric Hematology and Oncology*. 6th ed. London, United Kingdom: Academic Press; 2016:492.

Adrenocortical carcinoma is a rare adrenal malignancy in children that is associated with *p53* mutations and has a poor prognosis. Neuroblastoma is a malignancy of the sympathoadrenal axis. The prognosis for children with neuroblastoma varies greatly with the clinical and pathological features of the disease. Renal cell carcinoma is very rare in children and carries a poor prognosis.

PREP Pearls

- About 75% of cases of nephroblastoma are sporadic, with the remainder associated with an underlying syndrome.
- Approximately 90% of children with nephroblastoma will be cured of their disease, although the prognosis varies with the age of the child, the stage and histology of the tumor, and the presence or absence of 1p and 16q loss of heterozygosity.
- Nephroblastoma, also known as Wilms tumor, is the most common renal tumor in children.

American Board of Pediatrics Content Specification(s)/Content Area

- Understand the prognosis for a patient who has Wilms tumor
- Recognize the clinical findings associated with Wilms tumor

Suggested Readings

Davidoff AM. Wilms tumor. *Adv Pediatr.* 2012;59(1):247-67.

Friedman AD. Wilms tumor. *Pediatr Rev.* 2013;34(7):328-330.

PDQ Pediatric Treatment Editorial Board, National Cancer Institute. PDQ cancer information summaries: Wilms tumor and other childhood kidney tumors treatment. https://www.ncbi.nlm.nih.gov/books/NBK65842/.

Item 257   Preferred Response: C

The signs and symptoms present in the boy in the vignette are most consistent with the diagnosis of intussusception. Intussusception occurs when a segment of bowel telescopes into a more distal bowel segment. It is the most common cause of acute intestinal obstruction in young children, typically affecting children between 6 months and 3 years of age.

The typical presentation of intussusception involves an infant or toddler with intermittent episodes of colicky abdominal pain, often with vomiting (especially bilious vomiting). Between episodes of pain which are precipitated by bowel peristalsis, affected children may appear comfortable and even playful. When intestinal obstruction due to intussusception is prolonged, affected children may develop lethargy, pallor, altered mental status, and signs of frank peritonitis, shock, and gross blood per rectum ("currant jelly" stools) due to compromised perfusion to the affected segment of bowel. Abdominal examination may be significant for distention and a palpable "sausage-shaped" mass in the right upper quadrant; these findings are not present in many patients. The triad of bilious emesis, abdominal mass, and blood per rectum is seen in about 20% of children with intussusception. The absence of this triad does not rule out the

diagnosis. Children presenting early in the course of intussusception may have no history of bloody stools, though occult blood may be detected on rectal examination in 50% to 75% of patients.

Abdominal ultrasonography is the diagnostic study of choice for intussusception, with a positive study revealing a "target sign," reflecting a segment of bowel trapped within a distal segment of bowel. In most cases of intussusception, the recommended treatment is reduction by air contrast enema. In children with peritoneal signs, and those for whom attempts to reduce the intussusception by air contrast enema have failed, urgent operative management is indicated.

An inguinal hernia with incarceration may result in signs of intestinal obstruction with abdominal pain; however, a tender and red inguinal mass is commonly found. These findings are absent in the boy in the vignette. Furthermore, pain associated with an incarcerated inguinal hernia would typically be constant in nature rather than episodic.

Children may develop infectious enterocolitis due to infection with bacterial, viral, or parasitic pathogens. Signs and symptoms of infectious enterocolitis in children often include crampy abdominal pain, fever, nausea, and frequent watery stools (which may also contain blood and mucus, depending on the causative agent). Although the boy in the vignette has colicky abdominal pain and loose, heme-positive stools, he has no fever. Furthermore, his most predominant symptoms are episodic severe abdominal pain with progressive development of lethargy, rather than frequent profuse diarrhea. Intussusception is the diagnosis most consistent with his clinical presentation, though infectious enterocolitis should be included in his differential diagnosis.

Meckel diverticulum is a congenital abnormality of the small intestine arising from incomplete obliteration of the omphalomesenteric duct. Many children with this abnormality are asymptomatic. In symptomatic children, rectal bleeding is the most common presenting sign. This bleeding is typically painless, but some children may have pain before the onset of hematochezia. Intestinal obstruction is a potential complication of Meckel diverticulum. The clinical picture for the boy in the vignette is much more consistent with intussusception than Meckel diverticulum, and intussusception is a much more common reason for intermittent abdominal pain in a child his age.

PREP Pearls

- Intussusception should be included in the differential diagnosis for infants and young children with irritability, lethargy, and/or vomiting.
- Intussusception should be suspected in children with episodic abdominal pain and vomiting (particularly bilious vomiting).
- The triad of bilious emesis, abdominal mass, and blood per rectum can be seen in about 20% of cases in children with intussusception.

American Board of Pediatrics Content Specification(s)/ Content Area

- Recognize the clinical features associated with intussusception, and manage appropriately

Suggested Readings

Bachur RG. Abdominal emergencies. In: Shaw KN, Bachur RG, eds. *Fleisher and Ludwig's Textbook of Pediatric Emergency Medicine*. 7th ed. Philadelphia, PA: Lippincott Williams & Wilkins; 2016;chap 124

Ross A, LeLeiko NS. Acute abdominal pain. *Pediatr Rev*. 2010;31(4):135-144.

Item 258 — Preferred Response: D

The boy in the vignette has nephrotic syndrome (NS) most likely caused by minimal change disease. Nephrotic syndrome should be considered in any patient presenting with recurrent episodes of eye swelling and facial puffiness. Initially, these patients are often mistaken as having an allergic reaction and treated with a short course (3-5 days) of oral steroids or antihistamine. Nephrotic syndrome is characterized by edema (facial puffiness or generalized anasarca), proteinuria, hypoalbuminemia, and hyperlipidemia (elevated cholesterol and low-density lipoprotein cholesterol). In the pediatric population, NS is most commonly seen in school-aged children and adolescents. The worldwide prevalence of NS is approximately 16 cases per 100,000 children, with an incidence of 2 to 7 per 100,000 children. Overall, boys are more frequently affected than girls; however, this predominance does not persist into adolescence.

Nephrotic syndrome is categorized as 1) primary/ idiopathic, 2) secondary, or 3) congenital/infantile. Idiopathic NS is the most common form encountered in children. Based on renal biopsy findings, children with idiopathic NS are further characterized as having minimal change disease (most common), focal segmental glomerulosclerosis (FSGS), membranoproliferative glomerulonephritis (MPGN), or membranous nephropathy. Microscopic hematuria is present in nearly 20% of patients with minimal change disease and nearly 50% to 60% of children with FSGS or MPGN. In a child with NS, the presence of renal failure, hypocomplementemia or features of vasculitis (eg, joint pain and swelling, rash, oral ulcers, serologic evidence), gross hematuria, or infections (intrauterine, hepatitis B and C, human immunodeficiency virus) should prompt consideration of secondary NS. The congenital/infantile form of NS presents at birth or before the first year of age, and is associated with genetic abnormalities leading to increased permeability of the glomerular basement barrier.

Most cases of minimal change disease are diagnosed clinically and treated without kidney biopsy. These children typically present between 2 and 10 years of age, with the classic features of NS and a negative evaluation for secondary causes. Urinalysis will demonstrate nephrotic range proteinuria, defined as a spot urine (preferably a first-morning sample) protein-creatinine ratio greater than 2.0 (<0.2 is normal, 0.2-2 is non-nephrotic range). The initial episode of NS is treated with oral steroids (prednisone 60 mg/m^2 per day for 4-6 weeks, followed by 40 mg/m^2 per dose every other day for 2-5 months, with gradual tapering). The most important determinant of renal prognosis in idiopathic NS is steroid responsiveness. Patients with frequent relapsing or corticosteroid-dependent NS are treated with steroid-sparing medications to avoid the complications associated with long-term steroid therapy (eg, cushingoid features, cataracts, growth restriction, glaucoma, peptic ulcer disease, behavioral changes). Cyclophosphamide, an alkylating agent, is used as a steroid-sparing agent and can induce long-term remission. Patients resistant to initial steroid therapy or cyclophosphamide may be treated with other steroid-sparing therapies such as calcineurin inhibitors (cyclosporine, tacrolimus), mycophenolate mofetil, or rituximab.

Renal biopsy is recommended for patients with NS who are unresponsive to steroid therapy (steroid resistance), present outside the typical age range, have associated refractory edema, have features suggesting a diagnosis other than minimal change disease, or those starting calcineurin inhibitor therapy. Focal segmental glomerulosclerosis, membranous nephropathy, and membranoproliferative glomerulonephritis, each of which may present with NS, are diagnosed after renal biopsy.

Focal segmental glomerulosclerosis is characterized by renal fibrosis involving segments of some of the glomeruli along with features of mesangial hypercellularity, tubular atrophy, and tubulointerstitial fibrosis. In children, FSGS may be primary/idiopathic or secondary in etiology. Secondary FSGS is considered the final pathway of renal injury associated with glomerular inflammation and epithelial injury, glomerular hyperfiltration, and hypertension associated with significant nephron loss (congenital or acquired single kidney) or congenital glomerular basement membrane abnormalities. Up to 50% of patients with FSGS have associated microscopic hematuria, hypertension, steroid resistance, or progression to end-stage renal disease.

Chronic renal inflammation associated with mesangial hypercellularity and expansion is seen in MPGN. Glomerular inflammation associated with subendothelial electron-dense deposits is seen in type 1 MPGN, thickening and increased density of glomerular basement membrane is seen in type 2 MPGN, and type 3 MPGN has histopathologic features of both type 1 and type 2 MPGN. Membranoproliferative glomerulonephritis is frequently associated with hematuria (60%-100%), hypertension (40%-70%), elevated serum creatinine (20%-50%), and low C3 levels (60%-75%). Nephrotic syndrome is the initial presentation in up to 50% of patients with MPGN.

Membranous nephropathy is a rare cause of NS in children or adolescents; it is more frequently seen in adults. Children with membranous nephropathy usually present with NS (almost 80%), and frequently have associated hematuria (up to 80%) and hypertension. Progression to end-stage renal disease is seen in nearly 13% of the patients. Renal biopsy is characterized by diffuse thickening of capillary walls, and subepithelial electron-dense deposits and spikes seen on electron microscopy.

PREP Pearls

- Hematuria, hypertension, and elevated serum creatinine are more frequently seen in nephrotic syndrome associated with focal segmental glomerulosclerosis, membranoproliferative glomerulonephritis, and membranous nephropathy.
- Minimal change disease is the most common form of nephrotic syndrome in children, and most cases are initially treated with steroids without kidney biopsy.
- Nephrotic syndrome is characterized by edema (facial puffiness or generalized anasarca), proteinuria, hypoalbuminemia, and hyperlipidemia (elevated cholesterol and low-density lipoprotein cholesterol).

American Board of Pediatrics Content Specification(s)/ Content Area

- Identify the various etiologies of hyponatremia
- Recognize the clinical features associated with hypoproteinemia

Suggested Readings

Pais P, Avner EA. Nephrotic syndrome. In: Kliegman RM, Stanton BF, St. Geme J, Schor NF, eds. *Nelson Textbook of Pediatrics*. 20th ed. Philadelphia, PA: Saunders; 2016;2521-2528

Varade WS. Nephrotic syndrome. In: McInerny TK, Adam HM, Campbell DE, DeWitt TG, Foy JM, Kamat DM, eds. *American Academy of Pediatrics Textbook of Pediatric Care*. Elk Grove Village, IL: American Academy of Pediatrics; 2009; 2291-2303

Item 259   Preferred Response: D

Chest pain is a common chief concern in pediatrics, although an underlying cardiac condition is only rarely present. Chest pain that occurs with exertion or that is associated with abnormal cardiac examination findings is concerning and warrants a referral to a pediatric cardiologist. The patient in this vignette has chest pain with exertion and physical examination findings that are consistent with aortic stenosis. His chest pain may be associated with compromised coronary blood flow during exercise caused by the aortic stenosis. Therefore, for the patient in this vignette, referral to a pediatric cardiologist and exercise restriction until that evaluation is complete is the best next step.

Chest pain in children is far more commonly noncardiac in origin. Noncardiac causes of chest pain can be categorized into musculoskeletal, pulmonary/airway, gastrointestinal, and miscellaneous (Item C259A). Musculoskeletal etiologies are the most common cause of chest pain in children and adolescents.

Item C259A. Noncardiac Causes of Chest Pain in Children (4-6 Years).

Musculoskeletal
- Costochondritis/costosternal syndrome
- Nonspecific or idiopathic chest-wall pain
- Sickle cell vaso-occlusive crisis
- Slipping rib syndrome
- Tietze syndrome
- Trauma and muscle strain-overuse injury
- Xiphoid pain (xiphoidalgia)

Pulmonary or Airway-related
- Acute chest syndrome
- Bronchial asthma
- Bronchitis
- Exercise-induced or cough variant asthma
- Pleurisy
- Pneumonia
- Pneumothorax
- Pulmonary embolism

Gastrointestinal
- Cholecystitis
- Drug-induced esophagitis/gastritis
- Esophageal spasm
- Gastroesophageal reflux disease
- Peptic ulcer disease

Miscellaneous
- Breast-related conditions
- Herpes zoster
- Hyperventilation
- Panic disorder
- Spinal cord or nerve root compression

Reprinted with permission from Reddy SR, Singh HR. Chest pain in children and adolescents. *Pediatr Rev*. 2010;31(1):e2.

Cardiac causes of chest pain (Item C259B) are far less common. These causes can be categorized into inflammatory, increased myocardial demand/decreased cardiac output, coronary artery anomalies, drugs, and miscellaneous. Referral to a cardiologist is recommended for any child with chest pain associated with exertion, palpitations, syncope, abnormal cardiac examination findings (as seen in the patient in this vignette), abnormal electrocardiogram, personal history of cardiac disease or surgery, or family history of genetic syndromes, arrhythmias, sudden death, or premature coronary artery disease.

Item C259B. Cardiac Causes of Chest Pain.

Inflammatory: Pericarditis, Myocarditis

- Infective: viruses, bacteria
- Noninfective: SLE, Crohn disease, postpericardiotomy syndrome

Increased Myocardial Demand or Decreased Supply

- Arrhythmias
- Cardiomyopathy: dilated or hypertrophic
- LVOT obstruction: aortic stenosis, subaortic stenosis, supravalvar aortic stenosis

Coronary Artery Abnormalities

- Acquired: Kawasaki disease, postsurgical (after arterial switch operation, after Ross procedure), posttransplant coronary vasculopathy, familial hypercholesterolemia
- Congenital: ALCAPA, ALCA from right coronary sinus, coronary fistula

Miscellaneous

- Aortic dissection
- Herpes zoster
- Pulmonary hypertension
- Rupture of aortic aneurysm
- Spinal cord or nerve root compression

Drugs

- Cocaine
- Sympathomimetic overdose

Abbreviations: ALCA, anomalous left coronary artery; ALCAPA, anomalous origin of the left coronary artery from pulmonary artery; LVOT, left ventricular outflow tract; SLE, systemic lupus erythematosus

Reprinted with permission from Reddy SR, Singh HR. Chest pain in children and adolescents. *Pediatr Rev*. 2010;31(1):e4.

Regardless of the etiology of chest pain, a thorough history and physical examination are important first steps that then dictate whether reassurance or additional testing is needed. Chest radiography and pulmonary function tests are not the best next step given that this chest pain occurred with exertion. Referral to a cardiologist should be done first. Also, exercise restriction until a complete diagnosis is made is necessary based on the history. An exercise stress test may be revealing, but may also place the patient at unnecessary risk.

PREP Pearls

- A thorough history and physical examination significantly aid in the categorization of chest pain as cardiac or noncardiac in origin.
- Chest pain associated with abnormal cardiac examination findings or that occurs with exertion is a concerning finding that warrants referral for a cardiac evaluation.
- Chest pain in children and adolescents can be noncardiac or cardiac in nature. Noncardiac chest pain is far more common.

American Board of Pediatrics Content Specification(s)/ Content Area

- Recognize the cardiovascular and non-cardiovascular causes of chest pain in children of various ages

Suggested Readings

Angoff GH, Kane DA, Giddins N, et al. Regional implementation of a pediatric cardiology chest pain guideline using SCAMPs methodology. *Pediatrics*. 2013;132(4):e1010-e1017.

Reddy SR, Singh HR. Chest pain in children and adolescents. *Pediatr Rev*. 2010;31(1):c1-c9.

Saleeb SF, Li WY, Warren SZ, Lock, JE. Effectiveness of screening for life-threatening chest pain in children. *Pediatrics*. 2011;128(5):e1062-e1068.

Item 260   Preferred Response: D

The adolescent girl in this vignette has a classic presentation for primary dysmenorrhea, which is the most common gynecologic cause of abdominal pain in female adolescents, affecting 60% to 90% of adolescent girls. It is characterized by crampy lower abdominal pain that occurs with menses and may be associated with lower back pain, nausea, vomiting, diarrhea, bloating, headaches, and dizziness. It most commonly begins when a female starts to have ovulatory cycles 1 to 3 years after the start of menarche. The pain may begin 1 to 2 days prior to the start of the menstrual cycle and be most severe for the first 2 days after the start of a cycle.

Primary dysmenorrhea is thought to be caused by excess production of endometrial prostaglandins ($F_{2\alpha}$ and E_2). Prostaglandin $F_{2\alpha}$ increases smooth muscle contractility, and prostaglandin E_2 causes vasodilatation and platelet dysfunction. Prostaglandins can also have an activating effect on the gastrointestinal tract, causing the gastrointestinal problems associated with menstruation.

Secondary dysmenorrhea has similar symptoms to primary dysmenorrhea but is caused by pelvic pathology. It is more prevalent in older women, but adolescent girls may report menstrual pain that started with the onset of menses or have a time course or pattern that is unusual for primary dysmenorrhea. The history is crucial to differentiate the pain as acute or chronic and cyclic or noncyclic and to determine if the patient is sexually active. Adolescents with acute pelvic pain warrant an abdominal and pelvic examination (with bimanual examination) if they are sexually active and an external genital examination if they are not sexually active. The pelvic examination is helpful in assessing sexual maturity rating, identifying a patent hymen or vaginal bulge that may signify an obstructive anomaly, and identifying cervical motion tenderness or uterine/adnexal tenderness or masses.

For acute pelvic pain in the adolescent girl, medical emergencies must be ruled out first, including ovarian torsion and complications from pregnancy (ie, ectopic pregnancy or uterine rupture). Ovarian torsion (twisting of the ovary on its pedicle) may present with acute onset of sharp abdominal pain associated with nausea and vomiting. An ectopic pregnancy may present with crampy abdominal pain and vaginal bleeding, with a missed period of more than 6 weeks. Other conditions in the differential diagnosis for acute pelvic pain include endometritis, pelvic inflammatory disease, and endometriosis. The most common etiologies for acute pelvic pain in adolescent girls are dysmenorrhea, mittelschmerz (cyclic midcycle ovulatory pain), ruptured ovarian cyst, and pelvic inflammatory disease. It is important to consider other organ systems that may present with acute pelvic pain including appendicitis, urinary tract infections, renal stones, trauma (blunt trauma vs sexual abuse), or a foreign body.

Chronic pelvic pain, present more than 3 months, can be cyclic or noncyclic. The most common gynecologic causes of cyclic pain include outflow tract obstruction, endometriosis, and ovarian cysts. The most common causes of noncyclic pain include pelvic inflammatory disease and an ovarian cyst or mass with concern for torsion. The adolescent girl with an outflow tract obstruction usually has normal pubertal development, but is premenarchal. The differential diagnosis would include a complete transverse vaginal septum, vaginal agenesis, or an imperforate hymen, which would cause hematocolpos. These mullerian anomalies may present with urinary frequency or retention, constipation, and lower back pain. Endometriosis should be considered in the adolescent girl with chronic pelvic pain that is often crampy and is refractory to treatment with nonsteroidal anti-inflammatory drugs and combined oral contraceptive pills or other combined hormonal therapy. Ovarian cysts are commonly identified as incidental findings on pelvic ultrasonography during evaluations for abdominal pain. Cysts that are complex, loculated, solid, or larger than 5 cm require further evaluation to differentiate a benign process (eg, teratoma) from a malignancy (eg, germ cell tumor). Sequelae of untreated pelvic inflammatory disease are chronic pelvic pain and pelvic adhesions. Nongynecologic causes of chronic pelvic pain include interstitial cystitis, inflammatory bowel disease, and abdominal migraines. Psychosomatic symptoms are also on the differential diagnosis of chronic pelvic pain in a patient with normal results from laboratory and imaging studies who may have depression or a history of sexual abuse.

For the adolescent girl in this vignette, endometriosis would be a consideration if a trial of an appropriate dose of a nonsteroidal anti-inflammatory drug and/or combined hormonal therapy did not improve her symptoms. The definitive diagnosis of endometriosis is made by laparoscopy. Irritable bowel syndrome is less likely because this patient only experiences significant abdominal pain and gastrointestinal symptoms during the first 2 days of her period. Ovarian cysts can be painful if they grow quickly or rupture, and the symptoms are generally acute. A functional simple ovarian cyst is physiologic and a normal occurrence of the menstrual cycle. It is not usually associated with pain.

American Board of Pediatrics Content Specification(s)/Content Area

- Recognize the gynecologic etiologies of acute and chronic abdominal pain
- Recognize normal variations in the menstrual cycle in adolescent girls

Suggested Readings

Kaskowitz A, Quint E. A practical overview of managing adolescent gynecologic conditions in the pediatric office. *Pediatr Rev.* 2014;35(9):371-381.

Laufer MR. Gynecologic pain: dysmenorrhea, acute and chronic pelvic pain, endometriosis, and premenstrual syndrome. In: Emans SJH, Laufer MR, eds. *Emans, Laufer, and Goldstein's Pediatric and Adolescent Gynecology.* 6th ed. Philadelphia, PA: Wolters Kluwer; 2012:238-271

Powell J. The approach to chronic pelvic pain in the adolescent. *Obstet Gynecol Clin N Am.* 2014;41(3):343-355.

Item 261 **Preferred Response: C**

The boy in this vignette is receiving ceftriaxone and vancomycin to treat septic shock and meningitis resulting from an invasive gram-positive infection. The starting dose regimen is appropriate. The levels will not yet be in the therapeutic range because the steady state is not reached after 2 doses. Therefore, the most appropriate management is to continue the current antibiotic regimen.

The principles of pharmacokinetics and pharmacodynamics determine the efficacy and toxicity of drugs. Pharmacokinetics describe how a drug is absorbed, distributed, metabolized, and eliminated in the body. Pharmacodynamics describe the effects of the drug on the body. The rate and extent of absorption of the active form of the drug is known as bioavailability. Enteral, intramuscular, subcutaneous, and topical bioavailability can be affected by drug-specific chemical factors such as pH and solubility, as well as the patient-specific factors such as the local environment at the site of drug administration. Intravenous medications are considered to be 100% bioavailable, because they are injected directly into the circulation. Drug distribution is affected by drug-specific factors such as molecular size, degree of protein binding, and water and fat solubility as well as patient-related factors such as serum protein concentration, body composition of water and fat, and tissue perfusion. The volume of distribution determines the concentration of the drug:

Concentration = Dose/volume of distribution

Drugs that are lipophilic and low protein binding, and those that cross the blood-brain barrier have a higher volume of distribution, whereas hydrophobic and highly protein-bound drugs have a lower volume of distribution. Drug metabolism and excretion are also dependent on drug-related factors, such as whether they are substrates for hepatic enzymes or are renally eliminated, as well as patient-related factors such as organ function.

Vancomycin is a renally excreted antibiotic used to treat invasive and resistant gram-positive infections. If the vancomycin concentration reaches toxic levels, acute renal injury can occur. Close therapeutic monitoring of vancomycin and other drugs with a narrow therapeutic index is important to ensure efficacy and to limit toxicity. The elimination half-life of a drug is the time required to reduce the concentration by 50%. For drugs such as vancomycin which are subject to first-order kinetics, steady state concentration, in which the rate of elimination of the drug is equal to the rate of administration, is achieved after about 4 half-lives. A dosing interval approximating the half-life should be chosen. Therefore, steady state trough and peak levels can be obtained before and after the 4th or 5th dose (or later), respectively. For the boy in the vignette, although the peak and trough levels are lower than recommended, steady state has not been achieved by the second dose, so the regimen should be continued until steady state levels could be obtained. A higher dose or a shorter interval is not recommended, because it could lead to toxic levels when steady state is reached. Although dexamethasone has been used as an adjunctive therapy in children with bacterial meningitis, it is controversial, and does not have any benefit if initiated more than 1 hour after antibiotics.

PREP Pearls

- Drug concentration is the dose divided by the volume of distribution.
- Drugs that are lipophilic and low protein binding, and those that cross the blood-brain barrier have a higher volume of distribution, whereas hydrophobic and highly protein bound drugs have a lower volume of distribution.
- For drugs that undergo first-order kinetics, steady state concentration, in which the rate of elimination of the drug is equal to the rate of administration, is achieved after about 4 half-lives.

American Board of Pediatrics Content Specification(s)/Content Area

- Plan the appropriate timing for measurement of serum drug concentrations
- Recognize the association between half-life, therapeutic range, and drug toxicity
- Understand the number of half-lives required to reach steady-state serum drug concentrations

Suggested Readings

Cole TS, Riordan A. Vancomycin dosing in children: what is the question? *Arch Dis Child*. 2013;98(12):994-997.

Sandritter TL, McLaughlin M, Artman M, Lowry J. The interplay between pharmacokinetics and pharmacodynamics. *Pediatr Rev*. 2017;38:195.

Swanson D. Meningitis. *Pediatr Rev*. 2015;36:514.

Item 262   Preferred Response: D

The boy in this vignette has a cholesteatoma, which is a collection of squamous epithelial cells in the middle ear or mastoid. Because cholesteatomas typically continue to enlarge, can become infected, and can lead to hearing loss, cranial nerve palsies, vertigo, and rarely, venous thrombosis, meningitis, or brain abscess, referral to an otolaryngologist for removal is necessary. There is no indication for antibiotic-corticosteroid otic drops, oral antibiotics, or reassurance.

Cholesteatomas can be congenital or associated with recurrent middle ear infections and/or middle ear surgery. They are often asymptomatic and simply noted on routine physical examination, but cholesteatomas can also cause chronic ear drainage or new-onset hearing loss. The differential diagnosis includes tympanosclerosis, an inclusion cyst of the tympanic membrane, a white foreign body, and exostosis (outgrowth of bone into the external ear canal). Early and small cholesteatomas can be diagnosed on physical examination, but in some situations, imaging with computed tomography or magnetic resonance imaging may be necessary to evaluate the extent of involvement. All children with a suspected or confirmed cholesteatoma should undergo audiologic evaluation. The recurrence rate after surgical excision is high (up to 50%), so children must have regular follow up.

PREP Pearls

- A cholesteatoma is a collection of squamous epithelial cells in the middle ear or mastoid. Because cholesteatomas typically continue to enlarge, can become infected, and can lead to hearing loss, cranial nerve palsies, vertigo, and rarely, venous thrombosis, meningitis, or brain abscess, referral to an otolaryngologist for removal is necessary.
- After surgical excision, the recurrence rate for cholesteatomas is high (up to 50%) so children must have regular follow up.
- Cholesteatomas can be asymptomatic and simply noted on routine physical examination, or they can present as chronic ear drainage or new-onset hearing loss.

- Recognize the clinical findings associated with a cholesteatoma and the consequences if left untreated

Suggested Readings

Ching HH, Spinner AG, Ng M. Pediatric tympanic membrane cholesteatoma: systematic review and meta-analysis. *Int J Pediatr Otorhinolaryngol.* 2017;102:21-27.

Isaacson G. Diagnosis of pediatric cholesteatoma. *Pediatrics.* 2007;120(3):603-608.

Item 263   **Preferred Response: D**

Postexposure passive immunization with varicella-zoster immune globulin is indicated for the high-risk, immunocompromised adolescent in this vignette with significant exposure to varicella zoster virus (VZV). Individuals who receive hematopoietic stem cell transplantation (HSCT) should be considered nonimmune to varicella despite any previous history of disease or receipt of varicella immunization. With the exception of HIV-infected children with a CD4+ T-lymphocyte percentage of greater than or equal to 15%, live virus vaccines, such as varicella vaccine, are not routinely administered to patients with congenital or acquired T-lymphocyte immunodeficiency disorders, such as the patient in this vignette who is less than 1 year post HSCT.

Varicella (chickenpox) is a vaccine-preventable, highly communicable disease caused by primary infection with VZV. Transmission of VZV from person to person occurs most commonly through airborne respiratory droplets; it may also occur following direct contact with vesicular skin lesions, or less commonly, upon contact with infected respiratory secretions. Varicella zoster virus infects the susceptible host via the upper respiratory tract or conjunctivae. The usual incubation period is 14 to 16 days (range, 9-21 days). An infected individual is contagious 1 to 2 days before the appearance of rash until all cutaneous lesions have crusted. Primary varicella typically presents with fever, constitutional symptoms, and a generalized vesicular, pruritic rash that primarily involves the trunk and face; symptoms usually resolve within 7 to 10 days. In the United States, inclusion of varicella vaccine as part of the routine childhood immunization series has resulted in a dramatic decline in the incidence of varicella and its complications.

Severe or complicated disease is more common in infants, adolescents, pregnant women, and immunocompromised people. Management of exposure to VZV is based on an assessment of the extent of the exposure, followed by determination of evidence of immunity to varicella (Item C263). An individual is considered immune to varicella if 1 of the following criteria are met: health care provider diagnosis of varicella or zoster disease; health care provider–verified history of varicella or zoster disease; documentation of age-appropriate immunization; or laboratory evidence of immunity or laboratory confirmation of disease. Options for VZV postexposure immunoprophylaxis include passive immunoprophylaxis with varicella-zoster immune globulin, active immunization with varicella vaccine, or chemoprophylaxis with oral acyclovir or valacyclovir.

Postexposure prophylaxis using varicella-zoster immune globulin is recommended for exposed individuals without evidence of immunity to varicella who are at elevated risk for severe disease and in whom varicella vaccine is contraindicated. Candidates who should receive varicella-zoster immune globulin as postexposure prophylaxis include:

- Immunocompromised children without a history of varicella disease or varicella vaccination
- Susceptible pregnant women
- Newborns whose mothers have signs and symptoms of chickenpox within 5 days before delivery to 48 hours after delivery
- Hospitalized preterm infants ($\geq$ 28 weeks of gestation) whose mothers lack varicella immunity
- Exposed hospitalized preterm infants (< 28 weeks of gestation or $\leq$ 1,000 g birth weight), regardless of maternal history of varicella or VZV serostatus

In the case of an exposed, susceptible, immunosuppressed individual at risk for severe disease, varicella-zoster immune globulin should be administered as soon as possible after establishing VZV exposure (< 10 days). If varicella-zoster immune globulin is not available, an alternative is intravenous immunoglobulin (IGIV; 400 mg/kg once). However, data showing the effectiveness of IGIV for postexposure prophylaxis of varicella are lacking.

If neither varicella-zoster immune globulin nor IGIV is available, chemoprophylaxis with oral acyclovir or oral valacyclovir beginning 7 to 10 days after exposure, and continuing for 7 days, is an option for susceptible immunosuppressed individuals. Chemoprophylaxis with a 7-day course of oral acyclovir or oral valacyclovir may prevent or attenuate the disease in exposed, susceptible, immunocompetent children and may be considered if varicella vaccine cannot be used. However, no published evidence exists on the effectiveness of antiviral agents as postexposure prophylaxis in immunocompromised patients or adults.

The minimum age for routine administration of varicella vaccine for immunocompetent children is 12 months. Vaccination is not recommended as postexposure prophylaxis for exposed infants younger than 12 months. Varicella vaccine would be recommended to prevent or modify disease among exposed healthy individuals ($\geq$ 12 months of age) without evidence of immunity and should be given as soon as possible, preferably within 3 days and possibly up to 5 days after varicella or herpes zoster exposure.

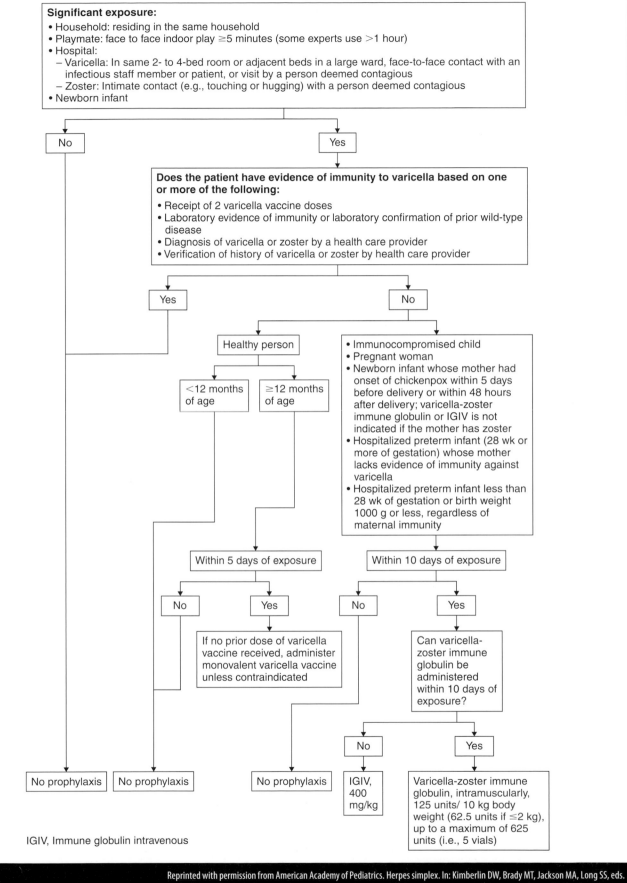

Significant exposure:
- Household: residing in the same household
- Playmate: face to face indoor play ≥5 minutes (some experts use >1 hour)
- Hospital:
  – Varicella: In same 2- to 4-bed room or adjacent beds in a large ward, face-to-face contact with an infectious staff member or patient, or visit by a person deemed contagious
  – Zoster: Intimate contact (e.g., touching or hugging) with a person deemed contagious
- Newborn infant

No → Yes

Does the patient have evidence of immunity to varicella based on one or more of the following:
- Receipt of 2 varicella vaccine doses
- Laboratory evidence of immunity or laboratory confirmation of prior wild-type disease
- Diagnosis of varicella or zoster by a health care provider
- Verification of history of varicella or zoster by health care provider

Yes → No

Healthy person

- Immunocompromised child
- Pregnant woman
- Newborn infant whose mother had onset of chickenpox within 5 days before delivery or within 48 hours after delivery; varicella-zoster immune globulin or IGIV is not indicated if the mother has zoster
- Hospitalized preterm infant (28 wk or more of gestation) whose mother lacks evidence of immunity against varicella
- Hospitalized preterm infant less than 28 wk of gestation or birth weight 1000 g or less, regardless of maternal immunity

<12 months of age | ≥12 months of age

Within 5 days of exposure

No | Yes

Within 10 days of exposure

No | Yes

If no prior dose of varicella vaccine received, administer monovalent varicella vaccine unless contraindicated

Can varicella-zoster immune globulin be administered within 10 days of exposure?

No | Yes

No prophylaxis | No prophylaxis

No prophylaxis

IGIV, 400 mg/kg

Varicella-zoster immune globulin, intramuscularly, 125 units/ 10 kg body weight (62.5 units if ≤2 kg), up to a maximum of 625 units (i.e., 5 vials)

IGIV, Immune globulin intravenous

Item C263: Exposures to varicella-zoster virus: evaluation and management.

Exposed immunocompetent individuals should also receive a second dose of the varicella vaccine at the age-appropriate interval. Patients should be advised that the vaccine may not prevent disease in all instances; however, receiving the vaccine as postexposure prophylaxis will confer immunity against future exposure.

PREP Pearls

- In exposed, susceptible, immunosuppressed individuals at risk for severe disease, varicella-zoster immune globulin should be administered as soon as possible following exposure but within 10 days.
- Individuals who receive hematopoietic stem cell transplantation should be considered nonimmune to varicella despite any previous history of disease or receipt of varicella immunization.
- Severe or complicated varicella is more common in infants, adolescents, pregnant women, and immunocompromised people.

American Board of Pediatrics Content Specification(s)/Content Area

- Plan appropriate antiviral therapy for normal and immunocompromised patients who have varicella-zoster virus infection
- Plan the appropriate management of an immunocompromised patient exposed to varicella

Suggested Readings

American Academy of Pediatrics. Herpes simplex. In: Kimberlin DW, Brady MT, Jackson MA, Long SS, eds. *Red Book: 2018 Report of the Committee on Infectious Diseases*. 31st ed. Itasca, IL: American Academy of Pediatrics; 2018:437-449.

Centers for Disease Control and Prevention. Prevention of varicella: recommendations of the Advisory Committee on Immunization Practices (ACIP). *MMWR Recomm Rep*. 2007;56(RR-4):1-40.

Centers for Disease Control and Prevention. Updated recommendations for use of VariZIG–United States, 2013. *MMWR Morb Mortal Wkly Rep*. 2013;62:574-576.

Item 264   Preferred Response: A

The girl in this vignette is having episodes of asthma triggered by allergens. Although the cat is not in the bedroom at night, it is a likely culprit. The immune response triggered by IgE-mediated allergy has both immediate and delayed components. The immediate response of watery eyes and sneezing when she holds the cat represents the release of preformed mediators from mast cells as inhaled cat antigen interacts with respiratory mast cell–bound IgE. A delayed response that occurs hours after the exposure, characterized by eosinophils and neutrophils that have responded to the chemotactic effect of the immediate-release mediators, is responsible for a longer, often more severe and refractory bronchospasm that may not be temporally related to the responsible antigen. The complex interactions of multiple inflammatory cell types in immediate and delayed asthma are shown in Item C264.

Bronchodilators are effective treatment for the immediate bronchospastic response to mast cell mediator release but are not adequate for the delayed inflammatory response. Chronic use of inhaled corticosteroids will prevent the delayed response when taken before exposure. Systemic corticosteroids may be needed for resolution of a well-established delayed allergic response.

Drying of the respiratory mucosa caused by breathing drier and cooler air through the mouth during exercise is one component of exercise-induced bronchospasm. Mouth breathing alone is not recognized as a trigger for wheezing. The immediate allergic response is associated with IgE-specific antibodies (not IgG-specific antibodies). Although allergy to house dust mite could be a contributor to the nocturnal symptoms, it is IgE (and not IgG) antibodies that are responsible for the allergic reaction. Overuse of short-acting bronchodilators has been associated with decreased pharmacologic response but not with a rebound phenomenon.

PREP Pearls

- Bronchodilators alone are not adequate to treat the delayed allergic response; anti-inflammatory drugs (inhaled daily steroids or systemic corticosteroids for well-established delayed allergic responses) are also required.
- The delayed response in allergic asthma may be more severe and refractory to management than the immediate, IgE-mediated allergic response.

American Board of Pediatrics Content Specification(s)/Content Area

- Recognize the early and late effects of an IgE-mediated allergen in a patient with asthma

Suggested Readings

Guill MF. Asthma update: epidemiology and pathophysiology. *Pediatr Rev*. 2004;25(9):299-305.

Hill VC, Wood PR. Asthma: epidemiology, pathophysiology, and initial evaluation. *Pediatr Rev*. 2009;30(9):331-336.

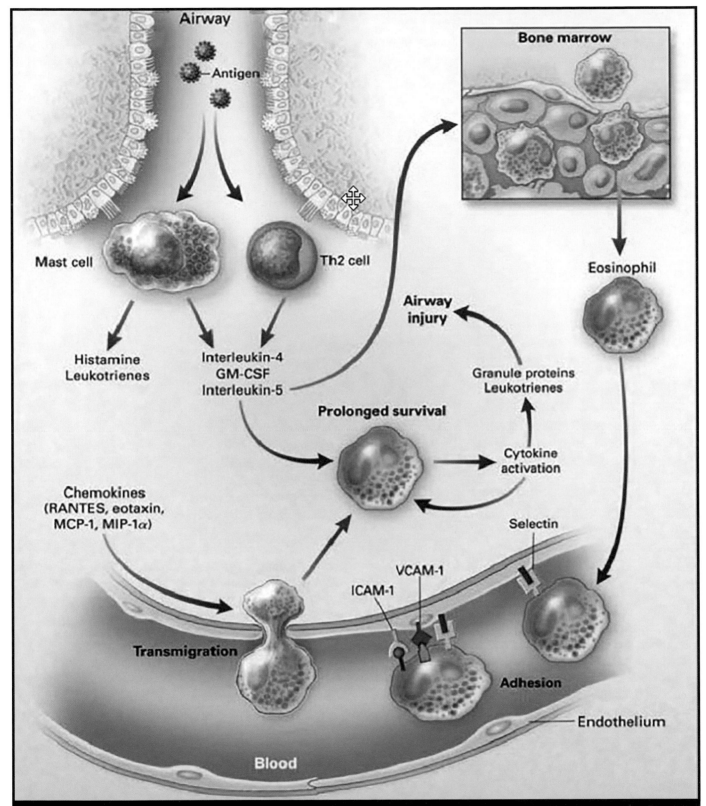

Reprinted with permission from Busse WW and Lemanske RF, Advances in Immunology. *N Eng J Med*. 2001; 344: 350

Item C264: Cellular mechanisms involved in immediate and delayed allergic response. Abbreviations: GM-CSF, granulocyte-macrophage colony-stimulating factor; ICAM-1, intercellular adhesion molecule 1; MCP-1, monocyte chemotactic protein; MIP-1a, macrophage inflammatory protein; MCP-1, monocyte chemotactic protein; VCAM-1, vascular-cell adhesion molecule 1.

The neonate in the vignette, born to a group B *Streptococcus* (GBS)–positive mother with fever, who received inadequate prophylaxis, is at risk for early-onset sepsis (EOS). Of the response choices, maternal fever is most predictive of EOS. Early-onset sepsis is defined as a positive blood or cerebrospinal fluid culture obtained within the first 72 hours after birth. It occurs in 0.57 per 1,000 deliveries of neonates with more than 34 weeks of gestation. In the United States, GBS and *Escherichia coli* are the most common causative organisms. Early-onset sepsis is thought to occur due to neonatal exposure to maternal microbes during labor and delivery. Risk factors for infection include gestational age and maternal GBS colonization. Early-onset sepsis with GBS typically presents with nonspecific signs of sepsis such as hypothermia and bradycardia.

In 1996, obstetricians began routinely screening pregnant women for GBS between 35 and 37 weeks of gestation. If GBS screening is positive, mothers should receive penicillin prophylaxis during labor to decrease GBS exposure to the neonate. If a mother has had a previous child with GBS sepsis, or had GBS bacteriuria during the pregnancy, she should receive penicillin prophylaxis irrespective of the results of GBS screening. The practice of culture-based screening and antibiotic prophylaxis has been extremely effective in reducing the rate of EOS, as described in Verani et al.

Since the implementation of GBS screening and prophylactic antibiotics for mothers who are GBS positive, risk factors for EOS have changed. Also, there is an increasing awareness of antibiotic resistance and changes in the microbiome due to unnecessary antibiotic exposure, with the potential for long-lasting health impacts.

Clinicians struggle to identify those neonates at highest risk for EOS. Any neonate who is symptomatic should be evaluated with a complete blood cell count, blood culture, chest radiography, and lumbar puncture. Antibiotic treatment should be tailored to reflect local antibiotic resistance patterns.

Determining the risk of infection for an asymptomatic neonate born to a mother with inadequate antibiotic prophylaxis is challenging. Puopolo et al examined the risk of EOS among asymptomatic neonates born at 34 or more weeks of gestation. Gestational age and maternal intrapartum fever were the risk factors most associated with EOS. Gestational age of less than 37 weeks or more than 40 weeks were the most predictive of EOS. Administration of intrapartum antibiotics decreased the risk of EOS in this cohort.

In this vignette, maternal fever higher than 39°C most closely correlates with risk of EOS. The neonate is at 38 weeks of gestation, making gestational age less important. Rupture of membrane for 22 hours is less predictive of EOS, and a birthweight less than 2.5 kg is not associated with EOS.

PREP Pearls

- All pregnant women with a positive screening culture for group B *Streptococcus*, obtained between 35 and 37 weeks of gestation, should receive penicillin prophylaxis during labor.
- For neonates born to group B *Streptococcus*–positive mothers who did not receive adequate antibiotic prophylaxis during labor and delivery, the strongest predictors of early-onset sepsis from group B Streptococcus are prematurity (<37 weeks of gestation), post-term gestation (>40 weeks of gestation), and intrapartum maternal fever.
- Group B *Streptococcus* is the leading cause of early-onset sepsis in neonates in the United States.

American Board of Pediatrics Content Specification(s)/Content Area

- Plan the management of a neonate whose mother is febrile at the time of delivery
- Plan appropriate antimicrobial therapy for suspected sepsis in the immediate newborn period

Suggested Readings

Puopolo KM, Draper D, Wi S, et al. Estimating the probability of neonatal early-onset infection on the basis of maternal risk factors. *Pediatrics*. 2011;128(5):e1155-e1163.

Randis TM, Baker JA, Ratner AJ. Group B streptococcal infections. *Pediatr Rev*. 2017;38;254.

Verani JR, McGee L, Schrag SJ; Division of Bacterial Diseases, National Center for Immunization and Respiratory Diseases, Centers for Disease Control and Prevention (CDC). Prevention of perinatal group B streptococcal disease: revised guidelines from CDC, 2010. *MMWR Recomm Rep*. 2010;59(RR-10):1-36. https://www.cdc.gov/mmwr/preview/mmwrhtml/rr5910a1.htm?s_cid.

Item 266   **Preferred Response: C**

Posttest probability can be determined by using the Fagan nomogram (Item C266), a tool that allows the determination of posttest probability given the pretest probability of disease and the likelihood ratio for the diagnostic test. The pretest probability of disease can be estimated based on disease prevalence.

Likelihood ratios provide information about diagnostic tests. The likelihood ratio of a positive test is defined as the probability that an individual with disease has a positive test result divided by the probability that an individual without disease has a positive test result. It combines the sensitivity and specificity of the test into a single measure. The likelihood ratio for a positive test can be calculated from the sensitivity and specificity as follows: sensitivity/(1-specificity), when sensitivity and specificity are expressed as decimals. The likelihood ratio of 32 for the tissue transglutaminase IgA antibody test means that individuals who have celiac disease are 32 times more likely to have a positive test than individuals who do not have celiac disease.

For the boy in this vignette, the pretest probability is 5%, the prevalence of celiac disease in individuals with type 1 diabetes. The posttest probability of celiac disease for the boy

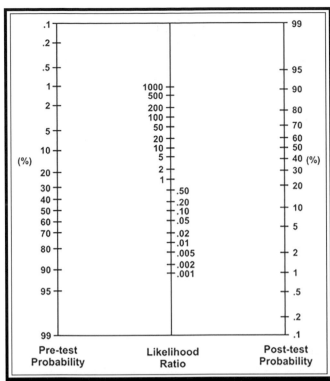

Item C266: Nomogram for pre- and posttest probabilities and likelihood ratios. A line can be drawn from the pretest probability estimate on the left side of the figure through the likelihood ratio to identify the posttest probability of disease.

Modified and reprinted with permission from Fagan TJ. Nomogram for Bayes's theorem. *N Engl J Med.* 1975;293(5):257.

in this vignette can be determined with a Fagan nomogram (Item C266) by drawing a line from a pretest probability of 5%, through a likelihood ratio of 32, to a posttest probability of about 60%. Thus the positive test result increases the boy's probability of having celiac disease from 5% to 60%.

The posttest probability of having celiac disease is 60%, so it is not certain that the boy has celiac disease. The boy is not 32 times more likely to have celiac disease. Rather, a positive test result is 32 times more likely to occur in someone with celiac disease than in someone without celiac disease. The posttest probability of celiac disease would not be the same if the boy did not have type 1 diabetes. The pretest probability would be lower, resulting in a lower posttest probability.

PREP Pearls

- By using the Fagan nomogram, posttest probability can be determined from the pretest probability and likelihood ratio of the test.
- Likelihood ratios provide information about diagnostic tests by combining sensitivity and specificity of the test into a single measure.
- The likelihood ratio of a positive test is defined as the probability that an individual with disease has a positive test result divided by the probability that an individual without disease has a positive test result.

American Board of Pediatrics Content Specification(s)/Content Area

- Understand likelihood ratio and when it might be useful to reach a diagnosis
- Understand relative risk analysis and odds ratio

Suggested Readings

Akobeng AK. Understanding diagnostic tests 2: likelihood ratios, pre- and post-test probabilities and their use in clinical practice. *Acta Paediatr.* 2007;96(4):487-491.

Crewe S, Rowe PC. Research and statistics: likelihood ratio in diagnosis. *Pediatr Rev.* 2011;32(7):296-298.

Item 267   Preferred Response: B

The boy in the vignette has Huntington disease (HD), an autosomal-dominant, trinucleotide repeat disorder that leads to progressive motor disability, cognitive decline, and psychiatric disturbances. The average age at onset is 35 to 44 years, with a survival of 15 to 18 years after the onset of symptoms. It can occur at later or earlier ages depending on the number of CAG trinucleotide repeats that are present. Motor symptoms include hypokinesia, chorea (Item C267), rigidity, ataxia, and dystonia. Psychiatric disturbances include agitation, anxiety, depression, apathy, disinhibition, delusions, and hallucinations. Suicidal ideation is common in individuals with HD. The cognitive decline is progressive, resulting in patients' inability to care for themselves, speak, swallow, or walk. There is no cure, only symptomatic management. Juvenile HD, characterized by symptom onset before age 20 years, occurs in 5% to 10% of cases. In juvenile HD, decline tends to be more rapid, with severe mental deterioration, prominent motor and cerebellar symptoms, and epileptic seizures. Initial manifestations are typically chorea and significant behavioral disturbances.

A multimedia element is available for this critique on PREP® SA Online at www.pedialink.org.

Reprinted with permission from Kruer MC. Pediatric movement disorders. *Pediatr Rev.* 2015;36(3):108.

Item C267: Intermittent chorea.

Trinucleotide repeat disorders are characterized by a phenomenon known in genetics as anticipation. With anticipation, a condition tends to become more severe and manifests at an earlier age as it is passed down from 1 generation to the next. This is because of expansion of an unstable trinucleotide repeat that is prone to errors during cell division. In HD, anticipation occurs when a normal premutation carrier, an individual with 27-35 CAG repeats in the *HTT* allele, transmits an unstable *HTT* allele to their child. This unstable allele is at risk for the parent's premutation to expand into a full mutation with more than 40 CAG repeats, leading to an individual being affected (because of full penetrance at this repeat number). If it expands to 36 to 39 CAG repeats, the individual is at risk for HD, but may not develop symptoms; this phenomenon is known as reduced penetrance. The mutation tends to expand through the father; it tends to be stable or remain at a similar number if passed down by the mother. Importantly, if the affected individual already has more than 40 CAG repeats, regardless of further expansion, he/she will have a 50% risk of passing the disorder to the offspring with full penetrance, male or female. Other trinucleotide repeat disorders with anticipation include myotonic dystrophy and fragile X syndrome.

Duchenne muscular dystrophy is an X-linked recessive disorder that is characterized by early childhood onset with delayed motor milestones, proximal weakness, waddling gait, and elevated creatine kinase levels (10 times normal). Progression inevitably leads to wheelchair dependency. Dilated cardiomyopathy typically occurs after 18 years of age, with very few surviving beyond the third decade.

Parkinson disease, typically an adult disorder, presents with tremor, rigidity, postural instability, and bradykinesia. Dementia occurs in 20% to 25% of individuals. The sporadic form of Parkinson disease occurs after age 60 years; however, juvenile presentations can be seen and are commonly due to mendelian forms. These cases can be inherited in an autosomal dominant, autosomal recessive, or, less commonly, X-linked manner. Chorea and dystonia are not common findings.

Spinal muscular atrophy is an autosomal recessive disorder that presents with proximal muscular weakness and atrophy, because of progressive neurodegeneration and loss of the anterior horn cells of the spinal cord and the brain stem nuclei. Symptoms include progressive motor difficulties with loss of skills, global hypotonia with sparing of the facial musculature, areflexia/hyporeflexia, and tongue fasciculations. Presentation can vary from infancy to adulthood depending on the subtype.

PREP Pearls

- Huntington disease is an autosomal-dominant, trinucleotide repeat disorder that leads to progressive motor disability, cognitive decline, and psychiatric disturbances, with an average age at onset of 35 to 44 years; however, because of CAG trinucleotide repeat expansion, clinical onset can occur in childhood, a condition known as juvenile Huntington disease.

- Trinucleotide repeat disorders are characterized by a phenomenon known in genetics as anticipation; the condition tends to become more severe and manifests at an earlier age as it is passed down from 1 generation to the next.

- Types of trinucleotide repeat disorders include Huntington disease, fragile X syndrome, and myotonic dystrophy.

American Board of Pediatrics Content Specification(s)/Content Area

- Understand the role of trinucleotide repeat analysis in the diagnosis of genetic disorders

Suggested Readings

American College of Medical Genetics/American Society of Human Genetics Huntington Disease Genetic Testing Working Group. Laboratory guidelines for Huntington disease genetic testing. *Am J Hum Genet.* 1998;62:1243-1247.

Committee on Bioethics, Committee on Genetics, and American College of Medical Genetics and Genomics Social, Ethical, Legal Issues Committee. Ethical and policy issues in genetic testing and screening of children. *Pediatrics.* 2013;131:620-622.

Warby SC, Graham RK, Hayden MR. Huntington disease. *GeneReviews.* https://www.ncbi.nlm.nih.gov/books/NBK1305/.

Item 268   Preferred Response: D

The mother in this vignette should call the pediatrician's office as soon as possible after the birth to arrange an evaluation within 24 hours. Because midwives and other health care professionals attending home births usually stay for only a few to several hours after the birth, an evaluation of the neonate within 24 hours of birth by a pediatric-trained clinician ensures monitoring for feeding problems and dehydration. Another evaluation within 48 hours of this initial visit is also recommended. Together, these evaluations ensure that the neonate receives screening for congenital heart defects, completes the state-required newborn screening for metabolic and other conditions, and is assessed for hyperbilirubinemia.

Planned home births represent less than 1% of all births in the United States. The American Academy of Pediatrics (AAP) agrees with the American College of Obstetricians and Gynecologists' position that it is safer to deliver in a hospital or birthing center, as compared to at home. Neonates born at home have a 2- to 3-fold increased risk of mortality in the United States. The 2013 AAP policy statement regarding newborn care during and following planned home births was, in part, an effort to reduce this risk by recommending standards for care. The AAP does not recommend a home birth over one in a health care setting.

A neonate born at home should be cared for by a certified health care professional trained in neonatal resuscitation. This provider should only be responsible for the neonate. There should be 2 providers attending the birth, one to care for the mother, and one to care for the neonate. The neonate should receive care according to AAP guidelines for perinatal care, including a physical examination, assessment of growth parameters, frequent assessment of vital signs, screening for hypoglycemia, prophylaxis against gonococcal ophthalmia neonatorum, administration of vitamin K, and vaccination against hepatitis B. The provider team should remain in the home long enough to ensure the mother and neonate are stable. Any neonate requiring more intense monitoring or treatment should be transferred to a medical facility. Examples include a neonate with persistent hypoglycemia despite feeding and a neonate born to a group B *Streptococcus*–positive mother showing signs of chorioamnionitis. Neonates thought to be less than 37 weeks' gestational age should also be transferred for monitoring and treatment of prematurity-associated conditions.

An initial evaluation by a pediatric-trained clinician within 24 hours of birth and another evaluation within 24 to 48 hours of that initial visit are needed to ensure that further screening and monitoring procedures are followed. In addition, these 2 visits allow for assessment of feeding problems and dehydration. Home visits with a nurse and a lactation consultant in the first days after birth can augment pediatric office visits but will not provide screening for hyperbilirubinemia and congenital heart conditions. Serum glucose monitoring, if indicated, should commence shortly after birth, not at 24 hours after birth. Waiting until 24 to 48 hours after birth to have a first evaluation by a pediatric provider will fail to capture some cases of severe hyperbilirubinemia, poor feeding, and dehydration. Although this is an appropriate age to perform screening for congenital heart defects, it should not be the initial visit.

PREP Pearls

- Hospitals and birthing centers are safer locations compared to the home for delivery of all neonates.
- Neonates born at home should be evaluated by a pediatric-trained clinician within 24 hours of birth, and again 24 to 48 hours after this initial visit.
- Neonates born at home should receive care that is as close to standard hospital care as possible, including having a dedicated provider trained in resuscitation who performs assessments, screening, monitoring, and treatment consistent with recommendations from the American Academy of Pediatrics.

American Board of Pediatrics Content Specification(s)/Content Area

- Plan appropriate evaluation and management of an infant who was born at home

Suggested Readings

Committee on Fetus and Newborn. Planned home birth. *Pediatrics.* 2013;131(5):1016-1020.

Roth P. Pulse oximetry and the neonate. *Pediatr Rev.* 2016;37(9):402-405.

Warren JB, Phillipi CA. Care of the well newborn. *Pediatr Rev.* 2012;33(1):4-18.

Item 269   Preferred Response: B

For the patient in this vignette, the best plan is to provide conjugate meningococcal vaccine today. Individuals with sickle cell disease are predisposed to invasive meningococcal infections given their functional asplenia and should be vaccinated as infants.

As of 2018, there are several licensed meningococcal vaccines in the United States: 3 vaccines for serogroups A, C, Y, and W135, one vaccine for serogroups C and Y (which is combined with vaccination for *Haemophilus influenzae* type B), and 2 vaccines for serogroup B. Quadrivalent conjugate meningococcal vaccine is recommended for all US children at the 11- to 12-year-old preadolescent visit, with a booster dose at age 16 years. Serogroup B vaccine can be considered in healthy adolescents and young adults. Quadrivalent conjugate meningococcal vaccines are recommended in infants

and children who have underlying conditions that predispose them to developing invasive meningococcal infections, including complement component deficiencies and functional (sickle cell disease) or anatomic asplenia. Additional vaccine recommendations exist for outbreak control, travel to endemic regions, and for high-risk occupational settings.

Children with underlying conditions can receive bivalent or quadrivalent conjugate vaccine as part of a multidose series starting at the 2-month-old health supervision visit. Boosters are given, typically at an interval of every 5 years for quadrivalent conjugate vaccine unless the initial series was given to a child younger than 7 years, in which case the first booster is recommended at a 3-year interval. Vaccination against serogroup B is also recommended for individuals with high-risk underlying conditions but not until 10 years of age.

Conjugate vaccine would be recommended at 11 years of age if the child had no underlying conditions. Serogroup B vaccines are recommended for children with underlying conditions and are licensed for children 10 years of age or older; thus, serogroup B vaccine should not be administered at today's visit or at the 2-year-old visit.

PREP Pearls

- Meningococcal vaccines are also recommended in infants and young children who have underlying conditions that predispose them to developing invasive meningococcal infections, including complement component deficiencies and functional (sickle cell disease) or anatomic asplenia.
- Quadrivalent conjugate meningococcal vaccine is recommended for all US children at the 11- to 12-year-old preadolescent visit, with a booster dose at age 16 years.
- Vaccination against serogroup B is also recommended for individuals with high-risk underlying conditions but not until 10 years of age and can be considered in healthy adolescents and young adults.

American Board of Pediatrics Content Specification(s)/Content Area

- Know which serotypes are included in the meningococcal vaccine
- Know the indications and schedule for the meningococcal vaccine

Suggested Readings

American Academy of Pediatrics. Meningococcal infections. In: Kimberlin DW, Brady MT, Jackson MA, Long SS, eds. *Red Book: 2018 Report of the Committee on Infectious Diseases.* 31st ed. Itasca, IL: American Academy of Pediatrics; 2018:550-561.

Vaz LE. Meningococcal disease. *Pediatr Rev.* 2017; 38(4):158-169.

Item 270   Preferred Response: D

The girl in the vignette sustained a lower extremity fracture and is wearing a hard splint. She is experiencing a sudden increase in pain that is not responding to an opioid medication. This scenario is concerning for acute compartment syndrome. Her parents should immediately loosen the splint and bring her to the emergency department for evaluation.

A 'compartment' is a group of limb muscles and their associated nerves and blood vessels, surrounded by fascia. Following an injury, bleeding and swelling can cause increased pressure in a given compartment. Acute compartment syndrome occurs when increased pressure, often as a result of injury, leads to compression of intracompartmental vasculature and ischemia, causing subsequent nerve and muscle damage. Acute compartment syndrome is a surgical emergency. Because the early signs can be subtle, and children may have difficulty articulating their symptoms, this condition can be difficult to diagnose.

Children most often present with compartment syndrome following forearm, distal humerus, or tibia fractures. The classic "5 Ps" of acute compartment syndrome are pain, pallor, pulselessness, paresthesia, and paralysis. With the exception of pain, these signs and symptoms are late findings. A child with a fracture who presents with agitation and increased pain that does not respond to medications should be urgently evaluated for compartment syndrome. Providers should remove casts or splints and palpate along the limb for pain and swelling. For severe fractures, a portion of the cast or splint can be left in place, but enough should be removed to allow for complete examination of the affected limb. Muscle stretch will often increase pain with acute compartment syndrome. The treatment of acute compartment syndrome is urgent fasciotomy surgery. Failure to recognize an acute increase in pain as a symptom of possible compartment syndrome can lead to delayed diagnosis and severe, permanent disability due to nerve and muscle damage. Therefore applying ice packs, ibuprofen, and evaluation in 24 hours would not be appropriate for the girl in the vignette.

Chronic exertional compartment syndrome (CECS) occurs when exercise leads to a mild increase in intracompartmental pressure. This condition almost always affects the muscle compartments of the lower leg. Athletes present with cramping pain, and sometimes with numbness and paresthesias, during exercise. Pain onset typically follows a predictable period of exercise, especially with running, and worsens as the athlete continues the activity. Definitive diagnosis requires measurement of compartment pressure. Because this measurement is invasive, a high index of clinical suspicion is enough to initiate conservative management of this condition. Initial treatment of CECS involves physical therapy and modification of the activity schedule. For intractable CECS, referral to orthopaedic surgery for elective fasciotomy surgery may be indicated.

PREP Pearls

- Acute compartment syndrome is a surgical emergency.
- Failure to recognize an acute increase in pain as a symptom of possible compartment syndrome can lead to delayed diagnosis and severe, permanent disability due to nerve and muscle damage.
- The classic "5 Ps" of acute compartment syndrome are pain, pallor, pulselessness, paresthesia, and paralysis. With the exception of pain, these signs and symptoms are late findings.

American Board of Pediatrics Content Specification(s)/ Content Area

- Recognize the clinical findings associated with compartment syndrome

Suggested Readings

Gresh M. Compartment syndrome in the pediatric patient. *Pediatr Rev.* 2017;38(12):560-565.

Sarwark JF, LaBella CR, ed *Pediatric Orthopaedics and Sports Injuries: A Quick Reference Guide.* 2nd ed. Elk Grove Village, IL: American Academy of Pediatrics; 2014.

von Keudell AG, Weaver MJ, Appleton PT, et al. Diagnosis and treatment of acute extremity compartment syndrome. *Lancet.* 2015;386(10000):1299-1310.

Item 271 **Preferred Response: B**

Although bicycle riding in an urban setting with few parks and limited bike paths is a safety challenge, it remains a good form of family exercise. Families should be made aware that riding a bicycle in the street with the vehicular traffic flow is the best practice recommendation. The other choices listed are associated with a greater risk of accidental injury to the bicyclist and/or pedestrians.

Pediatric health care providers play an important role in providing age-appropriate home safety information to families, which includes tips for accident prevention related to common recreational activities. It is the pediatric provider's role to ensure that parents and children receive guidance on how to safely use bicycles and other wheeled recreational devices. In addition to discussing the importance of protective gear (eg, a properly fitted helmet and pads when indicated), providers should counsel families on how and where to ride safely. Bicycle safety can be fostered by adhering to rules about the cycling environment.

- Always ride with the vehicular traffic flow.
- Use hand signals.
- Obey traffic signs.
- Ride in designated lanes when possible.
- Do not ride in the dark without proper lights and reflective apparel.
- Always use a properly fitted helmet
- Choose a bicycle size that is appropriate for height.
- Make sure the bicycle and its brakes are in good repair.
- Never ride when intoxicated.

PREP Pearls

- Bicycle safety can be fostered by following rules about the cycling environment.
- Properly fitted bicycle helmets should be worn and have been shown to decrease serious morbidity and mortality from accidents.
- Riding a bicycle with the vehicular traffic flow, in the street or in a designated lane when available, is the best practice to prevent accidental injury to the cyclist and/or pedestrians.

American Board of Pediatrics Content Specification(s)/ Content Area

- Provide age-appropriate home safety information

Suggested Readings

Embree TE, Romanow NTR, et.al. Risk factors for bicycling injuries in children and adolescents: a systematic review. *Pediatrics.* 2016;138(5):1-13.

Okun A. Bicycle safety. *Pediatr Rev.* 2015;36(3):138-139.

Sanders JE, Mogilner L. Child safety and injury prevention. *Pediatr Rev.* 2015;36(6):268-269.

The adolescent in this vignette has hypopigmented scaling macules with well-defined borders distributed on the chest and back. These findings are consistent with a diagnosis of tinea (pityriasis) versicolor, and treatment with topical selenium sulfide is appropriate. Second-line treatments might include oral fluconazole and itraconazole, but oral ketoconazole is not approved for the treatment of cutaneous fungal infections. Minocycline and ammonium lactate may be used to treat confluent and reticulated papillomatosis, an uncommon disorder that produces hyperpigmented papules, patches, or thin plaques on the trunk, especially the central chest. Individual lesions have a rough texture (Item C272A).

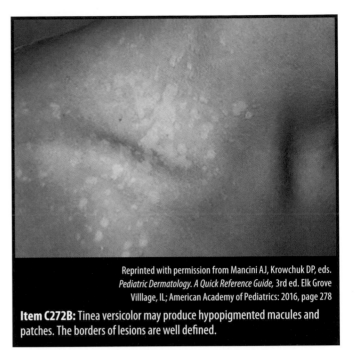

Reprinted with permission from Mancini AJ, Krowchuk DP, eds. *Pediatric Dermatology. A Quick Reference Guide*, 3rd ed. Elk Grove Villlage, IL; American Academy of Pediatrics: 2016, page 278

Item C272B: Tinea versicolor may produce hypopigmented macules and patches. The borders of lesions are well defined.

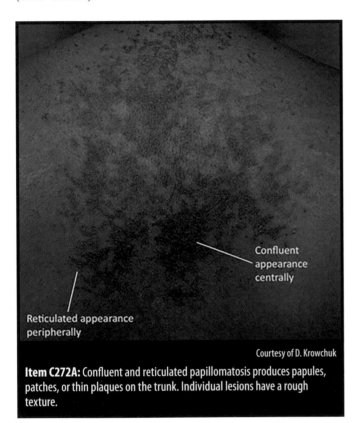

Confluent appearance centrally

Reticulated appearance peripherally

Courtesy of D. Krowchuk

Item C272A: Confluent and reticulated papillomatosis produces papules, patches, or thin plaques on the trunk. Individual lesions have a rough texture.

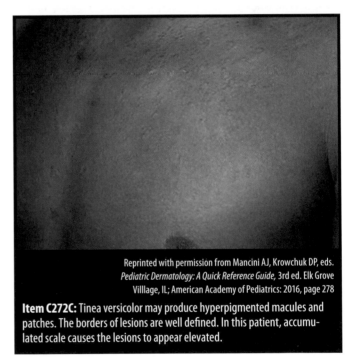

Reprinted with permission from Mancini AJ, Krowchuk DP, eds. *Pediatric Dermatology: A Quick Reference Guide*, 3rd ed. Elk Grove Villlage, IL; American Academy of Pediatrics: 2016, page 278

Item C272C: Tinea versicolor may produce hyperpigmented macules and patches. The borders of lesions are well defined. In this patient, accumulated scale causes the lesions to appear elevated.

Tinea versicolor is a common superficial infection with yeasts of the genus *Malassezia* (formerly *Pityrosporum*). Adolescents and young adults are commonly affected, likely because of the sebum-rich cutaneous environment that supports the organism's growth. Although *Malassezia* species are part of the normal skin flora, hot and humid weather, sweating, and use of oils on the skin may trigger a change from the yeast form to the hyphal form, resulting in appearance of the rash. Most patients are asymptomatic but some report pruritus. The eruption is composed of well-defined, round, hypo- or hyperpigmented macules that may coalesce into large patches; scale may be present (Item C272B and Item C272C). The trunk is the primary site of involvement but the proximal extremities and sides of the neck may be affected. Tinea versicolor usually is diagnosed clinically. If uncertainty exists, a potassium hydroxide preparation performed on scale from a lesion will demonstrate short hyphae and spores (ie, "spaghetti and meatballs," Item C272D), and a Wood lamp examination will reveal yellow-gold fluorescence of the affected areas.

Several options exist for treatment. First-line treatment usually employs a topical agent:

- Selenium sulfide lotion 1% (available without a prescription) or 2.5% (requires prescription): Apply a thin coat to affected and adjacent areas for 10 minutes then shower. Repeat daily for a total of 7 days. If a stinging or burning sensation occurs, wash off immediately.
- Ketoconazole shampoo: Apply for 5 minutes once daily for 1 to 3 days.
- Terbinafine spray: Apply twice daily for 2 to 3 weeks.

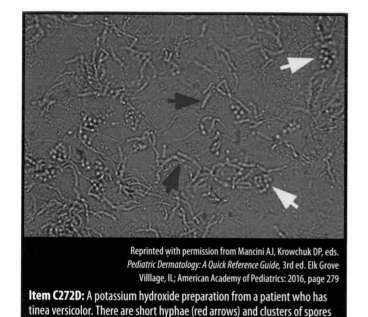

Reprinted with permission from Mancini AJ, Krowchuk DP, eds. *Pediatric Dermatology: A Quick Reference Guide*, 3rd ed. Elk Grove Villlage, IL; American Academy of Pediatrics: 2016, page 279

Item C272D: A potassium hydroxide preparation from a patient who has tinea versicolor. There are short hyphae (red arrows) and clusters of spores (yellow arrows).

- Imidazole creams (eg, clotrimazole, miconazole nitrate, ketoconazole): Effective for localized infection (not practical for the treatment of large areas).
- Oral agents are reserved for patients who have resistant infections or cannot tolerate or effectively use a topical agent. Options include itraconazole (400 mg once or 200 mg/day for 7 days) and fluconazole (400 mg once).

Because recurrence rates may be as high as 60%, regardless of the initial treatment used, it is prudent to advise once-monthly prophylaxis for 3 months using selenium sulfide (a single 8- to 12-hour application). Additionally, it is important to counsel patients that normalization of pigmentation may not occur for several months after treatment.

PREP Pearls

- First-line treatment of tinea versicolor is with a topical agent such as selenium sulfide.
- In tinea versicolor, the trunk is the primary area of involvement; occasionally lesions may be present on the sides of the neck or proximal extremities.
- Tinea versicolor is characterized by hypo- or hyperpigmented macules and patches that have well-defined borders; scale may be present.

American Board of Pediatrics Content Specification(s)/Content Area

- Recognize the clinical findings associated with pityriasis (tinea) versicolor

Suggested Readings

American Academy of Pediatrics Section on Dermatology. Tinea versicolor. In: Mancini AJ, Krowchuk DP, eds. *Pediatric Dermatology: A Quick Reference Guide*, 3rd ed. Elk Grove Village, IL: American Academy of Pediatrics; 2016:277-281.

Hu SW, Bigby M. Pityriasis versicolor: a systematic review of interventions. *Arch Dermatol*. 2010;146(10):1132-1140.

Kelly BP. Superficial fungal infections. *Pediatr Rev*. 2012;33(4):e22-e37.

The infant in this vignette is critically ill with a midgut volvulus, which is associated with heterotaxy syndrome in which failure of normal embryological rotation results in abnormally positioned organs in the chest and abdomen. In infants and children, a midgut volvulus is most commonly associated with intestinal malrotation, a congenital abnormality caused by incomplete in utero rotation of the bowel around the superior mesenteric artery. Intestinal malrotation is often associated with other congenital anomalies including heterotaxy syndrome, omphalocele, gastroschisis, congenital diaphragmatic hernia, esophageal atresia, renal anomalies, and cardiac anomalies.

With normal in utero intestinal rotation, the third portion of the duodenum crosses the midline of the abdomen. With malrotation, the duodenum is abnormally fixed, thus the third portion of the duodenum is positioned in the right upper quadrant of the abdomen. The abnormal duodenal positioning increases the risk for the bowel to twist on itself, resulting in a midgut volvulus. The twisting and subsequent obstruction can quickly progress to bowel ischemia and necrosis.

Midgut volvulus must be quickly diagnosed and treated, because sepsis and shock can rapidly ensue. Signs of midgut volvulus include bilious emesis, abdominal distention, hematochezia, and peritonitis. If the diagnosis is suspected clinically (ill- or toxic-appearing infant with bilious emesis and peritonitis), resuscitation and emergent laparotomy (without radiographic imaging) are indicated with operative correction of the volvulus and malrotation (Ladd procedure). Radiologic imaging may be used to diagnose malrotation and volvulus, particularly in an infant or child who is less toxic appearing. Plain abdominal radiographs may show signs of a small bowel obstruction; however, they may appear normal, even in the setting of malrotation with an acute volvulus. Upper gastrointestinal series is the gold standard for diagnosis of malrotation and volvulus, because this fluoroscopic study can evaluate the positioning of the duodenum. Item C273 demonstrates intestinal malrotation

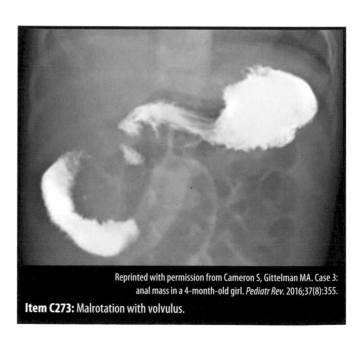

Reprinted with permission from Cameron S, Gittelman MA. Case 3: anal mass in a 4-month-old girl. *Pediatr Rev*. 2016;37(8):355.

Item C273: Malrotation with volvulus.

(the third portion of the duodenum does not cross midline) and volvulus ("corkscrew" sign).

Gestational diabetes, history of hemangiomas, and maternal tobacco smoke exposure are not associated with increased risk of midgut volvulus.

PREP Pearls

- Gold standard for diagnosis of malrotation and volvulus is an upper gastrointestinal series; however, surgical intervention may be warranted in toxic-appearing infants and children with suspected volvulus, even before radiologic testing confirms the diagnosis.
- Infants and children with heterotaxy syndrome and/or gastrointestinal, renal, or cardiac anomalies are at risk for intestinal malrotation.
- Midgut volvulus is a surgical emergency that requires quick diagnosis and treatment.

American Board of Pediatrics Content Specification(s)/ Content Area

- Recognize the clinical features associated with volvulus, and manage appropriately

Suggested Readings

Kapadia MR. Volvulus of the small bowel and colon. *Clin Colon Rectal Surg*. 2017;30(1):40-45.

Langer JC. Intestinal rotation abnormalities and midgut volvulus. *Surg Clin North Am*. 2017;97(1):147-159.

Shalaby MS, Kuti K, Walker G. Intestinal malrotation and volvulus in infants and children. *BMJ*. 2013;347:f6949.

Item 274 — Preferred Response: C

The boy in this vignette has multiple risk factors for substance use: academic failure, authoritarian parenting, early drug use, and low self-esteem. Early drug use is the strongest predictor of serious problems with substance use disorder. The younger the age, the higher the likelihood. Most people with substance use disorder began using substances (most commonly alcohol, tobacco, or marijuana) before the age of 18 years. Adolescents, whose brain reward pathways are active and whose decision-making pathways are still under development, are particularly vulnerable to risk-taking behaviors such as substance use.

Risk factors for substance use are manifold. Family, twin, and adoption studies support a genetic contribution to the development of alcohol use disorder, nicotine dependence, and, to a lesser degree, illicit substance use (eg, cannabis). Environmental factors such as low socioeconomic status, availability of substances in the community, and substance use/abuse by peers contribute to substance use by youth. Familial factors such as family substance use/abuse by parents, family conflict (eg, parent-child, parent-parent) and disruption (eg, divorce), family mental illness, family violence and abuse, poor supervision by parents, and permissive or authoritarian parenting style increase a child's risk of using substances. In addition, youth with mental health conditions (eg, attention-deficit/hyperactivity disorder, anxiety, depression, conduct disorder); school failure; poor social

and coping skills; low self-esteem; and impulsive, aggressive, and antisocial traits are at risk for substance use disorders.

Protective factors against substance use include high self-esteem; good emotional health; personal success; parental involvement; and engagement with family, school, or community. Community availability of evidence-based prevention programs, mentoring programs, and afterschool programs are also protective against substance use in children. The primary care physician can be instrumental in assisting patients by engaging with the community and schools to provide multidisciplinary care for individual patients and to partner in implementing preventative educational programs for the broader community and student body.

PREP Pearls

- Early drug use is the strongest predictor of serious problems with substance use disorder. The younger the age, the higher the likelihood.
- Familial factors such as family substance use/abuse by parents, family conflict and disruption, family mental illness, family violence and abuse, poor supervision by parents, and permissive or authoritarian parenting style increase a child's risk of using substances.
- Youth with mental health conditions (eg, attention-deficit/ hyperactivity disorder, anxiety, depression, conduct disorder); school failure; poor social and coping skills; low self-esteem; and impulsive, aggressive, and antisocial traits are at risk for substance use disorders.

American Board of Pediatrics Content Specification(s)/ Content Area

- Understand the risk factors associated with drug dependence
- Understand environmental/familial factors contributing to substance use/abuse
- Understand genetic factors contributing to substance use/abuse
- Understand the importance of the primary care physician's involvement in school- and community-based educational initiatives with regard to substance use/abuse and the value of such initiatives

Suggested Readings

Harrop E, Catalano RF. Evidence-based prevention for adolescent substance use. *Child Adolesc Psychiatric Clin N Am*. 2016;25(3):387-410.

Nackers KAM, Kokotailo P, Levy SJL. Substance abuse, general principles. *Pediatr Rev*. 2015;36(12):535-544.

Ocampo AMS, Knight JR. Substance use in adolescence. In: Augustyn M, Zuckerman B, Caronna EB, eds. *The Zuckerman Parker Handbook of Developmental and Behavioral Pediatrics for Primary Care*. 3rd ed. Philadelphia, PA: Wolters Kluwer; 2011:366-372.

Item 275 — Preferred Response: B

The adolescent in this vignette plans to use an indoor tanning bed. Tanning beds emit primarily ultraviolet A (UVA) rays, which penetrate the deeper layers of the skin causing damage (premature aging, sun spot, immune suppression). Ultraviolet B (UVB) rays are responsible for sunburns. Exposure to artificial UV rays may also cause skin dryness, pruritus, and photokeratitis. Both UVA and UVB rays contribute to the pathogenesis of skin cancer. Continuous use of indoor tanning beds may increase the risk of melanoma by 60%, especially in pediatric patients. Furthermore, long-term exposure to powerful, artificial UV rays from tanning beds may cause damage to the eyes, including cataracts. Chemical blocking sunscreens protect against UVB rays, but tanning beds emit mostly UVA rays.

The sun protection factor (SPF) rating system of sunscreens is a measure of UVB protection alone. For example, sunscreen rated SPF 30 filters 97% of UVB rays while SPF 50 blocks 98%. No sunscreen completely protects against sun damage. Despite marketing practices, indoor tanning is never safe given the risk of skin cancer. Because vitamin D may be obtained via dietary or pharmaceutical supplementation without the associated risks of UV exposure, tanning beds should not be used to attain adequate vitamin D levels. The American Academy of Pediatrics (AAP) recommends avoidance of indoor tanning devices.

Additional AAP recommendations regarding sun exposure include:

- Seek shade and avoid midday sun exposure (10 AM-2 PM)
- Wear dark, tightly woven clothing that covers the body.
- Wear a wide-brimmed hat and sunglasses with both UVA and UVB protection.
- Apply a broad-spectrum sunscreen that filters both UVA and UVB rays with an SPF of at least 15 on both cloudy and sunny days
- Reapply sunscreen every 2 hours and after swimming or sweating
- Infants younger than 6 months should avoid direct sunlight, stay in shaded areas, wear a protective hat and clothing, and have sunscreen applied to unprotected sun, including face and hands, when sun exposure is unavoidable

PREP Pearls

- Exposure to artificial ultraviolet rays may cause sunburn, skin dryness, pruritus, and photokeratitis; long-term exposure may cause cataracts, skin aging, and cancer.
- Pediatricians should counsel adolescents that any amount of artificial ultraviolet ray exposure is harmful.

American Board of Pediatrics Content Specification(s)/ Content Area

- Counsel parents and children regarding sunscreens and exposure to the sun

Suggested Readings

Balk SJ, Fisher DE, Geller AC. Teens and indoor tanning: a cancer prevention opportunity for pediatricians. *Pediatrics*. 2013;131(4):772-785.

Council on Environmental Health and Section on Dermatology. Ultraviolet radiation: a hazard to children and adolescents. *Pediatrics*. 2011;127(3):588-597.

Long M. Sun exposure. *Pediatr Rev*. 2017;38(9):446-447.

Item 276   Preferred Response: D

The girl in the vignette has spinal muscular atrophy (SMA). She has weak, hypotonic limbs, areflexia, and paradoxical breathing, which implies weakness of muscles of respiration. The muscles of her face are spared, but she has tongue fasciculations. An additional finding in SMA can be finger trembling. The girl's physical examination findings suggest a disorder of the peripheral nervous system. Electromyography/nerve conduction study would confirm dysfunction of the motor neurons. Genetic testing for SMA would confirm the diagnosis.

Congenital muscular dystrophy is a group of disorders that can also present with weakness, hypotonia, and hyporeflexia or areflexia. Affected infants may have bulbar weakness that causes poor feeding or choking. A high arched palate, joint contractures, or hyperflexibility may be noted on physical examination. Depending on the specific disorder, associated brain malformations, ophthalmologic abnormalities, or cardiomyopathy may be seen. The clinical presentation can have elements of both a central nervous system disorder and a peripheral nervous system disorder. Electromyography/ nerve conduction study can indicate that there is a primary disorder of the muscles. Serum creatine kinase is sometimes elevated. A specific diagnosis can be made with muscle biopsy or genetic testing. Although the girl in the vignette has profound limb weakness and hypotonia, she does not have other findings seen in congenital muscular dystrophies, and she has the typical findings of SMA, so congenital muscular dystrophy is not the best answer.

Cerebral palsy can cause hypotonia, in which case, it is usually referred to as "ataxic cerebral palsy." Ataxic cerebral palsy can be caused by prenatal or perinatal brain injury, especially to the cerebellum, or by cerebellar hypoplasia. There may be associated speech or language disorders and intellectual disability. Diagnosis is made based on history, physical examination, and abnormalities seen on brain imaging. Tongue fasciculations would not be present, so for the girl in the vignette, cerebral palsy is not the best answer.

Infant botulism presents with a prodrome of constipation, followed by ptosis, decreased facial movements, head lag, and choking or aspiration. Limb weakness and hypotonia are less prominent early in the course. Deep tendon reflexes are usually diminished. The infant can appear to be asleep or encephalopathic due to bilateral ptosis, but careful observation will show normal limb movements even when the eyes are closed. If the examiner opens the eyelids, the infant will appear alert and interactive. These findings suggest a disorder of the peripheral nervous system. Electromyography/nerve conduction study can confirm a disorder of the neuromuscular junction but can be technically difficult in an infant. Diagnosis is made by identification of botulinum toxin in the stool. The girl in the vignette has limb weakness and hypotonia, but her face is spared, so infant botulism is not the best answer.

PREP Pearls

- Infant botulism presents with a prodrome of constipation, followed by ptosis, decreased facial movements, head lag, and choking or aspiration. Limb weakness is less prominent early in the course.
- Spinal muscular atrophy presents in infancy with head lag; weak, hypotonic limbs; areflexia; paradoxical breathing; tongue fasciculations; and finger trembling. The muscles of facial expression are spared.

- Plan the appropriate evaluation of hypotonia in patients of various ages
- Differentiate the findings associated with central nervous system causes of hypotonia from those of peripheral nervous system causes

Suggested Readings

Beinvogl BC, Rosman NP, Baumer FM, et al. A 10-month-old with intermittent hypotonia and paralysis. *Pediatrics.* 2016;138(1):e20151896.

Lisi EC, Cohn RD. Genetic evaluation of the pediatric patient with hypotonia: perspective from a hypotonia specialty clinic and review of the literature. *Dev Med Child Neurol.* 2011;53(7):586-599.

Item 277   Preferred Response: B

The patient in this vignette is a young boy who has a significant iliopsoas bleed without a history of trauma and a past history remarkable for easy bruising and bleeding after circumcision. This presentation and history are consistent with a disorder of hemostasis. In particular, the iliopsoas bleed is most consistent with an abnormality of the coagulation cascade. After von Willebrand disease, factor VIII and IX deficiencies are the most common coagulation disorders. Both are inherited in an X-linked manner, so all male individuals who present with a nontraumatic, significant bleeding episode should be evaluated for factor VIII deficiency (hemophilia A) and factor IX deficiency (hemophilia B). One-third of cases of hemophilia A and B occur through spontaneous mutation and have no family history of bleeding.

Factors VIII and IX are in the intrinsic pathway of the coagulation cascade and will therefore prolong the partial thromboplastin time (PTT) when deficient (Item C277). The prothrombin time (PT) is unaffected by a deficiency in either factor.

Factor XIII deficiency is rare and does not typically present with intramuscular bleeds. Factor XIII stabilizes fibrin clots and does not influence the PT or PTT. Although it is possible that the child in this vignette could have a low platelet count, his history is more consistent with a coagulation factor defi-

Intrinsic
(contact activation pathway)

$XII \longrightarrow XIIa$

$XI \longrightarrow XIa$

Extrinsic
(tissue factor activation pathway)

$$IX \xrightarrow{VIIIa} IXa \qquad VIIa \xrightarrow{TF} VII$$

$$X \xrightarrow{Va} Xa \xleftarrow{Va} X$$

$$Prothrombin \longrightarrow Thrombin$$

$$Fibrinogen \longrightarrow Fibrin$$

Item C277. Coagulation pathways.

ciency. A low platelet count would more often present with petechiae and mucosal bleeding. The PT would be prolonged if there were a deficiency of factors in the extrinsic pathway, in particular factor VII. A deficiency of factors in the common pathway would prolong both the PT and PTT.

PREP Pearls

- One-third of cases of factor VIII or IX deficiency occur through spontaneous gene mutation and have no family history of bleeding.
- Young male children who have a history of nontraumatic severe bleeding should be evaluated for factor VIII and IX deficiencies.

**American Board of Pediatrics Content Specification(s)/
Content Area**

- Understand the genetic risks when a congenital bleeding or thrombotic disorder is suspected
- Understand the hematologic significance of a rapidly enlarging hematoma
- Recognize the clinical manifestations and complications associated with hemophilia, and manage appropriately
- Recognize laboratory findings associated with hemophilia

Suggested Readings

Rodriguez V, Warad D. Pediatric coagulation disorders. *Pediatr Rev.* 2016;37(7):279-291.

Sharathkumar AA, Pipe SW. Bleeding disorders. *Pediatr Rev.* 2008;29(4):121-129.

Zimmerman B, Valentino LA. Hemophilia: in review. *Pediatr Rev.* 2013;34(7):289-294.

Item 278   Preferred Response: A

The adolescent girl in the vignette presents with lethargy, tachycardia, hypotension, dry and flushed skin, mydriasis, and a widened QRS complex on electrocardiography (ECG) following a suspected medication overdose. Of the medications accessible to her, the one most likely responsible for her clinical picture is amitriptyline, a tricyclic antidepressant (TCA).

Tricyclic antidepressants include agents such as imipramine, amitriptyline, desipramine, and nortriptyline. Despite the availability of newer-generation antidepressants (including serotonin-specific reuptake inhibitors), TCAs are still commonly used in the management of a range of disorders including depression, nocturnal enuresis, anxiety, neuropathic pain, attention-deficit/hyperactivity disorder, and migraines. These medications remain a significant cause of morbidity and mortality related to poisoning in the United States, and can cause serious toxicity and death in children. Children have been reported to have a higher sensitivity to TCAs than adults, and often display symptoms of toxicity at lower dosages.

Children may develop TCA toxicity after ingesting toxic amounts of their own medication or medication(s) prescribed for a family member or even a pet. The ingestion of TCAs at a dose of 10 to 20 mg/kg generally represents a moderate to serious exposure in children, with central nervous system (CNS) depression and cardiovascular manifestations expected. Ingestion of TCA doses of 35 to 50 mg/kg and higher may be lethal to a child.

Tricyclic antidepressants have multiple pharmacologic effects, including inhibition of norepinephrine, serotonin, and dopamine in the CNS, and blockade of type Ia sodium channels in the cardiovascular system (which can lead to cardiac conduction delays and myocardial depression). They also have anticholinergic effects.

The most predominant signs and symptoms of TCA toxicity involve the cardiovascular system and CNS. Central nervous system effects include lethargy, delirium, ataxia, hallucinations, seizures, and coma (in severe cases). Cardiovascular effects may include sinus tachycardia, hypotension, cardiac conduction delays, and myocardial depression. A widened QRS interval on ECG can be observed, due to blockage of the type Ia sodium channels in the myocardium. Studies have demonstrated that a QRS interval of more than 100 milliseconds in patients with TCA toxicity is associated with significant morbidity and mortality; this conduction delay may lead to complete heart block, wide complex ventricular dysrhythmias, and cardiac standstill. Children with TCA toxicity may also display signs and symptoms of central and peripheral anticholinergic toxicity due to effects on M1-muscarinic receptors. These may include altered sensorium, tachycardia, flushed dry skin, mydriasis, decreased bowel sounds, delayed gastric emptying, and urinary retention.

Management of TCA toxicity includes aggressive supportive care (with emphasis on support of the airway, breathing, and circulation). An ECG should be obtained as early as possible in children with TCA toxicity, and intravenous sodium bicarbonate should be administered to those with signs of significant cardiovascular toxicity (prolonged QRS complex of ≥100 msec). Children presenting with seizures due to suspected TCA toxicity should be treated with benzodiazepines. Although physostigmine was previously recommended for the treatment of TCA poisonings, because of its effects on anticholinergic receptors, this therapy actually has the potential to lower the seizure threshold and worsen ventricular conduction abnormalities; physostigmine is now contraindicated for TCA overdoses, particularly in patients with abnormal ECG findings. All children with clinically significant TCA ingestions should undergo continuous cardiac monitoring and be admitted to an intensive care unit. Gastric decontamination with activated charcoal should be initiated in children with significant TCA overdoses, provided that a definitive airway is in place or it is certain that the child can protect his/her airway.

The key clinical findings of clonidine poisoning are similar to those seen with opioid toxicity: CNS depression, respiratory depression, bradycardia, hypotension, and miosis. Although the girl in the vignette has CNS depression, she is tachycardic (rather than bradycardic) and her pupils are large rather than constricted. Furthermore, a widened QRS complex would not be expected in patients with clonidine toxicity.

Children presenting in the initial stage of iron sulfate poisoning would typically have vomiting, diarrhea, and hematemesis, in addition to altered mental status and possibly hypotension. These gastrointestinal symptoms are not seen in the girl in the vignette.

Although acute metformin overdose is rare in children, doses of more than 5 g in an adolescent may result in lactic acidosis. Early symptoms of metformin poisoning may include abdominal pain, nausea, malaise, myalgia, and dizziness. Altered mental status, respiratory depression, hypotension, and hyperglycemia may be seen as lactic acidosis develops. QRS complex widening on ECG is not an expected finding in patients with metformin overdose.

PREP Pearls

- Electrocardiography should be performed early in children with suspected tricyclic antidepressant toxicity. A QRS duration of more than 100 milliseconds warrants intravenous sodium bicarbonate administration.

- Physostigmine is contraindicated in the treatment of children with tricyclic antidepressant overdose, because it has the potential to lower the seizure threshold and worsen ventricular conduction abnormalities.

- The signs and symptoms of tricyclic antidepressant toxicity involve the cardiovascular (sinus tachycardia, hypotension, cardiac conduction delays, and myocardial depression) and central nervous systems (lethargy, delirium, ataxia, hallucinations, seizures, and coma).

American Board of Pediatrics Content Specification(s)/Content Area

- Recognize the signs and symptoms of tricyclic antidepressant toxicity, and provide appropriate initial management

Suggested Readings

O'Donnell KA, Osterhoudt KC, Burns MB, Calello DP, Henretig FM. Toxicologic emergencies. In: Shaw KN, Bachur RG, eds. *Fleisher and Ludwig's Textbook of Pediatric Emergency Medicine.* 7th ed. Philadelphia, PA: Lippincott Williams & Wilkins; 2016;chap 110.

Shah RR, Ronak R. Toxicology. In: Shah BR, Lucchesi M, Amodio J, Silverberg M, eds. *Atlas of Pediatric Emergency Medicine.* 2nd ed. New York, NY: McGraw-Hill; 2013;chap 17. http://accessemergencymedicine.mhmedical.com.

Williams SR, Sztajnkrycer MD, Thurman R. et al. Toxicological conditions. In: Knoop KJ, Stack LB, Storrow AB, Thurman R, eds. *The Atlas of Emergency Medicine.* 4th ed. New York, NY: McGraw-Hill; 2016; chap 17. http://accessemergencymedicine.mhmedical.com.

Item 279　　　　　　　　　　**Preferred Response: D**

Vesicoureteral reflux (VUR) is the retrograde passage of urine from the bladder to the kidneys. Vesicoureteral reflux may present prenatally, as hydronephrosis on maternal ultrasound screening, or be diagnosed in children after an episode of urinary tract infection (UTI) (usually before 6-7 years of age). Vesicoureteral reflux is associated with an increased risk for pyelonephritis. Children with prenatally diagnosed VUR are usually male, and have increased risk for other congenital abnormalities of the kidney, such as renal hypoplasia or dysplasia. A short intravesical ureter, which may be genetically linked, has been implicated in the failure of the antireflux mechanism, and is associated with primary VUR in children. Primary VUR may resolve spontaneously with patient growth.

Secondary VUR occurs because of abnormally high pressures in the bladder leading to incompetence of the ureterovesical junction. The high pressure can be the result of anatomic obstruction, as seen in posterior urethral valves (in boys only), or bladder contraction against a closed urethral sphincter, as seen in dysfunctional voiding. Dysfunctional voiding may be associated with neurogenic (cerebral palsy, myelomeningocele) or non-neurogenic causes. Bladder or bowel dysfunction leading to dysfunctional elimination is frequently seen in patients with VUR and is associated with recurrent infections, increased time for spontaneous resolution of reflux, and reduced success of endoscopic surgery. Symptoms for voiding dysfunction include constipation, urgency, urge incontinence, infrequent voiding, or recurrent infections. Appropriate management of voiding dysfunction may increase the likelihood of spontaneous resolution of reflux and decrease the risk for UTI, thereby improving overall patient prognosis.

In more than 50% of patients, the reflux resolves spontaneously. Lower-grade reflux, unilateral reflux, prenatal hydronephrosis, and diagnosis before age 1 year have been favorably associated with spontaneous resolution of VUR. Spontaneous resolution has been reported in 60% to 80% of children with unilateral grade I to grade IV VUR. Although patients with grade I to grade II VUR also have high rates of bilateral reflux resolution, only 10% to 20% of patients with grade III to grade IV bilateral reflux experience spontaneous resolution. Grade V reflux rarely resolves spontaneously; these patients usually need surgical intervention.

Management of VUR involves antibiotic prophylaxis and surgical correction. Antibiotic prophylaxis is recommended for children with high-grade reflux, recurrent UTI, bladder bowel dysfunction, or obstructive uropathy. Prophylaxis is continued until spontaneous or surgical resolution of VUR. In older children, it is suggested that antibiotic prophylaxis may be stopped as the risk of recurrent UTI diminishes with age; however, the age for discontinuing antibiotics is not well-established because of the lack of studies.

PREP Pearls

- Antibiotic prophylaxis is recommended for children with high-grade reflux, recurrent urinary tract infection, bladder or bowel dysfunction, or obstructive uropathy.

- Bladder or bowel dysfunction leading to dysfunctional elimination is frequently seen in patients with vesicoureteral reflux and has been associated with recurrent infections, increased time until spontaneous resolution of reflux, and reduced success of endoscopic surgery.

- Low grade of reflux, unilateral reflux, prenatal hydronephrosis, and diagnosis before age 1 year have been favorably associated with spontaneous resolution of vesicoureteral reflux.

American Board of Pediatrics Content Specification(s)/Content Area

- Recognize the clinical findings associated with vesicoureteral reflux
- Understand the natural history of vesicoureteral reflux

Suggested Readings

Feld LG, Mattoo TK. Urinary tract infections and vesicoureteral reflux in infants and children. *Pediatr Rev*. 2010;31(11):451-463.

Jahnukainen TJ, Vats AN. Urinary tract infections. In McInerny KT, Adam HM, Campbell DE, DeWitt TG, Foy JM, Kamat DM, eds. *American Academy of Pediatrics Textbook of Pediatric Care*. Elk Grove Village, IL: American Academy of Pediatrics; 2009; 2607-2614.

Item 280	Preferred Response: B

The neonate in this vignette has a patent ductus arteriosus (PDA) that is shunting left to right, as expected. The neonate is on minimal continuous positive airway pressure with an FiO_2 of 21% and full enteral feeds. Given this level of support, as well as a lack of clinically significant hemodynamic instability (ie, an increasing oxygen requirement or increased respiratory support requirements), further monitoring would be the most appropriate management. There is no clinical indication for surgical or medical closure of the PDA at this time, and there is no clinical indication for repeat echocardiography in 48 hours.

When a PDA is shunting left to right (aorta to pulmonary artery), as the pulmonary vascular resistance drops, the amount of blood being shunted away from the body increases and in turn the amount of blood being shunted to the lungs increases. This leads to pulmonary overcirculation resulting in pulmonary congestion, edema, and worsening respiratory status. The body on the other hand, has an overall relative decrease in cardiac output that can compromise perfusion to the gut, kidney, and brain. Although the prolonged presence of a PDA has been associated with prolongation of mechanical ventilation, bronchopulmonary dysplasia, increased mortality, pulmonary hemorrhage, necrotizing enterocolitis, impaired renal function, and intraventricular hemorrhage, the data directly connecting all of these outcomes to a PDA are limited.

The "normal" course for a PDA in a term neonate is closure within 72 hours of birth. In preterm neonates, this course is delayed, and the PDA remains open in 10% of neonates born at 30 to 37 weeks' gestation, 80% born at 25 to 28 weeks' gestation, and 90% born at 24 weeks' gestation. By 7 days after birth, these rates decline to 2%, 65%, and 87%, respectively. The natural history of spontaneous closure of PDAs in neonates who are smaller and less mature is unknown because there is widespread use of medications and procedures to close them. Data from controlled studies indicate that spontaneous closure of PDAs frequently occurs. The Trial of Indomethacin Prophylaxis in Preterms study included neonates with birth weight from 500 to 999 g. In this study, 50% of placebo recipients never developed clinical signs of a PDA. In a trial of early vs late indomethacin treatment in neonates born at 26 to 31 weeks' gestation, the PDA closed spontaneously in 78% of neonates randomized to the late intervention group. Deferral of treatment may actually result in avoidance of treatment, at least in some neonates.

While individual studies and meta-analyses have demonstrated the ability to close a PDA, both medically and surgically, no study has shown that closing a PDA improves long-term outcomes. There is insufficient data to determine whether a subset of preterm neonates might benefit from early treatment. Clinically less aggressive management plans for PDA do not result in worse outcomes compared with more aggressive strategies.

Based on these findings, a conservative approach is appropriate in most neonates with a PDA. Some PDAs will warrant pharmacological or procedural-based intervention, especially if respiratory status is worsening. Some providers will approach a PDA with fluid restriction, diuretics, and increasing end-expiratory pressure (to increase the pulmonary vascular resistance and decrease the amount of shunting). Each of these therapies needs further investigation. Hemodynamics, blood pressure, pulse pressure, respiratory support, and echocardiogram findings should all be taken into consideration for management decisions.

PREP Pearls

- The management of a preterm neonate with a patent ductus arteriosus is a point of controversy. Depending on the clinical and echocardiographic data, management can include watchful waiting, nonpharmacological management, pharmacological management, and procedural closure.
- The natural history of a patent ductus arteriosus is spontaneous closure, and this process is delayed and disrupted in preterm neonates.
- The presence of a patent ductus arteriosus has been linked with the development of necrotizing enterocolitis, bronchopulmonary dysplasia, intraventricular hemorrhage, impaired renal function, and pulmonary hemorrhage.

American Board of Pediatrics Content Specification(s)/Content Area

- Plan appropriate initial management of patent ductus arteriosus in an infant born prematurely

Suggested Readings

Benitz WE; Committee on Fetus and Newborn. Patent ductus arteriosus in preterm infants. *Pediatrics*. 2016;137(1):e2-e6.

Jain A, Shah PS. Diagnosis, evaluation and management of patent ductus arteriosus in preterm neonates. *JAMA Pediatrics*. 2015;169(9):863-872.

Item 281   Preferred Response: D

Adherence to a medical regimen is the degree to which a person is able to follow medical advice. Children and adolescents with chronic medical conditions often have issues with adherence to medication regimens. Based on the health belief model, a patient's adherence is based on one's perception of the severity of their medical condition and the benefit of the treatment.

Depending on their stage of development, it can be difficult for an adolescent to understand the severity of a medical condition. In early adolescence (10-13 years of age), teenagers become more autonomous, start separating from family, begin adjusting to pubertal changes in their bodies, and tend to have concrete thought. In middle adolescence (14-17 years of age), they become more independent, their peer group can become more important than family, and conforming with peers is a priority. They also begin to develop abstract thought. Late adolescence (18-21 years) is characterized by comfort with one's identity, making plans for the future, further development of abstract thought, and a time of transition into a more adult role in society. The ability to think abstractly and factor in consequences is an important factor in an adolescent being able to follow medical advice.

Adherence to a medical regimen can be derailed by numerous factors. Adolescents who have strong support systems and parents who are actively involved in their care, check in if medication is being taken on a daily basis, and attend medical appointments have higher rates of adherence. However, if the adolescent is not experiencing any symptoms from their disease, does not understand the seriousness of their condition, has numerous medications to take multiple times per day, and has experienced negative adverse effects from medications or treatments, they are more likely to not follow medical advice. This lack of adherence can lead to a poor prognosis, increased emergency department visits/hospitalizations, and death.

The adolescent in this vignette has systemic lupus erythematosus and has not been adhering to her medication plan because of unwanted adverse effects from her medication. To provide the best care to this patient, it would be useful to get her perspective on her medical condition, why she has been prescribed certain medications, and the potential consequences if she does not follow instructions. Motivational interviewing can be a useful tool to engage this adolescent in her own care, as opposed to lecturing in a more authoritarian style. It is a nonconfrontational style of counseling that allows the patient to play a role in his or her care by deciding if changes will be made that are beneficial to their treatment, what the changes would be, and when the changes would be implemented. It forces the provider to listen so that he or she can highlight the patient's change talk. Change talk is when a patient mentions a desire, ability, reason, or need to make a change in their behavior.

The other options mentioned in this vignette are related to understanding one's disease process and support networks, but do not directly encourage the patient to take an active role in their own health care. Involving the patient's parent may help with medication compliance but does not encourage the patient to take responsibility for their actions. A psychiatrist can be useful if the patient is describing signs and symptoms suspicious for depression. Many children and adolescents with chronic disease may experience depression secondary to their medical condition. Lastly, it is always recommended to review medication dosing and assess how often a patient is missing or skipping doses. This review allows the provider an opportunity to address any information the patient might have misunderstood. However, motivational interviewing is more likely to highlight the best treatment plan to get an adolescent engaged in their care.

PREP Pearls

- Ascertain the adolescent's perspective about their medical condition, medication regimen, and support system to devise realistic plans of care.
- Motivational interviewing can be a useful tool in engaging adolescents with chronic illness to be more engaged in their own care.

American Board of Pediatrics Content Specification(s)/ Content Area

- Understand factors that can affect adherence to health maintenance activities by adolescents
- Understand how to improve adherence to medical regimens by adolescent patients, including those with chronic illness, and the barriers to such adherence

Suggested Readings

Arrington-Sanders A. Adherence, in brief. *Pediatr Rev.* 2009:30(2);e9-e10.

Mahan JD, Betz CL, Okumura MJ, Ferris ME. Self-management and transition to adult health care in adolescents and young adults: a team process. *Pediatr Rev.* 2017;38(7):305-317.

Schaefer MR, Kavookjian J. The impact of motivational interviewing on adherence and symptom severity in adolescents and young adults with chronic illness: a systematic review. *Patient Educ Couns.* 2017;100(12):2190-2199.

Item 282 — Preferred Response: C

The girl in the vignette has an anticholinergic toxidrome, indicated by altered mental status, fever, tachycardia, hypertension, dry mucous membranes, and rigidity. Of the answer choices, the best next step in management is intravenous lorazepam.

Acetylcholine is a neurotransmitter active in the central nervous system, autonomic nervous system, and neuromuscular junction. Anticholinergic agents are competitive antagonists of acetylcholine receptors. Although acetylcholine binds to both nicotinic and muscarinic receptors, most anticholinergic agents primarily block muscarinic receptors. The wide distribution of the subtypes of muscarinic receptors contributes to the heterogenous presentation of the anticholinergic toxidrome. A convenient mnemonic for the anticholinergic toxidrome is "mad as a hatter, blind as a bat, hot as a hare, dry as a bone, and red as a beet." Altered mental status manifesting as coma, delirium, or agitation can occur as a result of decreased central neurotransmission. Visual and/or auditory hallucinations are common. Impaired autonomic nervous system function from acetylcholine inhibition can cause dilated and poorly reactive pupils, anhidrosis, dry mouth, blurry vision, and photophobia. Dry skin, muscle rigidity from central disinhibition, and autonomic instability can lead to tachycardia and hyperthermia. Hypertension may also occur due to agitation. Drugs causing primarily antimuscarinic effects include atropine, scopolamine, and benztropine. Some anticholinergic agents may also affect other ion channels or receptors. For example, cardiotoxicity from tricyclic antidepressants, antihistamines, and some antipsychotics can cause hypotension, QT prolongation, and malignant arrhythmias.

The differential diagnosis for the anticholinergic toxidrome includes central nervous system infection, primary acute psychiatric conditions, and drug withdrawal. It must be distinguished from other poisonings, such as alcohol, sympathomimetics, and serotonin syndrome (Item C282). Serotonin syndrome, which can also cause muscle rigidity, hyperpyrexia, hyperreflexia, and central nervous system depression, can be distinguished from anticholinergic toxidrome by a predominance of gastrointestinal symptoms such as nausea, vomiting, and diarrhea.

Benzodiazepines are a mainstay of treatment for anticholinergic poisoning. Sedation can mitigate agitation, delirium, rigidity, hypertension, and tachycardia, and secondary hyperpyrexia can improve. A toxicology screen is important to rule out concomitant poisonings. Supportive care, such as cardiopulmonary monitoring, should be provided.

Naloxone, an opioid antagonist used to treat narcotic toxicity, would not be the appropriate treatment for the girl in the vignette, because she does not have symptoms consistent with narcotic toxicity, such as respiratory depression, hypotension, or constricted pupils. Fomepizole is an alcohol dehydrogenase inhibitor used to decrease the toxic metabolites of ethanol, methanol, and ethylene glycol. Haloperidol is used

Item C282. Toxic Syndromes.

Group	BP	P	R	T	Mental Status	Vital Signs			
						Pupil Size	Peristalsis	Diaphoresis	Other
Anticholinergics	–/↑	↑	±	↑	Delirium	↑	↓	↓	Dry mucous membranes, flush, urinary retention
Cholinergics	±	±	–/↑	–	Normal to depressed	±	↑	↑	Salivation, lacrimation, urination, diarrhea, bronchorrhea, fasciculations, paralysis
Ethanol or sedative-hypnotics	↓	↓	↓	–/↓	Depressed, agitated	±	↓	–	Hyporeflexia, ataxia
Opioids	↓	↓	↓	↓	Depressed	↓	↓	–	Hyporeflexia
Sympathomimetics	↑	↑	↑	↑	Agitated	↑	–/↑	↑	Tremor, seizure
Withdrawal from ethanol or sedative-hypnotics	↑	↑	↑	↑	Agitated, disoriented	↑	↑	↑	Tremor, seizure
Withdrawal from opioids	↑	↑	–	–	Normal, anxious	↑	↑	↑	Vomiting, rhinorrhea, piloerection, diarrhea, yawning

↑, increased; ↓, decreased; ±, variable; –, change unlikely; BP, blood pressure; P, pulse; R, respirations; T, temperature.

to treat acute psychosis. These medications would not be appropriate in this case, because the girl's symptoms of rigidity, dilated and poorly reactive pupils, and hyperpyrexia are not commonly seen in alcohol poisoning or acute psychosis.

PREP Pearls

- A convenient mnemonic for the anticholinergic toxidrome is "mad as a hatter, blind as a bat, hot as a hare, dry as a bone, and red as a beet."
- Sedation with benzodiazepines is a mainstay of therapy for anticholinergic toxidrome, because it can mitigate agitation, delirium, rigidity, hypertension, and tachycardia, and secondarily hyperpyrexia may improve.
- The differential diagnosis for the anticholinergic toxidrome includes central nervous system infection, primary acute psychiatric conditions, and drug withdrawal.

American Board of Pediatrics Content Specification(s)/ Content Area

- Recognize the signs and symptoms of ingestion of an anticholinergic drug, and manage appropriately

Suggested Readings

Dawson AH, Buckley NA. Pharmacological management of anticholinergic delirium—theory, evidence and practice. *Br J Clin Pharmacol.* 2016;81:516-524.

Gerardi DM, Murphy TK, Toufexis M, et al. Serotonergic or anticholinergic toxidrome case report in a 9 year-old girl. *Pediatr Emerg Care.* 2015;31(12):846-850.

Toce MS, Burns MM. The poisoned pediatric patient. *Pediatr Rev.* 2017;38:207.

Item 283   Preferred Response: D

The girl in this vignette has vitamin D–deficient rickets. Vitamin D is naturally found in liver and other organ meats; egg yolk; oily fish such as salmon, sardines, and mackerel; and cod liver oil. Many foods are fortified with vitamin D, including milk, juices, and infant formulas. Although breast milk is the best source of nutrition for neonates and infants, it typically contains insufficient concentrations of vitamin D for an infant to meet the recommended daily intake. Vitamin D can be produced by the human body when ultraviolet B radiation from the sun converts previtamin D to vitamin D_3 in the skin. Vitamin D_3 is hydroxylated in the liver to 25-hydroxyvitamin D (25[OH]-D), which is then converted to the active form, 1,25-dihydroxyvitamin D (1,25[OH]-D) by 1α-hydroxylase in the kidney. The 1,25[OH]-D increases plasma calcium and phosphorus concentrations by facilitating renal calcium reabsorption, increasing intestinal calcium and phosphorus absorption, and stimulating osteoblasts in the bone to become osteoclasts, which releases calcium and phosphorus. Production of 1,25[OH]-D is regulated by parathyroid hormone, calcium, and phosphorus levels.

The main circulating form of vitamin D is 25[OH]-D, and therefore, laboratory measurement of this form is the most accurate means of determining a patient's overall vitamin D status. There is ongoing disagreement about the definition of vitamin D deficiency in children, but most sources define vitamin D insufficiency as a 25[OH]-D level of 12 to 20 ng/mL (30 to 50 nmol/L) and vitamin D deficiency as a 25[OH]-D level of less than 12 ng/mL (< 30 nmol/L). Vitamin D deficiency can occur because of decreased synthesis in the skin, insufficient dietary intake, malabsorption, or maternal deficiency. Risk factors for vitamin D deficiency include exclusive breastfeeding without supplementation (especially if the infant's mother is deficient in vitamin D), vegetarian diet, dark skin, decreased sun exposure, higher latitude, and winter season.

Infants with vitamin D deficiency can be asymptomatic, or they may present with seizures and tetany caused by hypocalcemia, poor growth, widened cranial sutures, frontal bossing, or hypotonia. Older infants and children may have developmental delays and/or bony abnormalities including delayed dental eruption, valgus deformity of the leg, kyphosis, widening of the metaphysis of the wrists, and rachitic rosary (an enlarged costochondral junction along the anterolateral aspect of the rib cage). Radiographs will show widening of the epiphyseal plate with cupping, splaying, and stippling as the demineralization worsens. Long bones are osteopenic with thin cortices. Individuals with vitamin D deficiency have an increased risk of several types of cancer, autoimmune disease, cardiovascular disease, depression, and wheezing.

Vitamin D deficiency should be treated with daily oral supplementation with vitamin D, followed by maintenance therapy after levels normalize. While oral vitamin D_2 (ergocalciferol) and D_3 (cholecalciferol) are both absorbed well, supplementation with vitamin D_3 raises serum levels more rapidly. To prevent deficiency, the American Academy of Pediatrics recommends supplementing all breastfed infants and formula-fed infants who are consuming less than 1 L of vitamin D–fortified formula each day with 400 IU/day of vitamin D. Premature infants and infants with other risk factors may require higher doses. There is evidence that supplementing lactating mothers with high doses of vitamin D (6,400 IU/day) can provide sufficient dietary vitamin D for the breastfed infant and may be an alternative strategy for prevention. The Institute of Medicine recommends 600 IU/day for children and adolescents.

Rickets is caused by decreased bone mineralization with architectural disruption at the growth plate. Normal bone mineralization requires the presence of sufficient calcium and phosphorus; rickets can be caused by a deficiency of either. Calcipenic rickets is usually due to vitamin D deficiency or defects in the metabolism of vitamin D. Phosphopenic rickets is caused by renal phosphate wasting. Item C283 shows the laboratory findings typical for several subtypes of rickets.

The girl in this vignette has vitamin D–deficient rickets. She has risk factors of exclusive breastfeeding without vitamin D supplementation and dark skin. Her genu varum, low weight and height for age, delayed gross motor milestones, and radiographs showing widened, cupped, and irregular epiphysis are supportive of the diagnosis. The girl's low levels of calcium, phosphorus, and 25-hydroxyvitamin D and elevated levels of parathyroid hormone and alkaline phosphatase confirm the diagnosis.

Item C283. Types of Rickets.

Types of Rickets	Calcium	Phosphorus	Parathyroid Hormone	Alkaline Phosphatase	25[OH]-D	1,25[OH]-D
Vitamin D deficient	Normal or ↓	↓	↑	↑	↓	Variable
1α-hydroxylase deficiency (vitamin D–dependent rickets type 1)	↓	↓	↑	↑↑	Normal	↓
Hereditary resistance to vitamin D (vitamin D–dependent rickets type 2)	↓	↓	↑	↑↑	Normal	↑↑
Vitamin D resistant (X-linked hypophosphatemia)	Normal	↓↓	Normal or ↑	↑	Normal	Normal or ↓

Abbreviations: 1,25[OH]-D, 1,25-dihydroxyvitamin; 25[OH]-D, 25-hydroxyvitamin D.

Adapted and reprinted with permission from Sethuraman U. Vitamins. *Pediatr Rev*. 2006;27(2):50.

PREP Pearls

- Dietary sources of vitamin D include liver and other organ meats; egg yolk; oily fish such as salmon, sardines, and mackerel; and cod liver oil. Many foods are fortified with vitamin D, including milk, juices, and infant formulas.
- Vitamin D deficiency can be prevented by supplementing breastfed infants and infants consuming less than 1 L of vitamin D–fortified formula each day with 400 IU of vitamin D. Older children and adolescents need 600 IU of vitamin D daily.
- Vitamin D deficiency can lead to poor growth, developmental delays, and bony abnormalities (frontal bossing and widened cranial sutures in infants, delayed dental eruption, valgus deformity of the leg, kyphosis, widening of the metaphysis of the wrists, and rachitic rosary in older children). Individuals with vitamin D deficiency have an increased risk of several types of cancer, autoimmune disease, cardiovascular disease, depression, and wheezing.

American Board of Pediatrics Content Specification(s)/Content Area

- Recognize the signs, symptoms, and causes of vitamin A deficiency, and manage appropriately
- Recognize the laboratory and radiologic features of vitamin D-deficient rickets
- Recognize the effects of vitamin D deficiency in patients of various ages, including those who are breast-fed

Suggested Readings

Hollis BW, Wagner CL, Howard CR, et al. Maternal versus infant vitamin D supplementation during lactation: a randomized controlled trial. *Pediatrics*. 2015;136(4):625-634.

Lauer B, Spector N. Vitamins. *Pediatr Rev*. 2012;33(8):339-352.

Misra M, Pacaud D, Petryk A, Collett-Solberg PF, Kappy M. Vitamin D deficiency in children and its management: review of current knowledge and recommendations. *Pediatrics*. 2008;122(2):398-417.

Item 284 **Preferred Response: B**

The toxic-appearing, unimmunized young girl in this vignette, with acute onset of fever, inspiratory stridor, drooling, and severe respiratory distress, and evidence of markedly swollen epiglottis during endotracheal intubation, has the classic presentation of epiglottitis caused by *Haemophilus influenzae* type b (Hib) infection. Of the choices listed, the best initial antimicrobial treatment for this girl's illness is ceftriaxone.

Acute epiglottitis results from inflammation and swelling of the supraglottis; it has the potential to cause serious, life-threatening illness due to upper airway obstruction. *Haemophilus influenzae* type b, a gram-negative coccobacillus, is the most frequent cause of epiglottitis in unimmunized children, followed in order by group A *Streptococcus* (GAS), *Streptococcus pneumoniae*, and *Staphylococcus aureus*. Acute epiglottitis can also be caused by viruses (eg, herpes simplex virus), fungi (eg, *Candida albicans*), and noninfectious sources (eg, physical trauma, chemicals, and heat), especially in adults. The peak incidence of Hib epiglottitis in unimmunized children occurs between 2 and 4 years of age, but the disease may present in any age group, including neonates, older children, and adults.

The incidence of invasive Hib disease in children in the United States has declined dramatically since the introduction of the Hib conjugate vaccine in 1987. Historically, the peak incidence of invasive Hib disease occurred between 6 and 18 months of age; Black, Alaskan native, Apache, and Navajo children had a higher rate of disease. *Haemophilus influenzae* type b was the most common cause of acute bacterial meningitis in children in the pre-Hib vaccine era. Other serious Hib infections included pneumonia, bacteremia, cellulitis, and septic arthritis. Only 30 cases of invasive Hib disease occurred among US children younger than 5 years in 2012. Children with sickle cell disease, asplenia, HIV, and certain immunodeficiency syndromes remain at increased risk of invasive Hib disease.

Nontypeable *H influenzae* is implicated in approximately 50% of cases of acute otitis media and sinusitis in the pediatric age group. In the post-Hib vaccine era, the epidemiology of invasive Hib disease has evolved significantly. Currently, the majority of invasive *H influenzae* disease in children and adults is caused by nontypeable *H influenzae*; from 1999 to 2008, the annual incidence of invasive disease caused by nontypeable *H influenzae* was 1.73 per 100,000 in children younger than 5 years. Invasive *H influenzae* type a disease (Hia) has also emerged as an important disease among southwestern Alaskan native children, with a peak incidence of 72 per 100,000 annually.

Clinical manifestations of acute epiglottitis include abrupt onset of high fever, inspiratory stridor, drooling, and respiratory distress. Patients appear toxic and may prefer to sit up and lean forward (tripod position) to alleviate breathing difficulty. Other features may include sore throat, odynophagia, dysphagia, and cervical lymphadenopathy. Rapid progression to life-threatening upper airway obstruction and respiratory failure is a major concern. The differential diagnosis of acute epiglottitis includes croup, bacterial tracheitis, retropharyngeal abscess, and foreign body.

Acute epiglottitis is a medical emergency, and diagnosis is based on clinical criteria. For a toxic-appearing child with respiratory distress, securing the airway is a key priority. Interventions such as examination of the oropharynx, blood collection, intravenous line initiation, or neck radiography are not recommended, given the risk of potential respiratory arrest. Collaboration between the emergency department physician or pediatrician with the otolaryngologist and anesthesiologist is vital. The child should be transported to the operating room under the direct supervision of health care providers with expertise in airway management. Establishment of a secure airway as the first priority in cases of epiglottitis with impending airway obstruction is the standard of care.

Antimicrobial therapy is recommended for acute epiglottitis, but should be started only after securing the airway. Empiric antimicrobial therapy must cover Hib (especially in unimmunized children) and other potential pathogens (GAS, pneumococcus, and *S aureus*). Approximately 30% to 40% of *H influenzae* strains seen in the United States produce β-lactamase. Therefore, a third-generation cephalosporin (eg, cefotaxime or ceftriaxone) would be the preferred initial therapy for the suspected case of Hib epiglottitis illustrated in this vignette. A third-generation cephalosporin would also treat infection caused by GAS and pneumococcus.

Antistaphylococcal agents, such as vancomycin and clindamycin, may be added if *S aureus* epiglottitis is suspected (eg, trauma to the epiglottis). Ampicillin alone would not be an appropriate empiric antibiotic choice. The antibiotic regimen may be tailored based on isolation of an organism on culture (obtained at the time of direct laryngoscopy and endotracheal intubation) and antimicrobial susceptibility. The recommended duration of intravenous antibiotic treatment for Hib epiglottitis ranges from 7 to 10 days. Droplet precautions are indicated for hospitalized patients with invasive Hib disease until 24 hours after starting appropriate antibiotic therapy.

Rifampin chemoprophylaxis is recommended for all household contacts of children with invasive Hib disease, in the setting of at least 1 unimmunized or incompletely immunized contact younger than 48 months of age. In contrast, rifampin chemoprophylaxis is recommended for all household contacts of children with invasive Hib disease in the setting of at least 1 household contact who is immunocompromised, regardless of that contact's age or immunization status. Chemoprophylaxis is also recommended for preschool and child care center contacts of children with invasive Hib disease if 2 or more cases of invasive Hib disease occur at that site within 60 days. Chemoprophylaxis is not recommended for index patients with invasive Hib disease treated with cefotaxime or ceftriaxone. Chemoprophylaxis is also not recommended for contacts of children with invasive non–type b or nontypeable *H influenzae* disease, 24 hours after treatment with cefotaxime or ceftriaxone.

PREP Pearls

- *Haemophilus influenzae* type b is the most frequent cause of epiglottitis in unimmunized children; a third-generation cephalosporin (eg, ceftriaxone or cefotaxime) is the treatment of choice.
- Acute epiglottitis is a medical emergency. In a toxic-appearing child with respiratory distress, securing the airway is a key priority.
- Acute epiglottitis results from inflammation and swelling of the supraglottis, with a potential to cause serious, life-threatening illness due to upper airway obstruction.

American Board of Pediatrics Content Specification(s)/Content Area

- Recognize the clinical features associated with typable and nontypable *Haemophilus influenzae* infection
- Plan appropriate prophylaxis for individuals exposed to invasive *Haemophilus influenzae* type B
- Understand the epidemiology of *Haemophilus influenzae* infection
- Plan the appropriate management of a typable and nontypable *Haemophilus influenzae* infection

Suggested Readings

American Academy of Pediatrics. *Haemophilus influenzae* infections. In: Kimberlin DW, Brady MT, Jackson MA, Long SS, eds. *Red Book: 2018 Report of the Committee on Infectious Diseases*. 31st ed. Itasca, IL: American Academy of Pediatrics; 2018:367-375.

Butler DF, Myers AL. Changing epidemiology of *Haemophilus influenzae* in children. *Infect Dis Clin North Am*. 2018;32(1):119-128.

D'Agostino J. Pediatric airway nightmares. *Emerg Med Clin North Am*. 2010;28(1):119-126.

Item 285	Preferred Response: D

The infant in this vignette has necrotizing enterocolitis with persistent pneumatosis, thus enteral feeding is contraindicated. Because it is likely that she will require parenteral nutrition for several days to weeks, total parenteral nutrition (TPN) is indicated.

Parenteral nutrition (PN) should be considered when enteral nutrition is contraindicated or when enteral nutrition intake is insufficient to meet caloric needs. If a patient can tolerate a small amount of enteral nutrition, it should be continued but supplemented with PN. Indications for PN can include ileus or postoperative state, necrotizing enterocolitis, intestinal failure (from short bowel syndrome or chronic intractable diarrhea), or severe sepsis/multiorgan failure.

Peripheral PN could be an option for a child who needs very short-term and limited PN. Delivered through a peripheral intravenous catheter, peripheral PN is generally unable to meet all nutritional requirements because of osmolarity limitations.

For infants and children who cannot tolerate sufficient enteral nutrition and require substantial nutritional rehabilitation or prolonged intravenous nutrition, TPN is indicated. A central catheter (percutaneous nontunneled central catheter, tunneled central catheter, peripherally inserted central catheter, or implanted port) is required for TPN. Use of a central catheter allows for intravenous nutrition that will meet metabolic needs; however, substantial risks are present, particularly in infants and children requiring long-term TPN therapy. Risks can include infection/sepsis (related to the presence of the central catheter), PN-associated cholestasis (particularly in neonates and young infants), and specific macronutrient and micronutrient deficiencies, if nutritional status is not closely monitored.

PREP Pearls

- Parenteral nutrition should be considered in patients for whom enteral nutrition is contraindicated or in patients who cannot meet nutritional requirements with enteral nutrition alone.
- Peripheral parenteral nutrition may be considered for very short-term parenteral nutrition supplementation in patients who are not at significant nutritional risk.
- Total parenteral nutrition requires a central catheter and should be considered for patients who have anticipated long-term (days to weeks or more) parenteral nutrition needs.

American Board of Pediatrics Content Specification(s)/ Content Area

- Know the indications for total and peripheral alimentation

Suggested Readings

Hartman C, Riskin A, Shamir R. Parenteral nutrition. In: Duggan C, Watkins JB, Koletzko B, Walker WA, eds. *Nutrition in Pediatrics*. 5th ed. Shelton, CT: People's Medical Publishing House-USA; 2016:1035-1090.

Koletzko B, Goulet O, Hunt J, et al. Guidelines on paediatric parenteral nutrition of the European Society of Paediatric Gastroenterology, Hepatology and Nutrition (ESPGHAN) and the European Society for Clinical Nutrition and Metabolism (ESPR). *J Pediatr Gastroenterol Nutr.* 2005;41(suppl 2):S1-S87.

Item 286   Preferred Response: C

The neonate's most likely diagnosis is ophthalmia neonatorum, or neonatal conjunctivitis, following delivery at home without ocular prophylaxis with erythromycin ointment. In 1881, German obstetrician Dr Carl Crede reduced the incidence of ophthalmia neonatorum from 10% to 0.3% among his patients with prophylactic ocular administration of 2% silver nitrate. Historically, ophthalmia neonatorum was the leading cause of neonatal blindness, caused primarily by *Neisseria gonorrhoeae*. With improved treatment of maternal *N gonorrhoeae* infection, *Chlamydia trachomatis* has became the most common cause of ophthalmia neonatorum affecting 8.2 in 1,000 live births. Because of the risk of chemical conjunctivitis with the use of silver nitrate, in the United States neonates receive ocular prophylaxis with 0.5% erythromycin ointment.

Congenital nasolacrimal duct obstruction occurs because of abnormal formation of the nasolacrimal duct. Neonates often present with unilateral eye discharge and/or excessive tearing with normal conjunctivae. Parents may be instructed to provide gentle downward massage to help drain the duct.

Although a perfumed shampoo could cause a chemical conjunctivitis, it is not commonly seen in neonates. Other possible eye irritants include smoke, smog, and household cleaning sprays.

Saline irrigation of the eyes is recommended as part of the treatment of gonococcal ophthalmia, in conjunction with administration of ceftriaxone or cefotaxime. Saline irrigation should not cause or prevent the conjunctivitis seen in the neonate in the vignette.

PREP Pearls

- Erythromycin ocular prophylaxis after birth is indicated for all neonates.
- Ophthalmia neonatorum, neonatal conjunctivitis, may be caused by exposure to maternal *Chlamydia trachomatis* or *Neisseria gonorrhoeae* infection.
- When used as ocular prophylaxis against ophthalmia neonatorum, silver nitrate may cause a temporary chemical conjunctivitis.

American Board of Pediatrics Content Specification(s)/ Content Area

- Plan appropriate eye prophylaxis for a newborn infant

Suggested Readings

Olitsky SE, Hug D, Plummer LS, Stahl ED, Ariss MM, Lindquist TP. Disorders of the conjunctiva. In: Kliegman RM, Stanton BF, St Geme JW, Schor NF, eds. *Nelson Textbook of Pediatrics*. 20th ed. Philadelphia, PA: Saunders Elsevier; 2016:3036-3040.

Richards A, Guzman-Cottrill, JA. Conjunctivitis. *Pediatr Rev.* 2010;31:196.

Item 287   Preferred Response: C

The patient in this vignette has delayed puberty caused by Kallmann syndrome, which is hypogonadotropic hypogonadism associated with anosmia or hyposmia, the lack of or reduced ability to smell. The association results from disrupted migration of gonadotropin-releasing hormone and olfactory neurons in the developing brain. The patient's history of cryptorchidism was an early indicator of hypogonadism. Gonadotropin (luteinizing hormone [LH], follicle-stimulating hormone [FSH]) and testosterone levels are low in Kallmann syndrome. The patient's testes are prepubertal in size (sexual maturity rating 1) because of the lack of gonadotropin stimulation. His pubic hair development is a result of adrenal androgen production (adrenarche), which occurs normally in Kallmann syndrome.

Constitutional delay of puberty is the most common cause of delayed puberty, especially in boys. Short stature is commonly associated with constitutional delay, and adrenarche is also delayed. The pubertal growth spurt occurs later, duration of growth is longer, and final adult height is usually in the normal range. There is often a family history of delayed puberty in individuals who are affected. The adolescent boy in this vignette has normal stature, normal timing of adrenarche, and no family history of constitutional delay, making this diagnosis less likely.

Functional hypogonadism caused by excessive exercise may be considered for the patient in this vignette. However, his body mass index is normal and his clinical features are more consistent with Kallmann syndrome. Other common causes of functional hypogonadism include eating disorders and chronic systemic disease.

Klinefelter syndrome (47,XXY karyotype) is another cause of delayed puberty in boys. The delayed puberty is caused by primary testicular failure (primary hypogonadism). Small, firm testes on physical examination are characteristic. Adrenarche occurs normally, so pubic hair is usually present at the expected time. Other features of Klinefelter syndrome include language delay, learning problems, and tall stature with disproportionately long legs. Although the physical examination findings of the patient in this vignette can be consistent with Klinefelter syndrome, his history of anosmia makes Kallmann syndrome more likely.

Puberty is considered delayed if there is no breast development by age 13 years in girls or if there is a lack of testicular growth to at least 4 mL in volume or 2.5 cm in length by age 14 years in boys. The etiologies of delayed puberty can be classified based on gonadotropin (LH, FSH) levels. In constitutional delay, gonadotropin levels are low or early pubertal. Gonadotropin levels are also low in functional hypogonadism and hypogonadotropic hypogonadism. Hypogonadotropic hypogonadism may be isolated, as in Kallmann syndrome, or associated with other pituitary hormone deficiencies. Hypogonadotropic hypogonadism can be acquired when associated with a central nervous system abnormality, such as a craniopharyngioma.

Gonadotropin levels are elevated in hypergonadotropic hypogonadism. Etiologies of hypergonadotropic hypogonadism include Klinefelter syndrome (47,XXY) in male individuals, Turner syndrome (45,X and variants) and autoimmune ovarian failure in female individuals, and gonadal toxicity (eg, from chemotherapy or radiation).

The evaluation of an adolescent with delayed puberty should include a complete history and physical examination with special attention to signs and symptoms of underlying systemic disease, sense of smell, nutrition, exercise, history of cryptorchidism, and family history of pubertal timing. Examination of the growth charts, body mass index percentile, sexual maturity ratings, and testicular size and consistency should be performed. Features associated with Turner or Klinefelter syndrome should be identified. A bone age radiograph can be helpful because bone age often correlates better with pubertal status than with chronologic age. In constitutional delay, bone age can help predict catch-up growth, which is often a concern. Initial laboratory evaluation should include gonadotropins (LH, FSH) and either estradiol for girls or testosterone for boys. Other laboratory testing should be done as indicated by history and physical examination findings. Brain magnetic resonance imaging is indicated for unexplained hypogonadotropic hypogonadism or if a central nervous system abnormality is suspected.

Delayed puberty can cause significant psychosocial stress. For adolescents with constitutional delay and significant stress, a short course of sex steroid may trigger pubertal onset. Individuals with permanent hypogonadism require long-term treatment with sex steroid. For individuals with functional hypogonadism, correction of the underlying problem results in pubertal progression.

PREP Pearls

- Gonadotropin (luteinizing hormone, follicle-stimulating hormone) levels are important for narrowing the differential diagnosis of delayed puberty.
- Major categories of delayed puberty include constitutional delay, functional hypogonadism, hypogonadotropic hypogonadism, and hypergonadotropic hypogonadism.
- Puberty is considered delayed if there is no breast development prior to age 13 years in girls or if there is a lack of testicular growth to at least 4 mL in volume or 2.5 cm in length prior to age 14 years in boys.

American Board of Pediatrics Content Specification(s)/Content Area

- Understand the relationship between bone age and chronologic age
- Recognize the clinical features associated with a delay in sexual maturation of various causes
- Plan the appropriate evaluation of an adolescent boy or girl who has no signs of the onset of puberty
- Identify the causes of delayed puberty
- Recognize the psychosocial risks associated with delayed puberty

Suggested Readings

Kaplowitz PB. Delayed puberty. *Pediatr Rev*. 2010;31(5):189-195.

US National Library of Medicine. Kallmann syndrome. Genetics Home Reference website. https://ghr.nlm.nih.gov/condition/kallmann-syndrome.

Wolf RM, Long D. Pubertal development. *Pediatr Rev*. 2016;37(7):292-300.

Item 288 **Preferred Response: A**

The neonate in the vignette has phenylketonuria (PKU), detected via universal newborn screening based on the presence of hyperphenylalaninemia using tandem mass spectrometry on a heel stick blood spot. Phenylketonuria is a metabolic disorder resulting from an enzymatic deficiency of phenylalanine hydroxylase (PAH) that, without dietary restriction of phenylalanine implemented in early infancy, will result in irreversible and profound intellectual disability in most children.

Universal newborn screening can detect PKU in nearly 100% of cases, thus preventing significant cognitive deficits through early intervention and treatment. Additional testing is warranted to confirm a suspected diagnosis of PKU, which should include serum amino acids, red blood cell dihydropteridine reductase assay, and urine pterin analysis. This should be followed by molecular genetic testing for biallelic pathogenic variants in the *PAH* gene, given that this is an autosomal recessive disorder.

Treatment involves implementation of a Phe-free medical formula as soon as possible after birth. The goal is to normalize the concentrations of Phe (phenylalanine) and Tyr (tyrosine) in the blood. Blood Phe should be maintained between 120 and 360 µmol/L throughout the lifespan, which is achieved with a low protein/phenylalanine-free diet. Many individuals will also respond to sapropterin supplementation, an orally active form of tetrahydrobiopterin, with up to a 30% decrease in Phe plasma levels. This may allow some liberalization of the dietary phenylalanine restriction, provided normal levels of Phe can still be maintained.

Classic PKU is the most severe type, with plasma Phe concentrations typically greater than 1,000 µmol/L. Phenylalanine dietary tolerance of less than 500 mg/day is required to prevent clinical manifestations, thus warranting close management by a metabolic team consisting of a nutritionist, genetic counselor, and a biochemical geneticist. Pregnancy is a risky time for a mother affected with PKU and her unborn fetus. High maternal plasma Phe concentrations seen in maternal PAH deficiency are highly teratogenic, and can lead to intellectual disability, microcephaly, heart defects, and intrauterine growth restriction in the fetus, highlighting the importance of close monitoring of dietary phenylalanine intake and serum Phe levels during pregnancy.

The other options listed highlight other important types of biochemical screening. Serum ammonia is important in the detection of urea cycle defects and organic acidurias. Urine succinylacetone is a biochemical screen used to detect tyrosinemia type I. Very-long-chain fatty acids are a sensitive screen for peroxisomal disorders. If an inborn error of metabolism is suspected, an immediate referral to a metabolic genetics team is recommended for appropriate testing, management, and treatment.

PREP Pearls

- Individuals with untreated phenylketonuria present with a mousy body odor, developmental regression, light skin and hair, eczema, seizures, and irreversible intellectual disability.

- Phenylketonuria is a metabolic disorder caused by the enzymatic deficiency of phenylalanine hydroxylase that, without dietary restriction of phenylalanine implemented in early infancy, will result in irreversible and profound intellectual disability in most children.

- Women of childbearing age with phenylalanine hydroxylase deficiency warrant genetic counseling and close follow-up because of the teratogenic effects of elevated maternal plasma Phe concentrations on an unborn fetus potentially leading to intellectual disability, microcephaly, heart defects, and intrauterine growth restriction.

American Board of Pediatrics Content Specification(s)/ Content Area

- Understand the natural history of treated and untreated phenylketonuria
- Understand the long-term prognosis for patients who have phenylketonuria, including the importance of dietary adherence
- Recognize the clinical features associated with phenylketonuria

Suggested Readings

American College of Obstetricians and Gynecologists. Committee opinion no. 636: management of women with phenylketonuria. *Obstet Gynecol.* 2015;125:1548-1550.

Singh RH, Rohr F, Frazier D, et al. Recommendations for the nutrition management of phenylalanine hydroxylase deficiency. *Genet Med.* 2014;16:121-131.

Vockley J, Andersson HC, Antshel KM, et al; for the American College of Medical Genetics and Genomics Therapeutic Committee. Phenylalanine hydroxylase deficiency: diagnosis and management guideline. *Genet Med.* 2014;16(2):188-200.

Item 289   **Preferred Response: C**

For the 18-month-old child in the vignette, lack of pointing to something that interests him while looking to another to share that interest is concerning for an autism spectrum disorder. Joint attention, or a shared focus on an object between 2 individuals, is thought to be essential for learning language, gaining knowledge about the world, and developing social communication skills. It begins to develop around 8 months of age. Deficits in joint attention are associated with autism spectrum disorder, and improvements in joint attention are a target of therapy for autism. In contrast, children with a language disorder but not autism generally have normal joint attention.

The child in this vignette should undergo developmental screening at his upcoming health supervision visit involving a screening tool to identify concerns in the following domains: gross motor, fine motor, communication, problem-solving, and personal-social development. The American Academy of Pediatrics recommends this broad screening at 9 months, 18 months, and 24 or 30 months. A separate tool, such as the Modified Checklist for Autism in Toddlers–Revised with Follow-up, should be used to screen for autism spectrum disorder. Screening for autism is recommended at ages 18 and 24 months.

At today's visit, the clinician can help address the mother's concerns about autism and speech delay with a few questions and observations to identify "red flags" for these disorders. In addition to joint attention deficits, concerning signs would include: he does not copy others' actions, has fewer than 6 words, is not learning new words, and does not show distress when separated from a familiar caregiver. When a clinician detects a developmental concern through questions and observations, the child should be evaluated for the need for developmental services.

While a typically developing 18-month-old can scribble on his own, understand the purpose of common objects (eg, spoon), and say several single words, he cannot yet draw a circle, name objects in a book, or use 2 words together in a meaningful way (eg, "want ball"). These skills develop between 18 months and 2 years of age. Eighteen-month-old children also typically do the following: understand the word "no," have temper tantrums, display basic pretending (eg, feeding a stuffed animal), point to things they want, cling to familiar caregivers in new situations, drink from a cup, and walk well. However, observing these behaviors can be falsely reassuring and is not a substitute for more sensitive screening tools administered at recommended ages.

American Board of Pediatrics Content Specification(s)/ Content Area

- Evaluate the motor developmental progress/status of a child at 18 months of age, including recognition of abnormalities
- Evaluate the cognitive and behavioral developmental progress/status of a child at 18 months of age

Suggested Readings

Centers for Disease Control and Prevention. Learn the signs. Act early. https://www.cdc.gov/ncbddd/actearly/index.html.

Marks KP, LaRosa AC. Understanding developmental-behavioral screening measures. *Pediatr Rev.* 2012;33(10):448-458.

Simms MD, Jin XM. Autism, language disorder, and social (pragmatic) communication disorder: DSM-V and differential diagnoses. *Pediatr Rev.* 2015;36(8):355-363.

Item 290   **Preferred Response: D**

The boy in this vignette has expressive and receptive language delay, academic achievement below his peers, a preference for interacting with younger children, and lower than expected adaptive skills. This constellation of clinical features is concerning for possible mild intellectual disability (ID), and a psychoeducational evaluation from the boy's school would be the most appropriate next step in management because it would clarify his learning profile and needs.

Intellectual disability is a condition in which both intellectual and adaptive functioning are impaired. The first sign of ID can be language delay, with greater concern for possible ID if receptive language (ie, understanding of language) is problematic. Children with mild ID are typically identified when academic progress is behind expectations. Their problem-solving and self-care skills will be lower than that of their peers.

Language delay or differences are also present in autism spectrum disorder (ASD) and profound hearing loss. Autism spectrum disorder is defined by the fifth edition of the *Diagnostic and Statistical Manual of Mental Disorders* as a condition encompassing verbal and nonverbal social communication deficits and restricted and/or repetitive behaviors or interests. Social interactions and relationships are challenged by impaired language and conversational skills and difficulties in interpreting social cues and managing social situations. Motor movements, speech, or play may be repetitive or stereotypic (eg, rocking, spinning, echolalia, lining up objects), and interests may be unusual or intense (eg, natural disasters, maps, wires). There may be significant difficulties tolerating changes in schedules or situations and a preoccupation with or avoidance of certain sensory stimuli (eg, loud noises, lights, food textures). A deficit in joint attention (ie, shared interest in activities) and difficulty in viewing situations from another's perspective are characteristic of ASD. Severe or profound hearing loss occurs in 1 or 2 of 1,000 children. Children with this degree of hearing loss will coo and babble until 6 to 9 months of age and respond to loud sounds when they can feel the vibrations from the sounds. Because of the lack of further progress, speech and language development is then delayed when compared to same-age peers.

Similar to a child with ASD, a child with ID or profound hearing loss may present with language delay. However, ASD is suspected when there are atypical aspects to language (eg, echolalia, unusual tone of voice), social interactions (eg, lack of eye contact or gestures, lack of shared interest), or behaviors (eg, stereotypic motor mannerisms, behavioral rigidity, sensory seeking or sensory avoidance, intense or unusual interests). Although some stereotypic behaviors (eg, hand flapping) may be present in a child with ID, social engagement, nonverbal communication, joint attention, and play are intact and appropriate to the child's developmental level. Intellectual disability is suspected when problem-solving and life skills difficulties are present in addition to language delay. Autism spectrum disorder can coexist with ID and is diagnosed when social skills and restricted and repetitive behaviors are atypical for the child's developmental age. Like the child with ID, a child with profound hearing loss will also demonstrate developmentally appropriate social intent and interest, nonverbal communication, and joint attention. Hearing loss is suspected when speech production and comprehension of spoken language are impaired.

Although the boy in this vignette has occasional hand flapping, this stereotypic behavior can be seen in typically developing children as well as in children with ID. The boy lacks key features of ASD (eg, impaired social communication, behavioral rigidity, sensory issues) and therefore applied behavioral analysis therapy would not be indicated. At 6 years of age, the boy would not qualify for early intervention services, which are provided from birth to 3 years of age. Brain magnetic resonance imaging or electroencephalography may be considered if clinically indicated or as part of a medical evaluation for the etiology of developmental differences when there is macrocephaly, microcephaly, focal neurological abnormalities, or concern for possible seizures.

Suggested Readings

Harrington JW, Allen K. The clinician's guide to autism. *Pediatr Rev.* 2014;35(2):62-78.

Shea SE. Intellectual disability (mental retardation). *Pediatr Rev.* 2012;33(3):110-121.

Item 291   Preferred Response: A

The girl in the vignette has diabetic ketoacidosis (DKA) from newly diagnosed type 1 diabetes mellitus. She is encephalopathic and dehydrated, but hemodynamically stable and maintaining her airway, oxygenation, and ventilation. Among the response choices, the most appropriate next step in management is to slowly start intravenous fluid resuscitation with 10 mL/kg of 0.9% sodium chloride over 1 hour.

With normal physiology, the release of insulin after a dextrose-rich meal leads to the uptake of glucose into fat, liver, and skeletal muscle tissue, as well as cellular glycogen and fat synthesis. In DKA, insulin deficiency causes decreased glucose uptake, and increased glycogenolysis, and gluconeogenesis. Abnormal glucose metabolism leads to the release of counterregulatory hormones including glucagon, epinephrine, and growth hormone, all of which further increase glycogenolysis and gluconeogenesis. As another counterregulatory mechanism to provide cellular energy in DKA, free fatty acids are released from adipose tissue and converted via beta-oxidation into ketoacids (acetoacetate and beta-hydroxybutyrate). Clinically, this leads to an elevated anion gap metabolic acidosis (bicarbonate level <15 mEq/L [<15 mmol/L]), hyperglycemia (>200 mg/dL [11.1 mmol/L]), and the presence of serum or urine ketones. Hyperglycemia causes glucosuria, which in turn, leads to osmotic diuresis and dehydration. Polyuria and polydipsia are commonly seen. Hyperosmolarity is caused by ketoacidosis and hyperglycemia, as well as the hypernatremia and elevated urea nitrogen caused by dehydration from osmotic diuresis. Dehydration is treated with gradual fluid resuscitation, and this physiology is ultimately reversed by the administration of an insulin infusion.

Encephalopathy from cerebral edema is an important potential complication of DKA. In response to elevated serum osmolality, neurons produce organic osmolytes (also referred to as "idiogenic osmoles") to maintain osmolar equilibrium, thereby preventing cellular dehydration. As serum osmolarity decreases, cellular edema occurs because of shifting of water toward the higher intracellular osmolality caused by the organic osmolytes. This can occur before presentation from intake of hypotonic fluids. In DKA, administering 0.9% normal saline, which has an osmolality of 286 mmol/L, will lower serum osmolality. Although the girl in the vignette is dehydrated and needs correction of her fluid deficit, overaggressive fluid administration could worsen cerebral edema. The 2014 International Society of Pediatric and Adolescent Diabetes (ISPAD) guidelines recommend an initial normal saline bolus of 10 mL/kg over 1 hour, followed by initiation of an insulin infusion. Subsequently, the free water deficit should be corrected over 48 to 72 hours. For a patient in shock, more aggressive fluid administration is indicated, but should be balanced against potential neurologic complications.

If cerebral edema is severe, intracranial hypertension, herniation, and death can occur. Signs of severely elevated intracranial pressure and impending herniation include systemic hypertension, bradycardia, unreactive and/or unequal pupils, respiratory depression, and loss of cranial nerve function. Computed tomography of the brain is rarely indicated in the acute setting, because a patient's condition can deteriorate in the radiology suite where there is less monitoring, it can delay care, and the clinical examination is reliable enough to direct care.

Osmotherapy, which may include 3% saline or mannitol, can be used to treat the rare patient with severe cerebral edema. However, this is not indicated for the girl in this vignette because her clinical presentation does not support this diagnosis. Although she is somnolent, her Glasgow Coma Score is 9, and she does not have other clinical findings of impending herniation such as abnormal pupillary reactions, decorticate or decerebrate posturing, or bradycardia. The rapid increase in serum sodium level that would result from treatment with 3% saline can cause central pontine myelinolysis, and osmotic diuresis from mannitol can worsen dehydration and predispose to venous sinus thrombosis.

Normal respiratory compensation for metabolic acidosis follows the Winters formula:

$$PaCO_2 \text{ (predicted)} = 1.5 * HCO_3 + 8 \pm 2$$

If a patient with metabolic acidosis has a partial $PaCO_2$ higher or lower than the predicted range, there is a concomitant respiratory acidosis or alkalosis, respectively. The girl in the vignette has a $PaCO_2$ of 14 mm Hg, which falls within the range of her predicted $PaCO_2$ of 13.5 to 17.5 mm Hg, so she does not have a respiratory disorder. The girl in this vignette should not be intubated. Hypoventilation increases cerebral blood volume and intracranial pressure. During the intubation procedure of a child with DKA, the pause in ventilation can lead to herniation and death. After intubation, it can be difficult to match this high level of physiologic minute ventilation. A child with DKA should not be intubated as long as the airway is protected and oxygenation and ventilation are maintained.

Lastly, an insulin bolus should not be administered in DKA because the serum glucose and osmolality could fall too rapidly, risking cerebral edema.

PREP Pearls

- Early fluid management of diabetic ketoacidosis that is either excessive or hypotonic may worsen cerebral edema and neurologic outcomes.
- Patients with diabetic ketoacidosis rarely benefit from intubation. Indications include respiratory acidosis (using the Winters formula), and loss of respiratory drive and airway protective reflexes.
- Patients with diabetic ketoacidosis rarely benefit from mannitol or hypertonic saline. Indications include clinical findings of severe intracranial hypertension.
- Reversal of diabetic ketoacidosis occurs with the administration of intravenous normal saline 10 mL/kg over 1 hour, followed by correction of free water deficit and an intravenous insulin drip.

American Board of Pediatrics Content Specification(s)/ Content Area

- Recognize the complications associated with diabetic ketoacidosis

Suggested Readings

Cooke D, Plotnick L. Management of diabetic ketoacidosis in children and adolescents. *Pediatr Rev.* 2008;29:431-436.

Glaser NS, Wootton-Gorges SL, Buronocore MH, et al; International Society for Pediatric and Adolescent Diabetes. Subclinical cerebral edema in children with diabetic ketoacidosis randomized to 2 different rehydration protocols. *Pediatrics.* 2013;131(1):e73-80.

Wolfsdorf JI, Allgrove J, Craig ME, et al. ISPAD Clinical Practice Consensus Guidelines 2014: diabetic ketoacidosis and hyperglycemic hyperosmolar state. *Pediatr Diabetes.* 2014;15(suppl 20):154-179.

PREP® Self-Assessment 2019 Answer Sheet

To notify the American Board of Pediatrics (ABP) of completion of this activity or claim CME credit, you must enter all data electronically in PediaLink at: www.pedialink.org (click "answer sheet" tab). This form is provided as a convenient way to record your responses as you read through the questions. Do not send this form to the AAP or the ABP for processing. Please write in your answer next to the question number, and then go to the website to enter your answers online.

1. ____	43. ____	85. ____	127. ____	169. ____	211. ____	253. ____
2. ____	44. ____	86. ____	128. ____	170. ____	212. ____	254. ____
3. ____	45. ____	87. ____	129. ____	171. ____	213. ____	255. ____
4. ____	46. ____	88. ____	130. ____	172. ____	214. ____	256. ____
5. ____	47. ____	89. ____	131. ____	173. ____	215. ____	257. ____
6. ____	48. ____	90. ____	132. ____	174. ____	216. ____	258. ____
7. ____	49. ____	91. ____	133. ____	175. ____	217. ____	259. ____
8. ____	50. ____	92. ____	134. ____	176. ____	218. ____	260. ____
9. ____	51. ____	93. ____	135. ____	177. ____	219. ____	261. ____
10. ____	52. ____	94. ____	136. ____	178. ____	220. ____	262. ____
11. ____	53. ____	95. ____	137. ____	179. ____	221. ____	263. ____
12. ____	54. ____	96. ____	138. ____	180. ____	222. ____	264. ____
13. ____	55. ____	97. ____	139. ____	181. ____	223. ____	265. ____
14. ____	56. ____	98. ____	140. ____	182. ____	224. ____	266. ____
15. ____	57. ____	99. ____	141. ____	183. ____	225. ____	267. ____
16. ____	58. ____	100. ____	142. ____	184. ____	226. ____	268. ____
17. ____	59. ____	101. ____	143. ____	185. ____	227. ____	269. ____
18. ____	60. ____	102. ____	144. ____	186. ____	228. ____	270. ____
19. ____	61. ____	103. ____	145. ____	187. ____	229. ____	271. ____
20. ____	62. ____	104. ____	146. ____	188. ____	230. ____	272. ____
21. ____	63. ____	105. ____	147. ____	189. ____	231. ____	273. ____
22. ____	64. ____	106. ____	148. ____	190. ____	232. ____	274. ____
23. ____	65. ____	107. ____	149. ____	191. ____	233. ____	275. ____
24. ____	66. ____	108. ____	150. ____	192. ____	234. ____	276. ____
25. ____	67. ____	109. ____	151. ____	193. ____	235. ____	277. ____
26. ____	68. ____	110. ____	152. ____	194. ____	236. ____	278. ____
27. ____	69. ____	111. ____	153. ____	195. ____	237. ____	279. ____
28. ____	70. ____	112. ____	154. ____	196. ____	238. ____	280. ____
29. ____	71. ____	113. ____	155. ____	197. ____	239. ____	281. ____
30. ____	72. ____	114. ____	156. ____	198. ____	240. ____	282. ____
31. ____	73. ____	115. ____	157. ____	199. ____	241. ____	283. ____
32. ____	74. ____	116. ____	158. ____	200. ____	242. ____	284. ____
33. ____	75. ____	117. ____	159. ____	201. ____	243. ____	285. ____
34. ____	76. ____	118. ____	160. ____	202. ____	244. ____	286. ____
35. ____	77. ____	119. ____	161. ____	203. ____	245. ____	287. ____
36. ____	78. ____	120. ____	162. ____	204. ____	246. ____	288. ____
37. ____	79. ____	121. ____	163. ____	205. ____	247. ____	289. ____
38. ____	80. ____	122. ____	164. ____	206. ____	248. ____	290. ____
39. ____	81. ____	123. ____	165. ____	207. ____	249. ____	291. ____
40. ____	82. ____	124. ____	166. ____	208. ____	250. ____	
41. ____	83. ____	125. ____	167. ____	209. ____	251. ____	
42. ____	84. ____	126. ____	168. ____	210. ____	252. ____	

Answer Sheet